Principles of APPLIED BIOMEDICAL INSTRUMENTATION

Principles of
APPLIED BIOMEDICAL
INSTRUMENTATION

SECOND EDITION

L. A. GEDDES

Purdue University

L. E. BAKER

The University of Texas at Austin

A WILEY-INTERSCIENCE PUBLICATION

JOHN WILEY & SONS, New York • London • Sydney • Toronto

Library of Congress Cataloging in Publication Data:

Geddes, Leslie Alexander, 1921–
 Principles of applied biomedical instrumentation.

 "A Wiley-Interscience publication."
 Includes bibliographies and index.
 1. Medical electronics. 2. Physiological apparatus.
I. Baker, L. E., joint author. II. Title.

[DNLM: 1. Biomedical engineering. QT34 G295p]
R856.G4 1975   574'.028   74-34390
ISBN 0-471-29496-9

Printed in the United States of America

10 9 8 7 6 5 4 3

Preface to the Second Edition

Like the first edition, published some six years ago, this edition is written for the life scientist or the physical scientist who may be engaged in research, teaching, or patient care and has recognized the need for additional knowledge of the principles underlying many of the physical instruments he employs. This book is also intended to serve the needs of the physical scientist who feels that he has a contribution to make to the life sciences and is relatively unaware of what has been accomplished in the special area of bioinstrumentation used to measure physiological phenomena.

Although the philosophy of the second edition remains the same as the first, many changes have been effected: there have been more additions than deletions, and more emphasis has been placed in the area of the applications of the principles to measure physiological events. As in the first edition, an extensive bibliography has been included in each chapter to allow the reader to consult original sources. Two chapters (Chemical Transducers and Criteria for the Faithful Reproduction of an Event) remain essentially the same. Two chapters (The Mechanoelectronic Transducer Tube and Amplifiers) have been deleted completely. The former chapter was removed because the mechanoelectronic transducer tube is no longer available. The place it occupied is now filled by a new type of differential strain gauge (the deflection sensor cartridge) and the Pitran (a pressure-sensitive transistor); descriptions of the new devices are included. The chapter on vacuum tube and transistor amplifiers was deleted because investigators rarely wire their own circuits these days, and many contemporary biomedical electronics texts cover this area of technology. In place of information on amplifiers we have provided material on some semiconductor devices that are ideally applicable to the measurement of physiological events. Specifically, attention has been given to light-emitting diodes, optical-isolation devices, and the Pitran. Practical applications of solid-state strain gauge and Hall effect transducers have been added, along with a section on humidity-sensitive resistors, which the authors have designated "humistors."

To the chapter on inductive transducers, there has been added a section on the electromagnetic blood flowmeter, and the chapter on piezoelectric transducers now contains a short section on ultrasonic instruments.

This chapter devoted to the measurement of physiological events by impedance, a topic that has preoccupied both authors for many years, has been totally rewritten and expanded to include descriptions of new applications and to evaluate, whenever possible, the calibratibility of the impedance signal in terms of the physiological event that it reflects. The same chapter has been augmented by a section on electrical safety and a discussion of the problems associated with the use of electric current to provide a controlled painful stimulus.

Like the impedance chapter, the one on recording electrodes has been completely rewritten and expanded. In particular, coverage is given to the use of "dry" electrodes for the measurement of bioelectric events. In addition, a technique for measuring the impedance of a single electrode–electrolyte interface is presented, along with a method for the measurement of electrolytic resistivity which is free from electrode polarization-impedance errors.

The chapter on bioelectric events has also been totally rewritten and expanded to include broad coverage of electrocardiography, vectorcardiography, electromyography, electroencephalography, the electrodermal phenomena, electrooculography, electroretinography, and magnetography (which describes the magnetic component of a bioelectric event). These old and new sections contain information on the physiological meaning of the bioelectric events, to enable those who record them to know what the signals mean.

The authors are most indebted to a large number of colleagues who have verified the accuracy of many old and new sections. Useful criticisms on the impedance chapter were provided by Drs. W. Kubicek, E. Kinnen, and S. Markovich. Sections of the bioelectric events chapter were carefully reviewed by Drs. C. Vallbona, R. Edelberg, R. Borda, H. Ito, and M. Proler. A colleague, J. Bourland, was always willing to proofread and add very useful information that led to clarified presentations.

It would be an unjustifiable oversight to omit recognition of the National Heart and Lung Institute, which provided the senior author training funds for 18 years. It was from the lectures and course work presented during this period in the course "Classical Physiology with Modern Instrumentation" that much of the material in this book was drawn. Equal recognition must also be given to Dr. H. E. Hoff for his support and encouragement throughout our association with him (22 years for L. A. G., 16 years for L. E. B). We also recognize the support of several thousand medical and several hundred graduate students whom we have been fortunate enough to lead. In the teaching and research activities that involved these students, a great deal of equipment was constructed for the authors by A. G. Moore, J. Vasku, M. Hinds, J. Bourland, T. W. Coulter, G. Cantrell, E. Arriaga, and C. Martinez. These devices allowed the authors to demonstrate many of the principles of instrumentation and to obtain many of the records presented herein. Finally, because no manuscript of this magnitude comes to life by itself, we wish to recognize the tireless efforts of Toby Newman, Dixie Hahn, Marcia Williams, and Chris Crump, secretaries who converted illegible notes into a readable typed manuscript.

L. A. GEDDES
L. E. BAKER

Purdue University
W. Lafayette, Indiana

The University of Texas at Austin
Austin, Texas

Contents

11. THE BIOELECTRIC EVENTS   411

Principles of APPLIED BIOMEDICAL INSTRUMENTATION

1

The Transduction and Measurement of Physiological Events

Etienne Jules Marey, pioneer physiologist of the last century, called attention to an activity that many believe to be a modern innovation, namely, use of the latest tools of physics and engineering to investigate the phenomena of living organisms. The following statement (1878) was prophetic of the present-day application of these techniques in the biological sciences:

"In effect in the field of rigorous experimentation, all the sciences give a hand. Whatever is the object of these studies, that which measures a force or movement, or electrical state or a temperature, whether he [the investigator] be a physicist, chemist or physiologist, he has recourse to the same method and employs the same instruments."

In the biomedical sciences instrumentation for the purpose of quantification in measurement has not pervaded all areas, and a major task yet to be accomplished is to develop the tools and technology for solving the problems of detection and quantitative measurement of living processes. To do this, transducers must be created. In the chapters that follow many of the current methods for the conversion of physiological events to electrical signals are described. Although the term transducer is used here to denote the conversion of a physiological event to an electrical signal, it should be recognized that it has a broader meaning, applying also to the conversion of one type of energy to another.

When a physiological event is transformed to an electrical signal, there exists the opportunity of deriving the maximum amount of information from it by using appropriate processing and display devices. With the event available as an electrical signal, it is much easier to obtain the advantages of modern computing and display equipment to present the desired information in the most useful form. With an electrical analog of a physiological event, it is possible to store the event on magnetic tape and reexamine it at a later time. Replay and reproduction at different display rates, as by the use of a slow or a fast time scale, permits interrogation of the data for information missed when the event was being measured. This capability offers one means of obtaining the maximum amount of information from a single measurement.

Many methods are employed to convert a physiological event to an electrical signal. The event can be made to vary, directly or indirectly, electrical quantities such as resistance, capacitance, inductance, or the magnetic linkage between two or more coils. The use of piezoelectric and photoelectric transducers is also common. Chemical events can be detected through potentials developed by membrane electrodes or by measurement of current flow through electrolytes. Detectors for radiant energy occupy a prominent place in the detection of physiological events. In some instances changes in the electrical properties of biological material can be employed for transduction purposes. Practical application of the principles of transduction embraces all the phenomena of the flow of electrons or ions through solids, liquids, gases, or a vacuum. In practice, however, it is convenient to use only a few of these possibilities.

Before discussing the various methods employed to convert physiological events to electrical signals, it is important to distinguish between a transducible property and a method or principle of transduction. A transducible property is defined as that singular characteristic of an event to which a principle of transduction can be applied. A principle of transduction is any one of the many methods that can be employed to convert the transducible property to an electrical signal. In essence the transducible property is the characteristic, like a fingerprint, that is singularly different from those of all the others around it; that is, it is the property that makes the event recognizable. The principle of transduction employs the device that recognizes the property and converts it to an electrical signal. For example, if gaseous carbon dioxide is to be detected in a mixture of respiratory air (oxygen, nitrogen, and water vapor), a property that distinguishes carbon dioxide in this mixture is infrared absorption. Carbon dioxide absorbs radiation at wavelengths of 2.7, 4.3, and 14.7 microns (μ). Although water vapor absorbs a small amount of radiation near 2.7 μ, the use of an infrared source operating at either of the other two or all three of the principal absorption bands and a detector sensitive to the same spectrum constitutes a means for detecting carbon dioxide. Thus with the respiratory air passing between the infrared source and the detector, the output from the latter will decrease in proportion to the amount of carbon dioxide in the respiratory air. In this example the transducible property is infrared absorption, and the principle of transduction employs an infrared source and detector. Parenthetically, it is obvious that the maximum resolution obtainable is intimately related to the singularity of the transducible property and the selectivity of the principle of transduction.

A transducer is in reality the sense organ for the electronic processing equipment. By its very nature it is a highly specialized device ideally possessing sensitivity to but one type of energy. For this reason it is difficult to discuss the merits of these devices in a general manner. Nonetheless, a few characteristics of high-quality transducers can be stated which will serve as a basis for their evaluation.

Irrespective of the event being measured, the transducer, insofar as possible, must obey Kelvin's first rule of instrumentation; that is, the measuring instrument must not alter the event being measured. In biomedical studies this goal is not always realizable, and the degree of alteration must constantly be borne in mind. Frequently, indirect methods are employed which partially isolate the transducer from the event. For this reason it is essential that the transducer exhibit a high degree of selectivity for the phenomenon being measured so that adequate rejection of other events occurs.

The transducer should also obey the three criteria for the faithful reproduction of an event: amplitude linearity, adequate frequency response, and freedom from phase distortion. Because these criteria are discussed in detail in Chapter 13, only brief explanation of their meaning is made here.

Amplitude linearity refers to the ability of the transducer to produce an output signal that is directly proportional to the input amplitude. This requirement is presented graphically in Fig. 1-1 by the solid line 0–A. If a phenomenon under measurement increases in the opposite direction, the transducer must also linearly indicate this condition, as shown in Fig. 1-1 by the solid line 0–A′.

Although the input-output characteristic of a transducer is represented as a straight line, careful testing with known inputs usually reveals a small deviation from linearity. In high-quality transducers such a test reveals a series of values which distribute themselves on either side of a straight line. The exaggeration of a typical case is portrayed by the dashed line in Fig. 1-1. In such instances it is customary to describe the degree of linearity in terms of the percentage deviation. For example, a linearity of $\pm 1\%$ means that within the total operating range of the device, the deviation from linear response will not be greater than $\pm 1\%$.

Another quantity related to the linearity of a transducer is hysteresis, which is a measure of the ability of the transducer to produce an output that follows the input independently of the direction of change in the input. In a linear system with no hysteresis the input-output relationship is a

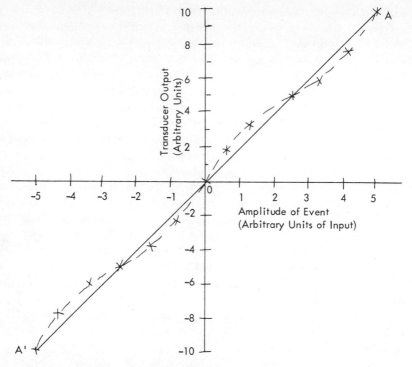

Figure 1-1. The meaning of amplitude linearity.

single straight line. If hysteresis is present, an open curve is obtained, as shown in Fig. 1-2. It is customary to express the amount of hysteresis in terms of the percentage of full-scale value. In the exaggerated example given, the hysteresis error is approximately 25%; in a well-designed device it would be less than 1%.

In connection with amplitude linearity it is pertinent to point out that the range of the event to be encountered should not exceed the range specified for the transducer. Large inputs may damage a transducer, hence decrease the linearity and increase the hysteresis error.

The overall *frequency response* and *freedom from phase distortion* refer to the ability of the transducer to provide a signal that will follow rapid and slow changes in the event presented to it. The overall frequency response must be equal to or greater than that dictated by harmonic analysis of the waveform of the event. Freedom from phase distortion requires that the transducer maintain the time differences in the sinusoidal frequency components revealed by harmonic analysis. Examples of the distortion encountered when these criteria are not fulfilled are described in Chapter 13.

Although it is highly desirable to obtain linear signals from all transducers, this is not always possible. Occasionally the transducer develops a signal that is not directly proportional to the event. For example, the resistance change of thermistors is not linear with temperature. Under such circumstances linearizing networks are necessary unless the event can be tolerated with a nonlinear calibration. Sometimes the signal is nonlinear by the nature of the physiological event itself; for example, the redness of the blood, reflecting the degree of oxygen saturation, is related to a logarithmic ratio of red and infrared transmissions. Under these conditions it is necessary to employ special processing devices to develop a signal linearly related to oxygen saturation.

The means for calibration of a transducer should be examined critically. A transducer which does not lend itself to calibration directly in terms of the physiological event has limited value; it serves to produce data that have meaning in the time domain. For example, waveform and time relation to another event form the basis for analyzing data that are acquired by transducers that cannot be calibrated.

Transducers can be expensive devices. For this reason selection of a particular type should be based in part on its ability to be incorporated into

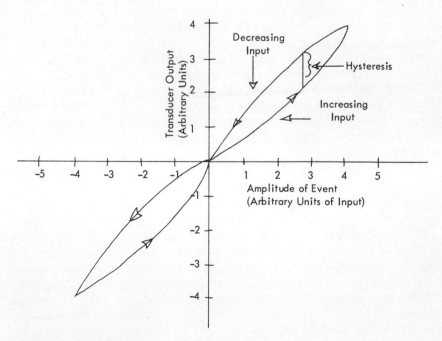

Figure 1-2. Hysteresis errors.

an existing processing or display system. Fulfilling such a requirement paves the way for the creation of a modular system that can accept a variety of transducers for many purposes.

Ultimately the transduced event is displayed by an indicating device. It is important to call attention to this fact because the type of display and use of the data frequently dictate the degree of precision required. Precision and cost are inextricably linked and often become the basis for bargaining. Perhaps the considerations in this regard were best expressed by Sir Thomas Lewis (1925), the pioneer of clinical electrocardiography, who wrote:

"Coal when weighed for sale is not thrown into a chemical balance, neither is coal placed on a coarse scale when submitted to fine analysis. Like these two machines, both classes of instruments have limitations; these should be recognized and, according to the circumstances of the case, one or the other is employed the more profitably."

In summary, it can be stated that the successful transduction of a physiological event requires the selection of an appropriate transducible property to which a selective principle of transduction is applied. Sometimes there are many suitable transducible properties and principles of transduction for a particular physiological event. In selecting a principle of transduction, a good criterion to bear in mind is Rein's (1940), which, although originally applied to an efficient blood pressure transducer, may be restated as follows: "maximum efficiency in the transducer, a minimum of electronics." In engineering terms the goal is to obtain the highest conversion efficiency, that is, electrical signal per unit of physiological event, while retaining all the criteria to achieve faithful conversion. Standardization, miniaturization, and financial compatibility with the use of the data are other obvious important considerations.

The field of electronics is replete with devices that will process and display electrical signals, but it has only a meager supply of transducers ideally suited to the measurement of physiological events. For this reason investigators in the biomedical sciences in the past, and to some degree at present, have borrowed and adapted industrial transducers or devised their own. No full-scale program has yet been launched to provide transducers for the biomedical science investigator. It should not be concluded, however, that transduction of the widest variety of physiological events cannot be accomplished. Each physiological event has many transducible properties, and there are several suitable principles of transduction already in existence. That industry has recognized and solved a similar problem can be deduced from a statement made by Carl Berkley (1950): "In nearly twenty years of oscillography, the Allen B. Dumont Laboratories has yet to find a phenomenon which is incapable of being converted to a suitable electrical signal."

Even with all the channel components (transducer, processor, and reproducer) functioning properly, repeated measurement of the same quantity will not produce exactly the same value. The question logically arising is, "Which is the correct value?" The question should really be rephrased to read "Which is the most representative value?" The answer requires the use of statistical techniques and forces a consideration of the terms precision, accuracy, and error. *Precision* refers to the degree of reproducibility of a measurement, *accuracy* is a measure of the closeness of the measurement to the true value, and *error* is the difference between the measured value and the true value. Although these terms are often used loosely, they convey different messages. For example, if a system has high precision, measurements of the same event under identical conditions differ little; that is, the scatter, spread, or range of values is small. In very many investigations, the accuracy and the error are never known, merely because the true value is not known.

Because a finite body of data contains a limited amount of information, it will be instructive to examine how a series of measurements can yield information about the quantity measured. The point can be well illustrated by the use of an example concerned with the measurement of systolic blood pressure by means of the auscultatory method. The example also illustrates the application of an indirect technique.

Let it be assumed that a human subject has a perfectly uniform heart rate and blood pressure and that an error-free transducer has been connected to the brachial artery just above the arm-occluding cuff. (The reading obtained from it will be taken as true blood pressure.) With the cuff pressure well above systolic pressure, no sound is heard in a stethoscope placed over the brachial artery just distal to the cuff. As the cuff pressure is reduced very slowly, a point is reached at which the arterial pressure exceeds the cuff pressure, the pulse breaks through, and a sound is heard. At the instant the sound occurs, the observer reads the cuff pressure and calls this value the systolic pressure. Repeated trials produce the values shown in Table 1-1. The observer naturally wants to know which value to select and how accurate that value is.

It is clearly evident that the measurements exhibit a scatter, spread, or range extending from 124 to 134 and that the most representative value lies somewhere in this range. Statistical analyses provide several methods to identify the tendency of the readings to cluster about a central value. Whenever data are encountered in this form, it is customary to plot a frequency distribution diagram. In other words, the range of the data is divided into a convenient number of equal steps, called class marks or in-

Table 1-1

Trial Number	Systolic Pressure (mm Hg)
1	131
2	128
3	130
4	131
5	134
6	128
7	130
8	133
9	129
10	132
11	129
12	132
13	130
14	125
15	129
16	130
17	126
18	124
19	127
20	131

tervals, and the number of values in each interval is tabulated. The width of the intervals is determined by the investigator. In Table 1-2 the data have been divided into intervals of 1 mm Hg, starting with 124 mm Hg. All values of 124 mm Hg and above (but below 125 mm Hg) are placed in this interval. The process is repeated for pressures up to 135 mm Hg. The number (frequency) in each interval is plotted in Fig. 1-3. When the points are joined by straight lines, the figure is called a frequency polygon; when they are joined by a smooth curve, it is called a curve of distribution. When the points are represented as rectangles (left), the figure is a bar graph; when horizontal lines fill the rectangles, a coin diagram is created; and when the points are displayed as steps (right), the figure is a histogram.

When the frequency-interval technique is employed, it becomes clear that certain values appear more often than others: that is, there is a central value about which the individual measurements appear to cluster. Many terms are used to describe the distribution of data about the central value. Perhaps the most familiar is the mean or arithmetic average, which is simply the sum of the individual values divided by the number of measure-

Table 1-2

Pressure Interval (mm Hg)	Number of Values in Interval
124–125	I
125–126	I
126–127	I
127–128	I
128–129	II
129–130	III
130–131	IIII
131–132	III
132–133	II
133–134	I
134–135	I

ments. Useful as the mean is, it does not identify the tendency of the measurements to cluster around a single value. Often the mean and the range are stated. In the example chosen, the mean is 129.4 (2589 ÷ 20), which, to the nearest integer, is 129; the range is 124 to 134 or 10 mm Hg. Another term that describes the central tendency is the mode, defined as the value in the table that occurs most frequently. In the example the mode is 130. Another useful term is the median, defined as that value which divides the group into two halves.

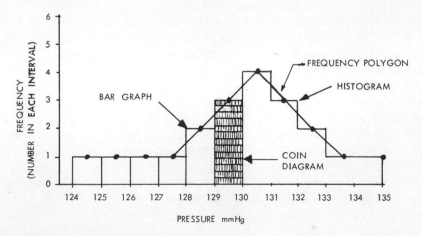

Figure 1-3. Frequency distribution diagram.

Because a vast number of measurement techniques produce data that fit what is called a normal (Gaussian) distribution curve, special terms have been developed to describe data falling into this pattern. The normal distribution curve, which gives equal weight to all measurements and assumes that small errors are more probable than large ones, is shown in Fig. 1-4. Note that the distribution of data plotted in Fig. 1-3 bears a resemblance to this curve.

If the measured data have a normal distribution, there are statistical methods for identifying the most representative value in the presence of a variation (dispersion) in magnitude. A single term that is sometimes used is the average deviation, defined as the sum of the deviations from the mean divided by the number of measurements. In the example cited the average deviation from Table 1-3 is $(+26 - 16) \div 20 = 0.5$. The most frequently used term to indicate variability is the standard deviation. This quantity is a measure of the dispersion of the data and, as will be shown, really informs about the reproducibility or precision of the measurement.

The standard deviation (σ) is defined as the square root of the sum of the squares of the deviations from the mean, divided by the number of measurements. If the distribution of data points is described by the normal distribution curve, it can be shown that 68.27% of the observations will fall between the mean ± 1 standard deviation. If the limits are widened to $\pm 2\sigma$, 95.45% of the observations will be found; 99.73% of the readings will fall within the limits of $\pm 3\sigma$.

Applying this information to the example presented, we see (Table 1-3) that the mean value of the blood pressure is 129 mm Hg and the value of one standard deviation is 2.6 mm Hg. Transferring this information to Fig.

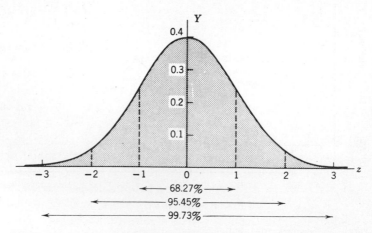

Figure 1-4.   The normal distribution curve.

Table 1-3

Pressure (mm Hg)	Deviation from Mean	Deviation Squared
131	+2	4
128	−1	1
130	+1	1
131	+2	4
134	+5	25
128	−1	1
130	+1	1
133	+4	16
129	0	0
132	+3	9
129	0	0
132	+4	16
130	+1	1
125	−4	16
129	0	0
130	+1	1
126	−3	9
124	−5	25
127	−2	4
131	+2	4

Total   2589   Total   138

20 $\overline{)2589}$

Mean   129.4 = 129

Standard deviation

$$\sigma = \left(\frac{138}{20}\right)^{1/2} = 2.63$$

$$= 2.6$$

1-5, we observe that the most representative value for the blood pressure is 129 mm Hg and that theoretically 68.27% of the readings will fall between 131.6 and 126.4 mm Hg.

It is now pertinent to recall that the true value of systolic blood pressure was measured by using a direct arterial error-free transducer. Thus the error in the blood pressure determined by the indirect method can be taken as the difference between the mean and the true value, bearing in mind that the precision of the measurement is indicated by the spread of values about the mean. If the direct arterial transducer read 134 mm Hg each time a de-

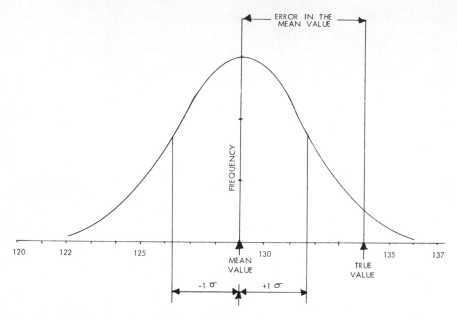

Figure 1-5.   Normal distribution curve of blood pressure measurements.

termination was made, it could be stated that the mean of the readings is −5 mm Hg in error.

In this example it was assumed that the direct arterial transducer yielded an accurate measure of systolic blood pressure. To the critical reader it should be apparent that although the direct arterial transducer measures the event as accurately as possible, it too has its own spread of values to which a statistical treatment must be applied. In connection with this statement there arises the question of ultimate accuracy. When the readings of a measuring instrument with a high reproducibility (i.e., σ is very small) are compared to an internationally accepted primary standard, the error of the mean can be ascertained and the accuracy of the measuring instrument can be specified. When such an instrument is used to measure a quantity, the standard deviation about the mean of the values obtained is descriptive of the constancy of the event being measured. The mean value of the readings can then be corrected to give the true value of the event.

REFERENCES

Berkley, C. 1950. A review of the design and application of transducers for oscillography. *Oscillographer* (A. B. Dumont Laboratories). **12**:9–22.

Lewis, T. 1925. *The Mechanism and Graphic Registration of the Heart Beat.* Shaw & Sons, London.

Marey, E. J. 1878. *La méthode graphique dans les sciences experimentales et principalement en physiologie et en medicine.* Masson, Paris.

Rein, H., A. A. Hampel, and W. A. Heinemann. 1940. Photoelektrische Transmissionmanometer zur Blutdruckschreibung. *Arch. Ges. Physiol.* **243**:329–335.

Thompson, S. P. 1910. *The Life of William Thomson, Baron Kelvin of Largs.* Macmillan, London.

2

Resistive Transducers

2-1. THERMORESISTIVE TRANSDUCERS

The variation of resistance has been used extensively to convert temperature and mechanical displacement to electrical signals. The resistance of a conductor, whether solid, liquid, or gas, is dependent on the material, the geometric configuration, and the temperature. Gaseous cells are used for the detection of radiant energy. Most of the transducers that operate on the resistance principle employ solids or liquids; the solid conductors, however, are more common.

Because the resistivity of most metals exhibits a considerable degree of temperature dependence, it is relatively easy to construct a temperature transducer. A resistor designed for such purposes is called a resistance thermometer. Although almost any metallic conductor can be used, choice of the material is based on either the linearity or the sensitivity of its resistance-temperature characteristic. The variation in resistance of most metals is approximately linear over a moderate temperature range near room temperature and is given by the relationship

$$R_t = R_0[1 + \alpha_0(T_t - T_0)],$$

where R_t = resistance at temperature T_t (°C),
            R_0 = resistance at temperature T_0 (°C),
            α_0 = temperature coefficient of resistivity at T_0.

Table 2-1 lists the temperature coefficients for some of the commonly encountered metals. From these data it can be seen that most metals exhibit an increase in resistance with rising temperature (positive temperature coefficient); typical values lie in the range of a 0.3 to 0.5% change in resistance per degree centigrade temperature change. Platinum has a temperature coefficient of 0.37% per degree centigrade and is frequently used because of its wide linear resistance-temperature relationship.

Resistance thermometers are usually low in resistance, varying from a

14

Table 2-1   Resistivities and Temperature Coefficients*

Material	Resistivity† ($\mu\Omega$-cm)	α = Temperature Coefficient† $[\Omega/(\Omega)/(°C)]$
Copper (annealed)	1.724	0.0039
Copper (hard drawn)	1.77	0.0038
Aluminum (commercial)	2.828	0.0036
Silver	1.629 (18°C)	0.0038
Platinum	10	0.00377
Nichrome	100	0.0004
Iron	10	0.005
Mercury	98.5 (50°C)	0.00089
Carbon	3500 (0°C)	−0.0005

*Handbook of Chemistry and Physics, Chemical Rubber Publishing Co., Cleveland, Ohio, 1962.
† At 20°C.

few ohms to a few hundred ohms. Because of their low thermal sensitivity, it is necessary to use a Wheatstone bridge (Fig. 2-1a) with a sensitive indicator to show the temperature of the thermal element (R_D). The bridge can be operated from either direct or alternating current.

To minimize errors caused by changes in resistance of the wires connecting the resistance thermometer to the bridge, it is necessary to employ compensating leads. The method of obtaining temperature compensation is

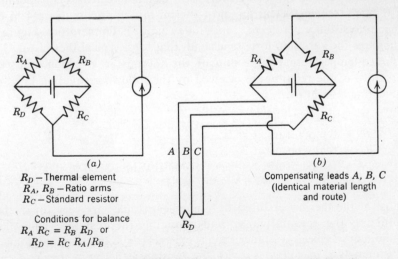

(a)

R_D —Thermal element
R_A, R_B —Ratio arms
R_C —Standard resistor

Conditions for balance
$R_A R_C = R_B R_D$ or
$R_D = R_C R_A/R_B$

A B C

R_D

(b)

Compensating leads A, B, C
(Identical material length
and route)

Figure 2-1.   Circuits for Wheatstone bridge (a) and compensated bridge (b).

shown in Fig. 2-1*b*. Initially R_D and R_C are made equal at the reference temperature. When R_D is then used to measure an unknown temperature and the temperature of the wires connecting R_D to the bridge changes, an equal amount of resistance is added to R_C and R_D, thereby minimizing errors caused by thermal gradients that exist along the wires. When this technique is employed, a temperature can be measured with an accuracy of a few hundredths of a degree centigrade. Miniature resistance elements that have a small thermal capacity and a short response time are available. Once calibrated, such detectors are remarkably stable.

Several precautions must be taken when using a resistance thermometer. If it is immersed in electrolytes, electrical shunting and fluid absorption must be prevented. Also, if the resistance of the thermal element is affected by magnetic fields (as is the case with some materials), its use in such environments may lead to error in temperature measurement. These effects are described in detail in this chapter. Perhaps the most important precaution to be observed is to avoid heating the resistance thermometer by the current employed to measure its resistance.

Because of its higher thermal coefficient, the thermistor is widely used to measure temperature. It is a hard ceramiclike device composed of a compressed and sintered mixture of metallic oxides of manganese, nickel, cobalt, copper, magnesium, titanium, and other metals. Molded into beads, rods, disks, washers, and many other forms, thermistors exhibit temperature coefficients many times larger than those of pure metals. Furthermore, the coefficient is negative: that is, with increasing temperature, the resistance of a thermistor element decreases considerably. The temperature coefficient for most thermistors approximates a 4 to 6% change in resistance per degree centigrade change in temperature. Figure 2-2 compares the variation for copper with that for a typical thermistor. The resistance-temperature relationship of the thermistor is exponential; the usual form of the relationship is given by the following equation [Victory Engineering (1955)]:

$$R_t = R_{t_0} e^{\beta(1/T - 1/T_0)},$$
R_t = temperature at $T°K$,
R_{t_0} = temperature at $T_0°K$,
β = temperature coefficient (typical values 3000 to 4000),
e = 2.71828.

Most of the thermistors used in biomedical studies are very small, thus minimizing the thermal mass and reducing the response time correspondingly. Typical resistance ranges extend from a few hundred ohms to approximately a megohm. As with the resistance thermometer great care must be exercised to limit the current through the thermal element, to

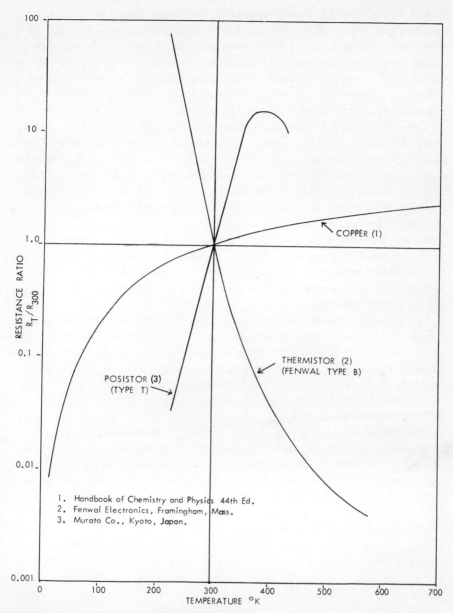

Figure 2-2. Resistance temperature characteristics of copper, a typical thermistor, and a posistor.

reduce errors resulting from self-heating. In many of the standard units, if the power dissipation is kept to the milliwatt level, measurement of a temperature difference of 0.01°C or smaller is easily possible. Because of the large temperature coefficient, compensating leads are not usually required with thermistors when making routine temperature measurements.

The thermistor is not, however, without its limitations; for example, the resistance-temperature characteristic of some of the earlier thermistors exhibited hysteresis. In addition, unlike pure metallic resistance elements, some thermistors tend to show a slight degree of long-term aging, which manifests itself as a small change in nominal resistance at a particular temperature. A comprehensive report on precautions in the use of thermistors in physiology was made by Fleming (1958). Modern manufacturing methods and improved quality control techniques have largely eliminated the defects present in the first thermistors.

A survey of the characteristics of many typical thermistors was presented by Van Dover and Bechtold (1960). In their comprehensive article they tabulated resistance range, maximum wattage dissipation, operating temperature, time constant, temperature coefficient, and dimensions of a variety of configurations.

The attractiveness of the high thermal coefficient is in part offset by the nonlinear nature of the resistance change, which becomes noticeable when large temperature changes are encountered. If a linear temperature scale is desired, it is necessary to employ linearizing techniques. One of the easiest methods of obtaining a linear scale is to connect a resistor of the appropriate value in parallel with the thermistor. A review of this technique was presented by Cornwall (1965).

One manufacturer[1] has devised a method of overcoming the nonlinear characteristics of thermistors by developing temperature sensors which contain pairs of thermistors. With these sensors employed in the circuits shown in Fig. 2-3, a linear voltage-temperature or resistance-temperature characteristic can be obtained over a range of temperature change of about 100°C. With these thermolinear[1] sensors the maximum departure from linearity is less than 0.2°C.

Recently, a new series of thermistors, called posistors,[2] has been announced. Made from barium titanate ceramic, these devices have remarkably high positive thermoresistive coefficients in the temperature range of −50 to +100°C. In one model the resistance at room temperature is multiplied tenfold by an increase in temperature of 60°C. The characteristics of the type T posistor are given in Fig. 2-2.

[1] Yellow Springs Instrument Co., Yellow Springs, Ohio 45387.
[2] Murata Manufacturing Co., Ltd., Kyoto, Japan.

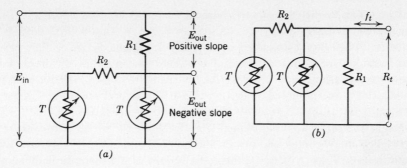

Figure 2-3. Circuits for obtaining linear temperature characteristics with thermolinear thermistors: (*a*) linear voltage versus temperature; (*b*) linear resistance versus temperature. (Courtesy of Yellow Springs Instrument Co., Yellow Springs, Ohio.)

Both resistance thermometers made of pure metals and thermistors have a variety of applications in biomedical studies. Quite apart from their obvious use as electrical transducers for measuring the temperature of the skin and of many regions inside the body, they see other service. For example, because the temperature of expired air is higher than that of inspired air, a temperature sensor (usually a hermetically sealed thermistor) placed in the airway will provide a signal that allows monitoring respiratory frequency. Simons (1962) used this technique to record respiration from aircraft pilots. Occasionally, heated thermistors are employed as hot-wire anemometers to measure flow velocity. Heated thermistors have been placed in the respiratory air stream to detect respiration and give a biphasic signal for a single breath, being cooled by both inspiration and expiration.

Ledig and Lyman (1927) used platinum resistance thermometers for transduction of carbon dioxide and oxygen to electrical signals by measurement of the thermal conductivities of these gases. By means of the same system, Lamson and Robbins (1928) measured the amount of carbon tetrachloride in respiratory air when a known amount of this substance was injected into the lumen of the gut.

There have been several applications of the thermoresistor that demonstrate the response time attainable. Hill (1920) showed that when an $11\text{-}\mu$ heated filament was laid across the lumen of a tube connected to a conical receiver placed over a pulsating vessel the rapid pulsations of the air stream modulated the temperature of the wire, hence its electrical resistance. The response time was short enough to show the notched transient (dicrotic wave) in the pulse curve. This pulse detector was used by Bramwell et al. (1923) in pulse wave velocity studies. The principle was improved upon by Tucker and Paris (1921) to construct a hot-wire microphone having a resonant frequency of 200 Hz. Anrep et al. (1927) used a hot wire to show the changes in coronary blood flow during the cardiac cycle. Blood collected in a reservoir displaced air, which passed over and cooled a heated thermal element. A somewhat different blood flow velocity transducer was described by Katsura et al. (1959); it used two thermistors, one mounted at the tip of a catheter and the other farther up the catheter. One thermistor detected the temperature of the blood, whereas the other was maintained slightly above the blood temperature. A change in flow cooled the hotter thermistor, and more current was sent through it to restore its temperature. A record of the increase in current to maintain the temperature difference was related to blood flow. An improved isothermal blood flowmeter was described by Mellander and Rushmer (1960). The improvement consisted of a spring arrangement which held the probe in the center of the vessel.

One manufacturer[3] has announced the availability of single- and double-lumen medical-grade catheters in which thermistors have been embedded. Standard units with nominal resistances of approximately 1250 Ω at body temperature (37°C) can be employed to measure temperatures in blood vessels, ducts, and hollow organs. In addition, the response times listed (0.1 to 4 sec) are short enough to follow rapid changes in temperature such as those encountered when the thermodilution method is used to determine cardiac output.

2-2. METALLIC STRAIN GAUGES

A more popular use of the resistance change principle is in the detection of a small mechanical displacement from which the force producing the displacement can be determined directly. Tomlinson (1876–1877) found that when conducting wires were stretched, the length increased and the diameter decreased, and these dimensional changes were effective in increasing the resistance. The opposite situation obtains when conductors are compressed. Resistance elements constructed from specially prepared alloys, which change their resistance more than an amount attributable to elongation or alteration in cross-sectional area, are called strain gauges. Although virtually any metallic conductor can be used as a strain gauge, highly desirable characteristics for the material are (a) a high resistance-elongation coefficient, (b) a low value of resistance change and dimension change per unit change in temperature, and (c) a high sensitivity to strain in the direction measured and a low sensitivity to perpendicular strain.

Two types of strain gauge are in popular use. One is the bonded gauge

---

[3] Victory Engineering Corp., Springfield Ave., Springfield, N.J.

(Fig. 2-4), in which the resistance element is cemented to a backing approximately the size of a postage stamp.[4] In the other type (unbonded) the resistance wire is stretched between supporting members. The bonded gauge was patented by Simmonds (1942). With both types the deformation to be measured is coupled to the strain gauge element, altering tension in the resistance wire.

Strain gauges are usually made of wire approximately 0.001 in in diameter. The term customarily employed to denote the change in resistance of the strain gauge material when stretched is the gauge factor, defined as the fractional change in resistance divided by the fractional change in length; that is,

$$G = \frac{\Delta R/R}{\Delta L/L},$$

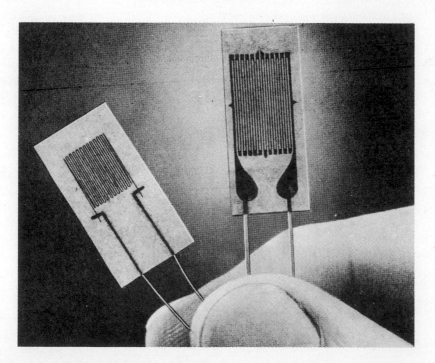

Figure 2-4. Bonded strain gauges. (Courtesy of BLH Electronics, Inc., a subsidiary of Baldwin-Lima-Hamilton Corporation, Waltham, Mass.)

---

[4] The methods of attaching strain gauges are described in *Bulletin* 4311A, Baldwin-Lima-Hamilton Corp., Waltham Mass.

where R and L are the resistance and the length, respectively. Although this ratio was discussed by Tomlinson, the term gauge factor is of more recent origin.

The gauge factors of various materials appear in Table 2-2. These data indicate that the gauge factor of most metals is approximately 2.0, whereas that of silicon is 60 times larger. For silicon the gauge factor depends entirely on the method of preparation and can be higher or lower than that shown; however, the slightly higher temperature coefficient often makes it difficult to take advantage of the high gauge factor if extremes in environmental temperature are to be encountered. In addition to the change in resistivity, Sanchez (1961) reported a slight decrease in gauge factor with increasing temperature.

In physiologic language the strain gauge is an isometric device, permitting measurement of only small displacements. The extension permissible is dependent on the material from which the strain gauge is made and can be calculated from the following expression:

$$\frac{\Delta L}{L} = \frac{f}{E},$$

where f is the tensile strength of the material, and E is Young's modulus.
Table 2-3 lists typical values for Young's modulus and the tensile strengths

Table 2-2 Characteristics of Strain Gauge Materials*

Material	Gauge Factor G	Temperature Coefficient † $[\Omega/(\Omega)(°C)]$	
Advance	2.1	0.00002	(25°C)
Constantan	2.0	0.000002	(25°C)
Isoelastic	3.5	0.00047	
Manganin	0.47	0.0000	(25°C)
Monel	1.9	0.002	
Nichrome	2.5	0.0004	
Nickel	12.1 to −20	0.006	
Phosphor bronze	1.9	0.003	
Platinum	6.0	0.003	
Silicon	120	0.005–0.007	(25°C)

* From LeGette (1958), Mason and Thurson (1957), Smith (1954), and Sanchez (1961); see also: *Shock and Vibration Handbook*, C. M. Harris and C. E. Crede, Eds., McGraw-Hill, New York, 1961, Vol. 1, Table 16.5.
† Values are for 20°C unless stated otherwise.

Table 2-3   Mechanical Characteristics of Strain Gauge Materials

Material	Ultimate Tensile Strength, f (psi = force/ area $\times$ 10^3)	Young's, Modulus, E (psi $\times$ 10^6)	Information Source
Constantan	60–125	24	International Nickel Co.
Isoelastic	85–155	26	International Nickel Co.
"R" Monel	85–100	26	International Nickel Co.
Nichrome	100–200	27	Driver Harris Co.
Nickel	60–135	30	Wilbur B. Driver Co.
Phosphor bronze	130	16	International Nickel Co.
Platinum	50–100	22	Wilbur B. Driver Co.
Silicon (P)	90	27	Kulite Semiconductor Prods.
479 (Pt-Rh)	200–300	34	Sigmund Cohn

for various materials. If large displacements are to be measured, their amplitudes must be reduced by suitable mechanical transformation.

Strain gauge elements are small and stiff; these characteristics together yield a rapid response time. In practice, the speed of response is more often determined by the device to which the strain gauge is affixed. The resistance of strain gauges is relatively low, ranging from about 100 to 2000 Ω. The resistance change is small with extension. By combining the expressions for length and gauge factor we can express the change in resistance as follows:

$$\frac{\Delta R}{R} = \frac{Gf}{E}.$$

The values for Young's modulus of elasticity E and the safe tensile stress f given in Table 2-3 can be used to calculate the maximum extension and resistance change expected. In practice, however, the change in resistance produced by the maximum safe extension is usually less than 1%.

Because temperature errors may be encountered, the use of single strain gauge element is uncommon. To reduce temperature errors, pairs of strain gauges are usually employed in a bridge circuit, with strains in the opposite directions applied to adjacent arms of the bridge, as in Fig. 2-5a. When strain gauges are employed in double pairs, strain in the same direction is applied to diagonal arms of the bridge, as in Fig. 2-5b. If a direct voltage is employed to energize the bridge, a galvanometer of resistance R_g is used, and the change in resistance of each gauge (ΔR) is small with respect to $R (= R_A = R_B = R_C = R_D)$; the galvanometer current I_g for an applied

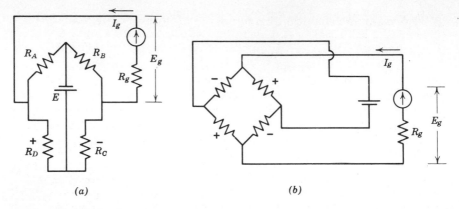

Figure 2-5. Strain gauge bridge circuits: (*a*) two strain gauge elements; (*b*) four strain gauge elements.

strain is given by the following expression:

$$I_g = \frac{\Delta R}{R}\left(\frac{E}{R + R_g}\right).$$

If, instead of a galvanometer, an a-c or d-c voltage-indicating device of very high resistance is employed in a bridge with two active strain gauges, as in Fig. 2-5*a*, the voltage obtained (E_g) for an applied strain is

$$E_g = E\,\frac{(\Delta R)}{2R}\,.$$

When two active strain gauges are employed, as indicated previously, temperature compensation is achieved. With four active gauges the voltage obtained is doubled. With either two or four strain gauges, alternating or direct current can be employed to energize the bridge, and signals in the low millivolt range are obtained in typical applications.

The strain gauge is frequently used in biomedical studies. One of the earliest applications appears to have been made by Grundfest and Hay (1945), who mounted a gauge on a stiff lever to create a nearly isometric myograph. Strain gauge elements were used by Lambert (1947) to construct a transducer in which the motion of a stiff diaphragm exposed to blood pressure was detected to obtain transduction of this physiological event. Many commercially available blood pressure transducers operate on this principle.

Physiologists have long been concerned with the force of contraction of cardiac muscle. To measure this parameter of cardiac function on an excised papillary muscle, Garb (1951) developed and employed a strain gauge

myograph. Boniface et al. (1953) devised an ingenious strain gauge arch
(Fig. 2-6a) which, when sutured to the wall of the left or right ventricle,
(Fig. 2-6b), provided an *in situ* means of continuously recording the force
developed by the cardiac fibers between the "feet" of the gauge unit. Encapsulated versions of the strain gauge arch have been permanently implanted in experimental animals to study the response of the heart to imposed workloads and to drugs. A larger transducer for measurement of the
same parameter of cardiac activity was described by Cotten (1957). With
this device (Fig. 2-7) it is possible to prestress the cardiac muscle fibers to

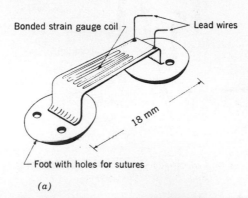

Bonded strain gauge coil — Lead wires

18 mm

Foot with holes for sutures

(a)

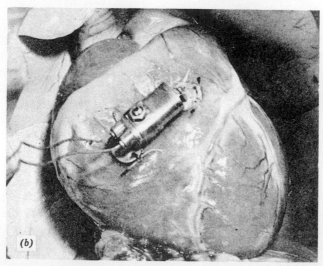

(b)

Figure 2-6. Strain gauge transducers for the measurement of contractile force of cardiac
muscle fibers: (a) strain gauge arch; (b) encapsulated strain gauge arch attached to ventricular
Wall. [From Brown, *Anesth. Analg. Curr. Res.* **39**:487–488 (1960).]

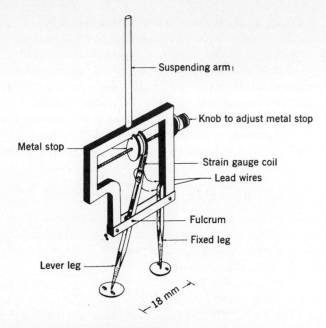

Figure 2-7. Strain gauge that permits application of an initial stress to muscle fibers. [From M. deV. Cotten, *Am. J. Physiol.* **189**:580–586 (1957).]

investigate the response to what is called diastolic loading, that is, the effect of an increased stretch to increase the force of contraction. This response is referred to as Starling's law of the heart.

Recognizing the potential of the strain gauge in biomedical studies, one manufacturer[5] has developed a universal transducer (Fig. 2-8) containing strain gauge elements, which, with interchangeable attachments, can be used as a pressure transducer, a sensitive myograph, and a stiff myograph. The compatibility of this device with basic strain gauge recording instruments should make it a useful general purpose transducer for events that can be converted to pressure or force.

Figures 2-9 and 2-10 present several strain gauge pressure transducers employed in biomedical research. Figures 2-9a illustrates one of the popular strain gauge bridge transducers employed for blood pressure measurement in man and animals; Fig. 2-9b shows a miniature version mounted in a stopcock. Figure 2-9c illustrates a strain gauge pressure-sensing element mounted in the plunger of a 20-cc syringe.

Recently the semiconductor materials (silicon and germanium) have been

[5] Statham Instruments, Oxnard, Calif.

employed in transducers. Despite the high thermoresistive coefficient of silicon, Angelakos (1964) was able to construct a practical four-element strain gauge microtransducer, which he affixed to the tip of a No. 7 catheter. Because of the small size of the device, the mass was low. The high gauge factor permitted use of a mounting possessing high stiffness. The net result was a frequency response in excess of 2000 Hz.

One of the most popular high-fidelity miniature catheter-tip strain gauge transducers was described by Millar and Baker (1973) and is illustrated in Fig. 2-10. Located on the side of the tip, which is 1.65 mm in diameter, is the pressure-sensitive silicone rubber diaphragm coupled to two silicon strain gauge elements (1500 Ω each). With the application of pressure, one element is stretched and the other is compressed. The strain gauges constitute a half-bridge, the other half of which is located in the electrical connector along with a calibrating resistor that provides a signal equivalent to 100 mm Hg. Freedom from drift due to temperature changes has been achieved by careful matching of the strain gauge elements for resistance and thermal coefficient. The back of the strain gauge detecting system is vented to atmospheric pressure at the connector.

The performance characteristics of the Millar MIKRO-TIP® catheter

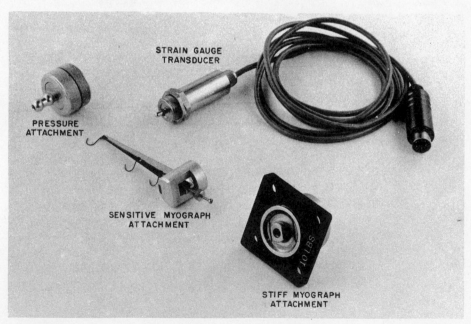

Figure 2-8.   Universal strain gauge element with attachments. (Courtesy of Statham Industries, Oxnard, California.)

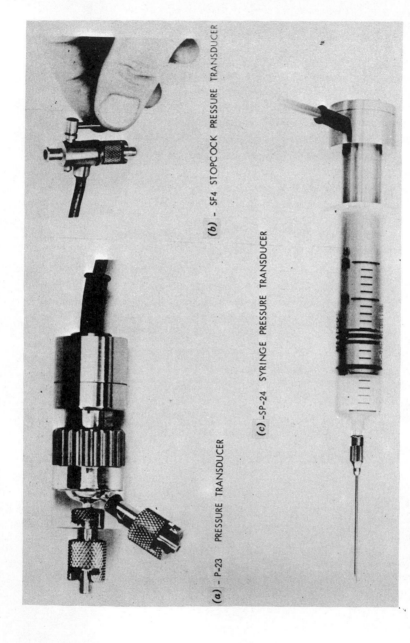

(a) - P-23 PRESSURE TRANSDUCER

(b) - SF4 STOPCOCK PRESSURE TRANSDUCER

(c) -SP-24 SYRINGE PRESSURE TRANSDUCER

Figure 2-9. Strain gauge pressure transducers: (*a*) P-23 pressure transducer; (*b*) SF4 stopcock pressure transducer; (*c*) SP-24 syringe pressure transducer. (Courtesy Statham Industries, Oxnard Cal.)

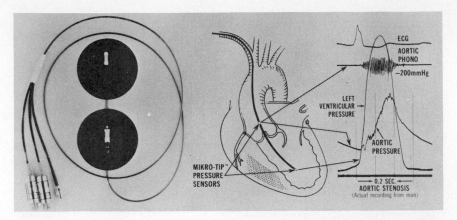

Figure 2-10. Millar MIKRO-TIP® transducer incorporating two miniature pressure sensors (*a*) with sampling lumen. (*b*) Double transducer used to record left ventricular and aortic pressure. From the aortic pressure signal, the sounds characteristics of aortic stenosis were detected. (Courtesy of Millar Instruments, Inc., Houston, Tex.)

transducer[6] are truly remarkable. For example, the typical output is 25 mV for a pressure change of 300 mm Hg, either positive or negative, using 3.5 V excitation (ac or dc). The maximum excitation voltage recommended is 10 V (ac or dc). The linearity and hysteresis are within ±0.5% of any selected range from −300 to + 400 mm Hg. The thermal stability is equivalent to ±0.1 mm Hg/°C change from 25 to 40°C. Typical overall stability is well within 1 mm Hg per hour, and its low mass makes the device relatively insensitive to acceleration forces and "catheter whip."

The dynamic response characteristics of the MIKRO-TIP® transducer permit high-fidelity recording of pressure transients anywhere in the vascular system. It is particularly useful for measuring the small pressure gradients across valves and along vessels. The volume displacement is 10^{-3} mm³/100 mm Hg, and the natural resonant frequency of the pressure-sensing system is typically 35 kHz in air and 30 kHz in water, which provides a response time short enough for the detection of intravascular sounds (see Fig. 2-10). Electrical safety is also an important feature; the leakage current rating is less than 0.5 μA for an applied voltage of 180 V dc. Thus the insulation resistance is in excess of 360 MΩ.

This type of transducer is ideally applicable for studies requiring accurate analyses of pressures and pressure waveforms and, particularly, first and second derivatives of waveforms. Signals from these transducers are suitable for storage on high-frequency-response data-acquisition systems or for on-line computer analysis.

[6] MIKRO-TIP is a registered trade mark of Millar Instruments, Inc., Houston, Texas.

2-3. THE DEFLECTION SENSOR CARTRIDGE

Disappearance of the RCA 5734 mechanoelectronic transducer tube, a device with a deflectable protruding anode, has been followed by the appearance of a worthy successor, the deflection sensor cartridge (DSC),[7] which has a protruding deflectable pin connected to a beam on which are mounted two semiconductor strain gauges. The new device, illustrated in Fig. 2-11, consists of a half-bridge, in which deflection of the protruding pin increases the resistance of one strain gauge (R_1) and decreases the resistance of the other (R_2). When these two active elements are combined with a potentiometer (R_b) to create a bridge circuit and excited with 10 V (E_{in}), a voltage of ± 300 mV is obtained for a deflection of $\pm$ 0.01 in., which is the maximum deflection obtainable. The force necessary to deflect the protruding pin to its maximum range is about 500 grams.

The deflection sensor cartridge is a low-cost device, and is ideal for the isometric measurement of force lending itself to a variety of transducing systems. As yet, it has seen relatively little service in the life sciences. However, one noteworthy application was described by Huntsman and his colleagues (1971, 1972). In their studies, the force developed by papillary muscle specimens was measured under a wide variety of experimentally

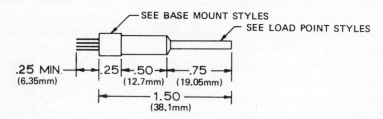

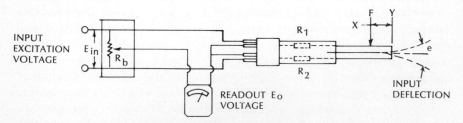

Figure 2-11. The deflection sensor cartridge (DSC) in which a pair of semiconductor strain gauges (R_1, R_2) detect that force applied to a protruding pin (input deflection). [Courtesy of DSC Inc. (Courtesy of Imperial Controls) Bellevue, Wash.]

---

[7] Imperial Controls, DSC, Inc., Bellevue, Wash.

controlled circumstances, to investigate the value of the various parameters used to describe contractility. Although there has been limited biological use of the deflection sensor cartridge, its low cost, high output, and short response time make it attractive for a variety of studies in which a physiological event can be converted to a mechanical force—as, for example, in pressure transducers.

2-4. POTENTIOMETER TRANSDUCERS

Wire-wound or carbon rotary or rectilinear potentiometers can be employed as high-efficiency transducers to detect movement when the moving object can develop a moderate force and when the movement is not rapid. Although there are few physiological applications of this type of transducer at present, the unusually high efficiency attainable will no doubt encourage wider application. Respiration was detected by Adams (1962), who measured changes in thoracic circumference by connecting a rotary potentiometer to a chest band on a monkey. Geddes et al. (1961) converted the rotation of a spirometer pulley to an electrical signal by using a low-torque potentiometer (Fig. 2-12). A device for recording the contraction of skeletal muscle *in situ* was also described by Geddes et al. (1966). In this transducer (Fig. 2-13), a low-torque potentiometer serves as the pivot for the caliper arms, which embrace the belly of the muscle. Contraction of the muscle causes the arms to be driven apart, and their motion is measured by the potentiometer.

A truly isotonic myograph for slowly contracting muscles could be constructed by passing a cord over a pulley mounted on the shaft of a low-torque potentiometer. One end of the cord could be connected to the muscle, the other to a weight. Contraction of the muscle would move the same weight through a height measured by the rotation of the pulley.

As previously stated, the unusually attractive feature of the potentiometer transducer is its high efficiency. With a large voltage applied across the potentiometer, the voltage appearing between the moving contact and one end terminal is related to the position of the moving contact. The amount of voltage that can be applied is limited by the wattage rating of the resistance element. Linear, logarithmic, sine, cosine, and other types of resistance proportional to rotation are available. Rotary units are available with 360-degree rotations, and rectilinear models can be obtained with strokes from a fraction of an inch up to almost 1 foot. With the rectilinear models a resistance-motion linearity of 1 to 2% is attainable. If the resistance element is a carbon film, the output is continuously related to the movement of the sliding contact. If the resistance element is wire-wound, the output versus movement is stepped; that is, the voltage changes

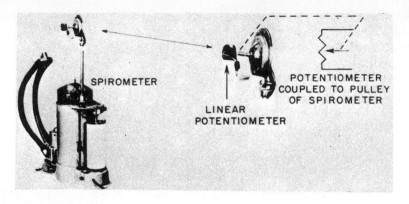

Figure 2-12. Potentiometer transducer applied to a spirometer.

abruptly with movement of the sliding contact as it passes from one wire to the next. With high-resistance units the number of wires is large and the steps are fine.

The force required to move the sliding contact depends on the design of the potentiometer. Between 0.2 and 0.5 oz in. is needed to move low-torque rotary potentiometers, compared to 0.5 to 6 oz in. for conventional potentiometers. The starting torque is slightly higher than the running torque.

In practical application the response time of a potentiometer transducer is difficult to describe quantitatively because it is intimately related to the mass, elasticity, and damping of the member to which the device is cou-

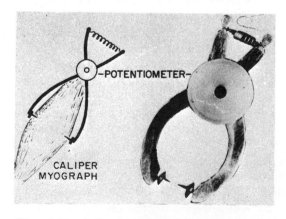

Figure 2-13. Caliper myograph.

pled. Nunn (1959) quoted a frequency response of up to 4 Hz for a potentiometer coupled to a Bourdon tube. In the experience of the authors,
potentiometric transducers can function at high efficiency for events which
change at rates less than a few Hz.

2-5.   MAGNETORESISTIVE TRANSDUCERS

Many substances exhibit a change in resistivity when exposed to a magnetic field. For example, the resistivity of most metals increases with
increasing field strength; with ferromagnetic metals the resistivity
decreases. The magnetoresistive effect is small in most metals; the resistivity of copper is increased by only 0.25% when exposed to a field of 200
kG. When bismuth is exposed to a magnetic field, however, a considerable
increase in resistivity occurs. At room temperature a field of 20 kG doubles
the resistivity. If the temperature is lowered, the effect is much more
pronounced. If the same field is presented to bismuth at the temperature of
liquid air, the resistivity is multiplied by 250. The relationship of increase in
resistivity with increasing magnetic field strength for 0 and $-50°C$ is plotted in Fig. 2-14.

The phenomenon of resistivity change with a change in magnetic field
has been employed in detectors for field strength. It was used by Hampel
(1941) in a blood pressure transducer. A double resistance coil was
mounted on an elastic diaphragm exposed to blood pressure; one-half of
the diaphragm entered a field while the other half moved out of the field
when the diaphragm was deformed. Thus the two coils became resistors
that varied in response to pressure. A record of the variation in resistance,
as measured by a Wheatstone bridge and galvanometer, reproduced the
blood pressure wave. A similar method was employed by Holzer (1940),
who constructed a myograph in which four coils (two of copper and two of
bismuth) were employed in a bridge circuit. The coils were mounted on a
tube and connected so that with movement, the bismuth coils were pulled
out of the magnetic field. The bismuth coils constituted one diagonal pair
of the bridge resistors; the copper coils, the other. The stiffness of the
system and the strength of the magnetic field combined to yield a rapid
response time and a high efficiency. To illustrate these characteristics,
Holzer recorded the twitch of a frog gastrocnemius muscle.

2-6.   THE HALL EFFECT

The Hall effect, discovered in 1879, is an interesting phenomenon
associated with a conductor that is exposed to a magnetic field. It cannot
be better described than in Hall's own words: "If the current of electricity

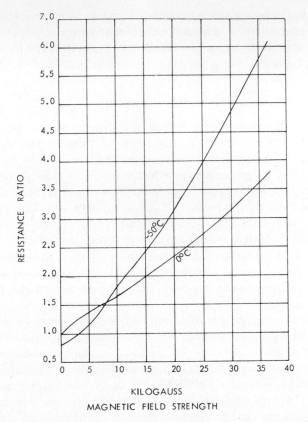

Figure 2-14. The effect of magnetic field intensity on the resistance of bismuth. (Redrawn from data by Graetz, *Handbuch der Elektrizität,* 1920.) Verlag J. A. Barth.

in a fixed conductor is itself attracted by a magnet, the current should be drawn to one side of the wire and therefore the resistance experienced should be increased." With this as his thesis, Hall proceeded to test the theory experimentally, using at first a thick conductor and finally a strip of gold leaf. Success rewarded his efforts, and he concluded, "It is perhaps allowable to speak of the action of the magnet as setting up in the strip of gold leaf a new electromotive force at right angles to the primary electromotive force."

To understand the nature of the Hall effect, consider a thin rectangular film of conducting material equipped with four electrodes, two at the ends (M, N) and two on the middle of the sides (P, Q). When current is led into and out of electrodes M and N, as in Fig. 2-15, there will be no potential E

measured between the side electrodes P and Q. If a magnetic field B is caused to pass through the conducting film at right angles to the plane of the film, the moving charges will be deflected toward the top or bottom of the film, depending on the directions of the field and current. Deflection of the charge carriers causes a potential to appear across electrodes P and Q, the magnitude and polarity of which depend on the direction and intensity of the magnetic field, the current, the type of charge carrier, and the dimensions of the film. The usual form of the relationship is

$$E = KIB/t$$

where E = the Hall voltage,
I = the excitation current in amperes through the film,
B = the field strength (G),
t = the thickness of the film (cm).

The Hall coefficient K depends on the material and temperature. It is small for most metals; the constants for bismuth, tellurium, and silicon, however, are approximately 100,000 times larger. N-type germanium, indium antimonide, and indium arsenide Hall devices are employed to obtain high outputs (Star, 1963), and are most frequently in Hall effect detectors for ac or dc magnetic fields. The outputs available are in the range of millivolts per kilogauss for typical models with rated excitation current. Although a linear voltage-field strength relationship can be obtained, with some materials the linearity is poor when low-intensity fields are used; with other materials the reverse is true. In addition, although it would appear that with a given field B, the Hall voltage can be increased by decreasing

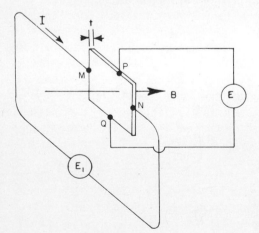

Figure 2-15.   The Hall effect.

the thickness of the film t and increasing the current I, a limit is soon reached at which the current density in the film is such that excessive heat is produced and the film changes its characteristics.

The output impedance of Hall effect generators depends on the resistivity and dimensions of the film. In commercially available probe detectors for magnetic fields, it extends from a few to a few hundred ohms.

Figure 2-16 illustrates two typical Hall-effect devices produced by one manufactuerer.[8] The transverse type is useful for measuring the field strength in a thin gap. The axial device finds applications in measuring the field strength inside a coil. The triaxial type contains three Hall devices mounted to be mutually perpendicular and serves for mapping magnetic fields.

Hall effect devices, sometimes called "chips," can be used in a variety of ways. Figures 2-17a–2-17c illustrate their application in transducers for displacement. In Fig. 2-17a(1) the Hall device occupies the null position; that is, each side is subjected to the same field intensity. Movement of either the magnets or the Hall device will produce a Hall voltage. In Fig. 2-17a(2) a field of varying strength exists between the magnets. The output of the Hall device is dependent on its position in this field. Thus movement along the direction of the arrow will give rise to an increase in the Hall voltage. In Fig. 2-17b and 2-17c, movement of the magnets past the Hall device produces a position-dependent voltage as shown. Use of the Hall device to detect rotary position is shown in Fig. 2-17d. Because the presence of ferromagnetic material alters the magnetic field passing through the Hall device, the assembly shown in Fig. 2-17e can serve as a detector for such materials. Figure 2-17f indicates how a Hall device can be used to measure current (I) by causing it to produce a magnetic field in an air gap in the magnetic circuit. The magnetic field strength is measured by the Hall effect chip as shown.

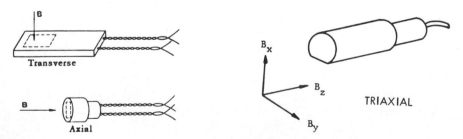

Figure 2-16.   Typical configurations of Hall effect devices.

[8] Bell, Inc., Columbus, Ohio.

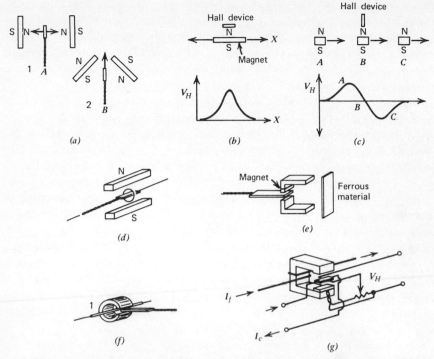

Figure 2-17. Applications of Hall effect devices. (a–f Courtesy of Bell, Inc., B56 North Ave., Columbus, Ohio.)

Although the technique as illustrated in Fig. 2-17*f* is adequate for the measurement of direct current, difficulties are encountered when alternating current or pulsating direct current is measured. Because the Hall chip and the wires leading from it that detect the Hall voltage constitute wholly or partly a single turn in the magnetic field, a voltage is induced by the changing current that is to be measured. This transformer voltage can be demonstrated by turning off the chip excitation current and varying the current to be measured. By careful arrangement of the wires carrying the Hall voltage, this transformer voltage can often be canceled. However, a more convenient method of eliminating the undesired signal (see Fig. 2-17*g*) consists of the purposeful detection of the transformer voltage by wrapping one or two turns of wire around the core and connecting the ends to a potentiometer. The Hall voltage is then connected in series opposition with the voltage derived from the potentiometer, as in Fig. 2-17*g*. Nulling of the undesired transformer voltage is accomplished by passing alternating current (I) through the current winding with the Hall chip excitation current turned off and adjusting the potentiometer. Once set, this adjustment need not be altered unless the physical arrangement of the wiring is changed. After this adjustment is made, the Hall chip current is applied and the Hall effect voltage (V_H) accurately reflects the current (I) being measured, provided the rate of change of current does not exceed the rise-time limit of the Hall chip.

Figure 2-17g diagrams the full potential of the Hall effect device as a circuit element. In reality, two variables, current and field strength, are related in the operation of the device. The variables may be alternating current or direct current or combinations thereof. The Hall voltage is proportional to the product of the two; thus the device functions as a multiplier.

Hall effect devices have been used relatively little in biomedical studies. They have obvious application in mapping the magnetic field produced by current from externally applied electrodes in studies of electroanesthesia and ventricular defibrillation. It is expected that Hall effect devices will find use in magnetobiology studies such as those reported by Valentinuzzi (1961, 1962) and Barnothy (1964), which describe the effects of magnetic fields on living specimens. The magnetic fields that accompany biological action currents may be detected by Hall effect transducers. (See Chap. 11).

2-7. GRANULAR STRAIN GAUGES

Another type of resistor used for transduction purposes consists of a capsule loosely packed with carbon granules. On one side of the capsule is a fixed electrode, and on the other is a movable one. When a force is applied, the granules are compacted and the resistance is reduced. Such capsules originated with the carbon button telephone transmitter, in which the diaphragm is coupled to the moving electrode. Small movements of the diaphragm change the resistance considerably and result in a high-efficiency conversion of sound pressure to an electrical signal.

In experimental physiology, the carbon button (granule) microphone was one of the first transducers to convert human heart sounds to an electrical signal. In 1895 Hurthle connected one in series with a battery and an inductorium, the secondary of which was connected to electrodes on a muscle attached in turn to a tambour that activated a writing lever. When the heart sounds occurred, the muscle was stimulated and the ensuing muscle twitches were recorded. Simultaneously, the movements of the chambers of the heart were detected and recorded by another tambour placed over the cardiac apex. The record did not illustrate the heart sound frequencies but did identify their temporal location in the cardiac cycle. About the same time Einthoven and Geluk (1894) recorded the heart sounds directly by connecting the carbon button microphone to a capillary electrometer. They were the first to record human, rabbit, and dog phonocardiograms. When electron tube amplifiers became available, the first amplifying stethoscopes used carbon button microphones.

To illustrate the efficiency of the carbon button microphone in detecting feeble sounds, the device was used by Falls and Rockwood (1923) to detect fetal heart sounds. Because of its high conversion efficiency, it is still employed in telephones today, but is infrequently used for research in acoustics because of its inferior frequency response and variable sensitivity. Perhaps the most serious defects in the carbon granule capsule are the inherently high hysteresis and high internal electrical noise, making it unreliable for the faithful registration of acoustic events.

Because of its high efficiency the carbon granule capsule still enjoys some popularity in biomedicine for detecting changing events. Using a carbon button in contact with an artery, Waud (1924) and Turner (1928) recorded the human pulse. No amplifier was employed in either study; the carbon button served to drive a recording pen directly in the former study and a string galvanometer in the latter. Gallagher and Grimwood (1953) included it in their indirect blood pressure-measuring system to detect the pulse in the caudal artery of the rat.

A variant of the carbon granule capsule was described by Clynes (1960). This device consisted of a distensible rubber tube filled with graphite. When wrapped around the chest, transduction of the respiratory movements was obtained.

Carbon-packed capsules are characterized by resistances in the hundreds of ohms and exhibit an appreciable and inconstant change in resistance with dimension change. High currents can be passed through them, resulting in high outputs—often sufficient to drive recorders directly. These devices, however, exhibit a poor baseline stability and, on occasion, tend to "freeze"; that is, the granules compact and must be loosened by vibration. If a high-gain system is employed with carbon granule capsules, the no-signal noise is quite high, a factor which caused the carbon button microphone to be abandoned in the early days of broadcasting.

2-8.   ELASTIC RESISTORS

By the appropriate addition of conducting material to rubber or to certain plastics, it is possible to make a resistor that increases its resistivity with strain ($\Delta L/L$), where L is the relaxed length and ΔL is the elongation. The addition of carbon to latex, which is then appropriately cured, produces a rubber with conducting properties which permits its use for the construction of elastic strain gauges. Badamo (1964) reported that one product, S-2086 electrically conducting carbon black loaded Silastic,[9] has been made to have a volume resistivity ranging from 8 to 60 Ω-cm. Another manufactuer[10] reported a standard product (UK 3032) with a resistivity of 7 Ω-cm. By varying the mixture, resistivities from 7 to 10^{16} Ω-cm were obtained. The elongation factor $(L + \Delta L)/L$ for UK 3032 is given as 2.1. The S-2086 conducting Silastic can be elongated by factors ranging from 1.4 to 2.5; the resistance of this material increases almost as an exponential function of elongation. The manufactuer reports that a 25% elongation more than triples the relaxed resistance. Figure 2-18 illustrates the resistance-elongation characteristic of a piece of this material measured by one of the authors. It shows that linearity is attainable only over a limited range of extension (10 to 20%). Although larger extensions can be tolerated by some conducting elastomers, with others, elongations greater than 25 to 30% result in appreciable resistance hysteresis.

Conducting rubber strain gauges have been used infrequently to detect force or movement; however, an application by Fromm (1967) is of more than passing interest. He fabricated an elastic strain gauge for detecting and telemetering uterine contractions in the unrestrained rabbit by using a

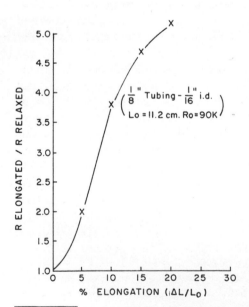

Figure 2-18.   Elastic resistor-resistance versus elongation.

[9] Dow Corning Center for Aid to Medical Research, Midland, Mich.
[10] Minor Rubber Co., Inc., Bloomfield, N.J.

$\frac{1}{16}$ in. diameter carbon-loaded Silastic cylinder around which he wrapped two electrodes of 35 gauge wire; the electrodes were separated by 1 mm. The elastic strain gauge was sealed in plastic tubing for waterproofing and implanted into a rabbit. This system was used to record uterine contractions for 6 weeks.

The elastic strain gauge used by Fromm exhibited a resistance of 200 Ω when relaxed. With stretch, the resistance increased by 1 Ω for one gram of applied force, the force-limit for linearity.

The attractive characteristics of elastic resistors recommended their use for the transduction of events associated with an appreciable dimension change. In practical applications, however, it is frequently difficult to establish a stable electrical contact with the material. Conducting paints, clamps, and nuts and bolts have all been employed. One of the authors has had success in making contact with conducting tubing by forcing the ends over short metal rods or tubes that served as electrodes.

2-9.   ELECTROLYTIC STRAIN GAUGES

Elastic strain gauges that employ liquid conductors are used to a limited extent in biomedical studies. As far back as the turn of the century Grunbaum (1898) described the first of such devices, an aqueous electrolytic pressure capsule 5 mm in diameter and 12.5 mm long, mounted on the end of a catheter. On the side of the capsule was a thin rubber window carrying an electrode. The other electrode was mounted on the inside wall of the capsule, which was filled with zinc chloride. Pressure applied to the distensible window decreased the interelectrode distance, thereby reducing the resistance between the electrodes. This device was certainly one of the first catheter-tip pressure transducers and must have produced blood pressure records of high fidelity for that time. However, no such records produced by this instrument have been found.

Successors to Grunbaum's transducer were described by Schutz (1931) and Wagner (1932). Schutz employed platinum electrodes and a copper sulfate solution as the electrolyte. Wagner's instrument also consisted of a capsule filled with copper sulfate solution mounted at the end of a catheter. Using this device, which exhibited a resonant frequency of approximately 60 Hz, he presented some of the earliest electrically transduced records of the pressures in the right ventricle of a rabbit.

For some reason the electrolytic strain gauge fell into disuse for many years, being revived by Müller (1942) and Dalla-Torre (1943) to record human digital volume pulses. Their strain gauges consisted of rubber tubing, a fraction of a millimeter in diameter, filled with an electrolyte. The ends of the tubing were plugged by the electrodes. When such tubes are stretched, the length increases and the diameter decreases, thereby raising the resistance appreciably.

Aqueous electrolyte strain gauges are lightweight, easy to make, and inexpensive. They are medium to high in resistance. Müller's units were 0.2 mm in diameter and 5 to 6 cm long. When filled with diluted Electroargol, the strain gauge had a resistance of 1 MΩ. After an initial elongation, the resistance increased nearly linearly with extension over a fairly wide range. Figure 2-19 presents the equation for the resistance increase and the degree of linearity that can be expected. Elongations to 50% of the relaxed length are often used to permit measurement of the large changes in circumference or length experienced by many organs and members. Although a large signal per unit of extension can be obtained, this advantage is partly offset by the errors introduced by temperature changes. The temperature coefficient for many aqueous electrolytes is -2% per degree centigrade but can be as high as -10%. Hence temperature compensation is necessary.

In an interesting electrolytic resistor strain gauge, described by Waggoner (1965), the electrolyte was an electrode paste contained in a rubber tube. Waggoner reported that the resistance of such gauges depends on the dimensions, and in practice, with tubing 0.2 to 3 mm in diameter, resistances varying between 1 and 400 kΩ were observed. The change in resistance varied as L^2/V, where L is the length and V the volume of the gauge. A small negative resistance-temperature coefficient was noted. Waggoner reported successful use of these strain gauges for recording respiration, cardiac contraction, kidney volume, and thumb pulse.

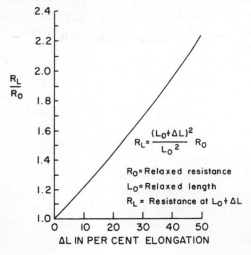

$$R_L = \frac{(L_0 + \Delta L)^2}{L_0^2} R_0$$

R_0 = Relaxed resistance
L_0 = Relaxed length
R_L = Resistance at $L_0 + \Delta L$

ΔL IN PER CENT ELONGATION

Figure 2-19. Electrolytic resistor-resistance versus elongation.

Aqueous electrolytic strain gauges usually have a relatively short life because electrolytic decomposition of the electrodes proceeds even when the devices are not in use. When direct current is passed through the element, the lifetime is further reduced. For maximum life, alternating current should be employed for excitation.

2-10. MERCURY STRAIN GAUGE

Whitney (1949) described the construction of strain gauges using small-bore rubber tubing filled with mercury. Like the aqueous electrolytic types, these gauges permit the measurement of small or large changes in elongation. Because they are lightweight, easy to construct, inexpensive, and available commercially,[11] they see considerable service in biomedical studies; for example, Whitney (1949, 1953, 1954) and Greenfield et al. (1963) employed them to measure the volume changes in body segments as blood entered and left the region encircled by the gauge. Rushmer (1955, 1965) selected similar gauges to measure the changes in circumference, hence the volume changes, of the rapidly beating canine left ventricle and aorta. Lawton and Collins (1959) used the mercury strain gauge to measure the pulsatile changes in aortic circumference. Maulsby and Hoff (1962) sutured similar strain gauges to the right ventricles of dogs and continuously measured the dimension changes that reflected the volume changes in that cardiac chamber. Shapiro et al. (1964) encircled the chests of human subjects with mercury-in-rubber gauges to detect the changes in thoracic circumference which accompany respiration.

When mercury is employed in small-bore (approximately 0.5 mm I.D.) elastic tubing, the resistance of typical gauges is in the vicinity of 0.02 to 0.20 Ω per centimeter of length. The force necessary to elongate a typical 35-mm gauge 6 mm was given by Lawton and Collins (1959) as 20 grams. The force-extension curve exhibited a slight nonlinearity. Rushmer (1955) noted that good linearity was obtained beyond a small initial extension. He also reported that his gauges performed satisfactorily with extensions up to 100% of the relaxed length.

The change in resistance with elongation can be determined from Fig. 2-19, whose values were calculated from perfect elasticity and constant-volume considerations; that is, an increase in length results in a corresponding decrease in diameter, the total volume remaining constant. For small extensions the coefficient is approximately 2% increase in resistance for a 1% increase in length. This value was quoted by Whitney, who employed rubber tubing. In a typical application, in which a low voltage was

---

[11] Parks Electronics Laboratory, Box 35, Beaverton, Ore.

applied to a Wheatstone bridge containing a 3.5-cm gauge, a signal of 0.24 mV was obtained per millimeter change in length per volt applied to the bridge (Lawton and Collins, 1959). Most investigators employ 2 to 6 V to energize the bridge.

Elsner et al. (1959) described a method of eliminating many of the difficulties encountered in using the mercury strain gauge with direct current. By coupling the gauge to a step-up transformer placed in one arm of an impedance bridge and by connecting balancing resistors to a transformer placed in the adjacent arm, they were able to operate the bridge on alternating current and obtain practical ease in balancing the bridge. The alternating current also permitted the use of conventional R-C coupled or carrier amplifiers to process the signal for ultimate recording. With this sytem these investigators reported obtaining an overall sensitivity of 1 mm of recorder deflection for 2 microns of extension of a mercury gauge 5 cm long.

In practical applications a rapid response time is attainable with the mercury strain gauge. Rushmer (1955) reported a value (0 to 100%) of less than 0.01 sec with his 35-mm gauges, and Lawton and Collins (1959), by applying a sinusoidal stretching force, carefully measured the frequency response and phase shift of similar gauges at various elongations. They found that the sine wave frequency response curve was essentially 100% to 20 Hz, increasing to 110% at approximately 50 Hz and reaching 150% at 100 Hz. The phase shifts at these frequencies were 10, 25, and 45°, respectively.

Because of its practical features, the mercury strain gauge will see continued application, despite its defects. As with the aqueous electrolyte strain gauge, temperature changes constitute a source of error in many applications. Although the temperature coefficient of resistivity for mercury is considerably less than that of the copper wires employed with the gauge, Whitney described the need for compensating resistors when mercury strain gauges are employed for peripheral plethysmography on human subjects. In biothermal plethysmographic studies the thermal resistance variation becomes objectionable. Eagan (1961) reported that a 22.5°C change in temperature is equivalent to a 2% change in resistance or a 1% change in length. Honda (1962) stated that a 25°C change in temperature of the mercury is equivalent to a 1% change in length. To compensate for this change, he mounted a compensating resistor made of copper wire in a rubber tube adjacent to the mercury strain gauge element. The compensating resistor was connected to the adjacent arm of the bridge. By using alternating current on the bridge and transformer coupling to the gauge and compensating resistor, he was able to adjust the bridge for full compensation for a 25°C temperature change.

Another factor worthy of attention is the short-term creep reported by Lawton and Collins (1959). However, they felt that this was unimportant in dynamic studies.

Perhaps one of the chief drawbacks to prolonged use of mercury gauges involves the corrosive nature of mercury. Some types of rubber tubing are attacked by mercury, and in nearly every case the elctrodes deteriorate after a period of time. Copper, brass, and platinum electrodes have been employed with some success. All who have made mercury strain gauges have called attention to the need to use clean mercury, perferably triply distilled.

Although latex rubber tubing was employed in the early gauges, silicone rubbers are now universally used. Whitney in the United Kingdom employed No. 1 surgical drainage tubing[12] (0.7-mm bore, 0.7-mm wall) and latex tubing[12] (0.5-mm bore, 0.8-mm wall). In the United States silicone[13] tubing can be readily obtained.

2-11. HUMISTORS

We define a humistor as any device in which there occurs a resistance change that depends on humidity; that is, a humistor is a humidity-sensitive resistor. A variety of names, including resistance or conductance hygrometer and resistance or conductance psychrometer, have been used to describe these transducers. The operation of all such devices relies on the moisture dependence of the resistivity and dielectric constant of many insulators, since changes in these properties are used to measure environmental humidity. In general, most materials exhibit a decrease in resistivity and an increase in dielectric constant with increasing moisture content. However, some materials increase their resistivity with increasing moisture content. The electrical recording of relative humidity is often designated electrohygrometry.

Before describing the various humidity-sensitive resistors, it is useful to give some definitions. Humidity is a measure of the water vapor present in a gas and is expressed in either relative or absolute terms. Relative humidity is defined as the ratio of the partial pressure of the water vapor present to the water vapor pressure required for saturation at a given temperature. Percent relative humidity is this ratio multiplied by 100. Absolute humidity is the mass of water vapor contained in a volume of moist gas; the units most frequently employed are grams per cubic meter.

Traditionally the moisture content of air is determined by a

[12] Dunlop Special Products, England.
[13] Dow Corning Center for Aid to Medical Research, Midland, Mich., Huntingdon Rubber Mills, Box 70, Portland, Ore.; Becton Dickinson (Vivosil 7002-012), Rutherford, N.J.

psychrometer, a device containing two thermometers; the bulb of one measures the environmental temperature (dry bulb), and around the bulb of the other is a wick from which water is evaporated to produce cooling. The relative humidity is related to the difference in temperature between the readings on the wet- and dry-bulb thermometers. Figure 2-20 presents this relationship. It is perhaps unnecessary to state that the wet- and dry-bulb thermometers could be suitably waterproofed thermistors.

Relative humidity is also measured by the dew-point technique in which the temperature of a polished metal container is reduced (usually by evaporation of a volatile liquid) until there is visible condensation of water vapor. The temperature of condensation is called the "dew point," and there is a relationship between the dew point, environmental temperature, and relative humidity. Figure 2-21 indicates this relationship.

A typical humistor consists of a dielectric film (often a plastic) that supports two electrodes. On the film is a hygroscopic salt such as lithium chloride, barium fluoride, potassium dihydrogen phosphate, or phosphorus pentoxide. Aluminum oxide and carbon have also been used. The resistance of such substances usually decreases nonlinearly with increasing relative humidity.

There are several biologic applications of humistors, and in all these the presence of sweat is detected. Hemingway (1944) pointed out the interesting fact that the appearance of "cold sweat" accompanied the oc-

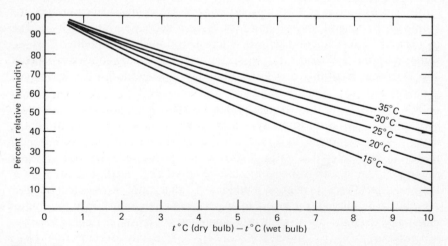

Figure 2-20. Percentage of relative humidity versus temperature difference between dry-bulb and wet-bulb thermometers and various environmental temperatures. (Plotted from data in *Handbook of Chemistry and Physics,* 44th ed., Chemical Rubber Publishing Co., Cleveland, 1962.)

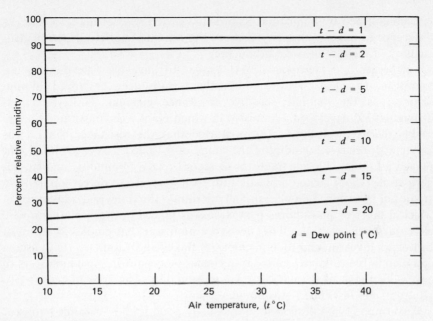

Figure 2-21. Relative humidity versus air temperature for various dew point depressions ($t -d$). (Plotted from data in *Handbook of Chemistry and Physics* 44th ed., Chemical Rubber Publishing Co., Cleveland, 1962.)

currence of motion sickness. To document the onset of motion sickness in subjects experiencing accelerative forces, Hemingway continuously recorded the resistance between two electrodes placed on the forehead. The secretion of cold sweat suddenly reduced the resistance and provided a definite index of the onset of motion sickness. This information was used in studies of the effectiveness of drugs designed to reduce sensitivity to motion sickness. The detection of cold sweat was described by Ackerman (1968) who developed a lithium chloride humistor having a short response time. Another application of humistors is concerned with measurement of the secretion of sweat that accompanies an emotional response to a stimulus. A very obvious application of humistors is in the measurement of thermal sweating.

Humistors are used to determine the rate of sweating by measurement of the relative humidity in the air passing over a circumscribed area of skin. The technique employs a small chamber applied securely to the skin where sweating is to be measured. Dry air (or air with a known moisture content) is admitted to the chamber and is moistened by the perspiration; hence there is an increase in the relative humidity of the air emerging from an exit port. Measurement of the difference in humidity of the inlet and outlet air is accomplished by humistors. Knowledge of the rate of air flow and the difference in relative humidity between the inlet and outlet air permits calculation of the rate of sweat production.

Sulzberger and Hermann (1954) appear to have been the first to use humistors to measure sweat rate; their transducer employed lithium chloride as the humidity-sensitive resistance element. Nakayama and Takagi (1959) developed a humistor in which plant pith constituted the humidity-sensitive substance. They reported that the resistance change was linear with relative humidity in the range of 5 to 25%. Bullard (1962) employed a lithium chloride humistor to record relative humidity, and Rosenberg et al. (1962) coated a plastic film with graphite to detect humidity in studies of sweating. Van Gasselt and Vierhout (1963) devised a humistor in which a layer of phosphorus pentoxide was placed between platinum-wire electrodes. Najbrt et al. (1964) devised a humistor that employed a film of bentonite, glycerin, and sodium chloride. Baker and Kligman (1967) used a commercially available[14] humidity recorder incorporating five humistors to cover the range of 0 to 100% relative humidity. The type of sensor employed in this instrument was not identified.

Ackerman (1968) described an unusually good lithium chloride humistor that was developed to have a short response time. His construction details are presented here since the device is easy to make and is quite temperature insensitive. The transducer consisted of two zigzag copper electrodes etched onto a circular polyvinyl chloride (PVC) printed-circuit board measuring 1.5 cm in diameter (see inset, Fig. 2-22). The humidity-sensitive coating, which bridged the electrodes, consisted of a hygroscopic substance (a mixture of lithium chloride and aluminum chloride) dissolved in a binder to which water was added. The binder was made with 0.7 gram of 98% hydrolyzed polyvinyl alcohol dissolved in 10 ml of distilled water under gentle heating until the solution became translucent. To this solution was added 0.1 ml of nonionic detergent (alkyl phenoxypolyethoxy ethanol) sold under the trade name Triton X-100. Ackerman's sensors were prepared by combining the desired volumes of saturated lithium chloride and aluminum chloride solutions with equal parts of binder and distilled water. The cleaned electrode assembly was then dipped into this solution, slowly withdrawn, and heat treated to 60°C for 30 min with the electrode surface in a horizontal position; then it was dried in a desiccator for at least 24 hr. Ackerman tested the performance characteristics of these sensors by varying the proportions of lithium chloride in the aqueous binder. A mixture of 0.2 vol % Li Cl · H_2O and 0.8 vol % $AlCl_3$ provided the shortest response time. Figure 2-22 presents typical data for such a sensor, which

[14] Sage Instruments, Inc., White Plains, N.Y. 10601.

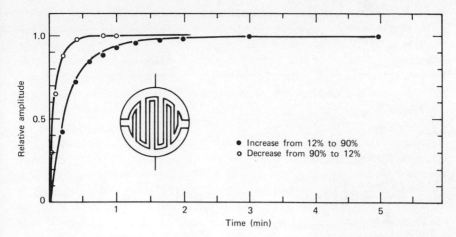

Figure 2-22. Response to a step change in relative humidity of a humistor consisting of a film of 0.2 vol % LiCl · H_2O and 0.8 vol % $AlCl_3$ applied to a zigzag electrode configuration (see inset). (Courtesy of U. Ackerman, Memorial University, St. John's, Newfoundland 1973.)

exhibited a resistance of about 25 Ω at 12% and 1 to 2 MΩ at 90% relative humidity. Ackerman used a current of 0.5 μA to measure the humidity-induced resistance change.

A simple method of measuring humidity employs organic material such as thread or hair. The shortening of human hair with increasing relative humidity is nonlinear and small in magnitude, amounting to about 2% change in length for a change in relative humidity of 0 to 100%. Small as this change is, it is nonetheless used in a number of familiar, low-cost dial instruments that indicate relative humidity directly. Although coupling a strain gauge element to a human hair, under moderate tension, ought to provide an easily-fabricated, low-cost electrical humidity sensor, the authors are unaware of the existence or use of such a device.

When sweating is measured, a skin chamber of about 4 cm² in area is employed; the air flow rate depends on the sweat rate. In practice, a typical air flow range is 0.1 to 1.0 l/min. Baker and Kligman (1967) presented the following expression for the water loss W, in milligrams per square centimeter per hour from a sweating surface S, in square centimeters.

$$W = \frac{60DA\,(\Delta RH)}{100S}.$$

In this expression ΔRH is the change in relative humidity between the outflowing and inflowing air, A is the air flow (l/min), and D is the density

Table 2-4   Rate of Sweating in Human Subjects

Authors	Site		Method	Average Value (mg/hr/cm²)
Baker and Kligman (1967)	Back	*in vivo*	Electrohygrometry	0.23
Baker and Kligman (1967)	Forearm	*in vivo*	Electrohygrometry	0.30
Baker and Kligman (1967)	Abdomen	*in vivo*	Electrohygrometry	0.36
Baker and Kligman (1967)	Shin	*in vivo*	Electrohygrometry	0.42
Burch and Winsor (1944)	Abdomen	*in vivo*	Gravimetric with air flow	5.8
	Abdomen	*in vitro*	Gravimetric with air flow	6.5
Feisher and Rothman (1945)	Abdomen	*in vivo*	Calcium chloride bag in closed chamber	1.1
Blank (1952)	Abdomen	*in vitro*	Diffusion chamber	0.1–0.2
Mali (1956)	Trunk	*in vitro*	Diffusion chamber	0.5–0.6
	Sole	*in vitro*	Diffusion chamber	3.0
Monash and Blank (1958)	Abdomen	*in vivo*	Calcium chloride bag in closed chamber	2.0–9.0
Rosenberg et al. (1962)	Abdomen	*in vivo*	Electrohygrometry, closed chamber	0.15–0.24
Onken and Moyer (1963)	Abdomen	*in vitro*	Diffusion chamber	0.3
Spruit and Malten (1965)	Forearm	*in vivo*	Electrohygrometry with air flow	0.5–1.7
Bettley and Grice (1965)	Abdomen	*in vivo*	Gravimetric with air flow	0.25

of water (mg/l of air) of saturated steam at the temperature of the flowing air stream. Values for A are obtained from standard tables.

Using the commercially available resistance hygrometer, Baker and Kligman (1967) obtained sweat-rate data for various sites on the bodies of typical human subjects. Their results are presented in Table 2-4 along with data obtained from their review of previous literature.

The measurement of sweat rate is not a clinical diagnostic test at present. There are, however, a variety of diseases in which sweating is enhanced or depressed. Whether the measurement of sweat rate will contribute to the early diagnosis of such diseases awaits future investigation.

REFERENCES

Ackerman, U. 1968. A detector for the outbreak of sweating. Institute of Biomedical Electronics. University of Toronto, Report 12, 19 pp.

Adams, R. 1962. Personal communication. School of Aerospace Medicine, Brooks, AFB, Texas.

Angelakos, E. T. 1964. Semiconductor pressure microtransducers for measuring velocity and acceleration of intra-ventricular pressures. *Am. J. Med. Electron.* **3**:260–270.

Anrep, C. V., E. W. H. Cruickshank, A. C. Downing, and A. S. Rau. 1927. The coronary circulation in relation to the cardiac cycle. *J. Physiol.* **14**:111–134.

Badamo, D. J. 1964. The silicones as bioengineering materials. *Proc. 17th Ann. Conf. Eng. Biol. Med.* McGregor and Werner, Washington, D. C., 129 pp.

Baker, H., and A. M. Kligman. 1967. Measurement of transepidermal water loss by electrical hygrometry. *Arch. Derm.* **96**:441–452.

Barnothy, M. 1964. *Biological Effects of Magnetic Fields.* Plenum Press, New York, 324 pp.

Boniface, K. H., D. J. Brodie, and R. P. Walton 1953. Resistance strain gauge arches for direct measurement of heart contractile force in animals. *Proc. Soc. Exp. Biol. Med.* **84**:263–266.

Bramwell, J. C., A. V. Hill, and B. A. McSwinney, 1923. The velocity of the pulse wave in man. *Heart.* **10**:233–256.

Brown, J. M. 1960. Anesthesia and the contractile force of the heart. *Curr. Res. Anesth. Analg.* **39**:487–498.

Bullard, R. W. 1962. Continuous recording of sweating rate by resistance hygrometry. *J. Appl. Physiol.* **17**:735–737.

Clynes, M. 1960. Respiratory control of heart rate. *IRE Trans. Med. Electron.* **ME-7**:2–14.

Cornwall, J. B. 1965. The matching and linearising of thermistor probes. *World Med. Electron.* **3**:233-234.

Cotton, M. de V., and H. M. Maling. 1957. Relationships among stroke work, contractile force and fiber length changes in ventricular function. *Am. J. Physiol.* **189**:580–586.

Dalla-Torre, L. 1943. Utilization d'une nouvelle méthode pour l'enrégistrement du sphygmogramme des artères digitales. *Helv. Physiol. Pharamcol. Acta.* **1**:C14-15.

Eagan, C. J. 1961. The mercury gauge method of digital plethysmography. USAF Tech. Note AAL-TN-60-15 (February 1961), TN, 60–16 (March 1961), TN–60–17 (February 1961). Alaskan Air Command.

Einthoven, W., and M. A. Geluk, 1894: Die Registreirung der Herztöne. *Arch. Ges. Physiol.* **57**:617–639.

Elsner, R. W., C. H. Eagan, and S. Andersen. 1959. Impedance matching circuit for mercury strain gauge. *J. Appl. Physiol.* **14**:871–872.

Falls, F. H., and A. C. Rockwood, 1923. Use of microphone stethoscope in demonstration of fetal heart sounds. *J. AMA.* **81**:1683–1684.

Fleming, D. G. 1958. Precautions in the physiological application of thermistors. *J. Appl. Physiol.* **13**:529–530.

Fromm, E. 1967. A miniature contractile force telemetering system. *Proc. 20th ACEMB* (Boston), vol. 9.

Gallagher, D. J. A., and L. H. Grimwood. 1953. A simple method for measuring blood pressure in the rat tail. *J. Physiol.* **121**:163–166.

Garb, S. 1951. The effects of potassium, ammonium, calcium, strontium, and magnesium on the electrogram and myogram of mammalian heart muscle. *J. Pharamcol. Exp. Therap.* **101**:317–326.

Geddes, L. A., H. E. Hoff, A. G. Moore, and M. Hinds. 1966. An electrical caliper myograph. *Am. J. Pharm. Educ.* **30**:209–211.

Geddes, L. A., H. E. Hoff, and W. A. Spencer. 1961. The Center for Vital Studies—A new laboratory for the study of bodily functions in man. *IRE Trans. Bio-Med. Electron.* **BME-8**:33–45.

Greenfield, A. D. M., R. J. Whitney, and J. F. Mowbray. 1963. Methods for the investigation of peripheral blood flow. *Brit. Med. Bull.* **19**:101–109.

Grunbaum, O. F. F. 1898. On a new method of recording alternations in blood pressure. *J. Physiol.* **22**:49–50.

Grundfest, H., and J. J. Hay. 1945. A strain gauge recorder for physiological volume, pressure and deformation measurements. *Science* **101**:255–256.

Hall, E. H. 1879. On a new action of the magnet on electric currents, *Am. J. Math.* **2**:287–292.

Hampel, A. 1941. Elektrisches Transmissionmanometer auf der Grundlage elektrischer Widerstandsänderungen des Wismuts im Magnetfeld. *Arch. Ges. Physiol.* **244**:171–175.

Hemingway, A. 1944. Cold sweating in motion sickness. *Am. J. Physiol.* **141**:172–175.

Hill, A. V. 1920–1921a. An electrical pulse recorder. *J. Physiol.* **54**:lii–liii.

Hill, A. V. 1920–1921b. The meaning of records with the hot wire sphygmograph. *J. Physiol.* **54**:cxvii–cxix.

Holzer, W. 1940. Über die Anwendung des galvano-magnetischèn Longitudinal-effektes des Wismuts zur elektrischen Fernübertragung von Bewegungsvorgängen. *Arch. Ges. Physiol.* **244**:176–180.

Honda, N. 1962. Temperature compensation for mercury strain gauge used in plethysmography. *J. Appl.-Physiol.* **17**:572–574.

Huntsman, L. L., G. L. Nichols, P. Verdugo, and G. H. Pollack. 1971. A new instrument for mechanical testing of tissues. *Proc. 24th Ann. Conf. Eng. Med. Biol.,* paper 7.9.

Huntsman, L. L., D. K. Stewart, and G. H. Pollack. 1972. An engineering approach to myocardial performance assessment. *Proc. 25th Ann. Conf. Eng. Med. Biol.,* paper 23–1.

Hurthle, K. 1895. Beiträge zur Hämodynamik. *Arch. Ges. Physiol.* **60**:263–290.

Katsura, S., R. Weiss, D. Baker, and R. F. Rushmer. 1959. Isothermal blood flow velocity probe. *IRE Trans. Med. Electron.* **ME-8**:283–285.

Lambert, E. H., and E. H. Wood. 1947. The use of resistance wire strain gauge monometer to measure intra-arterial pressure. *Proc. Soc. Exp. Biol. Med.* **64**:186–190.

Lamson, P. D., and B. H. Robbins. 1928. Thermal conductivity methods of gas analysis in the study of pharmacological problem. *J. Pharm. Exp. Therap.* **34**:325–331.

Lawton, R. W., and C. C. Collins. 1959. Calibration of an aortic circumference gauge. *J. Appl. Physiol.* **14**:465–467.

Ledig, P. C., and R. S. Lyman. 1927. An adaptation of the thermal conductivity method to the analysis of respiratory gases. *J. Clin. Invest.* **4**:494–565.

Le Gette, M. A. 1958. Strain gauge principles. *Instr. Automation* **31**:447–449.

Mason, W. P., and R. N. Thurston. 1957. Use of piezoresistive materials in the measurement of displacement, force and torque. *J. Acoust. Soc. Am.* **29**:1096–1101.

Maulsby, R. L., and H. E. Hoff. 1962. Hypotensive mechanisms of pulmonary insufflation in dogs. *Am. J. Physiol.* **202**:505–509.

Mellander, S., and R. F. Rushmer. 1960. Venous blood flow recorded with an isothermal flowmeter. *Acta Physiol. Scand.* **43**:13–19.

Millar, H. D., and L. E. Baker. 1973. A stable ultraminiature catheter-tip transducer. *Med. Biol. Eng.* **11**(1):86–89.

Müller, A. 1942. Über die Pulsform und Wellengeschwindigkeit in den Fingerarterien. *Arch. Krieslaufforsch.* **11**:198–206.

Najbrt, V. L., L. Rovensky, J. Pompeova, and B. Konrad. 1964. Studie o mereni dynamity bariéové funkce. *Cs. Derm.* **39**(2):88–93.

Nakayama, T., and K. Takagi. 1959. Minute pattern of human perspiration observed by a continuously recording method. *Jap. J. Physiol.* **9**:359–364.

Nunn, H. E. 1959. A guide to static pressure transducers that have a diaphragm, bellows or Bourdon pressure cell. *Prod. Eng.* **30**:48–49.

Rein, H., A. A. Hampel, and W. A. Heinemann. 1940. Photoelektrische Transmissionmanometer zur Blutdruckschreibung. *Arch. Ges. Physiol.* **243**:329–335.

Rosenberg, E. W., H. Blank, and S. Resnik. 1962. Sweating and water loss through the skin. *J.A.M.A.* **179**:809–811.

Rushmer, R. F. 1965. Pressure circumference relations in the left ventricle. *Am. J. Physiol.* **186**:115–121.

Rushmer, R. F. 1955a. Pressure-circumference relations in the aorta. *Am. J. Physiol.* **183**:545–549.

Rushmer, R. F. 1955b. Length-circumference relations of the left ventricle. *Cir. Res.* **3**:639–644.

Sanchez, J. C. 1961. Semiconductor strain gauges—a state of the art summary. *Strain Gauge Readings* **4**:3–16.

Schutz, E. 1931. Konstruktion einer manometrischen Sonde mit elektrisher Transmission. *Z. Biol.* **91**:515–521.

Shapiro, A., H. D. Cohen, E. Maher, and W. J. McAveney. 1964. On-line analog computation of volume of respired air. *Proc. 17th Ann. Conf. Eng. Med. Biol.* McGregor and Werner, Washington D.C., 129 pp.

Simmonds, E. E. 1942. U.S. Pat. 2,292,549.

Simons, D. G. 1962. Personal communication. School of Aerospace Medicine, Brooks AFB, Texas.

Smith, C. S. 1954. Piezoresistive effect of germanium and silicon. *Phys. Rev.* **94**:42–49.

Star, J. 1963. Hall effect transducers. *Instr. Control Syst.* **36**:113–116.

Sulzberger, M. B. and F. Hermann. 1954. *The Critical Significance of Disturbances in the Delivery of Sweat.* Charles C. Thomas, Springfield, Ill.

Swanson, C. A., and A. C. Emslie. 1954. Low temperature electronics. *Proc. IRE* **42**:402–413.

Tomlinson, H. 1876–1877. On the increase in resistance to the passage of an electric current produced on stretching. *Proc. Roy. Soc. (London)* **25**:451–453.

Tucker, W. S. and E. T. Paris. 1921. A selective hot-wire microphone. *Phil. Trans. Roy. Soc. (London)* Ser. A **221A**:389–430.

Turner, R. H. 1928. A sphygmograph using a carbon grain microphone and the string galvanometer. *Bull. Johns Hopkins Hosp.* **43**:2–13.

Valentinuzzi, M. 1961. *Magnetobiology*. North American Aviation, Los Angeles, 74 pp.

Valentinuzzi, M. 1962. A theory of magnetic growth inhibition. Chicago, Committee on Mathematical Biology, 58 pp.

Van Dover, J. and N. F. Bechtold. 1960. Survey of thermistor characteristics. *Electronics* **33**:58-60.

Van Gasselt, H. R. M., and R. R. Vierhout. 1963. Registration of the insensible perspiration and small quantities of sweat. *Dermatologica*. **127**:255-257.

Victory Engineering Corp., Union, N.J. 1955. *Thermistor Data Book*.

Waggoner, W. C. 1965. High-impedance elastic force gauge. *Am. J. Med. Electron.* **4**:175-177.

Wagner, R. 1932. Die Beeinflussung des Druckablaufes in verschiedenen Herzabschnitten bei wechselnden Bedingungen der Herztätigkeit. *Z. Biol.* **92**:55-86.

Waud, R. A. 1924. An electric polygraph. *JAMA* **82**:1203.

Whitney, R. J. 1949. The measurement of changes in human limb-volume by means of a mercury-in-rubber strain gauge. *J. Physiol.* **109**:5P-6P.

Whitney, R. J. 1953, 1954. The measurement of volume changes in human limbs. *J. Physiol.* 1953, **121**:1-27; 1954, **125**:1-24.

3

Inductive Transducers

3-1. SINGLE INDUCTOR

The inductance of a coil depends on its geometry, the magnetic permeability of the medium in which it is located, and the number of turns. The approximate low-frequency inductance in microhenries of a single-layer air-core coil can be calculated by the following formula, due to Wheeler (1928):

$$L = \frac{r^2 n^2}{9r + 10l},$$

where r and l are the radius and length in inches, and n is the number of turns. This expression is accurate when the length of the coil is much greater than the diameter. Wheeler stated that the accuracy is within 1% when l is greater than 0.8 times the radius. Although there are many other expressions for the inductance of single-layer coils in which a form factor (dependent on the ratio of length to diameter) is present, the important fact is that the inductance varies with the square of the number of turns and the geometry of the coil. Thus distortion of the coil, as by stretching or compressing, will alter its inductance. This method of inductance change is seldom used because of the small inductance and the even smaller inductance change occurring in coils that can be distorted. If a coil spring happens to be present in a system in which it is desired to detect motion, the changing dimensions of the spring can serve as an inductance transducer. If the spring is of ferromagnetic material, the inductance will be somewhat greater than that expected from calculations on the basis of coil geometry. If the coil surrounds a material having a magnetic permeability greater than that of air, the inductance is increased considerably.

Practically, control of the inductance can be gained by altering the magnetic permeability of the medium. A considerable increase in inductance can be obtained by inserting a magnetically permeable core into the coil.

Under these conditions the inductance will depend on the amount of core inside the coil, thereby affording a method of translating displacement to an inductance change.

Single inductors have frequently been employed to measure physiological events that can be converted to movement. One such transducer was described by Fuller and Gordon (1948), who fitted the diaphragm of a Marey tambour with a ferromagnetic ring. Inside the tambour was an iron-cored coil, the inductance of which was changed when the diaphragm was displaced by pressure. Müller et al. (1948) described a simple flowmeter consisting of a variable-inductance differential pressure tranducer connected to a Pitot tube. Their transducer consisted of an iron-cored coil placed close to an elastic diaphragm that carried a small soft iron disk. Movement of the disk, in response to pressure changes across the diaphragm, altered the inductance and unbalanced a 5-kHz bridge circuit, thereby producing an alternating voltage proportional to pressure, which was in turn proportional to blood flow. Rushmer (1954) described a truly remarkable application of the variable-inductance technique to measure continuously the diameter of the left ventricle of a dog as the heart was beating. He was able to suture a small coil to one ventricular wall and the core to the septum. As the diameter changed with each heart beat, the core moved within the coil, causing inductance changes that indicated, when recorded in the unanesthetized dog, alterations in the size of the ventricle during a variety of experimental conditions.

A commercially available[1] catheter-tip single-inductance blood pressure transducer is shown next to a sailmaker's needle in Fig. 3-1. A cutaway diagram of the variable-inductance sensor appears on the left. Pressure applied to the elastic membrane alters the position of the core in the inductor, which forms part of the frequency-determining circuit of an oscillator. As the core is displaced, the inductance is changed, giving rise to a frequency-modulated signal, which is recorded after suitable processing.

3-2. MUTUAL INDUCTANCE

The principle of mutual inductance, which employs two coils, is also used in the measurement of physiological events. When two coils are joined in series and their fields link, the inductance L is equal to $L_1 + L_2 + 2M$, where L_1 and L_2 are the inductances of the individual coils, and M, the mutual inductance between them, is dependent on the coupling between the coils. The coupling can be altered by inserting a magnetically permeable core or by moving one coil with respect to the other.

[1] Carolina Medical Electronics, King, N.C.

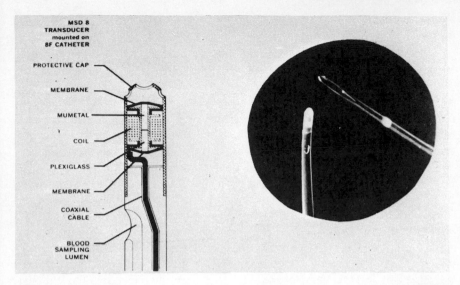

Figure 3-1. Catheter-tip inductance pressure transducer. (Courtesy of Carolina Medical Electronics, King, N.C.)

If the two coils are not joined electrically and an oscillator is connected across one of them, a voltage will be induced in the other. The arrangement constitutes a transformer. The two windings are designated the primary and the secondary, the energy source being connected to the primary winding. The magnitude of the voltage appearing across the secondary coil is dependent on the coupling, which can be varied by the insertion of a magnetically permeable core or by moving one coil with respect to the other.

There are many practical applications of two inductances connected in series opposition in which the coupling between them is altered by changing the position of a centrally mounted core. One such application is that of Gauer and Gienapp (1950), who built a unique catheter-tip blood pressure tranducer. A diaphragm having the diameter of the catheter actuated a small ferromagnetic core, which, moving in response to the pressure changes, altered the coupling between the coils and produced proportional changes in inductance. This early catheter-tip pressure transducer had a resonant frequency of 1000 Hz in fluid and for a considerable time stood alone as the highest-fidelity blood pressure tranducer.

A larger two-inductance pressure transducer, the "Clark Capsule," was described by Motley et al. (1947). In this device two coils were mounted on either side of a distensible, magnetically permeable, elastic diaphragm. The two coils constituted the two arms of an inductance bridge that was balanced in the absence of pressure on the diaphragm. When pressure was applied, the diaphragm was deformed and the bridge became unbalanced, producing a signal that was recorded after suitable processing. The performance was reported to be only slightly inferior to that of the Hamilton manometer, one of the highest-quality optical manometers and considered to be the standard instrument for blood pressure recording.

Scher et al. (1953) constructed an interesting inductance transducer for blood flow in which a ferromagnetic paddle in a flow tube was placed midway between two coils wrapped around the outside of the tube. The two coils formed the arms of a balanced inductance bridge. The flow of blood deflected the paddle and unbalanced the bridge. A recording of the unbalance voltage was calibrated in terms of volume flow per minute.

A pulse pickup using the two-winding variable transformer was developed by Benjamin et al. (1962). In their transducer the two coils were mounted in a small chamber, which was affixed to the skin over a pulsating artery. In the chamber facing the artery a rubber diaphragm carried the movable coil and the frame of the capsule carried the fixed coil. The coil on the rubber membrane was energized by a 100-kHz oscillator, and its position was modulated by the pulse. Amplification, rectification, and graphic recording of the signal produced a pulse tracing of high fidelity.

Blood flow was recorded by Pieper (1958), who constructed a catheter-tip velocity flowmeter employing the variable transformer. In this device a ferromagnetic sleeve carrying a small flange was displaced by the velocity of the blood stream. The displacement altered the coupling between the coils, thereby producing a recordable signal. A unique expandable, umbrella-type fixture served to maintain the transducer in the center of the vessel. Pieper reported a linear output with flow up to a velocity of 45 cm/sec and a frequency up to 25 Hz.

3-3. LINEAR VARIABLE DIFFERENTIAL TRANSFORMER (LVDT)

When three coils are used, the device is designated a differential transformer. The commonest of its many forms is an arrangement of two identical coils placed on either side of a third energizing coil (Fig. 3-2). This configuration was introduced by Schaevitz (1947) and is used extensively by industry. The center coil of the LVDT is excited by alternating current, which produces a field that induces equal voltages in the two adjacent coils. The outer coils are connected in series opposition so that the voltage generated in one cancels that from the other. In practice the residual voltage is in the order of 1% of the maximum output voltage. Insertion of a core unbalances the system so that the voltages generated in the outer coils are no longer equal. The imbalance voltage is proportional to the core

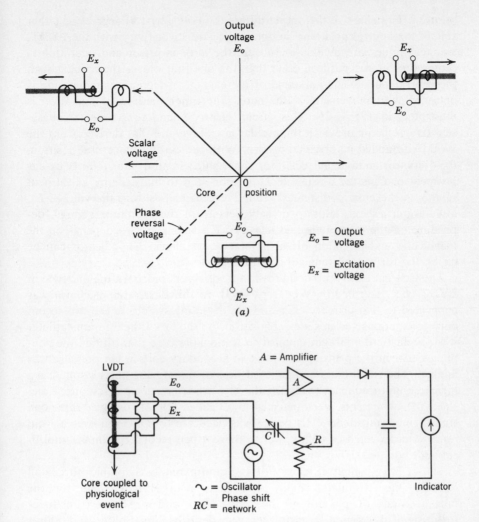

Figure 3-2. The linear variable differential transformer (LVDT): (a) output versus core position; (b) phase-sensitive detector for LVDT.

position. The relationship between the output voltage and the position of core in the differential transformer is shown in Fig. 3-2a. In comprehensive articles, Schaevitz (1947) and Heath (1958) have further analyzed the operation of the LVDT under a variety of practical measurement conditions.

It is to be noted that an output of the same magnitude is produced if the core is displaced an equal amount in either direction from its central position. The phase of the output differs, however, by 180 degrees on either side of the neutral position. To obtain direction sensitivity with the LVDT, two techniques are available. In one, the core is offset and operation is centered around a position other than the one that moves the core through the central point. Thus a signal of increasing or decreasing magnitude is obtained with movement of the core. The other method of operation is illustrated in Fig. 3-2b. This circuit arrangement constitutes a phase-sensitive detector in which the oscillator voltage and that derived from the LVDT are added before rectification. With the core in its central position, the oscillator voltage, corrected for phase shifts in all of the circuitry by adjustment of C, is fed to the indicator to bring it to midscale by adjustment of R. As the core is displaced from the central position, the voltage E_o, after amplification, adds to or subtracts from the oscillator voltage, depending on the magnitude and phase of E_o, which in turn depends on the magnitude and direction of the displacement. Thus the indicator can be calibrated for the full range of core motion.

The first catheter-tip blood pressure transducer incorporating one type of LVDT was described by Wetterer (1943). In this device the oscillator was connected to two primary coils and the detecting system to the two secondary coils, connected in series opposition. At the tip of the 3.5-mm catheter was an elastic diaphragm coupled to a movable core that altered the coupling between the primary and the two secondary coils when pressure was applied. The small mass and high stiffness of the moving parts resulted in a high resonant frequency (515 Hz), thereby producing a rapid response time.

Small movements were detected by Tucker (1952), using a three-coil transformer transducer. His device was accurate to 0.005 cm over a 1-cm range and provided enough power to drive a pen recorder without amplification.

The relatively high efficiency of the commercially available[2] three-coil LVDTs' has stimulated many investigators to employ them for the measurement of physiological events. A blood pressure transducer featuring a differential transformer was described by Shafer and Shirer (1949). In this device the core was affixed to a small circular elastic diaphragm exposed to blood pressure, and the whole assembly was mounted in a 2-cc syringe. The natural frequency of this transducer was 600 Hz; when it was connected to a 20-gauge needle, a frequency response flat to 100 Hz was obtained.

Erdos et al. (1962) described a truly isotonic myograph incorporating the LDVT. In this device the muscle specimen under study was connected to a beam-type balance. The motion of the balancing weight, which occurred

[2] Schaevitz Engineering Co., Camden, N.J.

with contraction of the muscle, was measured by variations in the position of the core in the LVDT.

Figure 3-3 illustrates the use of the LVDT to construct an efficient pressure transducer.[3] In this device movement of the tip of a Bourdon tube is detected by an LVDT. Linearity, rapidity of response, and a small volume displacement are achieved by means of a very stiff, short Bourdon tube. A very interesting electrical caliper incorporating the LVDT was described by Gow (1966). Employed for the continuous measurement of pulsatile arterial diameter changes, this device consisted of a jeweled-bearing, scissorlike, lightweight caliper; one end embraced the artery, while the other end was affixed to the LVDT. The small pulsatile changes in the artery modulated the position of the embracing ends of the caliper to provide (after four stages of amplification) an output of 1 to 1.5 V for changes in the diameter of the thoracic aorta and of the femoral artery, amounting to 500 and 80 μ, respectively. The low mass of the instrument resulted in a sinusoidal frequency response essentially uniform to 20 Hz measured on a segment of rubber tubing. When the device was tested for transient response, the natural resonant frequency was found to be in excess of 180 Hz, dramatically indicating the rapid response time available.

Because of the small size and low mass of the core of an LVDT, an insignificant load is imposed on the event being measured. No electromagnetic pull is imposed on the core in the null position. In practical units very little pull is encountered when the core is displaced from the null position. Although the transduction efficiency is moderate, the differential transformer is rugged and relatively insensitive to temperature changes, since the sensitivity alteration is almost entirely due to the resistance

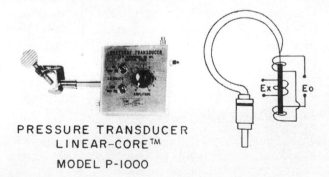

PRESSURE TRANSDUCER
LINEAR-CORE™
MODEL P-1000

Figure 3-3. LVDT pressure transducer, linear core model P-1000. (Courtesy of Narco Bio-Systems, Houston, Tex.)

---

[3] Narco Bio Systems, Houston, Texas.

change of the coils. Its ability to detect rapid changes is good, being limited to the characteristics of the moving system, the frequency of the excitation voltage, and the characteristic of the magnetic material. If extremely rapid rates of change are to be measured, high-frequency excitation and powdered magnetic materials must be used in the construction of the core.

Linear variable differential transformer units are relatively low in impedance and can be constructed to have almost any dimensions. Although many component manufacturers provide a standard line, they will construct special units to meet almost any particular need. *Engineering Bulletin* A2 of the Schaevitz Co. lists transformers having linear displacement ranges of ±0.005 to ±1.000 in., with a residual output (at balance) of 0.5% of that obtained with maximum displacement. The excitation voltage of many differential transformers is 3 to 10 V at frequencies ranging from 60 Hz to 20 kHz. The output per unit of displacement is dependent on the excitation voltage, its frequency, and the particular differential transformer model. Typical sensitivity figures for the miniature models are approximately 0.2 to 5 mV per thousandth inch per volt of excitation. The higher sensitivity figures are obtained with excitation voltages in the kilohertz range.

3-4. ROTARY VARIABLE DIFFERENTIAL TRANSFORMERS

Rotary variable differential transformers are also available commercially. Although rotation through a full 360 degrees is often possible, $\pm1\%$ linearity is obtained only over a range of ±40 degrees (Schaevitz R3B 1 S model). The nominal sensitivity of this particular unit is 1.8 mV per degree of rotation per volt of 2 kHz energy applied to the transfomer.

Perhaps one of the most desirable characteristics of the rotary variable differential transformer is that as a transducer for rotation, its output versus rotation is smooth or stepless. In many models, however, the maximum rotation is approximately 90 degrees. When continuous rotation is possible, the output voltage varies as the sine or cosine of the angle of rotation.

3-5. THE ELECTROMAGNETIC FLOWMETER

After Michael Faraday (1832) discovered the law governing magnetic induction, he speculated on the many possible ways of demonstrating this phenomenon which, at the time his discovery was made, was evidenced by the appearance of current flow in a conductor in a changing magnetic field. Faraday was well aware of the underlying practical details. For example, he knew that the magnetic field could be stationary and the conductor could move or the conductor could be stationary and the magnetic field could change; both situations give rise to a current induced in the conductor. Faraday knew that if a conductor moved in a magnetic field, the conductor, its direction of movement, and the direction of the magnetic field had to be mutually perpendicular to maximize the induced current; this fundamental requirement is sketched in Fig. 3-4. Most important, Faraday discovered that the magnitude of the induced current depended on the velocity and length of conductor in the magnetic field and the strength of the magnetic field.

Faraday realized that an aqueous electrolyte flowing in a constant magnetic field should give evidence of an induced current. He set about to verify the presence of such a current by calling attention to the fact that the Thames River in England is an electrolytic conductor that moves through the earth's magnetic field; therefore, the Thames ought to sustain a current proportional to the velocity of its flow. Faraday recounted his experiment (1832) as follows:

"I made experiments therefore (by favour) at Waterloo Bridge, extending a copper wire nine hundred and sixty feet in length upon the parapet of the bridge, and dropping from its extremities other wires with extensive plates of metal attached to them to complete contact with the water. The wire therefore and the water made one conducting circuit; and as the water ebbed or flowed with the tide, I hoped to obtain currents analogous to those of the brass ball.

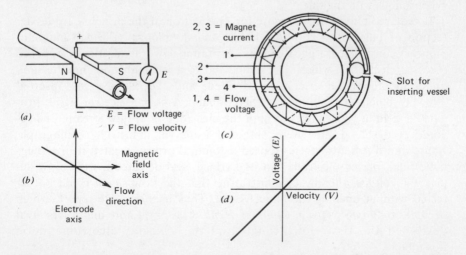

Figure 3-4. Basic principle of operation of an electromagnetic flowmeter: (a) and (b) direction of the electrodes and magnetic field with respect to flow; (c) practical arrangement for a perivascular flow probe; (d) linear relationship of the flow voltage, E to flow velocity, V.

I constantly obtained deflections at the galvanometer, but they were very irregular, and were in succession referred to other causes than that sought for. The different condition of the water as to purity on the two sides of the river; the difference in temperature; slight differences in the plates, in the solder used, in the more or less perfect contact made by twisting or otherwise; all produced effects in turn: and though I experimented on the water passing through the middle arches only; used platina plates instead of copper; and took every other precaution, I could not after three days obtain any satisfactory results."

Undaunted by this failure, Faraday insisted that a flow-dependent current ought to exist and stated: "Theoretically it seems a necessary consequence that when water is flowing, these electric currents should be formed."

Almost a century passed before Faraday's experiment to detect the flow of fluid by induction was executed successfully. Examining the problem more carefully, Young et al. (1920), also in England, calculated that tidal water moving in the earth's magnetic field at Dartmouth ought to provide a voltage of 0.215 μV per centimeter width of stream per knot velocity of flow. Accordingly, they placed chlorided silver electrodes, 1000 yd apart, into the water at the entrance to Dartmouth Harbor. The electrodes were connected to a Paul galvanometer, and the readings obtained were plotted against time. As Faraday had predicted, the investigators obtained a slow oscillation in potential, having a peak-to-peak value of 18.5μV and synchronous with the tide.

It required only a decade more for application of the principle to the detection of blood flow. In 1932 Fabre and d'Arsonval (the galvanometer pioneer) constructed a glass cannula containing two diametrically opposed recessed electrodes, which were connected to a vacuum tube amplifier and an oscillograph. An artery was divided, and the cannula was inserted allowing blood to flow through the cannula. A strong electromagnet provided a field at right angles to both the electrodes and flow stream, and recordings of blood flow were obtained using an industrial oscillograph. Fabre and d'Arsonval then exposed a femoral artery, located it in a magnetic field, placed electrodes on its surface, and detected a weak flow-dependent voltage, thereby demonstrating that the flow signal could be detected without opening the blood vessel. Thus in this single report, which occupies only two pages in *Comptes Rendus* (1932), Fabre and d'Arsonval described the first flowthrough and perivascular electromagnetic flowmeters.

The electromagnetic blood flowmeter became a practical instrument as the result of simultaneous, but independent, studies of Kolin (1936–1937) in the United States and Wetterer (1937, 1938) in Germany. Both men recognized that a blood vessel need not be opened to detect the flow-dependent voltage, and both placed "nonpolarizable" electrodes on the surface of the blood vessels and used strong constant-current (dc) electromagnets to obtain high-intensity magnetic fields. The voltage detected by the electrodes was found to be linearly proportional to blood flow velocity and the polarity was dependent on the direction of flow, as predicted by theory. In their initial studies, both investigators used sensitive galvanometers to display the flow signal. With stable electrodes, high-quality recordings were obtained; an example of one of these (Fig. 3-5) was published by Wetterer, who placed his flow probe around the aorta of a 4.5-kg dog.

Elegantly simple as the dc electromagnetic flowmeter was, two serious problems delayed its widespread use. One problem was related to the size of the signal, which in practical situations lies in the microvolt range and demands the use of stable, high-sensitivity direct-coupled display devices. The second difficulty was related to electrode instability, manifested by slow changes in electrode-electrolyte potential with time. In addition, if current flowed through the electrodes, the electrode potential became even more unstable; in these early instruments, moreover, the indicators used to display the flow voltage were galvanometers that required current for their operation. These two problems conspired to make it difficult to specify the zero-flow point in the flow record.

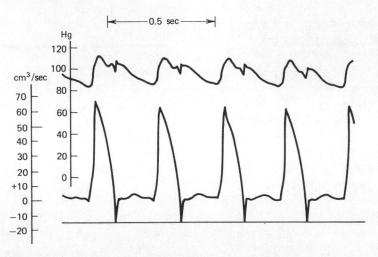

Figure 3-5.   Aortic blood pressure (upper) and flow velocity (lower) recordings in the aorta of a dog. [From E. Wetterer, *Z. Biol.* **99**:158–162 (1938). By permission.]

When the electromagnetic flowmeter was first introduced, stable, high-gain direct-coupled (dc) voltage amplifiers were not generally available, although Wetterer had built one for use with his flowmeter. However, stable, high-gain alternating current amplifiers having a high input impedance were readily available, and Katz and Kolin (1938) connected an interrupter (driven by a 50-Hz tuning fork) to the electrode terminals of the dc electromagnetic flowmeter and amplified the resulting "chopped" flow signal using a conventional resistance-capacitance coupled ac amplifier. This technique permitted attaining high sensitivity and dramatically reduced the flow of current through the electrodes, thereby increasing stability.

3-5-1.   The Sine Wave Flowmeter

A considerable advance in electromagnetic blood flowmeter technology was made by Kolin (1941), who used sinusoidal alternating current to excite the electromagnet applied to the blood vessel. The result was a mixed blessing, since now two sinusoidal voltages appeared across the electrode terminals. One voltage was large and independent of flow; the other was much smaller and its amplitude was linearly proportional to flow velocity within the blood vessel; Fig. 3-6a illustrates these waveforms. Fortunately, these two voltages differ in phase by 90 degrees and can be separated. The large flow-independent signal, or "transformer voltage," results because the electrodes, the conducting path through the vessel, and the wires attached to the electrodes (Fig. 3-4) constitute a single-turn coil in the changing magnetic field; therefore, it has an induced voltage that is 90 degrees behind the magnetic field that produces it. The flow-dependent signal is also sinusoidal, but is in phase with the magnetic field.

To remove the large flow-independent transformer voltage, Kolin (1941) developed a compensator that permitted subtraction of the transformer voltage, leaving only the flow-dependent sinusoidal voltage whose amplitude reflected the instantaneous blood flow velocity in the vessel.

The use of an alternating magnetic field yielded tremendous practical advantages. For example, since electrode-electrolyte potentials were not detected, ordinary metal electrodes could be applied directly to the unopened blood vessel, thereby reducing the overall size of the blood flow transducer. Also, because the desired flow-dependent signal was proportional to the amplitude of an alternating voltage, stable, high-gain, narrow-band ac amplifiers having a high input impedance could be used, thereby increasing the sensitivity and allowing measurement of blood flow in small vessels.

Two major improvements in the design of the sinusoidal electromagnetic flowmeter were made by Kolin and Kado (1959) and Westerstein et al. (1959). One improvement consisted of the use of higher frequency

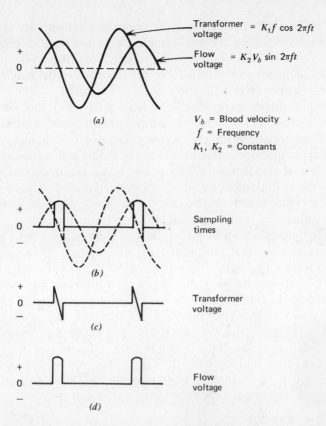

Transformer = $K_1 f \cos 2\pi f t$
voltage

Flow = $K_2 V_b \sin 2\pi f t$
voltage

V_b = Blood velocity
f = Frequency
K_1, K_2 = Constants

(a)

Sampling
times

(b)

Transformer
voltage

(c)

Flow
voltage

(d)

Figure 3-6. Waveforms associated with the sine wave electromagnetic flowmeter. (*a*) Blood-flow-dependent voltage (which is in phase with the sinusoidally varying magnetic field) and the induced (transformer) voltage, which is flow independent and 90 degrees out of phase with the flow voltage. (*b*) The technique of sampling the flow-independent voltage during the period when it is maximum and while the transformer voltage is passing through zero (*d* and *c*). Over the sampling period the average value of the transformer voltage is zero (*c*). The sampling technique is shown only for the positive phase of the flow signal; sampling could also be performed during the negative maximum of the flow signal. With this gating technique, the flow signal is recovered by synchronous detection and integration of the train of flow-dependent pulses.

sinusoidal current (400 Hz) instead of 60 Hz to excite the electromagnet, thus providing about a twentyfold reduction in weight of the transducer and a shorter response time, which allowed faithful reproduction of phasic flow. The second improvement consisted of the use of an electronic gating technique that permitted detection of the flow-dependent signal only at the time when the transformer signal was passing through zero; this situation is diagrammed in Figs. 3-6*b* through 3-6*d*. Thus the flow information is retrieved by continuously detecting the peak amplitude of the train of pulses, as in Fig. 3-6*d*. The amplitude of each pulse reflects blood flow velocity at that instant, and its polarity (with respect to the direction of the magnetic field) identifies forward or reverse flow.

Other improvements in the sine wave flowmeter were reported by Kolin (1945, 1952); these related to better methods of eliminating the transformer signal and improvements in the perivascular sleeve containing the electrodes. Of these many refinements it was the gating technique that permitted commercial production of the sine wave electromagnetic blood flowmeter. Most important, the problems solved during its long period of development were directly applicable to those encountered with its successors, the square wave and trapezoidal wave flowmeters.

Undoubtedly elimination of the bothersome, large-amplitude, non-flow-related transformer voltage prompted the development of the square and trapezoidal wave flowmeters. The magnitude of the transformer voltage depends on the rate of change of the magnetic field; therefore, with square wave excitation the transformer voltage is very large, but lasts only a very short time (see Fig. 3-7); after this time only the flow-dependent voltage is present. Trapezoidal wave excitation produces a small transformer voltage, appearing only during the slopes of the trapezoid, as in Fig. 3-8. During the flat part of the trapezoid, only the flow-dependent voltage is present. With both the square and trapezoidal wave flowmeters, the flow-dependent signal is repetitively sampled when the transformer voltage is zero.

3-5-2.   The Square Wave Flowmeter

The square wave electromagnetic flowmeter was developed by Denison and Spencer (1953), who employed at 30-Hz square wave to excite the magnet in the flow transducer. The flow-dependent voltage was sampled during the square wave after the transformer component had subsided, as in Fig. 3-7*b*. Choice of a 30-Hz frequency for magnet excitation meant that the response time was relatively long and only mean flow could be recorded. This limitation was removed by Denison and Spencer (1956), who used a square wave having a frequency of 240 Hz. These investigators made further improvements in the 240-Hz square wave flowmeter by sampling the flow signal during both the positive and negative portions of the square wave when only the flow signal was present; Fig. 3-7*c* illustrates the flow-dependent voltage. With this arrangement phasic blood flow could be recorded by sampling at the rate of 480/sec, each sample lasting about 1.9 msec. Thus the blood flow velocity signal was synthesized by detecting only the flow-de-

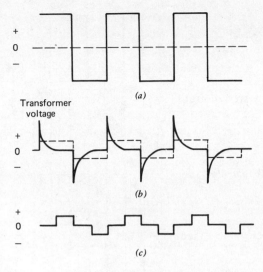

Figure 3-7. Waveforms associated with the square wave electromagnetic blood flowmeter. (*a*) Magnetic field waveform. (*b*) Induced transformer voltage (produced by the reversal in direction of the magnetic field) and flow-dependent voltage (dashed) which is proportional to flow velocity and the strength of the magnetic field. By sampling the flow-dependent signal when the transformer voltage is absent a train of pulses (*c*) is obtained; its amplitude is proportional to the flow velocity at that instant. The polarity of the pulses with respect to the direction of the magnetic field identifies with the direction of flow. Thus for unidirectional flow, a train of pulses of alternating polarity is obtained because the magnetic field alternates in direction. The flow signal is synthesized by synchronous detection of this pulse train.

pendent pulses (of alternate polarity) by a demodulator that smoothed out the pulse train and inserted a small filler signal (dependent on the average flow during sampling) between the sampling times. Figure 3.8 reconstructs the blood-flow velocity signal from the pulse train. The overall sinusoidal blood-flow frequency response obtained was 0 to 50 Hz. Stated another way, a response time (10 to 90%) of about 10 msec was attained.

Moody and his associates (1972) developed an interesting version of the squarewave flowmeter which incorporated automatic correction for zero flow. They employed a square wave in which there was an interval between the positive and negative phases when the perivascular probe excitation was turned off. Thus any potential appearing between the probe electrode terminals represented a no-flow signal, which was electronically subtracted from the flow signal by a high input impedance, direct-coupled, balanced amplifying system. To ensure that the zero-flow offset voltage would be as small as possible, recessed platinum-black electrodes were coupled to the

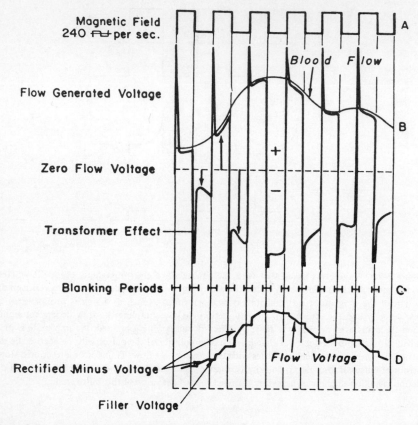

Figure 3-8. Synthesis of an arterial blood flow velocity wave by the square wave flowmeter. (*a*) The 240-Hz alternating square wave magnetic field; (*b*) voltage presented to the electrodes in the flow probe; (*c*) blanking periods (when sampling is not carried out); (*d*) synthesized flow signal using the timed sampling (gating) technique. [From Spencer and Denison, *IRE Trans. Med. Electron.* **ME-6**:220–227 (1959). By permission.]

vessel by a short column of saline. The saline column could be established or flushed at any time by means of a catheter leading to a saline-filled syringe.

Single- and multiple-channel versions of this novel flowmeter were described. Because of the unique design, it is characterized by high stability and accuracy. The frequency response attainable is inversely related to the number of channels, each being sampled sequentially. There is no doubt that the techniques employed in Moody's flowmeter will be incorporated in commercially available instruments.

3-5-3.   The Trapezoidal Wave Flowmeter

The trapezoidal wave electromagnetic blood flowmeter was developed by Yanof (1961) and Yanof et al. (1963). The excitation current for its perivascular electromagnet provided a trapezoidal wave magnetic field (Fig. 3-9a) alternating with a frequency of 1000/sec. The transformer signal is generated only during the changing magnetic field, that is, during the sloping parts of the trapezoid, as in Fig. 3-9b.

During the top and bottom of the trapezoid, the magnetic field is constant and no transformer signal is induced. During this interval the voltage across the electrodes is sampled and the amplitude (Fig. 3-9c) is proportional to the velocity of the blood flow. In Yanof's instrument a sampling time of 0.174 msec was chosen; therefore the blood flow signal is sampled 2000 times per second with pulses 0.174 msec long. When this pulse train of alternately positive and negative pulses (for a unidirectional

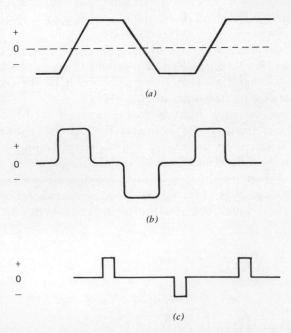

(a)

(b)

(c)

Figure 3-9.   Waveforms associated with the trapezoidal wave flowmeter. (a) Waveform of the magnetic field; (b) curve indicating that the transformer (flow-independent) voltage occurs during the ramps of the trapezoid; (c) the sampled voltage, whose amplitude is dependent on flow velocity. The polarity of the flow-voltage pulses in relation to the polarity of the magnetic field identifies the direction of flow. Synchronous detection of the pulse train provides a signal that describes the blood flow velocity.

flow) is fed into a demodulating circuit, the peak amplitude of the train is recovered and represents the phasic blood flow in the vessel. Yanof estimated (1961) that this flowmeter had an overall sinusoidal frequency response (for blood flow) ranging from 0 to 250 Hz, which is certainly adequate to show the most rapid changes in flow encountered in the vascular systems of most mammals.

3-5-4. Commercially Available Electromagnetic Flowmeters

Commercially available electromagnetic blood flowmeters, almost irrespective of type, have an adequately short response time to allow faithful reproduction of the range of blood flow velocities encountered in large and small vessels in animals and man. A study by Gessner and Bergel (1964) presented the hydraulic sinusoidal frequency response to two popular makes of flowmeter. The data indicated that the frequency response obtained hydraulically is essentiall the same as that measured for the electronic amplifying channel. Bandwidths extending to beyond 15 Hz were measured.

The output voltage provided by an electromagnetic flow probe is linearly proportional to flow velocity; the actual volume flow must be computed by obtaining the average flow ($\overline{V}_b$) and multiplying it by the cross-sectional area (A) of the flowing stream, as in Fig. 3-10.

Several important facts must be borne in mind in the practical application of the electromagnetic flowmeter. For example, to avoid detection of electrical interference, nearly all electromagnetic flowmeters require that the subject be grounded. It is important to recognize that there are two types of flow tranducers, the flow-through and the perivascular (Fig. 3-11). In the flow-through type (Fig. 3-11a), blood is caused to flow through a rigid plastic tube, which contains the electrodes and through which the

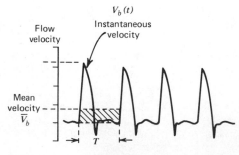

Blood flow = (mean velocity) × (vessel area) = $\overline{V}_b A$

$\overline{V}_b$ = area under $V_b\ (t)/T$

Figure 3-10. Method for computing average blood flow from a recording of instantaneous flow velocity $V_b(t)$.

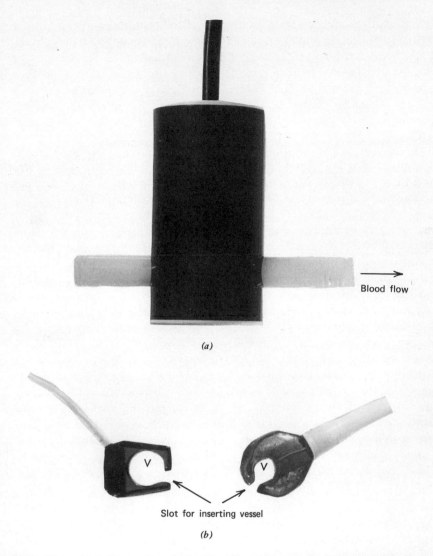

(a)

(b)

Slot for inserting vessel

Blood flow

Figure 3-11. Transducers (flow probes) for electromagnetic flowmeters: (*a*) flow-through type; (*b*) two perivascular probes (vessel occupies region *V*). (Courtesy of Carolina Medical Electronics, King, N.C.)

magnetic field also passes. This type of transducer is usually employed to measure large flows (e.g., the output of a heart-lung machine or cardiac bypass pump). Anticoagulants must be used because the blood comes into direct contact with plastic and metal surfaces. Since the diameter of the flow stream is known, simple processing of the transducer output voltage provides an accurate and linear display of volume flow per unit time. In addition, because the electrodes are in direct contact with the periphery of the flow stream, the flow-velocity signal is immune to resistivity errors; that is, variations in hematocrit (percentage of red cells) do not alter the calibration, which is easily accomplished by pumping saline through the transducer into a graduated vessel and timing the collection with a stopwatch.

The perivascular flow probe, illustrated in Fig. 3-11b, is placed around an unopened blood vessel; therefore no anticoagulant is necessary. To measure blood flow in vessels of differing diameters, a series of flow probes must be available. With nearly all commercially available electromagnetic blood flowmeters, the electronic processing circuity will accept the output from flow probes of all sizes, although probes are not necessarily interchangeable among instruments provided by different manufacturers. In deciding which probe size to use, the essential requirement is a snug fit with the vessel when short-term recordings are to be made; such a fit guarantees the presence of a stable flow measurement. In most instances the probe size is identified by the circumference of the vessel to which the probe is to be applied. To obtain a snug fit, a probe size of about 10% less than the vessel circumference is recommended. When a flow probe is to be implanted, a slightly looser fit is desirable to allow for the tissue growth that nearly always occurs in response to the presence of a foreign substance around the vessel. Adequacy of fit is also dependent on blood pressure. For example, with low blood pressure an artery is less distended; thus the probe fit may not be adequate, and a smaller size must be used.

Although the output voltage of a perivascular flow probe is linearly related to the flow velocity within the blood vessel, practical difficulties supervene when accurate calibration of the probe is desired. Since the electrodes are on the vessel surface, they are separated from the flow-induced voltage. Therefore, the voltage presented to the perivascular electrodes is slightly less than that developed within the vessel. Because the arterial wall consists of conducting tissue, the flow-induced voltage causes current to flow in the vessel wall and through any perivascular fluid that may be present. Wetterer pointed out in 1937 that such a current flows in the vessel wall. Figure 3-12a illustrates the pathways taken by these currents. Assuming either that perivascular fluid is not present or that its effect is eliminated by coating the vessel wall with mineral oil, the flow-induced voltage sends current around the vessel wall and through the bloodstream, as in Fig. 3-12b. The amount of current that flows depends directly on the magnitude of the flow-induced voltage (E) and inversely on the equivalent resistance of the vessel wall (R_v) and blood stream (R); the latter in turn is

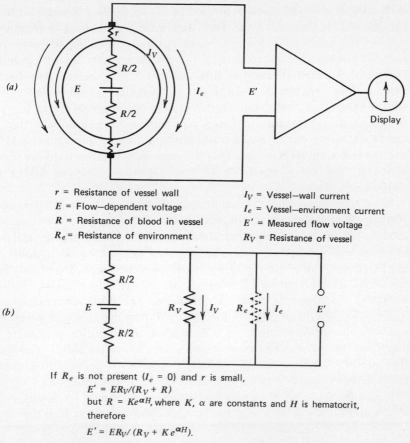

r = Resistance of vessel wall

E = Flow—dependent voltage

R = Resistance of blood in vessel

R_e = Resistance of environment

I_V = Vessel—wall current

I_e = Vessel—environment current

E' = Measured flow voltage

R_V = Resistance of vessel

If R_e is not present (I_e = 0) and r is small,

$E' = ER_V/(R_V + R)$

but $R = Ke^{\alpha H}$, where K, α are constants and H is hematocrit, therefore

$E' = ER_V/(R_V + Ke^{\alpha H})$.

Figure 3-12. Current pathways due to flow-induced voltage (E) and the effect of hematocrit (H).

dependent on the hematocrit (H)—the percentage of red cells. Because the resistivity of blood increases almost exponentially with hematocrit, the voltage (E') presented to the perivascular electrodes will decrease with increasing hematocrit; that is what is known as the "hematocrit error." Therefore, accurate flow calibration requires the *in vivo* timed collection of blood flowing through the vessel around which the flow probe is placed, or application of the flow probe to a vessel with the same dimensions and resistivity and the timed collection of flowing blood or saline with the same resistivity.

Roberts (1969) pointed out that the hematocrit error encountered with electromagnetic flowmeters is not entirely due to the conducting properties of the vessel wall. In a series of studies, using flowing blood of different hematocrits, he measured the true and indicated flow as a function of hematocrit, using several commercially available cannulated electromagnetic flowmeters. He found that all but one instrument tested exhibited a considerable underindication of flow with increasing hematocrit. The one that was free from this error employed an amplifier input impedance of 100 MΩ; all the others had input impedances in the range of 10 to 50 kΩ. If future studies substantiate these findings, it would appear that the hematocrit error due to vessel-wall shunting may be quite small and that existing electromagnetic blood flowmeters can be improved by merely increasing the input impedance of the amplifier connected to the flow transducer.

From the foregoing discussion it can be seen that accurate calibration of perivascular flow probes is difficult. At present, a variety of techniques is used to obtain reasonably accurate flow calibrations. Some investigators calibrate using preserved vessels or gut with dimensions comparable with the blood vessel in which the *in vivo* measurements were carried out. Some use blood as the calibrating solution; others use saline having the same resistivity as blood at body temperature. The technique employed is dictated by the type of information required from the flow measurement. If accurate volume-flow information is desired, a calibration procedure that duplicates the *in vivo* situation is necessary. However, if only changes in flow are of interest, calibration is often superfluous because flow changes are linearly indicated by electromagnetic blood flowmeters.

In conclusion, one very important practical fact must be noted in using electromagnetic flowmeters—namely, establishment of the zero flow point. With many instruments this point can be obtained only by cross-clamping the vessel distal to the flow probe. In newer instruments, in which the transformer voltage has been adequately eliminated, turning off the magnetic field provides a method of establishing an output from the flowmeter that corresponds to zero flow.

3-6. MAGNETORHEOGRAPHY

The method of detecting blood flow within the body or an appendage by passing a strong magnetic field through the body and using surface or needle electrodes to detect the flow voltage has been designated "magne-

Figure 3-13.   Magnetorheography: (*a*) application of the method to detect flow in the femoral artery of a dog; (*b*) comparison of flow signal (BF) with that obtained with an electromagnetic flowmeter; (*c*) flow-voltage relationship for this application. [From Okai et al., *J. Appl. Physiol.* **30**:564–566 (1971). By permission.]

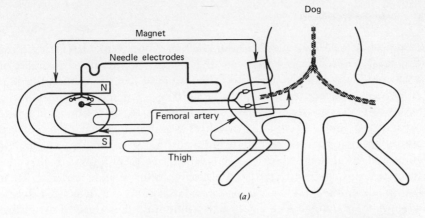

(a)

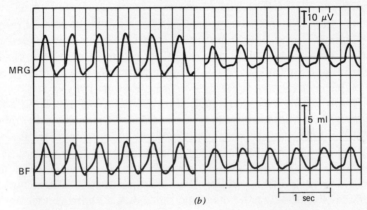

MRG

BF

10 μV

5 ml

1 sec

(b)

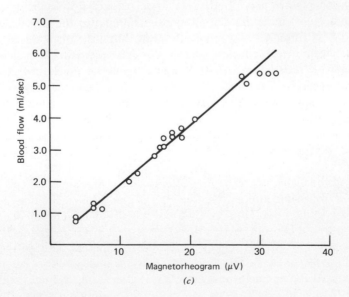

(c)

torheography" (MRG) by Okai et al. (1967). Kolin et al. (1941) described what must be credited as the first study in this area when he applied a sleeve containing two electrodes to a blood vessel. He then closed the skin and brought the leads out through a small incision. When blood flow in the vessel was to be recorded, the electrodes were connected to the amplifying-display device and a strong magnetic field was passed through the member containing the perivascular electrode assembly. The first successful demonstration of the method using body-surface electrodes was reported by Togawa et al. (1967), who passed a strong constant magnetic field (10,000 G) through a rabbit in the chest-to-back direction and detected a blood flow-dependent voltage with electrodes on the forelimbs (lead I). Although large amplitude ECG artifacts were present, the flow signal was confirmed by reversal of the direction of the magnetic field. Okai et al. (1967) applied the method to the human thorax with much more success using a field strength of 7000 G and electrodes on the thorax. Later Okai et al. (1971) applied the method to the femoral region of an anesthetized dog (see Fig. 3-13a). Using a field strength of 10,000 G, they verified the accuracy of their recordings by measuring blood flow in the same artery using an electromagnetic flowmeter. Flow changes, induced by the intravenous injection of noradrenalin, were displayed equally well by the magnetorheogram and electromagnetic flowmeter recording, as in Figs. 3-13b and 3-13c.

There are several important considerations in the use of magnetorheography to record blood flow. For example, the electrodes detect signals due to all fluid flow in the magnetic field; that is, both venous and arterial flow components are present. By and large, arterial flow velocity is much more rapid than venous flow and therefore dominates the signal. Because the blood flow voltage is very small, the recording instruments used to date have not been direct coupled; therefore, only pulsatile flow has been measured with resistance-capacity coupled systems having time constants of several seconds. The small flow voltage also favors the detection of bioelectric events such as the ECG and skeletal muscle action potentials, which are difficult to eliminate by filtering because their frequency spectrum is so similar to that of the flow signal. However, cancellation by electronic subtraction may be feasible when the ECG is the interfering signal.

Many of the difficulties encountered with constant magnetic fields can be eliminated by using alternating fields; however, this technique presents problems similar to those associated with the development of the perivascular electromagnetic blood flowmeter. One difficulty—not experienced yet with electromagnetic blood flowmeters because the magnetic field intensity is so low—may arise when high-intensity alternating fields are used for magnetorheography. The alternating voltage induced in the body tissues and electrolytes will cause alternating current to flow and may cause stimulation or tissue heating, which in turn may alter local blood flow. Therefore, when alternating fields are employed, care must be exercised to choose a field intensity low enough to exclude these effects.

REFERENCES

Benjamin, F. B., E. Mastrogiovanni, and W. Helveig. 1962. Bloodless method of continuous recording of pulse pressure in man. *J. Appl. Physiol.* **17**:844.

Denison, A. B., and M. B. Spencer. 1956. Square-wave electromagnetic flowmeter design. *Rev. Sci. Inst.* **27**:707–711.

Denison, A. B., M. P. Spencer, and H. D. Green. 1953. Square wave electromagnetic flowmeter for application to intact blood vessels. *Circ. Res.* **3**:39–46.

Erdos, E. G., V. Jackman, and W. C. Barnes. 1962. Instrument for recording isotonic contractions of smooth muscles, *J. Appl. Physiol.* **17**:307–8.

Fabre, P., and A. d'Arsonval. 1932. Utilisation des forces electromotrices d'induction pour enregistrement des variations de vitesse des liquides conducteurs: Un nouvel hemodromographe sans palette dans le sang. *C. R. Acad. Sci. (Paris)* **194**:1097–1089.

Faraday, M. 1832. Experimental researches in electricity. *Phil. Trans. Roy. Soc.* **122**:125–194.

Fuller, J. T., and T. M. Gordon. 1948. The radio inductograph. *Science* **108**:287–8.

Gauer, O. H., and E. Gienapp. 1950. A miniature pressure-recording device. *Science* **112**:404–5.

Geddes, L. A., and C. P. da Costa. 1973. The specific resistance of canine blood at body temperature. *IEEE Trans. Bio-Med. Eng.* **BME20**:51–53.

Gessner, U., and D. Bergel. 1964. Frequency response of electromagnetic flowmeters. *J. Appl. Physiol.* **19**:1209–1211.

Gow, B. S. 1966. An electrical caliper for measurement of pulsatile arterial diameter changes *in vivo. J. Appl. Physiol.* **21**:1122–1126.

Heath, J. H. 1958. The differential transformer as a sensitive measuring device. *Electrón. Eng.* **30**:631–633.

Katz, L. N., and A. Kolin. 1938. The flow of blood in the carotid artery of the dog under various circumstances as determined with the electromagnetic flowmeter. *Amer. J. Physio.* **122**:788–804.

Kolin, A. 1936. An electromagnetic flowmeter. *Proc. Soc. Exp. Biol. Med.* **35**:53–56.

Kolin, A. 1941. An AC induction flow meter for measurement of blood flow in intact blood vessels. *Proc. Soc. Exp. Biol. Med.* **46**:235–239.

Kolin, A. 1945. An alternating field induction flow meter of high sensitivity. *Rev. Sci. Inst.* **16**:109–116.

Kolin, A. 1952. Improved apparatus and technique for electromagnetic determination of blood flow. *Rev. Sci. Inst.* **23**:235–243.

Kolin, A., and R. Kado. 1959. Miniaturization of the electromagnetic blood flowmeter and its use for the recording of circulatory responses of conscious animals to sensory stimuli. *Proc. Nat. Acad. Sci. (U.S.)* **45**:1312–1321.

Kolin, A., J. L. Weissberg, and L. Gerber. 1941. Electromagnetic measurement of blood flow and sphygmomanometry in the intact animal. *Proc. Soc. Exp. Biol. Med.* **47**:323–329.

Motley, H. L., A. Cournand, L. Werko, D. Dresdale, A. Himmelstein, and D. W. Richards.

1947. Intravascular and intracardiac pressure recording in man: Electrical apparatus compared with the Hamilton manometer. *Proc. Soc. Exp. Biol. Med.* **64:**241–244.

Moody, N. F., D. L. Morrison, B. C. deKat, J. D. Henderson, A. M. Rappaport, and S. J. Lipton. 1972. A four-channel pulsed-field electromagnetic blood flowmeter system. *Digest of Papers,* Canadian Medical & Biological Engineering Society, September, Winnipeg, Man.

Müller, A., L. Laszt, and L. Pircher. 1948. Über ein Manometer mit elektrischer Transmission zur Druck und Geschwindigkeitmessung. *Helv. Physiol. Acta* **6:**783–794.

Okai, O., T. Togawa, and M. Oshima. 1967. Magnetorheography. Observation of blood flow emf in static magnetic field by surface electrodes. *Digest of 7th International Conference on Medical & Biological Engineering.* Paper 13-3, Stockholm.

Okai, O., T. Togawa, and M. Oshima. 1971. Magnetorheography: Nonbleeding measurement of blood flow. *J. Appl. Physiol.* **30:**564–566.

Pieper, H. P. 1958. Registration of phasic changes of blood flow by means of a catheter type flowmeter. *Rev. Sci. Instrs.* **29:**965–967.

Roberts, V. C. 1969. Haematocrit variations and electromagnetic flowmeter sensitivity. *Biomed. Eng.* **4:**408–412.

Rushmer, R. F. 1954a. Heart size and stroke volume. *Minn. Med.* **37:**19–29.

Rushmer, R. F. 1954b. Continuous measurements of left ventricular dimensions in intact unanesthetized dogs. *Circ. Res.* 1954, **2:**14–21.

Schaevitz, H. *Engineering Bulletin* A2 and R38. Schaevitz Co., Box 505, Camden 1, N.J.

Schaevitz, H. 1947. The linear variable differential transformer. *Proc. Soc. Stress Anal.* **4:**79–88.

Schafer, P. W., and H. W. Shirer. 1949. An impedance gauging system for measurement of biologic pressure variables. *Surgery* **26:**446–451.

Scher, A. M., T. H. Weigert, and A. C. Young. 1953. Compact flowmeters for use in the unanesthetized animal, an electronic version of Chauveau's hemodrometer. *Science* **118:**82–84.

Spencer, M. P., and A. B. Denison. 1959. The square wave electromagnetic flowmeter: Theory of operation and design of magnet probes for clinical and experimental applications. *IRE Trans. Med. Electron.* **ME-6:**220–227.

Togawa, T., O. Okai, and M. Oshima. 1967. Observation of blood flow emf in externally applied strong magnetic field by surface electrodes. *Med. Biol. Eng.* **5:**169–170.

Tucker, M. J. 1952. A linear transducer for the electrical measurement of displacement. *Electron. Eng.* **24:**420–422.

Westerstein, A., G. Herrold, E. Abbott, and N. S. Assali. 1959. Gated sine wave electromagnetic flowmeter. *IRE Trans. Med. Electron.* **ME-6:**312-316.

Wetterer, E. 1937, 1938. Eine neue Methode zur Registrierung der Blutstromungsgeschwindegkeit am uneröffneter Gefass. *Z. Biol.* **98:**26-36, 1938, **99:**162.

Wetterer, E. 1943. Eine neue manometrische Sonde mit elektrischer Transmission. *Z. Biol.* **101:**333–350.

Wheeler, H. A. 1928. Simple inductance formulas for radio coils. *Proc. IRE* **16:**1398–1400.

Yanof, H. M. 1961. A trapezoidal-wave electromagnetic blood flowmeter. *J. Appl. Physiol.* **16:**566–570.

Yanof, H. M., A. L. Rosen, and W. C. Shoemaker. 1963. Design of an unplantable flowmeter transducer based on the Helmholtz coil. *J. Appl. Physiol.* **18:**227–230.

Young, F. B., H. Gerrand, and W. Jevous. 1920. Electrical disturbances due to tides and waves. *Phil. Mag.* **40**(6th ser.):149–159.

4

Capacitive Transducers

4-1. SINGLE CAPACITOR

A capacitor or condenser consists of two conducting surfaces separated by a dielectric, which can be solid, liquid, gaseous, or a vacuum. The capacitance (coulombs per volt) is measured in farads. The magnitude of the capacitance depends on the nature of the dielectric and varies directly with the area of the conducting surfaces and inversely with their separation. The capacitance can be altered by changing any of these three factors.

A parallel-plate capacitor has identical plates, each of area A cm², which are separated by a distance d cm; between them is placed a material of dielectric constant K. The capacitance is given by the following formula:

$$C_{pF} = 0.0885 \frac{A}{d} K.$$

Because the dielectric constant of air is only very slightly higher than that of a vacuum, K can be given the value of unity for air capacitors. Thus a practical figure for rapid calculation of the capacitance of an air capacitor can be derived. A capacitor consisting of two plates 1 cm² in area separated by 1 mm has a capacitance of 0.885 pF, that is, slightly less than 1 pF. In inch dimensions a capacitor having plates 1 in.² in area separated by 0.1 in. exhibits a capacitance of 2.17 pF, or slightly more than 2 pF. Although the equation for a parallel plate capacitor indicates that the capacitance varies inversely with the distance between plates, this relationship holds only for distances that are small in comparison to the size of the plates. If the separation between the plates is large compared to their size, the capacitance-distance relationship deviates from that of a hyperbola.

Alternating current is usually employed to obtain a signal that reflects the value of a capacitance. Depending on the application, the voltage proportional to the static value of the capacitance is disregarded, and only the change is processed for ultimate reproduction. This method is illustrated in Fig. 4-1a. In this circuit the capacitance transducer is in series with a large resistance R. A small change in capacitance will produce a proportional change in the voltage across the capacitor and resistor.

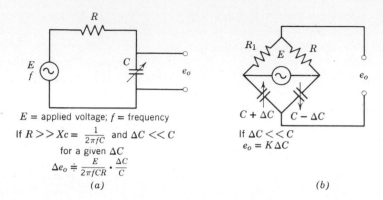

E = applied voltage; f = frequency

If $R \gg X_C = \dfrac{1}{2\pi fC}$ and $\Delta C \ll C$

for a given ΔC

$$\Delta e_o \doteq \frac{E}{2\pi fCR} \cdot \frac{\Delta C}{C}$$

(a)

If $\Delta C \ll C$

$e_o = K\Delta C$

(b)

Figure 4-1.   Capacitive transducer circuits: (a) series circuit; (b) bridge circuit.

A more convenient method of employing capacitance involves placing the capacitance transducer in a bridge circuit as shown in Fig. 4-1b. Frequently it is possible to create a differential capacitance transducer, each half being placed in adjacent arms of a bridge. The event being detected is caused to increase the capacitance of one side of the bridge and to decrease that of the other side. When this method is employed, the output signal is twice that obtainable by varying one capacitive element. This technique is characterized by a high degree of temperature stability.

When capacitance tranducers are employed in bridge circuits, two methods are available to obtain direction sensitivity. Either the bridge is operated slightly off balance, or a phase-sensitive detector is employed. With the first method the output of the bridge increases or decreases with a change in capacitance. The amount of initial unbalance chosen is dictated by the maximum expected change in C required to drive the bridge toward the balance point. With a phase-sensitive detector, direction sensitivity is automatically obtained.

Occasionally a single-element capacitive transducer is placed across a tuned circuit which is detuned by the change in capacitance, thereby causing a current change in the associated circuitry. Sometimes the tuned circuit constitutes the frequency-determining component in an oscillator. A change in the capacitance of the transducer alters the frequency of the oscillator, giving rise to a frequency-modulated signal that is detected and displayed with the aid of appropriate circuitry.

Capacitive transducers are frequently employed to detect mechanical displacement by movement of one or both of the capacitor plates, thereby producing a change in separation or effective area. Figure 4-2, composed by Foldvari and Lion (1964), illustrates many of the methods in which the capacitance change principle can be employed.

The capacitance method has often been applied to the measurement of physiological events, particularly the determination of blood pressure, for which the capacitive transducers has been extensively employed since the late 1930s. This transducer was developed because higher fidelity and sensitivity were needed than were available from optical manometers, which had been perfected to a remarkably high degree by reducing mass, increasing stiffness, and recovering the lost sensitivity by increasing the distance to the photographic recording surface. The practical inconvenience of the optical methods was a major factor in stimulating the application of electrical transduction systems.

In applying the capacitance method to measure blood pressure, an elastic member exposed to blood pressure constitutes one plate of the capacitor; the other plate is nearby and fixed. For high sensitivity each investigator using this technique has placed the distensible plate as close as possible to the fixed plate. To obtain a rapid response time the elastic member is made as small and as stiff as possible. This combination guarantees that only a small amount of fluid will be displaced when pressure is applied. The displacement is usually expressed in terms of cubic millimeters of fluid entering the transducer per 100 mm Hg of applied pressure. In practical terms this figure describes the ability of the transducer to measure transient pressure changes applied to interconnecting catheters and needles. Transducers having low-volume displacement figures can be employed to record faithfully pressure transients with small-bore interconnecting tubing.

Schutz (1937) appears to have been one of the first to use the capacitance method to measure blood pressure. In his tranducer the elastic member was a silvered glass membrane. The smallnesss and stiffness of the membrane he employed produced a natural frequency of 207 Hz. Following his lead, many other investigators constructed pressure transducers. Among these were Lilly (1942), Frommer (1943), Buchtal and Warburg (1943), and Hansen and Warburg (1947). In all these transducers the elastic members were small and stiff, providing a short response time and a small volume displacement. In all, the fixed and movable plates were in very close proximity. Ratios of area to separation varying from 10 to 10,000 have been employed.

An interesting application of the capacitive method to measure blood pressure is due to Beyne and Gougerot (1939), who converted the height of mercury in a U-tube manometer to an electrical signal. One "plate" of the capacitor was the mercury itself, whereas the other consisted of tinfoil wrapped around the outside of the glass tube forming the manometer. As the mercury column rose, the capacitance between the mercury and the tinfoil increased, causing a change in the current flowing through the capacitor. Although application of the principle in no way improved the fidelity of the manometer, it permitted remote location of the pressure-indicating device. It is to be noted that the fluid in such a manometer need not be mercury. Any solution of lower specific gravity can be used to produce a sensitive manometer or fluid level transducer. Beyne also used the same principle to convert small air pressure changes in the respiratory system of a dog to an electrical signal by fitting the diaphragm of a Marey tambour with an electrode of tinfoil which became the movable plate of a capacitor.

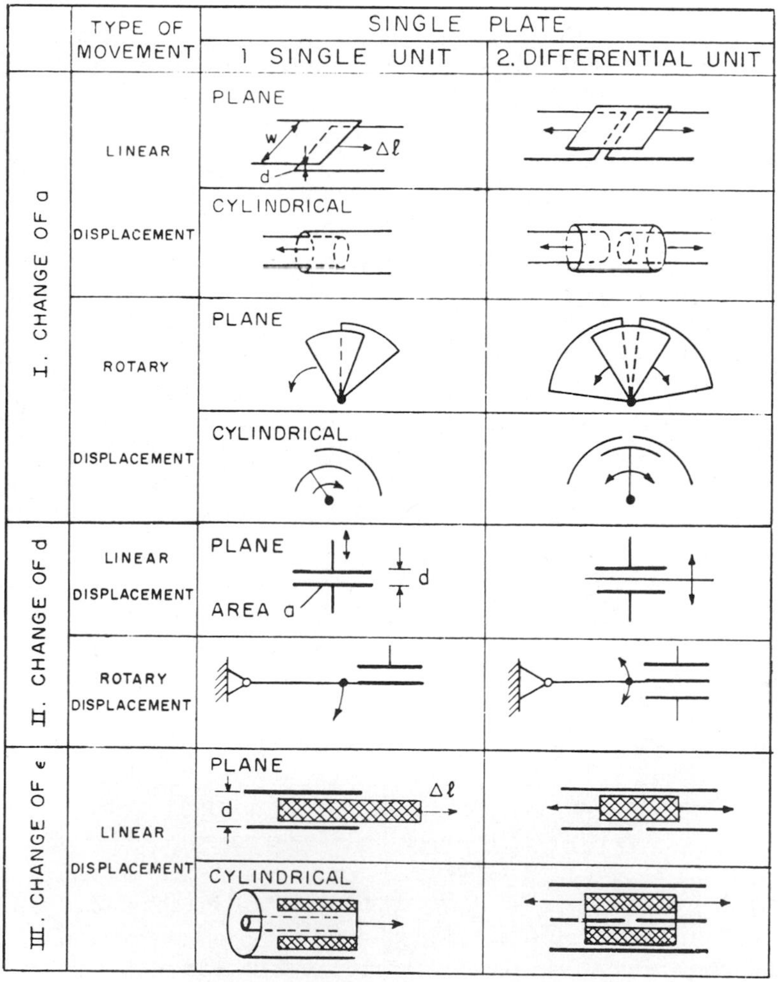

Figure 4-2. Synopsis of capacitive displacement transducers. [From Foldvari and Lion, *Instr. Contr. Syst.* **37**:77–85 (1964).]

The condenser microphone has seen service in physiology for the detection of heart sounds. Asher (1932) recognized its potential and used it to detect human heart sounds which, after amplification, were converted to variations in light intensity. A photographic record of the light beam produced phonocardiograms of high fidelity.

Liston (1950) employed a capacitive transducer to detect infrared radiation in his analyzer for gaseous carbon dioxide. The detector, sometimes referred to as a gas microphone, consisted of two carbon dioxide-filled

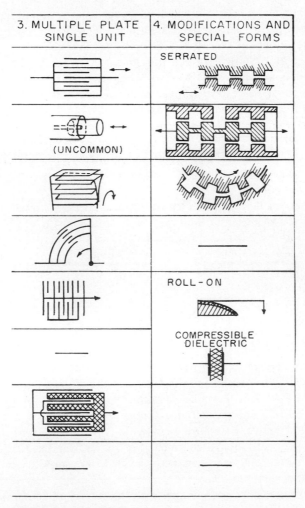

Figure 4-2. (*Continued*)

chambers, each with a window for the admission of infrared radiation. Between the chambers was a distensible diaphragm, which constituted one plate of the capacitive transducer. A second fixed plate was placed nearby. When carbon dioxide, which strongly absorbs infrared energy of characteristic wavelengths, is enclosed in a chamber, the pressure will rise in proportion to the amount of infrared radiation absorbed. The window of each detector was exposed to an infrared source. In front of one window was placed an infrared transparent tube containing the gas to be analyzed. Thus when a gas sample containing carbon dioxide was present, the amount of infrared radiation reaching one detector was reduced, creating an unbalance in the pressure in the two cells, which produced a deflection of the diaphragm between them. The change in capacitance so produced was calibrated in terms of the amount of carbon dioxide in the gas sample.

Adams et al. (1960) described the construction of a miniature capacitance microphone which they used as a high-fidelity pulse pickup. This device consisted of a small chamber containing a fixed electrode. Covering the chamber (and a short distance from the fixed electrode) was a metalized Mylar film, which constituted the other plate of the capacitor. In use the device was placed with the Mylar film applied to the skin over a pulsating vessel. The film tracked the skin motion and thereby modulated the capacitance. By means of a suitable processing apparatus, a recordable electrical signal was developed.

Calibration of the capacitance transducer applied to the radial artery was achieved first by occluding the artery at a point central to the transducer. This procedure established zero pressure. With the occlusion removed, the sensitivity was calibrated by requesting the subject to raise his arm 33.8 cm, which is equivalent to a change in pressure of 25 mm Hg.

An interesting use of the capacitance-change principle for the measurement of stroke volume in a diaphragm-type blood pump was described by Normann et al. (1973). In one application (see Fig. 4-3a), the blood within the pump and below the diaphragm was one "plate" of the capacitor (1); a metal foil in the air dome, into which positive and negative pressure was applied, constituted the other plate of the capacitor (2). The dielectric was therefore air and the plastic of the diaphragm. A capacitance change of slightly less than one picofarad was obtained for a pump stroke volume of 50 ml. The capacitance change varied the frequency of a 700-kHz oscillator, and the frequency change was processed to provide a signal that was linear with stroke volume. This system was used to monitor the amount of extracorporeal assistance provided to animals experiencing left-ventricular bypass.

Other configurations are possible with the capacitance method described by Normann. For example, in Fig. 4-3b, the blood could constitute the

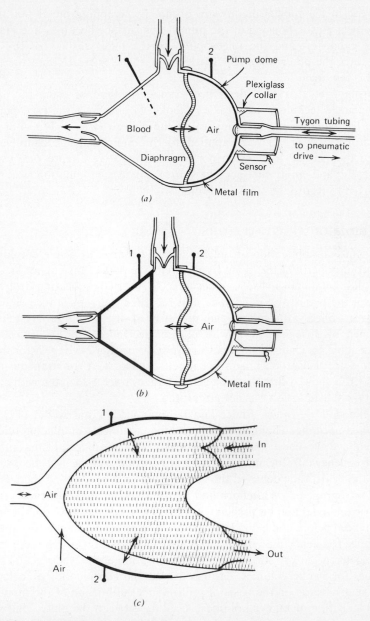

Figure 4-3. Three methods of using capacitance change to measure pump stroke volume. (*a*) Blood is one plate of the capacitor (1); metal film (2) in the air dome is the other. (*b*) Blood forms the changing dielectric between electrodes 1 and 2. (*c*) Blood in the sac (hatched area) forms the dielectric between the two electrodes 1 and 2. [Redrawn from Normann et al., *Cardiovasc. Res. Center Bull.* **12**:3–12 (1973).]

dielectric in the conical diaphragm pump. By wrapping metal foil around the conical plastic housing of the pump, this surface becomes one plate (1) of the capacitor, and the foil applied to the inner surface of the dome constitutes the other plate (2). In this way, no electrical contact with the blood is required.

Normann et al. (1973) described another method of using the capacitance-change technique to measure stroke volume in a sac-type pump in which the blood in the sac constituted the dielectric, as in Fig. 4-3c. Two capacitor plates (1, 2) were applied to the conical plastic chamber that housed the sac and into which positive and negative air pressure was applied to fill and empty the sac. The same frequency modulation system was employed to record the stroke volume.

4-2. BIOLOGICAL CAPACITORS

An unusual application of the capacitance-change principle employs the dielectric property of the living tissue itself as a part of the capacitor. A few examples are noteworthy. Cremer (1907) inserted a beating frog heart between the plates of a condenser and recorded the capacitance change as the heart filled with blood and emptied of it. A similar system was described by Joseph (1944), who placed electrodes over the thoraxes of human subjects. Using a 90-V battery in series with a 2-MΩ resistor, he was able to detect pulsatile changes in capacitive current. A simultaneous record of the ECG showed that the capacitive changes were associated with cardiac activity, but calibration was not attempted.

In blood flow studies Atzler and Lehman (1932) and Atzler (1935) applied a capacitance change method to human subjects by placing one electrode above the chest and one in contact with the back. Using an ultra-high-frequency current, modulated by respiration and the systolic discharge from the heart, they detected the capacitance changes, calling their method "Dielektrographie." Whitehorn and Pearl (1949) carried out studies similar to those of Atzler and his associates. Their electrodes were 15 cm square and were placed before and behind the thorax. The pulsatile changes in capacitive reactance frequency modulated a 10.7-MHz oscillator. Calling these records "cardioelectrograms," they attempted calibration of the tracings and stated, "Values for stroke volumes, cardiac output and cardiac indices, calculated from such records on the basis of preliminary calibration of the instrument by introduction of known volumes of saline between the plates, fall within the range of accepted normal values but conclusions as to the validity of this method are not yet possible."

Another application of the capacitance method was made by Fenning (1936–1937), who described an instrument he later called the "Oscillatocapacitograph." A rat was laid on one plate of the capacitor, and the other plate, 1 cm square, was placed 5 mm above the thorax of the animal. These plates were connected across the tuned circuit of a Hartley oscillator. Respiratory movements, changing the capacitance by varying the area, separation, and distribution of the dielectric, altered the anode current of the oscillator tube. By monitoring this current, a good record of respiration in the rat was obtained. In the hands of Fenning and Bonnar (1936–1937) the same instrument was used to record maternal respiration, uterine contractions, and fetal respiration in the rat. Employing a slight modification of this technique, Tomberg (1963, 1964) detected human respiration by placing electrodes on the thorax without making ohmic contact with the chest wall. Frequencies between 50 and 300 MHz were employed.

Heart sounds have been detected in an ingenious application of the capacitance-change principle. For example, Yamakawa et al. (1954) placed a metal electrode near the tip of a closed catheter, which was then advanced into the hearts of dogs and human subjects. When the changes in capacitive reactance, measured between the catheter tip and the body of the subject, were recorded, heart sounds were clearly identified. So sensitive was the system that the sounds of vocalization were clearly recordable.

A similar investigation of heart sounds was carried out by Groom et al. (1957, 1964), who constructed a monopolar electrode condenser microphone consisting of a chamber in contact with the thorax. Inside the chamber was the other electrode, mounted concentrically so that it did not contact the thoracic wall. Thus the heart sounds and all cardiac vibrations communicated to the thorax modulated the capacitance. The frequency response they attained extended from 0 to 50,000 Hz. In all probability cardiac vibrations had never been detected previously with such a large bandwidth.

When the capacitive method is applied by placing electrodes in, on, or near living tissue, it is often difficult to know whether capacitance changes are the only ones measured. Usually the circuit contains both resistive and reactive components, and what is measured is in reality an impedance change. The various physiological events that have been measured by impedance change are described in Chapter 10.

4-3. DIFFERENTIAL CAPACITOR

An ingenious application of the differential capacitance principle (Fig. 4-1b) was described by Boucek et al. (1959), who used it to construct a myograph for recording the contractions of the chick embryo heart at the 72-hr stage. At this time the heart is in a dynamic stage of development, changing from a tube to a four-chambered organ that a little while later exhibits an adult electrocardiogram. It is, however, incapable of exerting much force. To detect these feeble movements, Boucek and his colleagues placed the heart in a drop of plasma or saline solution. One end of a light lever was made to rest on the part of the heart from which movement was to be recorded; to the other was affixed a metal plate centrally placed between two other fixed plates. The assembly thus constituted a differential capacitor. As the heart beat, the lever was moved, and its recorded motion described the mechanical activity of the organ. The lever also constituted one of the electrodes for the ECG; the other electrode was a wire dipping into the plasma or saline solution. Thus these investigators were able to record and correlate the embryo ECG with the movement of the various chambers of the heart.

An interesting differential capacitor pneumotachograph was described by Krobath and Reed (1964). This device consisted of a circular aluminized Mylar membrane 0.0001 in. thick in which six equally spaced cuts were made, creating leaflets that moved backward and forward as air passed through. On either side were placed two circular plates having hexagonal holes. The metalized membrane constituted the movable plate; the plates with the hexagonal holes were fixed. When respiratory air flowed through the assembly, the capacitance changed in proportion to the flow velocity. With a 200-kHz voltage applied to the capacitor in a bridge configuration, a substantial signal reflecting the velocity of respiratory air was obtained. Time integration of the velocity signal produced an output reflecting the volume of air per breath.

4-4. DIODE TWIN-T CAPACITIVE TRANSDUCER

An ingenious method of employing the capacitance method has been described by Lion (1964). He pointed out that in a bridge circuit either the transducer or the oscillator must be operated above ground potential and that meeting this requirement frequently presents difficulties, surmountable only by the addition of special components and circuits. Instead of a bridge circuit he proposed the use of the diode twin-T circuit shown in Fig. 4-4. With this circuit configuration one side of the oscillator, transducing capacitor, and output signal are all at the same potential which can be ground.

In Lion's circuit S is a radio-frequency oscillator producing sine or square waves of an amplitude E_i. During the positive half-cycle diode D_1 conducts and charges C_1. During the next negative half-cycle D_1 does not conduct, and C_1 discharges through R_1 and R_L and also through R_2 and D_2. Similarly, during the first positive half-cycle D_2 does not conduct, but during the second negative half-cycle D_2 conducts and charges C_2. During

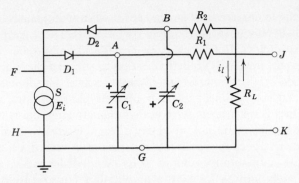

Figure 4-4. Diode twin-T circuit.

the following half-cycle C_2 discharges through R_2 and R_L and also through R_1 and D_1. If diodes D_1 and D_2 are identical, $C_1 = C_2$ and $R_1 = R_2$, the currents through R_1 and R_2 are equal in magnitude and opposite in sign, and when flowing through R_L the output circuit, the net current is zero. Any variation in C_1 and C_2 causes current to flow through R_L, the load, which can be a resistor or a direct-reading microammeter. If display by a rapidly responding recorder is desired, the voltage across R_L can be amplified and displayed appropriately.

Lion (1964) and Foldvari and Lion (1964) gave the following expression, in which $R = R_1 = R_2$, for the current through R_L:

$$I = E_i \frac{R + 2R_L}{(R + R_L)^2} \, \mathrm{Rf}(C_1 - C_2 - C_1 \, e^{-k_1} + C_2 \, e^{-k_2}),$$

where $\quad k_1 = \dfrac{R + R_L}{2\mathrm{Rf}C_1(R + 2R_L)} \quad$ and $\quad k_2 = \dfrac{R + R_L}{2\mathrm{Rf}C_2(R + 2R_L)}.$

Maximum sensitivity of the circuit occurs when $1/k_1 = 1/k_2 = 0.57$. In commercially available transducers[1] consisting of a two-plate capacitor with a separation of 0.005 in., a sensitivity on the order of 1000 V/in. can be obtained.

The output impedance of the diode twin-T circuit is determined by the choice of R_1 and R_L and is virtually independent of C_1 and C_2. By suitable choice of R_1 and R_2 an output impedance of 1 to 100 kΩ can be obtained. Optimum selection of these components will permit display of the capacitance change with a microammeter. If the output is to be displayed by means of a rapidly responding indicator, the rise time available is also de-

[1] Lion Research Corp., Cambridge, Mass.

pendent on the load resistance R_L and the oscillator frequency. With an R_L of 1000 Ω and an oscillator frequency of 1.3 MHz for an instantaneous change in capacitance a rise time of 20 μsec is attainable.

Foldvari and Lion (1964) called attention to some of the highly desirable characteristics of their interesting circuit. Because the diodes operate at high level and in the linear portion of their characteristic, selection of matched diodes is not necessary. Another attractive feature is that changes in oscillator frequency do not adversely affect the sensitivity of the circuit; for example, a 10% change in frequency results in only a 1% alteration in sensitivity to capacitance change. Extremely desirable also is the remarkably high output. For example, with 46 V (rms sinusoidal) for E_i at a frequency of 1.3 MHz, a capacitance change from -7 to $+7$ pF produces an output of -5 to $+5$ V across a 1-MΩ load (R_L).

4-5. CHARACTERISTICS OF CAPACITIVE TRANSDUCERS

The extreme flexibility of capacitive transducers is perhaps their most attractive feature. In many applications they can be employed to detect dimension change without direct mechanical contact with the moving member. For this reason capacitive transducers, which are often called proximity detectors, are free from loading, frictional, and hysteresis errors. By careful design of the capacitive element, extremely small or relatively large displacements can be measured. Another attractive feature of the capacitive transducer is the fact that the capacitance does not depend on the conductivity of its plates. Thus temperature errors from this source are extremely small, although not entirely absent, since the dimensions of the plates depend on temperature. The variation in the dielectric constant of air with temperature is small. Stability is achieved through the mechanical design of the capacitive transducer and the electrical circuitry connected to it. With efficient mechanical and electrical design, these sources of error can be reduced to insignificant levels.

Because the output impedance of a capacitive transducer is usually high, shielding is necessary, and a coaxial cable is frequently required to connect the transducer to the electronic equipment. In many applications the type of cable employed merits special consideration because its capacitance is in parallel with that of the transducing capacitor. Therefore a mechanically stable, low-capacitance coaxial cable is required. Often movement of the cable produces an undesirable capacitance change resulting from a slight displacement of the outer shield relative to the inner conductor, which produces a signal indistinguishable from that made by the transducer. The use of special coaxial cables, in which a layer of conducting powder has been applied to the dielectric directly below the shielding and in contact with it, greatly attenuates this source of error. In many instances the problems presented by the high output impedance can be eliminated by locating some of the processing circuitry at the capacitive transducer. With this technique it is usually possible to incorporate an impedance transformer that provides a low output impedance, permitting location of the transducer at a distance from the processing equipment.

REFERENCES

Adams, R., B. S. Corell, and N. H. Wofesboro, 1960. Cuffless, noncannula, continuous recording of blood pressure. *Surgery* **47**:46–54.

Asher, A. G. 1932. Graphic registration of heart sounds by the argon glow tube. *Arch. Intern. Med.* **50**:913–920.

Atzler, E. 1935a. Dielektrographie. *Hand. biol. Arbeitsmethoden* **5**:1073–1184.

Atzler, E. 1935b. Neues Verfahren zur Funktionsbeurteilung des Herzens. *Deut. Med. Wochenschr.* **59**:1347–1349.

Atzler, E., and G. Lehman. 1932. Über ein neues Verfahren zur Darstellung der Herztätigkeit. (Dielektrographie). *Arbeitsphysiologie* **5**:636-680.

Beyne, J., and L. Gougerot, 1939. Une méthode de transmission électrique et d'enregistrement à distance de la pression artérielle et du débit respiratorie. *C. R. Biol.* **131**:700–774.

Boucek, R. J., W. P. Murphy, and G. H. Paff. 1959. Electrical and mechanical properties of chick embryo heart chambers. *Circ. Res.* **7**:787–793.

Buchtal, F., E. Warburg. 1943. A new method for direct electrical registration of intraarterial pressure in man with examples of its application. *Acta Physiol. Scand.* **5**:55–70.

Cremer, H. 1907. Über die Registrierung Mechanischer Vorgänge auf Menschen. *Med. Wochenschr.* **54**:1629.

Fenning, C. 1936–1937. A new method for recording physiologic activities. I. Recording respiration in small animals. *J. Lab. Clin. Med.* **22**:1279–1280.

Fenning, C., and E. B. Bonnar. 1936–37. A new method of recording physiologic activities. II. The simultaneous recording of maternal respiration intrauterine fetal respiration and uterine contractions. *J. Lab. Clin. Med.* **22**:1280–84.

Foldvari, T., and K. Lion. 1964. Capacitive transducers. *Inst. Control Syst.* **37**:77–85.

Frommer, J. C. 1943. Detecting small mechanical movements. *Electronics* **16**:104–105.

Groom, D., and Y. T. Sihvonen. 1957a. High sensitivity pickup for heart sounds and murmurs. *IRE Trans. Med. Electron.* **PGME-9**:35–40.

Groom, D., and Y. T. Sihvonen. 1957b. A high sensitivity pickup for cardiovascular sounds. *Am. Heart J.* **54**:592–601.

Groom, D. L. H. Medena, and Y. T. Sihvonen. 1964. The proximity transducer. *Am. J. Med. Electron.* **3**:261–265.

Hansen, A. T., and E. Warburg. 1947. An improved manometer for measuring intra-arterial and intra-cardiac pressures. *Am. Heart J.* **33**:709-710.

Joseph, N. R. 1944. Direct current dielectrograph for recording movements of the heart. *J. Clin. Invest.* **23**:25–28.

Krobath, H., and C. Reed. 1964. A new method for the continuous recording of the volume of inspiration and expiration under widely varying conditions. *Am. J. Med. Electron.* **3**:105–109.

Lilly, J. C. 1942. The electrical capacitance diaphragm manometer. *Rev. Sci. Inst.* **13**:34–37.

Lion, K. 1964. Non-linear twin-T network for capacitance transducers. *Rev. Sci. Inst.* **35**:353–356.

Liston, M. 1950. Performance of a double-beam infra-red recording spectrophotometer. *J. Opt. Soc. Am.* **140**:93–101.

Normann, N. A., M. E. DeBakey, G. P. Noon, and J. N. Ross. 1973. Monitoring and closed-loop control of pneumatic blood pumps. *Cardiovasc. Res. Center Bull.* **12**:3–12.

Normann, N. A., G. P. Noon, and J. N. Ross, 1973. Monitoring and automatic control of pneumatic blood pump. *Proc. 26th Ann. Conf. Eng Med. Biol.* **15**:334.

Schutz, E. 1937. Konstruktion einer manometrischen Sonde mit elektrischer Transmission. *Z. Biol.* **91**:515–521.

Tomberg, V. T. 1963. The high frequency spirometer. *Proceedings of the International Congress on Medical Electronics,* Liège, Belgium.

Tomberg, V. T. 1964. Device and a new method of measuring pulmonary respiration. *17th Annual Conference on Engineering in Biology and Medicine.* McGregor and Werner, Washington, D. C.

Whitehorn, W. V., and E. R. Pearl. 1949. The use of change in capacity to record cardiac volume with human subject. *Science* **109**:262–263.

Yamakawa, K., Y., Shionoya, K. Kitamura, T. Nagai, T. Yamamoto, and S. Ohta. 1954. Intracardiac phonocardiography. *Am. Heart. J.* **47**:424–431.

5

Photoelectric Transducers

In the measurement of physiological events in living subjects, photoelectric transducers are employed in two ways. The photosensor functions in the first method as a detector of the changes in the intensity of light of a given wavelength, as in conventional colorimetry or spectrophotometry; in the second method it serves as a detector of changes in the intensity of light in which wavelength is relatively unimportant. There are numerous applications in both categories.

There are three basic types of photoelectric transducers: (1) the photoemissive (phototube), in which electrons are released from a metallic surface (usually alkali), (2) the photovoltaic (barrier-layer cell), in which a potential difference is produced between two substances in contact, and (3) the photoconductive (photoresistor), in which a change in conductivity occurs. Although there is some overlap in applicability, each is recommended for certain tasks because of its particular spectral response, light sensitivity, output current, and voltage characteristics. The following sections describe the principles of operation, characteristics, and applications of each type.

5-1. PHOTOEMISSIVE TUBES

The photoemissive tube consists of an evacuated or gas-filled bulb with two electrodes. On one, the cathode, is a coating of a specially prepared material that releases electrons when illuminated. The other electrode, the anode, usually consists of a thin rod or loop of wire. For electron emission to occur, there are certain restrictions on the type of surface and the wavelength of the impinging light. Electron emission is possible only if the wavelength is shorter than a certain threshold value, which depends on the amount of energy required to release an electron from the metal (work function). Thus there is a long-wave limit of sensitivity.

The electrode materials most frequently employed for the emissive surface are cesium, antimony, silver, and bismuth in combination with trace amounts of other substances. Each type of surface exhibits its own spectral characteristics. Some surfaces are designed to be highly sensitive to narrow spectral regions; others are designed to have a fairly broad spectral sensitivity.

Photoemissive tubes come in a variety of configurations and sizes. In general they, like other photodetectors, are described in terms of the direction of the light with respect to the location of the terminals connected to the internal electrodes. For example, if the terminals are on one end or on both ends of the device and the light enters at right angles, the device is designated as a "side-on" photodetector. If the electrode terminals are on one end or on both ends and the light enters at one end, the term "end-on" photodetector is employed. Typical configurations for the photoemissive tube are illustrated in Fig. 5-1, which illustrates side-on and end-on types.

With the photoemissive detector, a relatively high voltage (10–200 V) must be applied between the two electrodes. The electrons released by the light quanta are attracted to the anode. The electron flow constitutes a cur-

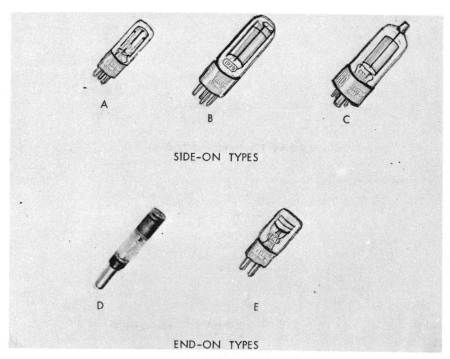

Figure 5-1. Photoemissive tubes: (a), (b), (c) side-on types; (d), (e) end-on types. (Courtesy of Radio Corporation of America, Lancaster, Pa.)

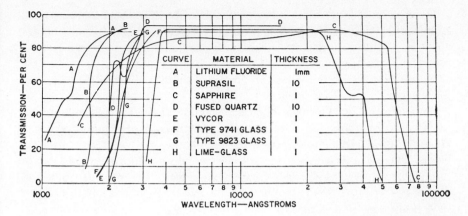

Figure 5-2. Transmission characteristics of various substances used in phototube windows. (From "RCA Phototubes and Photocells," Radio Corporation of America, Lancaster, Pa., 1963. By permission.)

rent that is linearly proportional to the intensity of the incident light. In the vacuum type the current produced is small and is not used to operate an indicator directly; it is usually led through a high resistance, and the voltage thus developed is applied to an amplifier having a high input impedance.

When higher currents are required, gas mixtures are often incorporated into the photoemissive detector. With this technique the primary electrons released by the incident light collide with gas molecules and produce secondary electrons and positive ions, thereby increasing the available current. To avoid the occurrence of a glow discharge, lower anode-to-cathode voltages must be employed. Although the current intensity is increased about tenfold, the linear current-light relationship is compromised at higher intensities.

Both vacuum and gas-filled photoemissive photodetectors respond quickly to changes in light intensity. The response time of the former is approximately 10^{-9} sec, whereas that of the latter is much longer, approximating 10^{-3} sec. Both exhibit a small current flow with no light (dark current). Typical values are 10^{-8} to 10^{-9} A for vacuum phototubes and 10^{-7} to 10^{-8} A for gas-filled phototubes.

Although photoemissive surfaces respond to ultaviolet radiation, unless special materials that transmit ultraviolet energy are used in constructing the bulb, the spectral sensitivity of photoemissive tubes seldom extends below 200 mμ. The use of a special bulb will permit operation further into the ultraviolet spectrum. Figure 5-2 illustrates the transparency of the various materials used as windows in photodetectors.

Most photoemissive tubes are sensitive to visible light, and a few respond to infrared radiation down to 800 mμ. The spectral sensitivity of a photoemissive surface is designated by the letter S and a number. This designation refers to a spectral curve recognized by all manufacturers. Data showing some of the spectral characteristics described by the various S-numbers are presented in Fig. 5-3 and Table 5-1.

By incorporating additional anodes (dynodes), each at a higher potential, a currrent amplification can be obtained through secondary electron emission. Photoelectrons emitted from the photoelectric surface are drawn to and strike the first dynode, releasing secondary electrons which are attracted to the second anode at a higher potential (75–150 V); there the process is repeated. With ten or more stages, a current amplification of several million can be obtained.

The spectral sensitivity of such a device, called a photomuliplier, is determined by the emitting surface. The response curves for typical tubes are S1, 4, 5, 8, 10, 11, 13, 17, 19, 20. Thus photomultipliers are available for almost the whole of the visible region and parts of the ultraviolet and infrared regions.

As with other members of its family, the photomultiplier tube has a small dark current of about 10^{-7} A. The response time is extremely short, on the order of 10^{-8} to 10^{-9} sec. Because of its very high sensitivity and

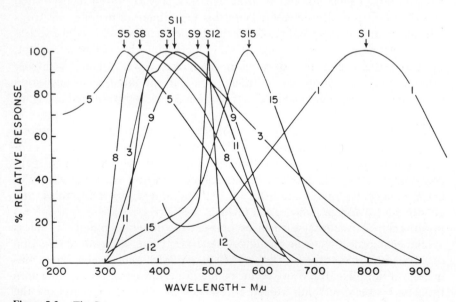

Figure 5-3.   The S curves.

Table   5-1   Spectral   Characteristics   of   the
S-Numbers*

Spectral Designation	Wavelength for Maximum Response (mμ)	50% Points
S1	800	620–950
S3	420	350†–640
S4	400	320–540
S5	340	230†–510
S8	370	320–540
S9	480	350–580
S10	450	350–590
S11	440	350–560
S12	500	Narrow band
S13	440	260–560
S14	1500	760–1730
S15	580	500–660
S17	490	310–580
S19	330	190–460
S20	420	325–595
S21	450	260–560

* Data derived from *RCA Photosensitive Devices and Cathode Ray Tubes*. Radio Corp. of America, Electron Tube Division, Harrison, N.J., 1960.
† Interpolated values.

short response time, the photomultiplier is an ideal detector for brief flashes of light of low intensity, such as those produced when radiation strikes the specially prepared crystals employed in scintillation counters.

5-2.   PHOTOVOLTAIC CELLS AND JUNCTION CELLS

The photovoltaic (photogalvanic) cell is encountered frequently in biomedical studies. Unlike the photoemissive tube, which requires a relatively high voltage and produces a small current when illuminated, the photovoltaic cell develops a voltage that can drive a substantial current through a galvanometer or other low-impedance circuit.

One of the most popular of the photovoltaic cells consists of a sandwich of a thin coating of selenium on an iron or steel backing. Above the selenium is a thin transparent film of metal. The film and selenium are insulated from each other, and this region constitutes the barrier layer. When the barrier layer is illuminated, light quanta are absorbed, electrons are released, and a potential difference appears across the barrier. The transparent metal film becomes negative and the selenium positive. Completion of a circuit between the two electrodes causes a current to flow. It is interesting to note that the resistance between the electrodes decreases with illumination. This feature makes it possible to parallel photovoltaic cells; only those that are illuminated will supply current; those not illuminated do not load the others. In the solar power supplies used on board satellites, a diode is placed in series with group of photodetectors to eliminate possible loading by partially illuminated or damaged photocells. This technique guarantees maximum current (Acker et al., 1960).

Other substances are used in voltaic cells. Cuprous oxide in contact with gold or platinum is sometimes employed in barrier layer cells. Although these devices are available, they are not common because, compared to the selenium cell, they have low sensitivity to light. The spectral peak of the cuprous oxide cell is around 560 mμ.

Selenium photocells cover the visible spectrum (300–700 mμ) with a spectral sensitivity curve peaking around 550 to 570 mμ. With an inexpensive filter it is easy to obtain a spectral curve closely resembling that of the human eye. For this reason these devices are used in illumination meters, exposure meters, and simple colorimeters, all of which operate without electronic amplification. The spectral sensitivity curves of many of the photovoltaic cells commercially available are plotted in Fig. 5-4.

The relationship between light intensity and the voltage developed by the photovoltaic sensor is not linear if the device is operated without a resistive load. At saturation a typical open-circuit voltage is in the vicinity of 200 to 600 mV. If a resistive load is placed across the device, the current flow becomes more linearly related to light intensity as the resistance is decreased. Hence it is necessary to employ a low-resistance galvanometer or measuring circuit to indicate light intensity if a linear scale is to be obtained. When a galvanometer having an internal resistance of approximately 100 Ω is employed, a current of 0.5 mA can be obtained from many standard photovoltaic cells when adequately illuminated.

Because of the large capacitance of the barrier layer, the response time of a typical photovoltaic cell is seldom less than 5 msec, although a few miniature types exhibit response times of 0.1 msec. Perhaps the most undesirable feature of the photovoltaic cell in biomedical application is its sensitivity to temperature changes as the load resistance is varied. Many cells have an optimum value for the resistance that can be connected across the device to minimize the sensitivity change with temperature. This resistance value is not necessarily the one that yields the maximum power transfer or linearity of current with light intensity.

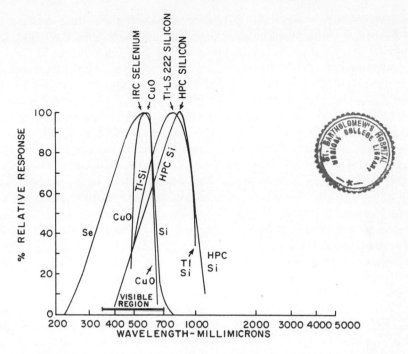

Figure 5-4. Spectral characteristics of photovoltaic cells, Redrawn from data in manufacturers' bulletins. (TI = Texas Instruments; HPC = Hoffman Electronics Corp., IRC = International Rectifier Corp.)

The absorption of light quanta by a semiconductor (P–N) junction results in the creation of hole-electron pairs and a voltage across the junction. Connection of an external load resistance produces a flow of current, hence the delivery of power. Thus the junction photocell is a photovoltaic device that converts light (electromagnetic radiation) to electrical energy.

The most interesting photodiode is the solar battery that is used to convert sunlight into electrical power. It consists of a layer of boron diffused on to the surface of N-type silicon. When illuminated with bright sunlight, a voltage of about 0.5 V is developed. Connection of a load resistor across its terminals results in a current flow.

When a junction photocell is operated as a photovoltaic device, the current-voltage characteristic reveals that the device is nonlinear. Decreasing the value of the load resistor (R_L) increases the output current but decreases the voltage (see Fig. 5-5). The optimum value of load resistance is that value for maximum power output (i.e., when the area of the rectangle $0–I_q–Q–V_q$ is maximum). The power available from a given unit is dependent on the area of the photojunction that is illuminated and the intensity of the illumination. The conversion efficiency is on the order of 5 to 10%.

The junction photocell can also be operated with forward or reverse bias applied to the P–N junction. Figure 5-6*b* illustrates the manner in which the current-voltage characteristic is altered when the cell is illuminated. To operate the device as a photoconductor, the P–N junction is reverse biased (i.e., P to negative, N to positive). The current-voltage characteristic of such a device is plotted upward, as in Fig. 5-6*c*. Thus by placing a battery (E_{bb}) in series with a load resistor (R_L) and the junction photocell, an output voltage (ΔV) and current (ΔI) can be obtained for an increase in illumination from 0 to ϕ, as indicated by movement of the operating point up the load line (slope $1/R_L$) as in Fig. 5-6*c*.

There are many different types of junction photovoltaic cell, each designed to have a desired spectral sensitivity. In general, junction photocells tend to have their spectral peak sensitivity toward the red and infrared regions. For example, silicon cells exhibit their peak around 800 mμ, whereas germanium units exhibit their maximum sensitivity around 1550 mμ. Indium arsenide and indium antimonide exhibit response peaks at 3200 and 6800 mμ, respectively. Frequently the later types are cooled with liquid air to increase their sensitivity and to reduce their thermal noise voltage.

The response time of junction photocells to light is short enough (micro-

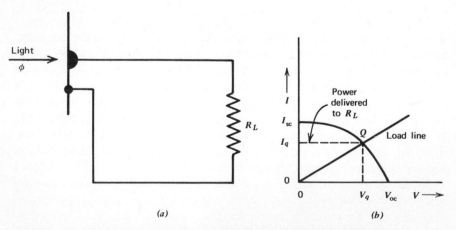

(a)   (b)

Figure 5-5. (*a*) The photojunction photocell; (*b*) the current-(I) voltage (V) characteristics in response to illumination: I_{sc}, is the short-circuit current; V_{oc}, is the open-circuit voltage. The power delivered to the load resistor (R_L) for the illumination ϕ is equal to the area of the rectangle represented by the dashed line. The load line has a slope equal to $1/R_L$.

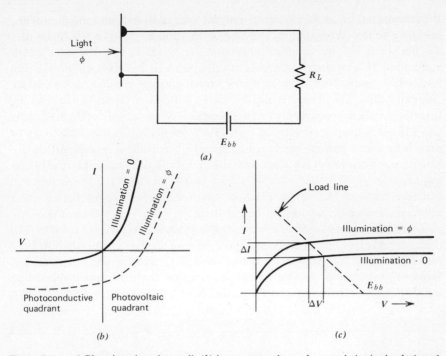

Figure 5-6. (a) Photojunction photocell; (b) its current-voltage characteristics in the dark and when illuminated; (c) illustrates operation of the device with a polarizing voltage (E_{bb}) to obtain an output voltage (ΔV) and current (ΔI). (Redrawn from Phototubes and Photocells. Technical Manual PT60. Radio Corporation of America. Lancaster, Pa. 1963.)

seconds to nanoseconds) to be used as light detectors in which there is rapid modulation of illumination. Because of their small size, high sensitivity, and short response time, junction photocells see a wide variety of uses as light detectors. One use, becoming increasingly important in the life sciences, is in optically coupled isolators. In these devices, which are discussed in Chapter 12, a photojunction cell is used to detect the light produced by a light-emitting diode (LED), mounted a few millimeters away. Thus the desired signal modulates the light produced by the LED, and the light is detected by a junction photocell. In this way, a signal is coupled from one circuit to another without any electrical interconnection, thereby providing excellent electrical isolation.

5-3.   PHOTOCONDUCTIVE CELLS

The photoconductive or photoresistive cell consists of a thin film of a material such as selenium, germanium, silicon, or a metal halide or sulfide.

When exposed to certain types of radiant energy, it exhibits the photoconductive phenomenon, that is, a decrease in resistance. When light quanta
are absorbed by the material, electrons are released into the conduction
band and, if a voltage is applied to the film, a current will flow. The
resistance change with illumination is considerable. In most photoconductive cells the conductance is nearly linear with high intensity. Resistance
therefore varies reciprocally with intensity. Most photoconductive cells
will exhibit a drop in resistance from many megohms in the dark to a few
hundreds ohms when highly illuminated. Such devices are extremely
sensitive photodetectors and are often employed as light-controlled
switches.

The resistance (R) versus illumination intensity (ϕ) characteristic of a
photoconductive cell is usually of the form $R = K/\phi^{\alpha}$ where K and α are
constants depending on the type of photoconductor; Figure 5-7 presents the
data for a typical unit. This logarithmic relationship with illumination (i.e.,
$\log R = \log K - \log \phi$) is useful in many colorimetric applications.
However, when it is desired to obtain a signal that is linearly related to
light intensity, obvious difficulties arise. Nonetheless, over a limited range

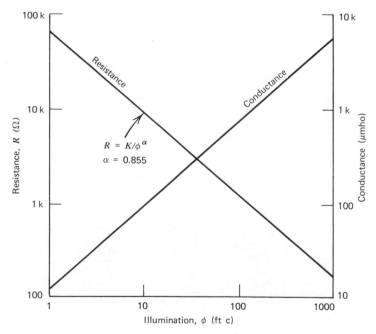

Figure 5-7. Resistance and conductance versus illumination for a typical photoconductive
cell.

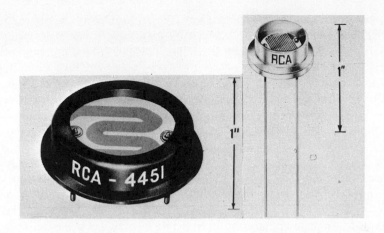

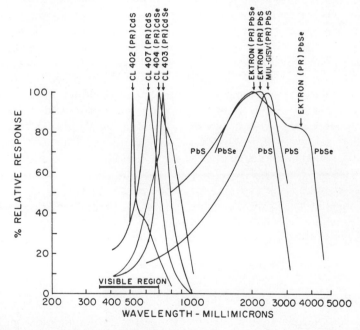

Figure 5-8. (*a*) Photoconductive cells. (Courtesy of Radio Corporation of America, Lancaster, Pa.) (*b*) Spectral characteristics of photoconductive cells: PR = Photoresistive; CL = Clairex Corp.; EKTRON = Kodak Corp.; MUL = Mullard Corp.

of illumination intensity, a reasonably linear current-light relationship can be obtained by connecting the photoresistor across a low-impedance voltage source (E) and measuring the current through the photoconductor with a current-measuring device having a resistance many times lower than the lowest resistance of the photoconductive cell with the maximum illumination to be employed. Since in many photoconductive cells α is not far from -1.0, the current (I) in the circuit is E/R, and if $R = K/\phi$, the current is equal to $EK'\phi$. If a low-resistance current-measuring device is not available, a low value of resistor can be employed and the voltage across it can be measured using an amplifier.

Figure 5-8a illustrates two of the standard configurations of photoconductive cells. A wide range of diameters is available; some card-reading cells are as small as 5 mm; others used in photoelectric relays are as large as 25 mm. Many manufacturers supply the same photosensitive material in side-on and end-on models.

Many of the photoconductive cells show good sensitivity to visible light; a few are sensitive to the ultraviolet and x-ray spectra. A large number, however, are exquisitely sensitive to the infrared region, a characteristic which prompted their development for spectroscopy and self-guiding infrared-seeking missiles. The sensitivity peaks of many units can be shifted by cooling; for example, Moss (1949) showed that the spectral peaks of lead sulfide, lead selenide, and lead telluride can be shifted farther into the infrared region by cooling to 20°K. The spectral characteristics of several of the photoconducting surfaces operated at room temperature are shown in Fig. 5-8b. Jacobs (1960) has listed the characteristics of many of the commercially available photoconductors when operated at reduced temperatures.

The response and decay times vary widely with the type of material and are not independent of the illumination level. In general, the response time is shorter with a high light level. Typical response times for photoconductors operated at room temperatures vary between 0.1 and 30 msec.

5-4. THE PHOTOTRANSISTOR

With the photodiode, the current change for an illumination change is small, although the response time is very short. If some response time can be sacrificed, a considerable increase in current sensitivity can be obtained by using a phototransistor (see Fig. 5-9). In such a device, the base (b)-collector (c) area is large and the base (b)-emitter (e) area is small. The incident radiation is caused to strike the base region which is intentionally left unconnected. With this arrangement, the holes generated in the base

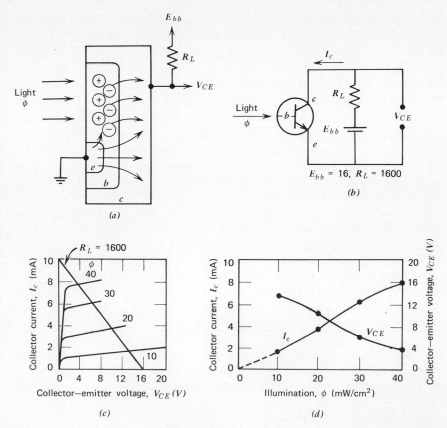

Figure 5-9. (*a*) Principle of operation of the phototransistor; (*b*) circuit employed with it; (*c*) and (*d*) operating characteristics in response to light flux ϕ.

region by the radiation cause the base potential to rise, forward biasing the base-emitter junction. Electrons then flow into the base from the emitter to neutralize the excess holes. Because of the close proximity of the collector junction, the probability of an electron combining with a hole is small, and most of the electrons are immediately drawn into the collector region, which is at a high positive potential. As a result, the total collector current is much larger than the photogenerated current; in fact, it is β times as large.

Since the base is left unconnected, there are only three variables associated with operation of the phototransistor: collector-to-emitter voltage (V_{CE}) collector current (I_c) and illumination intensity (ϕ). The operational characteristics of such a device can be predicted by knowing the collector characteristics; a typical example appears in Fig. 5-9c. The current-voltage characteristic thus resembles that of a conventional transistor, the parameter being illumination intensity ϕ rather than base current.

To employ the phototransistor as a light detector, it is merely necessary to connect it in series with a load resistor (R_L) and power supply (E_{bb}), as in Fig. 5-9b. By choosing a supply voltage and plotting the load line (slope $1/R_L$) on the collector characteristics, it is possible to predict the change in collector current and collector-emitter voltage in response to illumination (see Fig. 5-9c). The complete collector circuit response to light from 10 to 40 mW/cm² is plotted in Fig. 5-9d for a supply voltage of 16 and a load resistance of 1600 Ω. Clearly the device is linear over a considerable range of illumination.

The phototransistor is a high-gain photodetector whose spectral peak sensitivity lies in the red and infrared regions of the spectrum. The high collector-base capacitance causes the device to have a longer response time than a photodiode. Nonetheless the response time is on the order of 5 μsec, which allows operation up to 100 kHz in many models. Because of the flatness of the current-voltage characteristic, the output impedance is high, being on the order of many kilohms. The temperature sensitivity of phototransistors is comparable to other semiconducting devices.

Despite their small size, high efficiency, and reasonably short response time, phototransistors have found little application in the biological sciences. They also see limited industrial application, primarily because of their inferiority of response time when compared with a photodiode. It would appear that the combination of a photodiode, with an appropriately designed amplifier, provides a better light-detection system.

5-5. COMPARISON OF PHOTOELECTRIC TRANSDUCERS

With such an array of photodetectors, it is worthwhile reviewing the prominent characteristics of each type. The most important characteristics of photosensors are spectral sensitivity, response time and type of output provided (e.g., current or voltage) and linearity with illumination intensity.

Figure 5-10 illustrates the spectral characteristics of the human eye along with those of the photosensors described in this chapter. The photoemissive tubes tend to exhibit their peak spectral sensitivity in the visible and blue regions of the spectrum, possessing a rather short response time (microseconds). The response time is slightly longer, but the light sensitivity is higher in the gas-filled photoemissive tubes; both types require a fairly high polarizing voltage. The current-light relationship is very nearly linear with illumination intensity, but there is a small residual dark current. Only a small output current is produced with illumination. However, when the

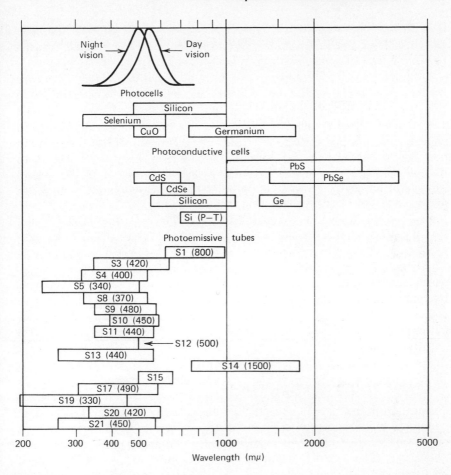

Figure 5-10. Spectral response of the human eye for night and day vision, along with the spectral sensitivities of photocells, photoconductors, and photoemissive tubes. The numbers in parentheses identify the spectral peaks for the S curves; P-T denotes a phototransistor.

small current is passed through a high resistance, a large output voltage is obtained. The fragility of the glass envelope restricts operation of the device to situations in which only small acceleration forces are encountered. Photomultiplier tubes are photoemissive tubes in which auxiliary electrodes (dynodes) are required to achieve electron multiplication.

Photovoltaic cells (photocells and photojunction cells) tend to have their peak spectral sensitivity in the visible and infrared regions. The response time depends on the type, the shortest response times being found in the photojunction cells. No polarizing voltage is needed, and current is delivered to the load resistor when the photovoltaic cell is illuminated. Photovoltaic cells are temperature sensitive, rugged and can be used as low-efficiency energy converters.

Photoconductive cells (photoresistors, biased junction photocells, and phototransistors) tend to be red and infrared sensitive. The response times depend on the type of device; the biased junction photocell exhibits the shortest response time, the phototransistor has a longer response time, and the photoresistor has the longest response time. All types require a polarizing voltage, and the resistance of the photoconductive cell varies almost inversely with illumination. The current-illumination relationship of the biased junction photocell and phototransistor is quite linear. All types are temperature-sensitive and rugged.

In choosing a photodetector for a particular colorimetric task, it is highly desirable to choose a device having a spectral peak at the wavelength of interest. If there is no photosensor with a spectral peak at the desired wavelength, a filter is chosen so that the combined spectral response of the photodetector and the transmission characteristics of the filter provide maximum spectral sensitivity at the desired wavelength. It is important to note that the use of filters decreases the efficiency of the photodetector; however, this price frequently must be paid to obtain the desired spectral sensitivity.

5-6. COLORIMETRIC APPLICATIONS

Apart from their use in colorimeters and spectrophotometers to analyze biological fluids, photoelectric transducers see service in the measurement of physiological events in the living subject Two applications are determination of the oxygen saturation in the blood as it circulates and measurement of cardiac output by the dye-indicator method. In both applications photodetectors are employed with appropriate filters to detect color density changes.

The determination of oxygen saturation by measuring the "redness" of the blood in the living subject is accomplished by transillumination of a web of tissue richly endowed with a capillary bed, such as the lobe or pinna of the ear. The emergent light is detected by two photovoltaic detectors, each one being covered with a filter. The first detects radiation in the red portion of the spectrum at 640 mμ and the second in the infrared at 800 mμ. The red channel provides a signal that contains information on the amount of oxygen in the blood and the amount of blood and tissue in the optical path. The infrared channel signal is independent of oxygen saturation and carries information on the amount of the blood and tissue in the optical path.

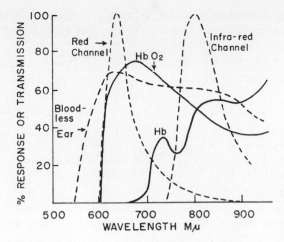

Figure 5-11.   Spectral data employed in oximetry.

Figure 5-11 illustrates the spectral characteristics of fully oxygenated blood (HbO_2) and blood without oxygen (Hb). Also shown are the spectral response of the bloodless ear (Elam et al., 1949) and the approximate bandpass characteristics of the red and infrared channels of a typical oximeter earpiece employing iron-selenium photovoltaic cells covered by appropriate red and infrared filters.

Oxygen saturation is determined by calibrating the photodetector against chemically analyzed blood samples. The calibration curve is a plot of oxygen saturation versus the ratio of the logarithm of the transmission in the red to the logarithm of the transmission in the infrared band. When such a calibration curve has been constructed on a well-flushed ear, 95% of the readings can be expected to fall within $\pm 5\%$ of the true value (Wood and Geraci, 1949).

The first practical oximeter was developed by Millikan (1942). In it the photodetectors were mounted in a small fixture that fitted over the pinna of the ear. In an improved instrument described by Wood and Geraci (1949), the photocell assembly was equipped with a pressure capsule that permitted rendering the optical path bloodless to make initial settings. Figure 5-12 shows a commercial version[1] of the Wood-Geraci ear oximeter.

It has been possible to determine oxygen saturation by reflectance colorimetry. After finding that the amount of light in a narrow band in the red spectrum reflected from a film of blood 3.5 mm or more thick was propor-

[1] Waters Co., Box 529, Rochester, Minn.

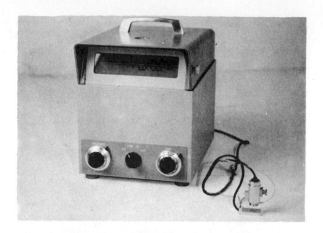

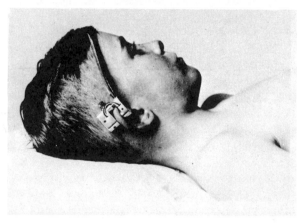

Figure 5-12.   Oximeter and earpiece. (Courtesy of Waters Co., Rochester, Minn.)

tional to oxygen saturation, Zijlstra (1951) set about to construct a
reflectance-type oximeter for human use. He employed a barrier layer
photocell in which was mounted concentrically a small lamp covered by a
red filter transmitting light of 600 to 680 mμ. A small box held the photocell
and light bulb a short distance from the forehead of the subject. To obtain
adequate stability in his first model, Zijlstra had to cool the photocell with
a water chamber mounted behind it. In a second model two photocells were
used and a differential circuit was employed, thereby eliminating the need
for a cooling chamber. In a later model two spectral bands (red and green)
were utilized, and a third photocell was added for compensation purposes.

The output of the photocells was calibrated in terms of oxygen saturation by chemically analyzed blood samples. Zijlstra stated that if the oximeter was employed without calibration, the output of the photocells reflected only changes in saturation. He recommended use of the device for monitoring saturation during surgery.

An outstanding intravascular reflectance oximeter using fiber optics was described by Enson et al. (1962). It was applicable to the measurement of oxygen saturation or cardiac output by means of the dye-indicator method. In this device beams of red (660 mμ) and infrared (805 mμ) light were transmitted 20 times per second down a fiber bundle in one lumen of a double-lumen catheter. The diffusely reflected light from the blood at the tip of the catheter was conducted to the external photodetector via a second fiber bundle in the other lumen of the catheter. The photodetecting apparatus consisted of a photomultiplier and oscilloscope, whose screen showed the red and infrared signals. The ratio of these signals was found to vary linearly with oxygen saturation. The calibration graph presented showed a standard deviation of $\pm 1.9\%$ around the regression line.

A high-efficiency intravascular fiberoptic catheter oximeter, which was described by Johnson et al. (1971), is now commercially available.[2] Two light-emitting diodes alternately transmit red (600–700 mμ) and infrared (800–900 mμ) light down fiberoptic bundles at a rate of 200/sec. The reflected light is transmitted up a third fiber bundle and detected by two silicon photodiodes that are sensitive to the red and infrared radiation. It was learned that the ratio of the two reflective signals very nearly cancels reflectance variations due to blood flow and that this ratio is inversely related to oxygen saturation. A very careful *in vitro* evaluation of the accuracy of this oximeter was presented by Woodroof and Koorajian (1973), who found that it exhibited its highest accuracy when the hematocrit was in the normal range. The standard error on this range was about 2%. Larger errors were obtained with hematocrit values below 25 and above 90%.

It is possible to measure the output of the heart per minute by injecting a known amount of indicator into the venous system and measuring its passage in the arterial system with a calibrated detector. With a stable flow for the period of measurement, the prime requisities are that the indicator mix uniformly with the blood and that it does not become lost from the circulation in the time between injection and measurement. A variety of indicators has been employed, the most popular being dyes.

The dye-injection method was widely accepted after Hamilton et al. (1948) demonstrated that results obtained thereby agreed with those ob-

[2] Physio Control, Redmond, Wash.

tained with the Fick technique. After recording densitometers for arterial blood became available, the method was widely accepted. Although many dyes have been employed. the three that appear to be the most popular at present are Evans blue (T1824), indocyanine green (cardio-green), and Coomassie blue. These dyes are nontoxic and nonstimulating. Each has its own characteristics that recommend it for certain purposes. Table 5-2 summarizes the two most important characteristics of each dye: the wavelength for maximum absorption, and the retention time in the vascular system.

A few comments will help to identify the relative advantages of each dye. Those that are retained in circulation for a long time yield the highest accuracy. Because of the long retention time, however, the circulation soon becomes loaded with the dye if repeated determinations are made. Such dyes, although they may be harmless, often discolor the skin if large amounts are injected. On the other hand, dyes that disappear rapidly permit more frequent measurements, but because they soon leave the circulation, accuracy is compromised.

The wavelength for measurement of the dye concentration merits special consideration. Oxygenated blood transmits maximally around 640 mμ; blood without oxygen (reduced blood) and fully oxygenated blood transmit equally well around 800 mμ. Measurements with dyes that absorb around 640 mμ are subject to errors with changes in oxygen saturation. Dyes with maximal transmission around 800 mμ are immune to such errors.

The type of dilution curve following the injection of a dye appears in Fig. 5-13. Cardiac output is calculated by measuring the area under the first time-concentration curve as shown. Because recirculation usually obscures identification of the end of the first pass, the falling phase is extrapolated to the baseline, or, as was proposed by Kinsman et al. (1929), a semilogarithmic plot of this portion of the curve and linear extrapolation to a negligible concentration (ca. 1% of maximum) are carried out to de-

Table 5-2   Characteristics of Dyes

Name	Absorption Wavelength (mμ)	50% Retention Time	Reference
Evans Blue (T1824)	640	5 days	Connolly and Wood (1954)
Indocyanine (cardiogreen)	800	10 min	Fox (1960), Wheeler et al. (1958)
Coomassie blue	585–600	15–20 min	Taylor (1959)

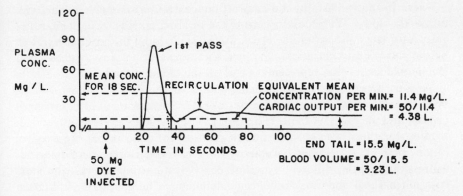

Figure 5-13.   Dye dilution curve. (Details on extrapolation technique in Section 5-10.)

termine the end of the first pass.[3] The area under the first pass is then determined, and the mean concentration for that time is calculated. The mean concentration for 1 min is then determined, and cardiac output per minute is calculated by dividing this figure into the amount initially injected. Sample calculations are shown in Fig. 5-13.

When the optical transmission of flowing blood is recorded continuously, scattering and reflection from blood cells cause variations. The transmission varies therefore with the velocity of the blood stream. For this reason it is often difficult to obtain a stable baseline in the recording. A method of overcoming some of these difficulties was reported by Sutterer (1960), who described a compensating densitometer for dye-dilution studies using indocyanine green. In this instrument he placed two photodetectors, one sensitive to a wavelength of 800 mμ, the other to all wavelengths except 800 mμ. By combining the outputs of the two photocells, he was able to compensate for changes in flow.

If the dye is retained in the circulation, after several circulations a stable concentration called the "end-tail" is obtained and is often utilized for calibrating the densitometer by withdrawing a sample of blood and analyzing it for the dye concentration existing at this time. This calibration technique is frequently employed when ear oximeters are used to determine cardiac output. It is apparent that calibration by this technique is inaccurate if the dye is cleared rapidly. Because the end-tail calibration point is low on the concentration scale, high accuracy can be attained only if the sample is carefully analyzed and corrected for indicator loss.

[3] The technique for processing an indicator-dilution curve is described in Chapter 10, Section 14-1.

There is another use for the end-tail concentration, namely, calculation of blood volume. With total mixing of the dye and no loss from the cardiovascular system, blood volume is calculated by dividing the amount injected by the end-tail concentration. The figure obtained in this way assumes that the sample analyzed is representative of all the blood in the body.

Various penetrating mathematical studies of the dilution method have been carried out by Meier and Zierler (1954), Stephenson (1958), Grodins (1962), and Zierler (1962a, 1962b, 1963). These studies are recommended reading for those who wish to investigate current concepts of the dye-dilution method. A number of investigators have developed mathematical expressions for the different types of concentration-time curves obtained with normal and abnormal circulatory dynamics. The goal in these studies has been to assign numerical values to the symbols in the equations, thus quantitating the factors underlying the development of the concentration-time curve. An excellent review of the work in this area was presented by Thompson et al. (1964). From their own studies, they developed the following expression for the concentration versus time curve $C(t)$:

$$C(t) = \frac{K(t - T)^\alpha}{e^{(t-T)/\beta}},$$

where t = time after injection,
  K = the scale factor constant,
  T = appearance time,
  α, β = system parameters.

After evaluation of α, β, it was found that this equation very closely fitted the concentration-time curves obtained on a group of normal subjects and patients.

Another *in vivo* colorimetric application of a photodetector is due to Baker (1961), who used the high infrared-sensitivity characteristics of a lead selenide photoresistor to construct a rapidly responding carbon dioxide analyzer to record breath-by-breath changes in the concentration of this gas in expired air. The $4.26\text{-}\mu$ absorption band of carbon dioxide was employed to detect the amount of this component in a gas sample passing between an infrared source and the photoconductive detector. The response time obtained was limited by the speed of admission of the gas sample and the frequency of the chopper amplifier. In practice an overall response time of about 50 msec was obtained.

5-7. NONCOLORIMETRIC APPLICATIONS

There are numerous instances in which photodetectors have been used noncolorimetrically for the transduction of physiological events. One of the earliest was due to Rein et al. (1940), who constructed a blood pressure transducer by affixing a shade to the free end of a Bourdon tube. On one side of the shade was a photovoltaic cell, and on the other was a ⅓-W exciter lamp. Pressure applied to the Bourdon tube moved the shade and exposed the photodetector to the light bulb, thereby producing a voltage that was recorded by a rapidly responding galvanometer. The response time reported was 12.5 msec, and the volume displacement was 13.5 mm³/100 mm Hg.

There have been other interesting applications of photodetectors to measure blood pressure; for example, Feitelberg (1942) described an in-genious servosystem with a phototube and light source in an assembly that was mounted on a lead screw and driven by a reversible motor. Between the phototube and light bulb was placed one arm of a mercury manometer, which displayed mean blood pressure. In operation, the phototube and exciter lamp assembly was made to track the level of mercury. Mechanically coupled to the photodetector assembly was an ink-writing recorder that displayed changes in mean blood pressure. The advantage of this early servosystem was the elimination of stylus friction, so bothersome in the smoked-drum kymographic recording systems. Feitelberg reported that the system worked well and achieved a tracking rate of 20 mm Hg/sec.

Gilson (1943) described the application of the photoelectric principle to detect the movement of the light beam of a Wiggers membrane manometer and the movement of a myograph lever. This method of transduction added sensitivity to an already high-quality photographic recording pressure transducer. His myograph was one of the first to produce an electrical signal from muscle pull. An ingenious method of using the photoelectric principle to develop a catheter-tip blood pressure transducer was described by Clark et al. (1965). In this device a tiny reflecting diaphragm was mounted at the tip of a catheter (0.11 in. diameter) which contained two concentrically mounted bundles of optical fibers. Light was transmitted down one bundle of 3-mil fibers and reflected back to a silicon photocell af-fixed to the end of the other. Pressure applied to the tiny diaphragm changed the curvature and altered the amount of light reflected to the photocell. With a silvered Mylar diaphragm of appropriate thickness (1 to 3 mils), the change in output was 200 μV for 0 to 50 mm Hg change in pressure. The resonant frequency of the diaphragm was reported by these investigators to be 10 kHz, indicating that the device had an extremely high frequency response and was capable of recording the briefest of transients in the cardiovascular system.

Figure 5-14 summarizes several applications of the photoelectric prin-ciple described by Geddes et al. (1961, 1957). Figure 5-14a illustrates a

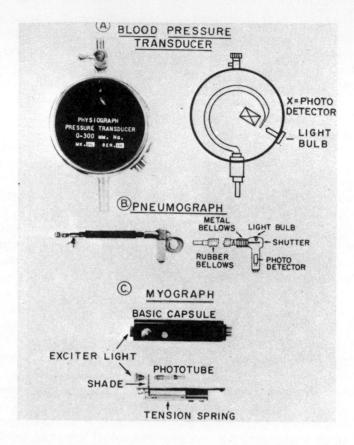

Figure 5-14. Photoelectric transducers: (*a*) blood pressure transducer; (*b*) pneumograph; (*c*) myograph.

blood pressure transducer that resembles Rein's except that a high-efficiency miniature photoemissive vacuum tube is employed instead of a photovoltaic cell. With a 15-psi Bourdon tube, a response time of 20 msec is easily attainable when the tube is filled with saline. Below the blood pressure transducer is a pneumograph (Fig. 5-14*b*), which detects respiration by measuring changes in chest circumference. When the closed rubber bellows is wrapped around the chest, the pressure in it decreases with inspiration. The reduced pressure, sensed by the metal bellows, causes a shade to alter its position between a photoemissive tube and light bulb. Figure 5-14*c* shows a photoelectric myograph. The stiff member with the hook carries the shade. When the muscle force is applied to the hook, the elastic member is deflected and the shade is made to move parallel to the face of the phototube by means of a parallelogram arrangement of springs. A series of different elastic members is employed to extend the range of the basic transducing element.

Photodetectors, particularly photovoltaic cells and photoresistors, are extremely practical for detecting pulsatile blood volume changes. For detecting the pulse the two techniques diagrammed in Fig. 5-15 are employed. Sometimes the vascular bed is placed between the light bulb and the photodetector; at other times the exciter lamp is adjacent to the photodetector. In the first technique the capillary pulse modulates the optical density; in the second, the pulse alters the amount of reflected and scattered light.

The reflectance transducer was introduced by Hertzman (1938). With this device connected to an amplifier and recorder having a time constant longer than 2 sec, excellent pulse tracings can be recorded from human and small animal subjects. The pulsatile signal recorded reflects the difference in the instantaneous inflow and the outflow of blood. Hertzman standardized the sensitivity of his system with clear glass filters. He computed an approximate relationship between one filter unit and the volume pulse derived from other plethysmographic techniques. It is to be emphasized that the volume pulse when so calibrated yields only information on the temporal changes in blood flow in the skin below the transducer. Although the photoelectric plethysmograph does not indicate total flow, it produces a signal which immediately shows changes in flow.

With photoelectric pulse pickups, detection of stray light sometimes produces artifacts in the recordings. Adequate shielding will eliminate much of this interference. Sensitivity to stray lighting can be decreased considerably if a photodetector which is responsive only to the infrared region near 800 mμ is employed. When the detector is covered with an infrared gelatin filter that passes this wavelength, variations in ambient visible light are not detected. An added advantage is that changes in oxygen saturation do not affect the detector.

When employing photoelectric pickups, an important consideration is the amount of heat produced by the exciter lamp. Heat causes dilatation of blood vessels, hence alters the state of the vascular bed under examination.

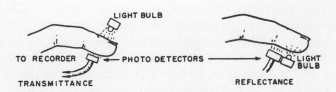

Figure 5-15. Photoelectric pulse transducers.

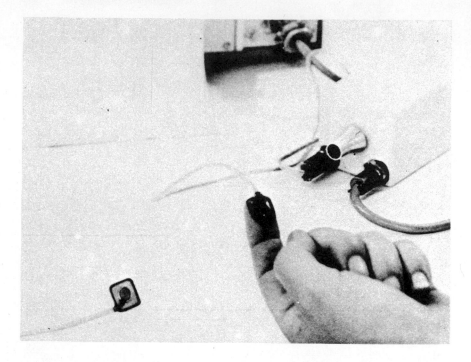

Figure 5-16.   Cold light pulse pickup. (Courtesy of Statham Medical Instruments, Oxnard.)

Although the heat aids in the production of a large signal from the pulse detector, in some instances this may not be desirable. One solution to the problem has been the creation of a reflectance pulse pickup which employs cold light.[4] In this interesting device, illustrated in Fig. 5-16, an electroluminescent panel emits light at 640 mμ and illuminates the vascular bed. In the center of this panel is mounted a photoconductive cell that detects the variations in reflected and scattered light caused by changes in blood flow under the transducer. Because it weighs little, is easily attachable, and measures only 0.5 × 0.5 × 0.1 in., this device should see considerable service in monitoring the pulse.

A photoelectric pulse pickup can be employed in systems that measure blood pressure, heart rate, and blood flow in the region examined by the photodetector. Capacitance coupling with a relatively short time constant (1 sec for human subjects) can be used in the former cases; direct coupling is necessary in the latter. If an artery central to a photoelectric pulse pickup is occluded by a pressurized cuff,[5] the pulse disappears. As the pressure is

---

[4] Statham Medical Instruments, Oxnard, Calif.
[5] The width of the cuff merits special consideration (see Geddes et al., 1966).

reduced, the pulse appears when the pressure in the cuff is slightly below systolic. If the pressure is read at the first appearance of the pulse, the value obtained is very close to the systolic blood pressure in the artery under the cuff. As the pressure in the cuff is further decreased, the pulse increases in amplitude and reaches a stable level. There is no consistently identifiable transitional point as the cuff pressure passes through mean or diastolic pressure.

An ingenious use of the photoelectric method to obtain a good approximation of systolic and diastolic pressures was described by Wood et al. (1950). With their method an oximeter earpiece with a pressure capsule was employed. A continuous record of the capsule pressure and the optical pulse was made. With a capsule pressure above systolic pressure, the optical pulse record showed no oscillations. As the capsule pressure was reduced, the pulse appeared at a pressure just below the systolic value. As the pressure was further reduced, the amplitude of the photoelectric pulse increased, passed through a maximum, and then stabilized at a reduced amplitude. When the pulses were maximal, the capsule pressure was taken as diastolic pressure. A simultaneous recording of direct blood pressure in the radial artery revealed a good degree of correspondence for systolic and diastolic pressures.

Geddes et al. (1961) employed the photoelectric transduction principle to obtain an electrical signal related to the partial pressure of oxygen in a gas sample by the method represented in Fig. 5-17. In this illustration the detector is the Pauling (1946) paramagnetic oxygen analyzer, which is now available commercially.[6] By replacing the scale with a photodetector having a triangular aperture and replacing the light source with an illuminated slit, the position of the mirror-carrying sensor in the analyzer was converted to an electrical signal.

When fluids flow at low rates, it is advantageous to count drops. Although the size of a drop depends on many factors, in most situations 15 to 30 drops constitute 1 cc of fluid. With a given orifice, drop size is fairly constant. Drop counters in which the fluid strikes a pair of contacts have never been dependable. To eliminate direct contact with the drops of fluid, the photoelectric principle has been employed with considerable success. In some instances the drop interrupts the beam of light to the photodetector; in others the drop reflects and scatters the light sensed by the photodetector. Among the investigators who have described such drop counters are Goetz (1948), Clementz and Ryberg (1949), Hilton and Lywood (1954), Lindgren and Unvas (1954), Peiss and McCoole (1958), and Geddes et al. (1969).

Another interesting use of the photoelectric principle is in the recording

---

[6] Beckman Instruments, Scientific and Process Instruments Division, Fullerton, Calif.

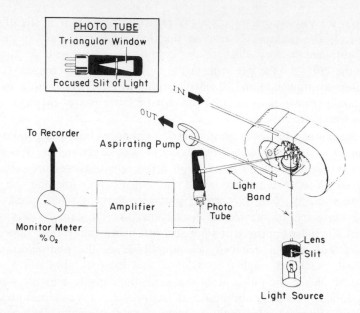

Figure 5-17. Photoelectric transducer applied to paramagnetic Beckman oxygen analyzer, model C (modified). [From Geddes et al., *IRE Trans. Bio-Med. Electron.* **8**:38 (1961). By permission.]

of the movements imparted to the body when the heart beats. Such a recording is called a ballistocardiogram, and from it may be derived body displacement, velocity, and acceleration. To record body movements directly rather than those of a table on which a subject was placed, Dock and Taubman (1949) developed a photoelectric transducer that was coupled to the shins or head of a supine subject. Body movements altered the position of a shade placed between a photodetector and a light source. For a time it was hoped that this signal could be calibrated directly in terms of the systolic discharge from the heart, but this has not been possible to date. In a given subject, however, ballistocardiograms do indicate changes in stroke volume.

As a practical and efficient transducer for large or small mechanical movements, the photodetector is difficult to surpass. A wide range of photodetectors is available with small or large photosensitive surfaces. By suitable masking, a variety of output versus shade motion relationships is available. Figure 5-18 illustrates a few of the types of transfer characteristics attainable by masking a circular photodetector with simple geometric shapes. When a light source is chopped by rotating a disk with a hole in it, various useful waveforms can be generated. For example, a curve closely approximating a sinusoid can be obtained when a square aperture passes over a circular photosensitive area having its diameter equal to the diagonal of the square. The same waveform can be obtained if the photosensitive surface is circular and the aperture is square. The direction of motion is such that the diagonal of the square moves coincidently with and along the diameter of the circle. A sinusoidal variation in light can also be obtained by rotating an eccentrically mounted circular mask made to vary the length of a slit exposed to light. This technique was used by Geddes (1951) to generate a variable-frequency sine wave with a notch fixed at its positive peak. This complex waveform was employed for testing phase distortion in amplifiers.

Another practical method of using the photoelectric method to detect motion features a pair of polarizing filters. One filter is used to polarize the light from a source and the other is placed between the source of polarized light and a photodetector. The amount of light reaching the photodetector

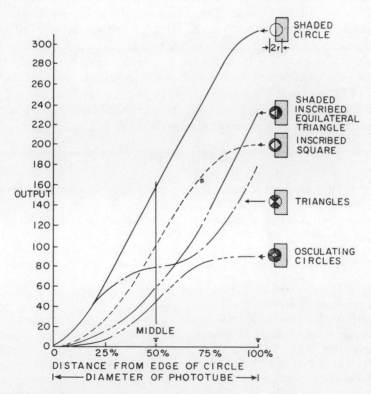

Figure 5-18.   Photodetector curves by masking.

depends on the relation between the planes of polarization of the filters. Rotation of either filter from the position of maximum or extinction will allow the frictionless detection of angular movement photoelectrically.

In using photoelectric transducers suitable choice of the type of photodetector will produce an appreciable voltage or current for a small change in light level. Thus a high conversion efficiency is easy to obtain. Because the mask mounted on a moving member usually can be made small and lightweight, it adds little inertia to the system. Freedom from contact also eliminates frictional and hysteresis errors. With a proper choice of photodetector, the response time is determined by the mechanical characteristics of the moving element. Alternating and direct current can energize exciter lamps. If alternating current is employed, the photodetector output contains a ripple signal with twice the frequency of the current used to excite the lamp.

There are disadvantages in using phototransducers. In most applications it is necessary to provide shielding to prevent stray light from entering the transducer; in nearly all, a constant-intensity light source is required. In addition, the light output of many lamps varies nearly as the square of the applied voltage; hence the lamp voltage must be well regulated. One way of reducing the need for regulation is to use two identical photodetectors in a differential configuration. In such a circuit arrangement one photodetector monitors the light intensity and the other senses the changes in light produced by the event being transduced. In practice, a signal derived from the difference in the outputs of the two photodetectors is immune to changes in light intensity over a considerable range.

REFERENCES

Acker, R. M., R. P. Lipkis, R. S. Miller, and P. C. Robinson. 1960. Solar cell power supplies for satellites. *Electronics* **33**:167–172.

Baker, L. E. 1961. A rapidly responding narrow-band infrared gaseous CO_2 analyzer for physiological studies. *IRE Trans. Bio-Med. Electron.* **BME-8**:16–24.

Clark, F. J., E. M. Schmidt, and R. F. De La Croix. 1965. Fiber optic blood pressure catheter with frequency response from DC into the audio range. *Proc. Nat. Electron. Conf.* **21**:213–216.

Clementz, B., and C. E. Ryberg. 1949. An ordinate recorder for measuring drop flow. *Acta Physiol. Scand.* **17**:339–344.

Connolly, D. C., and E. H. Wood. 1954. Simultaneous measurement of the appearance and disappearance of T1824 (Evans Blue) in blood and tissue after intravenous injection in man. *J. Appl. Physiol.* **7**:73–83.

Dock, W., and F. Taubman. 1949. Some techniques for recording the ballistocardiograph directly from the body. *Am. J. Med.* **7**:751–755.

Elam, J. O., J. F. Neville, W. Sleator, and W. N. Elam. 1949. Sources of error in oximetry. *Ann. Surg.* **130**:755–773.

Enson, Y., W. A. Briscoe, M. L. Polanyi, and A. Cournand. 1962. *In vivo* studies with an intravascular and intracardiac reflection oximeter. *J. Appl. Physiol.* **17**:552–558.

Feitelberg, S. 1942. A photoelectrical recorder for biological purposes. *Proc. Soc. Expl. Biol. Med.* **49**:177–178.

Fox, I. J., and E. H. Wood. 1960. Indocyanine green: Physical and physiologic properties. *Proc. Staff Meetings Mayo Clinic* **35**:732–744.

Geddes, L. A. 1951. A note on phase distortion. *EEG Clin. Neurophysiol.* **3**:517–518.

Geddes, L. A., H. E. Hoff, and A. S. Badger. 1966. Introduction of the auscultatory method of measuring blood pressure. *Cardiovascular Res. Center Bull.* **5**:57–74.

Geddes, L. A., H. E. Hoff, and W. A. Spencer. 1957. The Physiograph—An instrument in teaching physiology, *J. Med. Educ.* **32**:181–198; also: 1956. *IRE Conv. Record* **9**:29–37.

Geddes, L. A., H. E. Hoff, and W. A. Spencer. 1961. The center for vital studies—A new laboratory for the study of bodily functions in man. *IRE Trans. Bio.-Med. Electron,* **BME-8**:33–45.

Geddes, L. A., A. G. Moore, J. Bourland, J. Vasku, and G. Cantrell. 1969. An efficient drop transducer. *Med. Res. Engng.* **8**(4):27–29.

Gilson, W. E. 1943. Applications of electronics to physiology. *Electronics* **16**:86–89.

Goetz, R. H. 1948. A photoelectric drop recorder. *Lancet* **1**:830–831.

Grodins, F. 1962. Basic concepts in the determination of vascular volumes by indicator dilution methods. *Circ. Res.* **10**:429–446.

Hamilton, W., R. L. Riley, A. M. Attyah, A. Cournand, D. M. Powell, A. Himmelstein, R. P. Noble, J. W. Remington, D. W. Richards, N. C. Wheeler, and A. C. Witham. 1948. Comparison of the Fick and dye injection methods of measuring the cardiac output in man. *Am. J. Physiol.* **153**:309–321.

Hertzman, A. 1938. The blood supply of various skin areas as estimated by the photoelectric plethysmograph. *Am. J. Physiol.* **124**:328–340.

Hilton, S. M., and D. W. Lywood, 1954. Photoelectric drop counter. *J. Physiol.* **123**:64.

Jacobs, S. F. 1960. Characteristics of infra-red detectors. *Electronics* **33**:72–73.

Johnson, C. C., R. D. Palm, and D. C. Steward. 1971. A solid-state fiberoptic oximeter. *J. Am. Assoc. Adv. Med. Instr.* **5**:77–83.

Kinsman, J. M., J. W. Moore, and W. F. Hamilton. 1929. Studies on the circulation. *Am. J. Physiol.* **89**:322–330.

Lindgren, P., and B. Unvas. 1954. Photoelectric recording of the venous and arterial blood flow. *Acta Physiol. Scand.* **32**:259–263.

Meier, P., and K. L. Zierler. 1954. On the theory of the indicator-dilution method for measurement of blood flow and volume. *J. Appl. Physiol.* **6**:732–744.

Millikan, C. A. 1942. The oximeter, an instrument for measuring continuously the oxygen saturation of arterial blood in man. *Rev. Sci. Instr.* **13**:434–444.

Moss, T. S. 1949. The temperature variation of the long wave limit of infra-red conductivity in lead sulphide and similar substances. *Proc. Phys. Soc. (London)* **B62**:741–748.

Pauling, L., R. E. Wood, and J. H. Strudivant. 1946. An instrument for determining the partial pressure of oxygen in a gas. *Science* **103**:338.

Peiss, C., and R. D. McCoole. 1958. Simple optically recording flowmeter for drop or integrated flow measurement. *J. Appl. Physiol.* **12**:137–139.

RCA Phototubes-Photocells. *Bulletin* 1G1018. Radio Corporation of America, Electron Tube Div., Harrison, Pa.

Rein, H., A. A. Hampel, and W. A. Heinemann. 1940. Photoelectric Transmission-manometer zur Blutdruckschreibung. *Arch. Ges. Physiol.* **243**:329–335.

Stephenson, J. L. 1958. Theory of measurement of blood flow by dye dilution technique. *IRE Trans. Med. Electron.* **PGME-12**:82–88.

Sutterer, W. F. 1960. A compensated densitometer for indocyanine green. *Physiologist,* **3**:159.

Taylor, S. H., and J. P. Shillingford. 1959. Clinical applications of Coomassie blue. *Brit. Heart J.* **21**:497-504.

Taylor, S. H., and J. M. Thorp. 1959. Properties and biological behavior of Coomassie blue. *Brit. Heart J.* **21**:492–496.

Thompson, H. K., C. F. Starmer, R. E. Whalen, and H. D. McIntosh. 1964. Indicator transit time considered as a gamma variate. *Circ. Res.* **14**:502–515.

Wheeler, H. O., W. I. Cranston, and J. I. Meltzer. 1958. Hepatic uptake and biliary excretion of indocyanine green in the dog. *Proc. Soc. Exp. Biol. Med.* **99**:11–14.

Wood, E. H., and J. E. Geraci. 1949. Photoelectric determination of arterial oxygen saturation in man. *J. Lab. Clin. Med.* **34**:387-401.

Wood, E. H., J. R. B. Knutson, and B. E. Taylor. 1950. Measurement of blood content and blood pressure in the human ear. *Proc. Staff Meetings Mayo Clinic* **25**:398-405.

Woodroof, E. A., and S. Koorajian. 1973. *In vitro* evaluation of an *in-vivo* fiberoptic oximeter. *Med. Instr.* **7**:287-292.

Zierler, K. L. 1962a. Circulation times and the theory of indicator-dilution methods for determining blood flow and volume. *Handbook of Physiology,* Vol. 1, Sec. 18. Washington, D.C., American Physiological Society.

Zierler, K. L. 1962b. Theoretical basis of indicator-dilution methods for measuring flow and volume. *Circ. Res.* **10**(Part 2):393-407.

Zierler, K. L. 1963. Theory of use of indicators to measure blood flow and extracellular volume and calculation of transcapillary movement of tracers. *Circ. Res.* **12**(Part 1):464-471.

Zijlstra, W. G. 1951. *Fundamentals and Applications of Clinical Oximetry.* Van Gorcum and Co., Assen, The Netherlands.

6

Piezoelectric Transducers

6-1. PIEZOELECTRICITY

The piezo- (pressure)- electric effect, discovered in 1880 by Pierre and Jacques Curie, is a property of some natural crystalline substances to develop electrical potential along certain crystallographic axes in response to the movement of charge as a result of mechanical deformation. Figure 6-1 diagrams the method of designating crystallographic axes in some of the more familiar crystals. A necessary condition for the presence of the effect is the absence of a center of symmetry of charge distribution. Of the 32 crystal classes, 21 lack this symmetry, and crystals in all but one class can exhibit the piezoelectric phenomenon. Although about 1000 crystalline substances have been observed to have the property, for only about 100 are quantitative data available. The magnitude of the effect is of practical value in about 10 substances.

Since the application of an electric field to a piezoelectric crystal distorts it, the phenomenon is reversible. These two features of piezo crystals are responsible for their widespread application in industry and in biomedical studies.

To observe the piezoelectric effect, electrodes must be placed on specific faces of the crystal and the deforming force applied in the appropriate direction (Fig. 6-2). The voltage appearing between the electrodes is linearly related to the deformation. In practice, piezo elements are slabs removed from the parent crystal by cutting along appropriate crystallographic axes. The magnitude of the piezoelectric effect is dependent on the axis of the cut. The unit employed to designate the magnitude of the effect is the picocoulomb per square meter per newton per square meter $[pC/(m^2)/(N)/(m^2)]$. Table 6-1 lists the constants for some of the more common piezoelectric materials.

The slabs cut from the parent crystal can be mounted to permit the development of a piezoelectric voltage in response to bending, twisting, or

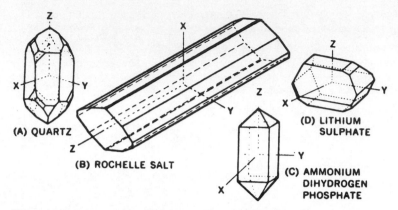

Figure 6-1.   Crystals and axes. (Clevite Corp., Bedford, Ohio. By permission.)

shearing forces. Frequently the slabs are assembled in pairs or in stacks. One configuration, the bimorph,[1] is particularly useful because it permits a greater range of motion than is attainable with a single plate. Some of the typical mounting arrangements are illustrated in Fig. 6-2.

In addition to the naturally occurring crystals, certain ceramics, notably barium titanate, can be induced to acquire the piezoelectric property. With the application of a high voltage to electrodes on the material, there is a reorientation of the crystalline structure that persists after removal of the polarizing voltage. Often the induction process is carried out at an elevated temperature. This technique, in addition to producing a material with a high piezoelectric constant, removes the geometrical constraints of crystallographic axes and makes it possible to cast piezo crystals having any desired form.

A piezo crystal need be distorted only a tiny amount to obtain a potential in the fractional volt range. For this reason it may be called an efficient isometric transducer. The stiffness of piezo crystals is high, and the permissible deformations are small. Donaldson (1958) stated that the deformation of crystals used in phonograph pickups is 10 μ per gram of force and that crystals used in accelerometers are distorted only 1 μ per kilogram force.

A close electrical analog to the piezo crystal is a condenser which is charged by the application of mechanical force. Figure 6-3 illustrates the simplest equivalent circuit. Typical phonograph crystals develop signals in the fractional volt range. With very large crystals and high forces, it is possible to develop many hundreds of volts. Materials lose their pie-

---

[1] Clevite Corp., Bedford, Ohio.

zoelectric property if heated. The temperature at which this occurs is called the Curie point. Most piezoelectric materials have an upper and a lower temperature limit for retention of the property. The safe operating range is usually much smaller than these two temperature extremes indicate. The upper temperature limits for many piezo crystals are shown in Table 6-1. With an increase in temperature, a slight deterioration of the piezoelectric effect occurs in the piezoelectric ceramics. Although the effect is small, it is nonetheless present and must be considered if techniques involving high accuracy are employed. Some natural crystals are deliquescent, and therefore their performance is adversely affected by high humidity.

Piezo crystals, being high-impedance devices, can deliver only very small

Table 6-1   Characteristics of Piezoelectric Materials*

Piezoelectric Material	Piezoelectric Constant [pC/(m²)/ (N)/(m²)]	Maximum Humidity Range (%)	Dielectric Constant†	Temperature (°C)
Rochelle salt (30°C)	$d14 + 550$ ⎫		350	−18 to +24
Rochelle salt (30°C)	$d25 - \ \ 54$ ⎬ 40–70		9.2	45
Rochelle salt (30°C)	$d36 + \ \ 12$ ⎭		9.5	45
Quartz	$d11 + \ \ \ \ 2.3$		4.5	550
Quartz	$d14 - \ \ \ \ 0.7$		4.5	550
Ammonium dihydrogen phosphate (ADP)	$d14 - \ \ \ \ 1.5$ ⎫		56	120 to 125
		0–94		
Ammonium dihydrogen phosphate (ADP)	$d36 + \ \ 48$ ⎭		15.5	120 to 125
Barium titanate (XTAL)	$d31 - \ \ 34$		170	125
Barium titanate (XTAL)	$d33 + \ \ 86$		170	125
Barium titanate (XTAL)	$d15 + 392$		2900	125
Barium titanate (ceramic)	$d31 - \ \ \ \ 7.8$		1700	
Barium titanate (ceramic)	$d33 + 190$		1700 ⎫	70 to 100
Barium titanate (ceramic)	$d15 + 260$		1450 ⎭	

* *Encyclopaedia Britannica* 1963, Encyclopaedia Britannica, Chicago, London, Toronto, Geneva. 24 vols.
† Relative to air.

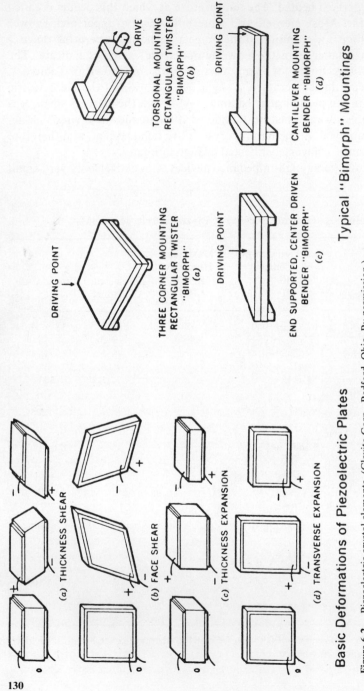

Basic Deformations of Piezoelectric Plates

Typical "Bimorph" Mountings

DRIVE

TORSIONAL MOUNTING
RECTANGULAR TWISTER
"BIMORPH"
(b)

DRIVING POINT

CANTILEVER MOUNTING
BENDER "BIMORPH"
(d)

DRIVING POINT

THREE CORNER MOUNTING
RECTANGULAR TWISTER
"BIMORPH"
(a)

DRIVING POINT

END SUPPORTED, CENTER DRIVEN
BENDER "BIMORPH"
(c)

(a) THICKNESS SHEAR

(b) FACE SHEAR

(c) THICKNESS EXPANSION

(d) TRANSVERSE EXPANSION

Figure 6-2. Piezoelectric crystal elements. (Clevite Corp., Bedford, Ohio. By permission.)

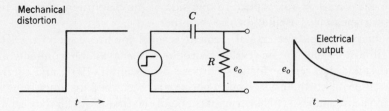

Figure 6-3. Piezoelectric crystal equivalent circuit.

currents. Connecting a resistive load across them reduces the output voltage and the time constant markedly. A more serious drawback is that because of leakage resistance, the voltage cannot be maintained when a sustained force is applied. Therefore piezo crystals are only suited to the measurement of changing mechanical forces. They can develop a voltage for changes in mechanical deformation having a frequency of a few hertz to many megahertz. The upper limit is determined by the total mass and stiffness of the moving system. Because of the high stiffness and low mass of such crystals, they see service as the transducing unit in phonograph pickups, microphones, and vibration detectors. A survey of these industrial uses was presented by Siegel (1959).

6-2. BIOMEDICAL APPLICATIONS

In biomedical studies there have been numerous applications of the piezoelectric crystal. Because of its low cost, small size, isometric nature, and large electrical output, the crystal is most useful for the transduction of a variety of time-varying events. A survey of some of the typical uses in physiology was presented by Malcolm (1946), who described a piezo crystal, in a holder of unique design, which served as a general-purpose transducer for ballistocardiography, heart sounds, pulse wave recording, drop counting, muscle pull, and respiration.

The piezoelectric transducer is particularly well suited to the detection of the pressure pulse and of low-energy acoustic phenomena such as heart and Korotkoff sounds. Just after the piezo crystal appeared in industry, Gomez and Langevin (1937) recognized its value for pulse wave recording in the human subject and discussed this application extensively. Miller and White (1941) employed a crystal microphone air-coupled to a chamber placed on the skin to measure arterial and venous pulses. The small pulsations seen in blood pressure cuffs were recorded with good fidelity by Rappaport and Luisada (1944) and Lax et al. (1956). Both teams rebuilt crystal microphones to operate as differential pressure transducers in which the mean cuff pressure was applied to one side of the diaphragm and the total pressure (mean plus oscillations) to the other.

In many respects the crystal element is ideal for heart sound transduction; almost as soon as the crystal microphone was available commercially, it was called into service for this purpose. Sachs et al. (1935) and Bjerring et al. (1935) used the crystal microphone and described an amplifying device for heart sounds. This instrument, one of the first of its kind to become available commercially, was described in more detail by Lockhart a few years later (1938). Narat (1936) eliminated the air coupling from the surface of the body to the microphone diaphragm by developing a contact crystal microphone for the transduction of all vibrations produced by the heart; however, this technique did not attract much attention. Nearly all subsequent workers have used the air-coupling method, probably to attenuate the large amount of low-frequency vibrational energy generated by the beating heart. Boone (1939) employed a crystal microphone with a cathode ray oscilloscope to guarantee maximum fidelity in reproduction of all the cardiac vibrations. Mannheimer (1941) used the high-efficiency and high-fidelity qualities of the crystal microphone in an attempt to calibrate phonocardiography by separating the sounds into four frequency bands. Rappaport and Sprague (1941, 1942) also selected the crystal microphone for their extensive studies on the nature of heart sounds and the frequency response of stethoscopes. The high-efficiency feature of the crystal microphone showed itself again in the transduction of fetal heart sounds. Wood and Gunn (1953) recorded, counted, and monitored these feeble sounds with the aid of an amplifying system with variable frequency tuning.

Contact crystal transducers are beginning to serve more frequently in biomedical investigations. One interesting application is due to Wallace et al. (1957) and Lewis et al. (1957), who constructed miniature phonocatheters by mounting hollow tubular barium titanate crystals on the ends of catheters to detect the intracardiac sounds during heart catheterization studies. Geddes et al. (1974) developed a catheter-tip unit containing a piezoelectric crystal transducer for monitoring breath and respiratory sounds in the esophagus. This device permits audible presentation of these sounds to an audience with very little interference from acoustic feedback.

Among the feeblest of auscultatory phenomena are the Korotkoff sounds, and the high-efficiency feature of the piezo crystal has been put to use in their detection. Omberg (1936) used a crystal microphone to control the cycling of a pump connected to a blood pressure cuff. As the cuff pressure decayed, the systolic sounds detected by the microphone restarted the pump; when they disappeared the pump stopped, thereby maintaining the cuff pressure very nearly equal to systolic blood pressure. Gilson et al. (1941, 1942) recorded human blood pressure indirectly by presenting two channel records of cuff pressure and Korotkoff sounds detected by a crystal microphone. These sounds, as they appeared in a smaller cuff located below the blood pressure cuff on the subject's arm, were detected by Rappaport and Luisada (1944). Like Omberg, Gilford and Broida (1954) used a crystal microphone as the primary detector in their fully automatic recording machine that plotted and indicated both systolic and diastolic human blood pressures. Detection of the Korotkoff sounds by crystal elements and their superimposition on the occluding cuff pressure was described by Currens et al. (1957) and Geddes et al. (1959).

For experimental purposes piezo crystals are readily obtained in a variety of inexpensive commercially available devices such as crystal microphones, phonograph cartridges, earphones, and loudspeakers. The crystal elements are easily removed and are readily adaptable to a wide variety of tasks. Figures 6-4 through 6-6 illustrate some of the uses for such piezoelectric elements. A piezoelectric pulse pickup constructed by Geddes

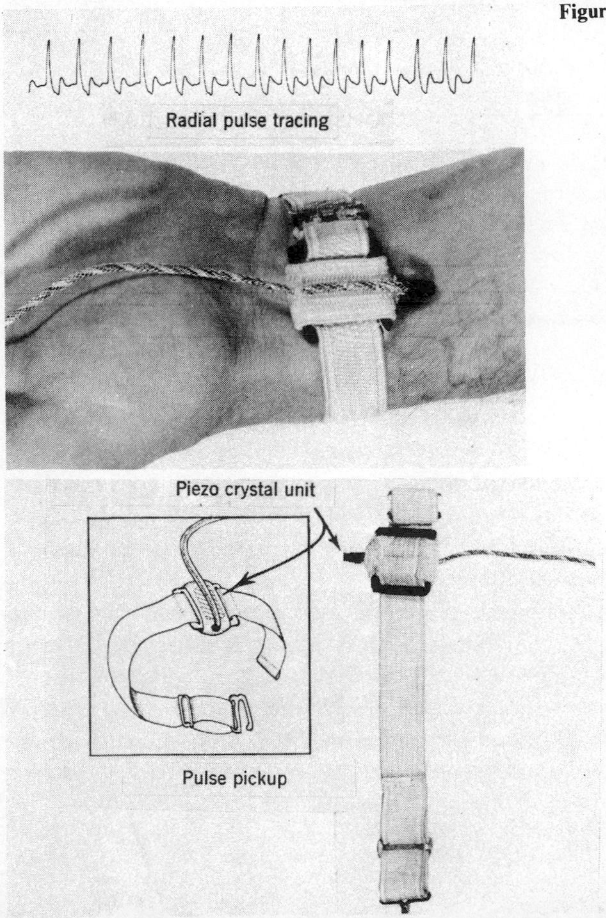

Figure 6-4.   Piezoelectric pulse pickup.

Radial pulse tracing

Piezo crystal unit

Pulse pickup

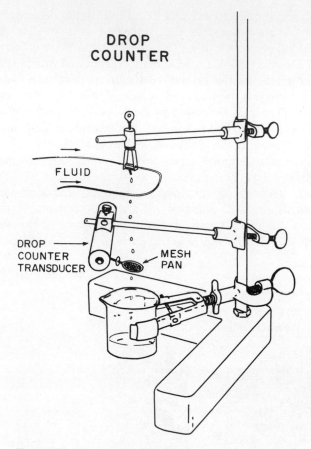

DROP COUNTER

FLUID

DROP
COUNTER
TRANSDUCER

MESH
PAN

Figure 6-5. Piezoelectric drop counter.

and Hoff (1960; see Figure 6-4) uses a piezo crystal removed from a phonograph cartridge. The element was first coated with an insulating spray and then wrapped with aluminum foil for electrical shielding. A coating of flexible insulation (Insul-X)[2] was then applied, and the element assembled in the bracelet.

A piezoelectric drop counter (Fig. 6-5) is merely a phonograph pickup mounted in a metal case; in place of the needle is a mesh pan. Drops striking the pan twist the piezo element and give rise to a voltage pulse of approximately 100 mV.

Figure 6-6 shows a piezo element from a phonograph cartridge mounted in the lower third of a blood pressure cuff (Geddes, 1959) to detect the

[2] Insul-X Products Corp., Yonkers, N.Y.

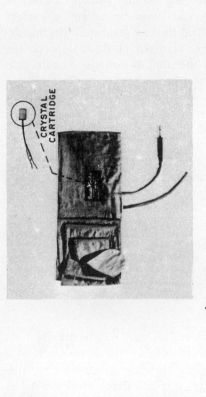

CRYSTAL
CARTRIDGE

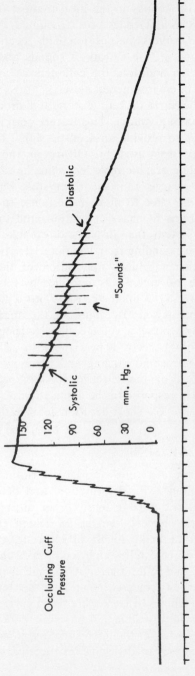

Diastolic

"Sounds"

Systolic

Occluding Cuff
Pressure

150
120
90
60
30
0

mm. Hg.

Time Marks – 1 Second

Figure 6-6. Korotkoff sound detector.

Korotkoff sounds in the measurement of blood pressure. In a subsequent report (1968) Geddes et al. mounted the piezoelectric crystal within the bladder in the same position. This technique maintains the crystal close to the source of the Korotkoff sounds and provides good coupling with the tissues. In addition, the cuff acts as an acoustic shield and reduces detection of environmental noise.

Piezoelectric crystals distort and produce force in response to the application of a voltage. This feature permits their use in earphones and loudspeakers to provide an acoustic signal from a varying voltage. The same property was used by Offner in the mid-1940s to create a rapidly responding graphic recorder, which he called the "crystograph." In this device two large, thin square crystals were clamped at three corners; the fourth was free to move in response to the applied voltage. The crystals were driven in phase opposition, and the free corners were coupled to a pulley system that drove a direct-inking recording stylus. A frequency response extending from less than 1 Hz to well above 60 Hz was achieved.

Another ingenious application of the ability of the piezo crystal to produce movement was described by Pascoe (1955). He faced the problem of advancing a microelectrode into a nerve cell that was enveloped in a tough membrane. By mounting the microelectrode on a piezo crystal and applying a pulse of voltage, the electrode was suddenly advanced 20 μ, and the tip of the electrode penetrated the cell without damage.

The ultrasonic ranging and imaging devices to be described use both properties of piezoelectric crystals because of their ability to distort rapidly in response to the application of a voltage and to develop a voltage in response to a short-duration deformation.

6-3. ULTRASONICS

The two attributes of piezoelectric materials—namely, the development of a voltage with deformation, and deformation by the application of a voltage—are used extensively in ultrasonic instruments. Now that piezoelectric elements can be fabricated easily in a variety of shapes, it is possible to make highly efficient detectors and radiators for ultrasonic energy which can be employed to measure position and movement by transmission and reflectance of ultrasonic energy traversing living tissues. Blood flow velocity measurement and the imaging of stationary and moving subcutaneous soft tissues are being carried out with increasing frequency in biomedical research and in clinical practice. The following paragraphs describe a few of the interesting and important applications of piezoelectric elements used in ultrasonic instruments.

6-3-1. Ultrasonic Blood Flowmeters

Kalmus (1954) described a 100-kHz ultrasonic flowmeter in which the velocity of water was detected by measuring the phase shift between an upstream and downstream transducer. A switching system, operating at 10 Hz, permitted interchanging the transmitting and receiving transducers; this method was used extensively in later instruments. The technique was soon applied to the measurement of blood flow by Herrick and Anderson (1959). The practical difficulties associated with this method were reduced by later investigators, who developed two different types of blood flowmeter—the transit-time and Doppler frequency shift instruments. With the transit-time method, short bursts of ultrasonic energy are carried by the bloodstream. An upstream transducer and a downstream transducer, placed outside a blood vessel, are used to produce and detect the ultrasonic pulse, as in Fig. 6-7a. An electronic switch (EE) allows interchanging the transmitter and receiver and permits measurement of the difference between upstream (t_u) and downstream (t_d) transit times. From this time difference ($t_u - t_d$), it

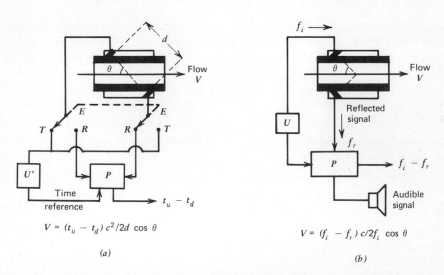

$$V = (t_u - t_d) c^2/2d \cos \theta$$

(a)

$$V = (f_i - f_r) c/2f_i \cos \theta$$

(b)

Figure 6-7. Ultrasonic blood flowmeters: (a) pulse-transit time instrument; (b) Doppler frequency-shift flowmeter. U' provides pulses of ultrasonic energy, U delivers a continuous output of ultrasound, EE is an electronic switch that permits rapidly alternating the piezoelectric elements so that they alternately function as a transmitter (T) and receiver (R), θ is the angle of the incident beam, V is the flow velocity, d is the separation of the piezoelectric elements, and c is the velocity of ultrasound in blood; t_u and t_d are the upstream and downstream transit times; f_i and f_r are the frequencies of the incident and reflected sound; P represents the signal-processing circuitry.

is possible to obtain a signal that is linearly proportional to flow velocity (V). Volume flow is obtained by multiplying the flow velocity signal by the area of the vessel. With the Doppler shift method (Fig. 6-7b), an incident beam of ultrasonic energy of frequency f_i is directed into the blood stream from a transducer outside the vessel, and the cellular elements in it reflect a portion of the energy back in the direction of the incident beam. The frequency of the reflected beam (f_r), which is different from that of the incident beam, is lower when the blood is flowing away and higher when it is flowing toward the transducer assembly. From the difference in frequency ($f_i - f_r$) between the incident and reflected beams, a signal can be obtained that is linearly proportional to blood flow velocity. As in the previous case, volume flow is obtained by multiplying the velocity flow signal by vessel area.

6-3-1-1. Pulsed Ultrasonic Blood Flowmeter. The pulsed (transit-time) ultrasonic flowmeter (Fig. 6-7a) was described by Franklin et al. (1959). In this device, 3 MHz ultrasound was applied to a barium titanate piezoelectric crystal mounted in a 1.3-cm lucite sleeve. The ultrasound pulse consisted of 8 cycles of the 3-MHz ultrasound repeated 12,000 times/sec; a similar piezoelectric transducer located downstream detected the arrival of the ultrasound. Electronic switching (EE) permitted the downstream receiver to become the transmitter (T) and the upstream transmitter to become the receiver (R). The switching rate for measurement of upstream and downstream times was 800/sec. A time difference on the order of nanoseconds was obtained with the transducer assembly applied to the dog aorta. An overall flow-velocity frequency response extending from 0 to beyond 15 Hz was obtained, which allowed high-fidelity recording of the contour of the velocity-flow wave at rest and during exercise.

6-3-1-2. Doppler Frequency-Shift Flowmeter. Measurement of the small time difference encountered with the pulsed ultrasonic flowmeter caused practical difficulties in many attempts to measure blood flow. To circumvent these, Franklin et al. (1961) developed the Doppler frequency-shift blood flowmeter. In this device, whose principle is illustrated in Fig. 6-7b, a continuous beam of 5-MHz (f_i) ultrasound was directed toward the center of the flowing stream by a piezoelectric crystal mounted in a perivascular sleeve. Also in the sleeve, and diametrically opposite, was another piezoelectric crystal which detected the back-scattered ultrasound with a frequency spectrum related to the velocity (V) of the moving cellular elements that provided the reflecting surfaces. An electronic processor (P) computed the difference in frequency between the incident (f_i) and reflected (f_r) beams of ultrasound. It was found that the mean Doppler frequency shift provided a signal linearly proportional to blood flow velocity and ideal for analog recording. According to Roberts (1973), mean flow is accurately reproduced by the frequency shift when the flow profile is uniform over the diameter of the vessel. When the profile is parabolic, Roberts stated that the indicated flow is expected to be 16% above true flow.

With the ultrasonic flowmeter, it is possible to listen to the Doppler shift in frequency by applying the incident and reflected signals to an appropriate circuit. In a typical instrument, a change in flow velocity from 0 to 100 cm/sec provides an audible signal with a frequency ranging from 0 to 3500 Hz. Aural monitoring of flow velocity is found to be very convenient.

The Doppler frequency-shift technique was developed further by Baker (1964) to accomplish detection of blood flow in subcutaneous vessels by constructing a transducer assembly in which the transmitting and receiving ultrasound transducers were mounted side by side. With the transducer applied to the skin (usually with a little moisture or oil to provide adequate coupling of the ultrasonic energy), graphic recording and aural monitoring of arterial and venous blood flow can be accomplished. It is extremely easy to distinguish between the arterial and venous flow by listening to the Doppler frequency shift. Arterial flow produces rhythmically fluctuating and whistling-like increase and decrease in frequency; venous flow is represented by a low-pitched rumbling sound having little variation in frequency.

Baker (1970) combined the pulse and Doppler shift techniques in a single instrument that provided a velocity profile of blood flow across the diameter of an unopened artery. Figure 6-8 is an isometric projection sketch of the flow profile.

Since the measurement of flow can be made in unopened vessels, the ultrasonic flowmeter enjoys considerable popularity. However, accurate calibration of both types is not possible because the signals obtained are dependent on the velocity profile. For this reason, ultrasonic flowmeters are best suited to measure changes in blood flow or to compare flow in one vessel with that in another.

Of the two types of ultrasonic blood flowmeter, the Doppler instrument is the most popular for a variety of practical reasons, including ease of application, simplicity of construction, and the availability of an audible signal related to blood flow. In most low-cost intruments, however, reverse flow cannot be identified. In addition, the quality of the returning echo depends on the presence of cellular elements in the bloodstream, and it is anticipated that lower intensity echoes will be encountered in subjects with low packed-cell volumes. Therefore, it is important to note that the Doppler instrument requires the presence of suspended reflectors (blood cells). The transit-time instrument does not have this requirement, but since in blood flow measurement, the very small time difference is difficult to

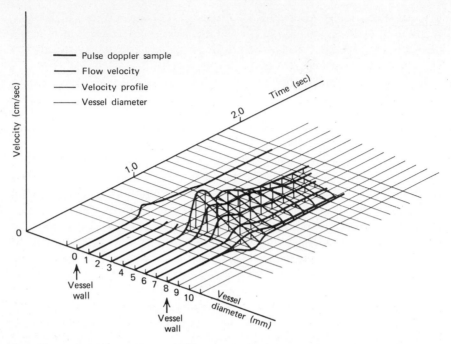

Figure 6-8. Blood flow velocity profile across the diameter of a blood vessel determined with a pulsed ultrasonic Doppler blood flowmeter. [From D. W. Baker, *IEEE Trans. Sonics and Ultrason.* **SU-17**:170–185 (1970). By permission.]

measure, this instrument is applicable to the measurement of flow only in the major vessels. At present, however, it is not possible to apply a transducer assembly to a vessel and obtain an accurate readout in terms of ml/min of blood flow in the vessel.

6-3-2.   Ultrasonic Imaging

There is no doubt that introduction of the diagnostic x-ray at the turn of the century dramatically changed the practice of medicine; Dibner (1963) has presented an interesting account of this event. The ability of the x-ray to "peer inside" the body permits the acquisition of information about the state and functioning of internal tissues and organs that absorb, reflect, refract, and scatter x-rays. However, the price paid for this valuable feature is exposure of the subject to radiation hazard. Since the effect of x-rays is cumulative, the hazard increases with the number and duration of exposures. A second difficulty with the use of x-rays relates to the way they interact with living tissue. In general, x-ray visualization of soft tissues within the body is difficult and often impossible. Because soft tissues exhibit different properties to ultrasound, visualization is possible with this type of energy. Moreover, ultrasonic examination of soft tissues can be performed using power levels that are nonhazardous to the subject. At present there is no evidence that repeated exposure to ultrasound, at the power levels presently used for visualization, constitutes a hazard. In addition, repeated exposure does not appear to produce a cumulative effect.

6-3-2-1. Safety Considerations. An excellent review of the ultrasonic power density levels for tissue injury was presented by Ulrich (1974); his data are summarized in Fig. 6-9. From these data it can be concluded that the use of low-level ultrasonic energy constitutes a nonhazardous method of visualizing soft tissues and offers a means of complementing, rather than competing with, conventional diagnostic x-ray techniques.

Virtually all the ultrasonic imaging techniques employ the pulse-echo technique, in which a short-duration pulse of ultrasonic energy is applied to tissue by way of a piezoelectric transducer. The ultrasonic beam enters the tissue and experiences absorption, reflection, refraction and scattering. Table 6-2 lists representative values for the velocity of propagation and absorption, expressed as attenuation in nepers (Np), of ultrasound in biological tissues. Fortunately the amount of energy reflected by tissue interfaces and the attenuation is such that a detectable signal is returned to the source of application of the ultrasonic energy when low incident power levels are used. The magnitude of the reflected signal depends on the type of tissue encountered and the angle with which the beam strikes the tissue. The strongest echoes are produced when the incident beam is perpendicular to the tissue and fluid interfaces. Wells (1970) stated that the percentages of energy returned by soft tissues and bone are 0.02 and 40%, respectively.

Table 6-2   Propagation Constants for Ultrasound in Biological Materials*

Material	Velocity (cm/sec)	Frequency (mHz)	Absorption per Centimeter (Np)		
Muscle	1.568×10^5	$f = 1.8$	0.1	$f = 0.8$	MHz
Liver	1.570×10^5	$f = 1.8$	0.15	$f = 1$	MHz
Fat	1.476×10^5	$f = 1.8$	0.05	$f = 0.8$	MHz
Skull bone	$3.36 \ \times 10^5$	$f = 0.8$	3.7	$f = 1.6$	MHz
Sciatic nerve			0.35	$f = 3.4$	MHz
Brain			0.075	$f = 2.4$	MHz
Blood			0.02	$f = 1.0$	MHz

* From J. E. Jacobs, *Ultrasonics in Biology, Advances in Bioengineering and Bioinstrumentation*, Vol. 1, J. Alt (ed.), Plenum Press, New York, 1960.

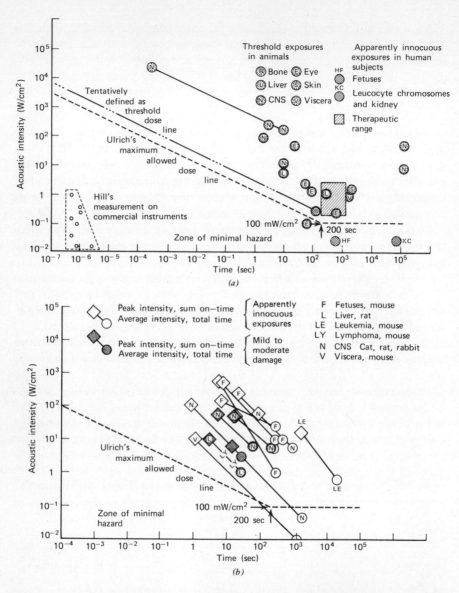

Figure 6-9. Power-density levels versus exposure times: (*a*) safe and hazardous levels for a single continuous wave exposure of 0.5 to 6 MHz energy; (*b*) same information for pulsed exposure to 0.5 to 15 MHz energy. [From W. D. Ulrich, *IEEE Trans. Biomed. Eng.* **BME-21**:50–51 1974. By permission.]

The frequency presently used for ultrasonic imaging ranges from 1 to 10 MHz. The choice of frequency is not critical, but there exists a tradeoff between resolution and intensity of returned echo. For example, the higher the frequency, the better the resolution but the greater the attenuation of the ultrasound.

6-3-2-2.   A- and B-Scan Displays.   In some imaging techniques a second piezoelectric transducer is used to detect the echo signal; in many instruments, however, the transmitter is used as a receiver to detect the echo that returns after the burst of ultrasound has been applied. An echo consists of a series of signals, produced by reflections from the underlying tissues. The time between the onset of the incident pulse of ultrasound and a returning echo pulse identifies the distance of the tissue interface below the transmitter and receiver. In most tissues the velocity of propagation of ultrasound is about 1.5×10^5 cm/sec; therefore a target 1 cm below the transducer assembly will return an echo in 13.3 μsec.

There are two principal techniques for displaying images obtained using the pulse-echo technique; these are designated the A- and B-scan presentations. Both display methods (see Fig. 6-10) present echo information that returns along a narrow beam extending below the transducer assembly.

The A-scan display employs a standard oscilloscope in which the time base (X axis) is triggered by the onset of the pulse of ultrasound (U') applied to the transducer. The echo signals are detected by the transmitting (T) piezoelectric element, which is electronically switched (E) to allow it to act as a receiver (R). The echo signals are displayed on the oscilloscope, as in Fig. 6-10a. With this type of display, the transmitter (T) is electronically switched (E) to act as a receiver (R), and the echo signals appear on the oscilloscope, as in Fig. 6-10a. With this type of display, the time between the start of the sweep and the onset of the various echoes represents the distances to the underlying structures. Therefore the X axis of the oscilloscope can be calibrated in centimeters of depth, rather than microseconds, to identify the depths of the echo-returning structures. The amplitudes of the echoes represent the reflecting and absorbing properties of the various tissues in the go-and-return paths. A continuous display is accomplished by repetitive pulsing the ultrasound at a rate of a few hundred to several thousand per second.

6-3-2-3.   Echoencephalography.   The A-scan presentation is used in echoencephalography (Leksell, 1955–1956) in which the midline structures of the brain are located by ultrasound. In the original application, separate transmitting and receiving transducers were placed on the same side of the head, and the echo pattern was displayed on an oscilloscope screen and photographed. Then the test was repeated with both the transmitter and the

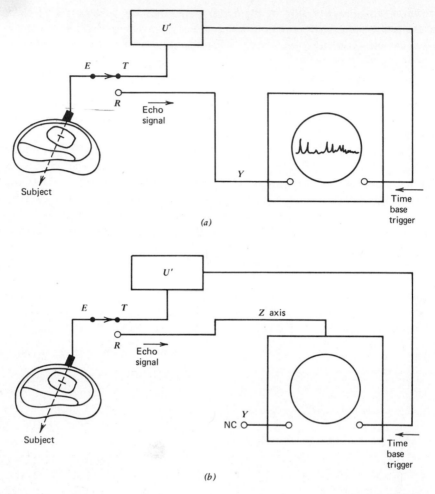

Figure 6-10. The A- and B-scan display techniques. (*a*) The A-scan method: the echo signals derived from reflections of the pulsed ultrasound (*U'*) are applied to the *Y* axis of a conventional oscilloscope, where sweep is triggered by the pulse of ultrasound. Thus the peak amplitude of an echo is related to the reflecting and attenuating properties of an underlying structure. The position of a peak indicates the depth of the underlying reflecting structure. (*b*) The B-scan method: the cathode ray tube beam is extinguished and the echo signals are applied to the *Z* axis to brighten the trace. Thus the brightness of a spot is related to the reflecting and absorbing properties of the underlying tissues. The position of the bright spot indicates the depth of the reflecting structure. (NC = not connected.)

receiver on the other side of the head. By comparing the echoes obtained from the two tests, as in Fig. 6-11, any deviation in the midline structures was easily identifiable and provided a diagnostic sign for surgical intervention.

6-3-2-4. B-Scan Imaging. In many instances, the position of the underlying structures is of more importance than the amplitude of the returned echoes; therefore the B-scan, or brightness-modulation presentation, becomes more meaningful. The arrangement of equipment for the B-scan presentation (Fig. 6-10*b*) is almost the same as that for the A-scan method except that the time base, which triggers the pulsed ultrasonic generator, does not illuminate the screen of the cathode ray tube. The returning echo signals are applied so that they modulate the intensity (*z* axis) of the display by reducing the negative grid bias of the cathode ray tube. Thus the display consists of a series of spots, whose brightness describes the reflecting and absorbing properties of the underlying tissues. The positions of the bright spots identify the distances of the reflecting structures below the transducer.

The B (or brightness) -scan presentation is employed in two ways. In one the display is moved while the transducer assembly is in a fixed location,

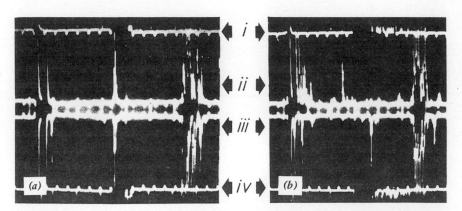

Figure 6-11. A-scan presentation of the ultrasonic reflections of structures within the head (Echoencephalography). The time markers (top and bottom) correspond to 1 cm distance. In I and IV the transmitter and receiver are placed on opposite sides of the head; in II and III, the transmitter and receiver were on the same side of the head; the multiple echoes from the skull (left and right) can be seen in (*a*) and (*b*). In (*a*), which is a recording from a normal subject, the midline-structure echoes are in the center of the illustration, and both the transmitter and receiver were placed first on one side, then on the other. The pattern in (*b*) is from a patient with an intracranial hemorrhage, which caused deviation of the midline structures. Note the separation of the echoes from the deviated midline-structures. [From P. N. T. Wells, *Bio-Med. Eng.* **5**:378–385 (1970). By permission.]

thereby showing location and any temporal variation in position of the underlying structures. With the other type of B-scan display, the transducer assembly is moved slowly across a body segment, and the position of the oscilloscope display tracks the transducer position. Thus a cross-sectional view of the underlying structures is presented on the oscilloscope screen.

6-3-2-5. Echocardiography.   The B-scan presentation is used to follow the movements of the leaflets of the mitral valve in human subjects. In mitral valve stenosis, the valve area and leaflet motion are reduced, thereby impairing filling of the left ventricle, the main cardiac pumping chamber. Ultrasonic visualization of the motion of the mitral valve is noninvasive and therefore constitutes an attractive clinical diagnostic test.

To visualize mitral valve action, the ultrasonic transmitter-receiver assembly is placed on the chest wall (Fig. 6-12a) and is manipulated carefully to guide the ultrasonic beam between the ribs so that it encounters the mitral valve (Fig. 6-12b). The optimum location for the transducer is over the third, fourth, or fifth left interspace, 1 to 4 cm lateral to the sternum. The echoes returning from the underlying structures brighten the oscilloscope display, which is arranged so that the time base is applied to the Y axis. Therefore, echoes returning from structures immediately under the transducer assembly appear at the top of the cathode ray tube. If the cathode ray display were stationary, the underlying structures would

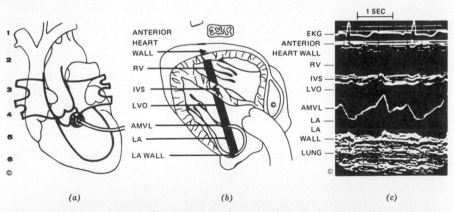

(a)   (b)   (c)

Figure 6-12.   Echocardiography: (a) sagittal view of the heart in the thorax; (b) identification of the structures illuminated by the ultrasound (U), beam; (c) typical echocardiogram, showing the echoes displayed by a brightness (B-scan) presentation that is moved slowly across the face of a cathode ray tube with the electrocardiogram (EKG) used as a timing reference for the cardiac cycle. When the ultrasound transducer is placed appropriately, the movements of the interior leaflet of the mitral valve are displayed (AMVL). (Courtesy of the Unirad Corp., Denver, Colo.)

produce a vertical line of bright spots. Underlying structures that move will, of course, produce bright-spot echoes that move up and down the vertical line. To show the temporal nature of the moving echo-producing structures, the display on the cathode ray tube is moved at a uniform rate across the tube, producing a tracing whose amplitude describes the excursion of the moving target. Movement toward the chest wall is shown by an upward motion of the echo-produced bright spot. To facilitate directing the ultrasonic beam to locate the mitral valve and its motion, the electrocardiogram is displayed along the top of the cathode-ray tube with the conventional A-scan presentation.

Figure 6-12c illustrates a typical echocardiogram, the name given to the record that displays motion of the heart using ultrasound. In this display the transducer has been adjusted to optimize detection of the anterior mitral valve leaflet (AMVL). By referring to the electrocardiogram, motion of the mitral valve can be followed. Just after the P wave, active ventricular filling occurs because of atrial systole. Descent of the leaflet motion is interrupted by the onset of ventricular systole, which accompanies the S wave of the ECG, and bulges the mitral valve into the left atrium. Rapid ventricular filling occurs after the end of ventricular systole, which follows the T wave of the ECG. At that time, there is a rapid descent in the record showing mitral valve movement, indicating free passage of blood from the left atrium into the left ventricle. Because this presentation is one of millimeters excursion and seconds, the velocity of movement of the valve leaflet can be calculated from the echocardiogram. In some echocardiographs, the signal that corresponds to the valve-movement display is brought out for graphic recording.

In sketches of echocardiograms from a normal subject (Fig. 6-13a), rapid movement of the anterior mitral valve leaflet in early diastole can be seen. Figure 6-13b presents the echocardiogram of mitral valve motion in a subject with mitral valve stenosis. Note that the rate of descent of the valve is considerably reduced, as shown by the slope of the dashed line following the E wave. The fact that the rate of motion of the anterior mitral valve leaflet (in mm/sec) is related to the mitral valve area has been adequately confirmed by Joyner and Reid (1963) and Segal et al. (1966). The type of correlation was presented by Segal and is shown in Fig. 6-13c.

Directing the ultrasound beam to intercept the mitral valve clearly requires skill. Although there was some early doubt about whether the structure actually was being tracked by the ultrasonic beam, these uncertainties have now been largely removed. It is interesting to note that in his early studies, Edler (1955, 1956) stated that the motion recorded was that of the anterior surface of the left atrial wall. In the paper by Effert et al. (1957), which confirmed Edler's work, only atrial wall movement was discussed. In

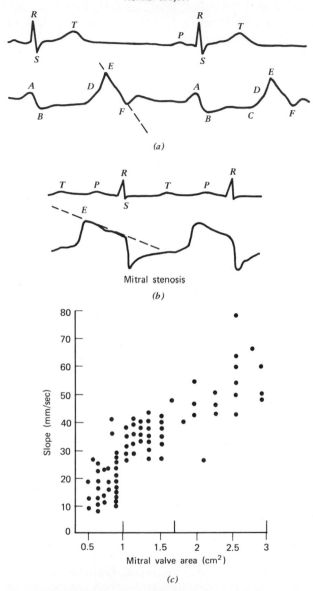

Figure 6-13. Echocardiograms of (*a*) a normal subject, (*b*) a subject with mitral valve stenosis; (*c*) correlation between velocity of movement of the anterior mitral valve leaflet (mm/sec), as shown by the dashed lines, and the mitral valve area (cm²). [(*a*) and (*b*) redrawn from B. L. Segal and D. C. Kilpatrick, *Engineering in the Practice of Medicine,* Williams & Williams Co., Baltimore 1967. (*c*) redrawn from B. L. Segal et al., *JAMA,* **195:**99–104 (1966).]

1961 Edler et al. reported on carefully conducted studies confirming that the echocardiogram, when carefully obtained, can represent movement of the anterior mitral valve leaflet.

6-3-2-6.   Tomography.   By moving the transmitter and receiver (transducer) assembly, it is possible to use the B-scan display method to obtain a cross-sectional view or an ultrasonic tomogram of a subject. Several ingenious methods have been described to obtain such a presentation, the principle of which is shown in Fig. 6-14.

The specimen to be imaged in cross section is immersed in a fluid to obtain adequate coupling of the ultrasonic energy (see Fig. 6-14). With the transducer located below the surface of a coupling liquid, and above the subject, a series of echoes will be obtained, appearing as bright spots along the sweep when the B-scan display is employed. In this particular case, it is convenient to apply the sweep to the Y axis of the oscilloscope, as in echocardiography. However, with ultrasonic tomography, the position of the X axis of the cathode ray tube indicates the position of the transducer assembly; thus as the transducer scans the subject, the bright-spot echoes represent the distances to the underlying reflecting tissues and organs, and

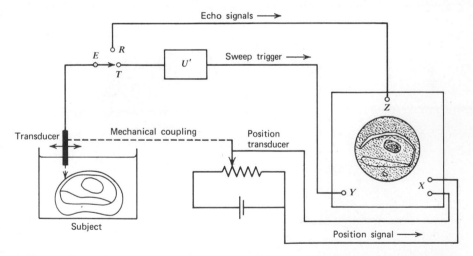

Figure 6-14.   Ultrasonic tomography. The pulsed ultrasound (U') is delivered to the transducer assembly and at the same time triggers the sweep, which is applied to the Y axis of the oscilloscope. The echoes returned from the reflecting surfaces in the subject are applied to the Z axis of the cathode ray tube to brighten the beam when an electronic switch (E) allows the transducer to act as a receiver, nanoseconds after the initial pulse of ultrasound is delivered. Repetitive ultrasonic pulsing and electronic switching are carried out while the transducer is moved to examine a cross section of the subject. The horizontal position of the transducer is displayed on the X axis of the oscilloscope.

their positions along the horizontal axis display their lateral locations. Therefore a single scan across a subject will display a cross-sectional view of all the reflecting structures intercepted by the scanning ultrasonic beam.

Numerous ingenious methods have been developed to achieve a fluid-coupling between the transducer assembly and the subject without requiring total immersion of the subject. For example, Ebina et al. (1967) developed the system represented in Fig. 6-15a, in which a water-filled plastic sac in a metal housing contained the transducer assembly. The part of the sac in contact with the chest was coated with olive oil to obtain adequate coupling of the ultrasonic energy. Figure 6-15b is an ultrasonic tomogram of the heart and great vessels obtained using this method. To obtain the images with the maximum clarity, it was necessary to use the ECG as a gating signal to control the instant when imaging was carried out.

Omoto (1967) called attention to the improvement in detail obtainable when the ultrasonic transducer assembly is located within the vascular system. To prove his point, he developed a miniature ultrasonic transducer mounted in a long catheter with a lateral window to allow passage of the ultrasound. The catheter was advanced into the vena cava to image the cardiac structures in front of it, using the brightness modulation presentation. Figure 6-16 gives the principle employed. Rotation of the

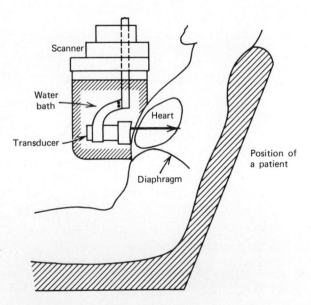

Figure 6-15. (a) Ultrasonic tomography in the human; (b) a tomogram showing the major structures of the heart. [From T. Ebina et al., *Japan. Heart J.* **8**:331–353 (1967). By permission.]

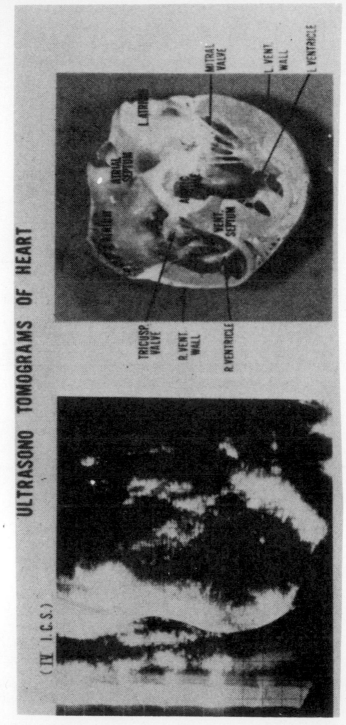

Fig. 6-15. (b)

151

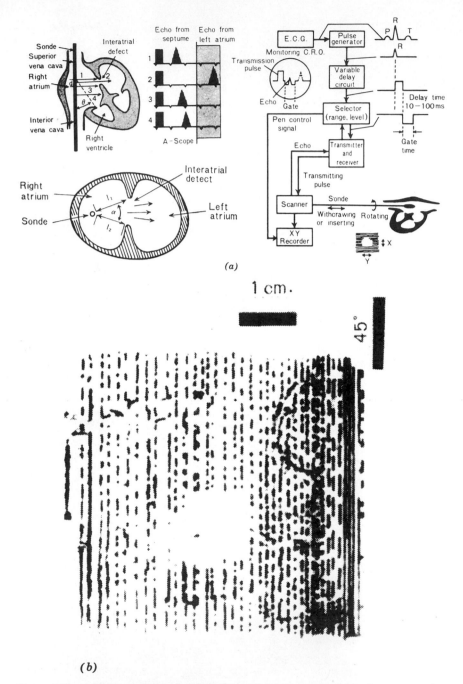

Figure 6-16. (*a*) Ultrasonic imaging of the interatrial septum using a transducer mounted on the side of a venous catheter that can be rotated to image the structures at a fixed head-foot level and can be placed at different head-foot levels to produce an ultrasonic tomogram of the heart and its chambers. (*b*) Ultrasonic tomogram of the interatrial septum in which there is a hole measuring 25 × 15 mm. [From R. Omoto, *Japan. Heart J.*, **8:**569–581 (1967). By permission.]

transducer allowed imaging in different directions. To obtain a spatial display, the angular position of the transducer was coupled to the Y axis of an oscilloscope in which the X axis identified the head-foot position of the transducer. An X-Y plotter, in which the pen could be lifted electronically, was also used as a display device. Thus by choosing a point in the vena cava (e.g., 1 in Fig. 6-16) and rotating the transducer through ± 90 degrees, the structures at the level of the transducer were imaged. Then the catheter-borne transducer assembly was moved to a new position and rotated again ± 90 degrees, thereby imaging at a new level. The procedure was repeated until the region of interest was completely examined.

The method developed by Omoto (1967) was used to identify the presence of a hole in the interatrial septum. Figure 6-16b presents an ultrasonic tomogram, displayed with an X-Y plotter, revealing a hole measuring 25×15 mm. At the time of surgery, the size of the hole was found to be 27×16 mm.

These few examples of ultrasonic imaging clearly indicate the considerable potential of the method and invite the development of new techniques for processing and display of the echo signals. There is no doubt that such techniques will appear, allowing the full potential for ultrasonic imaging to be realized. Journals are devoting an increasing amount of space to coverage of medical ultrasonics and an excellent survey of this field was presented by Jurgen (1974).

REFERENCES

Baker, D. W. 1964. A sonic transcutaneous blood flowmeter. *Proc. 17th Ann. Conf. Med. Bio. Eng.* 76.

Baker, D. W. 1970. Pulsed ultrasonic Doppler blood-flow sensing. *IEEE Trans. Sonics Ultrason.* SU17:170–185.

Bjerring, W. L., H. C. Boone, and M. L. Lockhart. 1935. Use of electrostethophone for recording heart sounds. *JAMA* 104:628–637.

Boone, B. R. 1939. An amplifier for recording heart sounds through use of the cathode ray tube. *J. Lab. Clin. Med.* 25:188–193.

Currens, J. H., G. L. Bramwell, and S. Aronow. 1957. An automatic blood pressure recording machine. *New Engl. J. Med.* 17:780–784.

Dibner, B. 1963. *The New Rays of Professor Roentgen.* Burndy Library, Norwalk, Conn.

Donaldson, P. E. K. 1958. *Electronic Apparatus for Biological Research.* Butterworth's, London.

Edler, I. 1955. The diagnostic use of ultrasound in heart disease. *Acta Med. Scand.* 152 Supp. 304–309:32–36.

Edler, I. 1956. Ultrasound-cardiogram in mitral valvular disease. *Acta Chir. Scand.* 111:230–232.

Edler, I., A. Gustafson, T. Karlefors, and B. Christensson. 1961. Ultrasound cardiography. *Acta Med. Scand.* Supp. 370:68–82.

Effert, S., H. Erkens, and F. Grosse-Brockhoff. 1957. The ultrasonic echo method in cardiological diagnoses. *German Med. Monthly,* 2:325–328.

Farrall, W. R. 1959. Design considerations for ultrasonic flowmeters. *IRE Trans. Med. Electron.* ME-6:198–201.

Franklin, D. L., D. W. Baker, R. M. Ellis, and R. F. Rushmer. 1959. A pulsed ultrasonic flowmeter. *IRE Trans. Med. Electron.* ME-6:204–206.

Franklin, D. L., W. Schlegel, and R. F. Rushmer. 1961. Blood flow measurement by Doppler frequency shift. *Science* 134:564–565.

Geddes, L. A., J. Bourland, and E. Arriaga. 1974. Recording esophogeal heart sounds with a catheter-tip microphone. *Cardiovasc. Res. Center Bull.* 13:3–7.

Geddes, L. A., and H. E. Hoff. 1960. Graphic recording of the pressure pulse wave *J. Appl. Physiol.* 15:959–960.

Geddes, L. A., and A. G. Moore. 1968. The efficient detection of Korotkoff sounds. *Med. Biol. Eng.* 6:603–609.

Geddes, L. A., W. A. Spencer, and H. E. Hoff. 1959. Graphic recording of the Korotkoff sounds. *Am. Heart J.* 57:361–370.

Gilford, S. R., and H. P. Broida. 1954. Physiological monitoring equipment for anesthesia and other uses. *Natl. Bur. Std. (U.S.) Ann. Rept.* 3301, Project 1204-20-5512.

Gilson, W. E. 1942. Automatic blood pressure recorder. *Electronics* 15:54–56.

Gilson, W. E., H. Goldberg, and H. Slocum. 1941. Automatic device for periodically determining and recording both systolic and diastolic blood pressure in man. *Science* 94:194.

Gomez, D. M., and A. Langevin. 1937. *La piézographe directe et instantanée.* Paris, Hermann.

Herrick, J. F., and J. A. Anderson. 1959. An ultrasonic flowmeter. *IRE Trans. Med. Electron.* ME6:195–197.

Jacobs, J. E. 1966. *Advances in Bioengineering and Bioinstrumentation.* F. Alt (ed.). Plenum Press, New York.

Joyner C. R., and J. M. Reid. 1963. Applications of ultrasound in cardiology and cardiovascular physiology. *Prog. Cardiovasc. Dis.* 5:482–497.

Jurgen, R. K. 1974. Ultrasonics in medicine. *IEEE Spectrum* 11(8):62–66.

Kalmus, H. P. 1954. An electric flowmeter. *Rev. Sci. Instr.* 25:201–206.

Lax, H., A. W. Feinberg, and B. M. Cohen. 1956. Studies of the arterial pulse wave. *J. Chronic Dis.* 3:618–631.

Leksell, L. 1955–1956. Echo-encephalography. *Acta Chir. Scand.* 110:301–315.

Lewis, D. H., G. W. Dietz, J. D. Wallace and J. R. Brown. 1957. Intracardiac phonocardiography in man. *Circulation* 16:764–775.

Lockhart, M. L. 1938. The stethograph. *Am. Heart J.* 10:72–78.

Malcolm, J. L. 1946. A piezoelectric unit for general purpose physiological recording. *J. Sci. Instr.* 23:146–148.

Mannheimer, E. 1941. Calibrated phonocardiography. *Am. Heart J.* 21:151–162.

Miller, A., and P. D. White. 1941. Crystal microphone for pulse wave recording. *Am. Heart J.* 21:504–510.

Narat, J. K. 1936. New electronic stethoscope and stethograph. Preliminary Report. *Illinois Med. J.* 70:131–134.

Omberg, A. C. 1936. Apparatus for recording systolic blood pressure. *Rev. Sci. Instr.* 7:33–34.

Pascoe, J. E. 1955. A technique for introduction of intracellular electrodes. *J. Physiol.* 128:26P-27P.

Rappaport, M. B., and A. Luisada. 1944. Indirect sphygmomanometry. *J. Lab. Clin. Med.* 29:638–565.

Rappaport, M. B., and H. B. Sprague. 1941. Physiologic and physical laws that govern auscultation and their application. *Am. Heart J.* 21:257–318.

Rappaport, M. B., and H. B. Sprague. 1942. Graphic registration of normal heart sounds. *Am. Heart J.* 23:591–623.

Roberts, V. C. 1973. The measurement of flow in intact blood vessels. *Crit. Rev. Bioeng.* 1:419–447.

Sachs, H. A., H. Marquis, and B. Blumenthal. 1935. A modification of the Wiggers-Dean system measuring heart sounds using audio amplification. *Am. Heart J.* 10:965–8.

Segal, B., W. Lekoff, and B. Kingsley. 1966. Echocardiography. *JAMA* 195:99–104.

Siegel, J. J. 1959. Piezoelectric transducers measure fluctuating forces, pressures, accelerations. *Prod. Eng.* 30:61–63.

Ulrich, W. D. 1974. Ultrasound dosage for non-therapeutic use in human beings— Extrapolation from a literature survey. *IEEE Trans. Bio-Med. Eng.* BME 21:48–51.

Wagai, T. 1965. Diagnostic application of ultrasound. *Japan Electron. Eng.* 2:25–30.

Wallace, J. D., J. R. Brown, D. H. Lewis, and G. W. Dietz. 1957. Phonocatheters: Their design and application. Part 1. *IRE Trans. Med. Electron.* PGME-9:25–30.

Wells, P. N. T. 1970. The present status of medical ultrasonic diagnostics. *Bio-Med. Eng.* 5:376–385.

Wood, M. C., and A. C. Gunn. 1953. The amplification and recording of foetal heart sounds. *Electron. Eng.* 25:90–93.

7

Thermoelectric Transducers

7-1. THERMOELECTRICITY

When two metals are joined, a temperature-dependent potential, called the contact potential, develops. First demonstrated in 1821 by Seebeck, the phenomenon has been used extensively for the measurement of temperature for more than a century. The contact potential is related to the differences in work function of the two metals. Although a single junction of two metals can be employed to develop the potential, such a simple arrangement is often impractical; the usual configuration for utilization of the thermoelectric effect is illustrated in Fig. 7-1a. The two metals (1, 2) constitute the thermocouple, and the potential developed is dependent on the temperature difference between the two bimetal junctions J_{1-2} and J_{2-1}. In practice, it is customary to keep one junction at a reference temperature, employing the other to measure the unknown temperature. Usually the reference point chosen is 0 or 100°C, although ambient temperature is sometimes employed.

Because the measuring junction often must be located some distance from the reference junction and the indicating instrument, it is usually impractical to choose the same metal for both the interconnecting cable conductors and the thermojunctions. For this reason conducting wires of a different material are introduced into the circuit. Under these conditions the thermodetector takes the form shown in Fig. 7-1b. Thus there are really three important thermal junctions: J_{1-2}, J_{1-3}, and J_{2-3}. The temperature $T_{J_{1-2}}$ can be measured only if the temperatures of the two remaining junctions are kept constant. Usually the connecting wires are made of materials chosen so that the thermal voltages between junctions J_{1-3} and J_{2-3} are small. Thus minor variations in the temperature of J_{1-3} and J_{2-3} will contribute only insignificant error voltages, and the voltage presented to the indicator is largely a function of $T_{J_{1-2}}$.

The potential developed by thermojunctions depends on the temperature of the metals and not on the size of their junctions. However, it is im-

156

$$E = f(T_{J_{1-2}} - T_{J_{2-1}})$$
$$\doteq K\Delta T$$

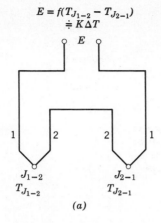

$$J_{1-2}$$
$$T_{J_{1-2}}$$
$$J_{2-1}$$
$$T_{J_{2-1}}$$

(a)

$$E = f(T_{J_{1-2}}, T_{J_{1-3}}, T_{J_{2-3}})$$
$$\text{If } T_{J_{1-3}} = T_{J_{2-3}}$$
$$E \doteq K T_{J_{1-2}}$$

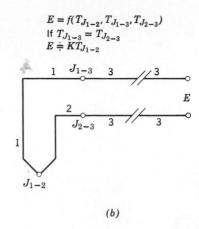

$$J_{1-2}$$

(b)

Figure 7-1.   Thermojunctions.

portant to note that the resistance of the circuit does depend on the size of the metallic conductors; if the thermo-electric voltage is to be employed to drive a current-drawing indicator, total circuit resistance must be considered. Another factor, the Peltier effect, is also involved and is discussed later.

The ability of a particular thermojunction to develop a voltage is specified by its thermoelectric power, an old term now of dubious merit. The voltages developed by couples of various metals are usually small. Certain special alloys that produce a large voltage per degree of temperature difference between the reference and exploring junctions have been developed. Typical values for some familiar thermocouples are given in Table 7-1. Over a limited range, the voltage is linear with temperature difference.

From these data it is apparent that the thermocouples produce a small voltage per degree of temperature difference between the junctions. For accurate determination of temperature, the voltage must be measured with a potentiometer. If current is passed through the junctions, one is warmed and the other cooled. This phenomenon is known as the Peltier effect, and although its magnitude is small, it must be considered in terms of both changing the resistance of the ciruit and adding heat to or abstracting heat from what is being measured.

7-2.   BIOMEDICAL APPLICATIONS

Although the thermocouple has been somewhat overshadowed by the thermistor as a temperature sensor, new techniques of fabrication indicate that it may see wider application in biomedicine. For example, Reed and Kampwirth (1964), Reed (1966), and Cain and Welch (1974) described

Table 7-1   Thermoelectric Sensitivities*'†

Thermojunctions	Thermoelectric Sensitivity ($\mu v/°C$)
Nickel-platinum	15
Lead-platinum	4
Silver-platinum	6.5
Copper-platinum	6.5
Iron-platinum	18.5
Nichrome-platinum	25
Platinum/rhodium-platinum	6
Chromel-Alumel	40–55
Copper-constantan	40
Iron-constantan	53
Germanium-platinum	300
Silicon-platinum	440
Selenium-platinum	900

* From K. S. Lion, *Instrumentation in Scientific Research*, McGraw-Hill, Book Co., New York, 1959.
† Reference junction, 0°C.

thermocouples of micron dimensions (Fig. 7-2) which could easily be inserted into single living cells to measure the temperature of the cytoplasm.

The response time for miniature thermocouples (25 μ) was given by Gelb et al. (1964) as 116 msec for 95% response. Thermocouples made from 40-gauge wire by a commercial firm[1] are advertised as having a time constant of 0.1 sec, and the time constant of its ultraminiature couples is given as 0.05 sec. Another supplier[2] has advertised fine wire (0.002–0.005 in.) iron-constantan thermocouples having time constants in the range of 0.002 to 1 sec. Such devices merely await application.

In biomedical studies thermocouples find a variety of other uses as detectors of temperature which reflect circulation in the regions measured. Scott (1930) described the use of four couples in series (a thermopile) for measuring skin temperature. Hardy (1934) measured radiant heat from the body with such a device. Miniature thermocouples for determining the temperatures of deep tissues and blood have been constructed and placed in hypodermic needles by Clark (1922), Bazzett and McGlone (1927), Sheard (1931), and Foster (1936). Bazzett and McGlone have reminded investigators that thermocouples were used to measure the temperature in human

[1] High Temperature Instruments Corp., Philadelphia, Pa.
[2] Omega Engineering Inc., Springdale, Conn.

muscle as long ago as 1835. In all probability the thermocouple was the first electrical transducer in physiology. In the hands of Hill (1932) the thermocouple showed that the temperature rise in nerve during the passage of an impulse was 7×10^{-8} degrees centigrade.

Rein (1928) described his blood flow transducer, the thermostromuhr, which employed a pair of small thermocouples and a heating element to measure blood flow. The apparatus consisted of a tube with the heating element located in the axial stream; proximal and distal to the heating element were mounted the thermocouples. Blood flowing past the heating element was warmed. The upstream couple detected the temperature of the blood before heating, and the downstream unit monitored the temperature of the warmed blood. The temperature difference was thus dependent on blood flow. By improving Rein's instrument, Baldes et al. (1933) were able to measure very tiny blood flows. Their contribution consisted of warming the blood with dielectric heating instead of using a heating element in the blood stream.

For a considerable time the thermostromuhr was a standard blood flow transducer. Burton (1938) analyzed the theoretical considerations underlying the functioning of the device. Applications, advantages, and limitations were set forth by Gregg (1948) and Linzell (1953).

Thermocouples can be small or large; the smaller they are, the more rapidly they respond to temperature changes. Furthermore, because small

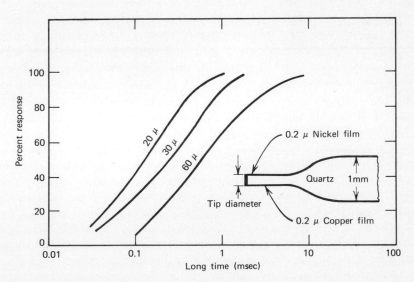

Figure 7-2. Copper-nickel thermojunctions and their response times. (Illustration by courtesy of A. J. Welch, U. of Texas, Austin, Tex. 1974.)

units have a low thermal mass, they will not appreciably alter the temperature of whatever is being measured. It is well to remember that the use of any temperature sensor always raises the problem of heat transfer by conduction along the wires connecting the device to the indicating apparatus.

Certain precautions must be observed in the construction of thermocouples. The material from which the junctions are made must be homogeneous, and considerable attention is needed to the fusing of the elements to form the active junction. Bulletin 15A-RP 1.4 of the Leeds and Northrup Co. covers the important details of construction and describes gas, electric arc, and resistance welding of the thermojunctions.

An ingenious laboratory method of arc welding thermocouple junctions electrically, described by Riley (1949), employs a metal cup in which is placed a small quantity of mercury covered with mineral or motor oil to a depth of 2 to 3 cm. The metal cup and the mercury within it constitute one electrode connected to the 115-V powerline. The ends of the thermocouple wires are cleaned and twisted tightly together for a distance of several millimeters. The distal end, which is to become the thermojunction, is then cut, leaving only a little more than a single turn of the twisted wires. The other ends of the wires are then joined and connected by way of a variable resistor to the other side of the power line. The resistor that Riley used consisted of a 400-W heating element to fabricate a 0.3-mm thermocouple. Welding is accomplished by lowering the twisted ends of the thermocouple wires into the oil to make contact with the surface of the mercury. The assembly is then withdrawn; as contact is broken, the high-temperature arc formed between the wires and the pool of mercury fuses the ends to form the thermojunction. Iron-constantan, platinum, platinum-rhodium, chromel-alumel, and copper-constantan wires have been welded by using this easily mastered technique. Riley reported that the magnitude of the resistor is dictated by the diameter of the wires chosen for the thermocouple. In his experience wires ranging from 0.1 to 4 mm were successfully welded.

By virtue of its ability to generate an electrical potential that can drive a current through a load and so produce power, the thermocouple is a thermoelectric converter. Although efficiency is low, it may permit the heat of metabolism to be employed as a source of electrical energy.

Thermojunctions are beginning to be used in biomedical research as heat pumps. Yamazaki (1965) and Hayward (1965) have reviewed many of the applications in which the Peltier effect has been used to cool tissues and fluids. Because the cold produced by thermojunctions is easily controlled, precise temperatures can be maintained. Small size, quietness of operation, freedom from moving parts, and ability to switch over instantly from cooling to heating are properties that make these devices attractive for biothermal studies.

REFERENCES

Baldes, E. J., J. F. Herrick, and H. E. Essex. 1933. Modification in thermostromuhr method of measuring flow of blood. *Proc. Soc. Exp. Biol. Med.* **30**:1109–1111.

Bazzett, H. C., and B. McGlone. 1927. Temperature gradients in tissues in man *Am. J. Physiol.* **82**:415–451.

Burton, A. C. 1938. Theory and design of the thermostromuhr. *J. Appl. Physics.* **9**:127–131.

Cain, C. and A. J. Welch. 1974. Thin-film temperature sensors for biological measurement. *IEEE Trans. Bio. Med. Eng.* **BME21**:(5):421–423.

Clark, H. 1922. The measurement of intravenous temperatures. *J. Exp. Med.* **35**:385–389.

Foster, P. C. 1936. Thermocouples for the medical laboratory. *J. Lab. Clin. Med.* **22**:68–81.

Gelb, G. H., B. D. Marcus, and D. Dropkin. 1964. Manufacture of fine wire thermocouple probes. *Rev. Sci. Instr.* **35**:80–81.

Gregg, D. E. 1948. *Thermostromuhr: Methods in Medical Research,* Vol. I. Chicago, Year-book Publishers.

Hardy, J. D. 1934. The radiation of heat from the human body. *J. Clin. Invest.* **13**:593–620.

Hayward, J. N., L. H. Ott, D. G. Stuart, and F. C. Cheshire. 1965. Peltier biothermodes. *Am. J. Med. Electron.* **4**:11–19.

Hill, A. V. 1932. A closer analysis of the heat production of nerve. *Proc. Roy. Soc. (London)* **BIII**:106–164.

Leeds and Northrup Co. Bulletin 15A-RP 1.4. Pittsburgh: The Instrument Society of America.

Linzell, J. L. 1953. Internal calorimetry in the measurement of blood flow with heated thermocouples. *J. Physiol.* **121**:390–402.

Reed, R. P. 1966. Thin-film sensors of micron size and application in biothermology, Ph.D. dissertation, University of Texas, Austin Texas.

Reed, R. P., and R. T. Kampwirth. 1964. Thermocouples of micron size by vapor deposition. *Direction,* **10**:8.

Rein, H. 1928. Die Thermo-Stromuhr. *Z. Biol.* **87**:394–418.

Riley, J. A. 1949. A simple method for welding thermocouples. *Science* **109**:281.

Scott, W. J. M. 1930. An improved electrodermal instrument of measuring the surface temperature. *JAMA* **94**:1987–1988.

Sheard, C. 1931. The electromotive thermometer, an instrument for measuring intramural, intravenous, superficial and cavity temperatures. *Am. J. Clin. Pathol.* **1**:209–226.

Yamazaki, Z. 1965. Medical application of thermoelectric cooling. *Japan. Elect. Eng.* **2**:32–35.

8

Chemical Transducers

8-1. INTRODUCTION

The survival of a living cell and of a whole organism depends entirely on the existence of chemical reactions that are precisely ordered and controlled by biological catalysts called enzymes. To understand the processes characterizing life, there is a need to measure the molecular and ionic concentrations of the materials that participate in these reactions. Accordingly, the measurements of pH, pCO_2, and pO_2 are of prime importance in understanding the chemical energy exchanges called metabolism. This chapter is a study of the methods of transduction of these quantities, as they appear in solution, into an electrical signal. Attention is devoted also to the detection of other important ions, such as sodium, calcium, potassium, and to the oxygen content of blood.

8-2. ELECTRODE POTENTIAL

The concept of electrode potential is fundamental to an understanding of the measurement of the concentration of ions in solution. Electrode potential is the potential produced at the interface between two material phases. For example, in the case of a metal-solution interface, an electrode potential results from the differences in rates between two opposing processes: (*a*) the passage of ions from the metal into the solution, and (*b*) the combination of metallic ions in solution with electrons in the metal to form atoms of the metal. When equilibrium is reached, a layer of charge is formed in proximity to the electrode; that next to the electrode is of one sign; that in the solution is of the opposite. The charge distribution is called the electrical double layer. Although diffuse, the layer in its simplest form was considered by Helmhotz to be a uniform layer of charge. This double layer of charge constitutes a capacitance that is important in determining the electrical impedance of the interface, as discussed in Chapter 9. The

162

potential appearing across the metal-electrolyte interface at equilibrium is the electrode potential. Table 8-1 lists various ion-to-metal potentials.

A potential is also developed if an interface is created by imposing a semipermeable barrier (membrane) between two liquid phases so that the membrane allows reversible transfer of a particular ion. After equilibrium has been established, the potential created is proportional to the logarithm of the ratio of the concentrations of the ion to which the membrane is selectively permeable. For a membrane that is ideally selective, the potential developed is given by the Nernst equation:

$$E = -\frac{RT}{nF} \ln \frac{C_1}{C_2} = -2.303 \frac{RT}{nF} \log_{10} \frac{C_1}{C_2},$$

where n = valence of the ion,
   R = gas constant (8.315×10^7 ergs per degree per mole),
   T = absolute temperature (degrees Kelvin),
   F = number of coulombs transferred (96,500 coulombs, i.e., 1 faraday, is required to convert one equivalent of an element to an equivalent of ions)
C_1 and C_2 = concentration of the selected ion on the two sides of the membrane.

This form of the Nernst equation is based on ideal thermodynamic considerations and is valid only for very dilute solutions. It has been found to be in error as the ionic concentrations are increased. This departure from ideal thermodynamic behavior is expressed in terms of the ionic activity, which is related to the ionic concentration in accordance with the expression

$$a = C \times \nu,$$

where a = the activity of a specific ion,
   C = the concentration of the ion,
   ν = the activity coefficient.

The Nerst equation is usually written in terms of ion activity as follows:

$$E = -\frac{RT}{nF} \ln \frac{a_1}{a_2} = -2.303 \frac{RT}{nF} \log_{10} \frac{a_1}{a_2}.$$

The activity of an ion species is a measure of the effective concentration rather than the actual concentration. For very dilute solutions ν approaches unity, and the ideal situation in which the potential developed is proportional to the logarithm of the ratio of concentrations more nearly holds. Activity coefficients must be known if the ion concentration is to be determined in terms of the electrical potential developed. The Debye-Hückel

Table 8-1   Half-Cell Potentials*

Material	Potential (V)
Aluminum^{3+}/aluminum	-1.66
Iron^{2+}/iron	-0.44
Nickel^{2+}/nickel	-0.250
Lead^{2+}/lead	-0.126
Hydrogen^{+}/hydrogen	0.0 (Reference)
Copper^{2+}/copper	$+0.337$
Copper^{+}/copper	$+0.521$
Silver^{+}/silver	$+0.799$
Platinum^{2+}/platinum	$+1.2$
Gold^{+}/gold	$+1.68$
Gold^{3+}/gold	$+1.50$

* *Handbook of Chemistry and Physics*, 45th ed., Chemical Rubber Publishing Co., Cleveland, Ohio, 1958.

NOTE: These potentials are listed in the reference as oxidation potentials and accordingly carry a sign opposite to that shown here.

equations have been found to yield accurate values for the activity coefficients of dilute solutions, such as those encountered in living systems. For a discussion of the application of the Debye-Hückel theory of electrolytes to biological systems, a textbook such as that of Bull (1964) is recommended.

The availability of a membrane that exhibits selective permeability for a particular ion provides, therefore, a means of creating a transducer for that species of ion.

8-3.   THE HYDROGEN ELECTRODE

Knowledge of the behavior of the hydrogen electrode is fundamental to an understanding of the determination of pH and pCO$_2$ by electrometric methods. It is impossible to measure the potential of a single interphase boundary because in the measuring process an additional interface is introduced. Therefore, it is necessary to specify one electrode or interface as the standard to which others may be compared. The hydrogen electrode has been chosen as the standard and its potential specified as zero, as shown in Table 8-1; the potentials of other metal-to-ion interfaces are measured with reference to it.

Of the interfaces listed in Table 8-1, hydrogen^{+}/hydrogen is the only one that does not consist of a solid metal in equilibrium with its ion. It is appropriate to inquire how electrical connection can be made to a gas. Because platinum adsorbs hydrogen readily and is itself a good conductor, electrical connection to the hydrogen is accomplished by electrolytically coating a platinum wire or plate with finely divided platinum (platinum black) to increase its surface area. The wire or plate is then said to be platinized. When such an electrode with its adsorbed hydrogen is placed in a solution containing hydrogen ions, a difference of potential, depending on the tendency of the gas to go into solution and on the concentration of hydrogen ions in solution, will develop. The platinum black must remain in external contact with hydrogen gas to ensure that the supply of gas will not be depleted. Hydrogen electrodes have been made in many forms, one of which is the Hildebrand type (see Fig. 8-1). In using this electrode, the platinized plate is submerged to one-half its height in the solution. Hydrogen gas is admitted through the tube as shown and completely surrounds the upper half of the plate. The gas escapes through the holes at the level of the middle of the plate.

Because the potential of the hydrogen electrode is dependent on the concentration of hydrogen ions in solution, it has been possible to design intracardiac catheters with single and double platinum electrodes for detecting and localizing left-to-right heart shunts (Vogel et al., 1962). In this method the catheter containing the hydrogen electrode is placed in the main pulmonary artery. A single breath of hydrogen gas is then administered to the patient, and this results in the almost immediate appearance of hydrogenated blood in the left side of the heart. If a left-to-right shunt is present, it is detected by the change in electrode potential. The shunt is then localized by repeating the single breath inhalation of hy-

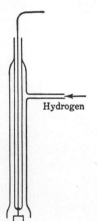

Hydrogen

Figure 8-1.   The Hildebrand hydrogen electrode. (From Glasstone, *The Elements of Physical Chemistry,* D. Van Nostrand Co., Princeton, N.J., 1946.)

drogen and searching for the maximum developed potential as the catheter is moved about the right heart while monitoring the position of the catheter with a fluoroscope.

The hydrogen electrode could be used (in theory at least) to measure the pH of solutions. It does, however, possess certain practical inconveniences, obvious from the foregoing description, which limit its everyday use both as a pH-determining electrode and as a practical standard electrode in the laboratory. Accordingly, electrodes of high stability and convenience (called standard or reference electrodes) are normally used to measure and compare potentials. Perhaps the two most practical reference electrodes are the calomel and the silver-silver chloride electrodes.

8-4. THE CALOMEL ELECTRODE

The calomel electrode (Fig. 8-2) is one of the most stable of the practical reference electrodes. The potential is developed across a junction of pure mercury and potassium chloride solution, which is saturated with calomel (mercurous chloride). The potential of the calomel electrode is dependent on the concentration of the potassium chloride solution used. Measurement of potential by means of the calomel electrode (or calomel half-cell, as it is

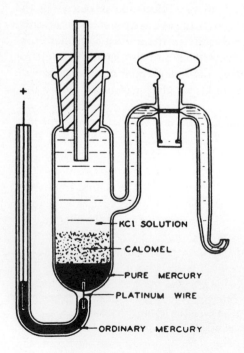

KCl SOLUTION

CALOMEL

PURE MERCURY

PLATINUM WIRE

ORDINARY MERCURY

Figure 8-2. The calomel electrode. (From Wellard, Merritt, and Dean, *Instrumental Methods Analysis*, D. Van Nostrand Co., Princeton, N.J., 1951.)

often called) and other half-cells, which may likewise possess a fluid boundary, gives a rise to a potential between the two liquid junctions. Such liquid-to-liquid junction potentials are minimized by the use of a "salt bridge," which usually consists of a saturated solution of potassium chloride held in an agar gel in a glass tube and serves as a liquid conductor to connect one liquid with the other. Potassium chloride is especially useful for this purpose because the potassium and chloride ions possess approximately the same mobilities, hence minimize the formation of concentration gradients and resulting electrical potentials. If potassium chloride cannot be used because the presence of certain ions (such as silver) in one or both solutions may produce undesirable chemical reactions, ammonium nitrate may be substituted.

Apart from the practicality of the calomel cell, its chief advantage lies in the stability of its potential over long periods. Because it is a chemical cell, temperature influences the mobility of the ions and hence a small temperature correction is necessary. The EMFs of typical calomel cells are listed in Table 8-2.

8-5.   THE SILVER–SILVER CHLORIDE ELECTRODE

Silver-silver chloride (Ag-AgCl) is widely used as a reference electrode because such electrodes are easy to prepare, reproducible, and small. A most complete summary of the preparation, characteristics, and application of this type of electrode was presented by Janz and Taniguchi (1953). Although there are many techniques for preparing these electrodes, one of the easiest methods consists of placing the cleaned silver specimen to be chlorided in a solution of sodium chloride. The specimen is then made positive with respect to a silver plate or wire also in the solution. The silver ions combine with the chloride ions to produce neutral silver chloride molecules, which coat the silver anode. For general purpose Ag-AgCl electrodes, Cooper (1963) recommended chloriding at the rate of about 2.5 mA/cm^2 for several minutes in bromide-free sodium chloride solution. The strength of this solution is not critical but should be at least that of physiological saline (0.9%). Copper pointed out further that contrary to general belief, the properties of the chloride layer are not materially changed by continued exposure to light, although Ag-AgCl is photosensitive and produces photovoltaic potentials that can be troublesome in some cases, such as recording the EEG while employing photic stimulation. The potential of the Ag-AgCl electrode is dependent on the solution which it contacts and the temperature. Typical values are presented in Table 8-2. Additional information regarding use of the Ag-AgCl electrode for recording bioelectric events is found in Chapter 9.

Table 8-2 The EMFs of Reference Cells*

Cell Type	EMF† (V)	Correction (V/°C)
Mercury-calomel		
Hg/HgCl$_2$/0.01 MKCl	+0.388	+0.00094
Hg/HgCl$_2$/0.1 MKCl	+0.333	+0.00079
Hg/HgCl$_2$/1.0 MKCl	+0.280	+0.00059 avg.
Hg/HgCl$_2$/3.5 MKCl	+0.247	+0.00047
Silver-silver chloride		
Ag/AgCl/0.01 MKCl	+0.343	+0.000617
Ag/AgCl/0.1 MKCl	+0.288	+0.000431
Ag/AgCl/1.0 MKCl	+0.235	+0.000250

* From *Encyclopedia of Electrochemistry*, C. A. Hampel (ed.), Reinhold Publishing Corp., New York, 1964.
† Referred to standard hydrogen electrode at 25°C.

8-6. THE pH ELECTRODE

Because it is impractical to use the standard hydrogen electrode to determine pH, the glass electrode is ordinarily employed. A typical glass electrode is illustrated in Fig. 8-3. According to Bull (1943), the glass electrode was discovered by Cremer and was developed by Haber and Klemensiewicz. It consists of a thin glass membrane that permits the passage of only hydrogen ions (in the form H_3O^+). The usual configuration consists of a spherical bulb 0.25 in. in diameter. On the inside of the pH-responsive glass bulb is placed a buffer solution, usually of pH = 1, in which is immersed an Ag-AgCl electrode. The other side of the glass bulb is exposed to the solution of unknown pH. The connection to the potential-measuring circuit and the solution being tested is completed through a potassium chloride salt bridge and a calomel cell.

The mechanism underlying the operation of the glass electrode is far from simple, and several theories have been proposed to explain the origin of the pH-dependent potential. According to Eisenman (1967), opinion regarding the origin of the glass electrode potential was for many years divided into two schools of thought. One view held that the potential was exclusively a phase-boundary potential produced at the membrane-solution interfaces. The other view attributed it to a diffusion potential arising within the membrane. These views have been reconciled, and Eisenman states, "It now seems virtually certain that the glass electrode is nothing more or less than a perfect cation-exchange membrane, whose electrode potential represents a sum of contributions from both diffusion and phase-boundary processes.'' The total glass electrode potential is therefore expressed as the sum of the two boundary potentials produced at the membrane-solution interfaces and the diffusion potential arising within the glass. The interested reader is referred to Eisenman (1967) for detailed theoretical and practical information pertaining to glass electrodes.

The potential developed across the glass membrane is about 60 mV per unit of pH at 30°C. Operation at a different temperature requires the application of a small correction.

The glass electrode made the determination of pH in the laboratory a simple and routine procedure. Bull (1943) listed the following advantages of the glass electrode as compiled by Dole et al. (1941):

1. The glass electrode is independent of oxidation-reduction potentials.
2. It is not necessary to pass a gas through the solution or to add any material to it.
3. It is possible to use very small quantities of solution.
4. The electrode can be used in colored or turbid solutions.
5. The electrode gives accurate values in unbuffered solutions.
6. Equilibrium is reached rapidly.

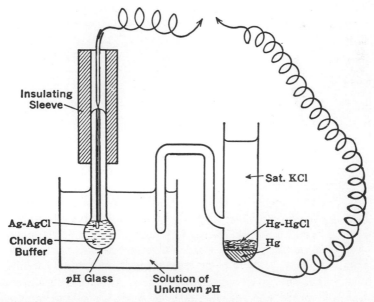

Figure 8-3.   The glass electrode used with the calomel half-cell to measure pH. (From H. B. Bull, *Physical Biochemistry,* Wiley, New York, 1943. By permission.)

The glass electrode does, however, possess some limitations. The range of pH over which accurate response is obtained may be restricted unless special glasses are used. For example, some error often exists in both highly acidic solutions (near pH = 0) and alkaline solutions (above pH = 9). Figure 8-4 shows the error in pH for both acid and alkaline solutions for electrodes constructed from the classical Corning 015 glass; the amount of error encountered because of sodium and potassium ion concentration can be seen. Errors in pH measurement in the range above pH = 9 are known as "salt" or "alkaline" errors. It is now possible to purchase pH electrodes constructed from special glass for use over the range pH = 0 to 14 with only a slight correction required above pH = 13.

Because the pH is determined in terms of the potential developed by the pH electrode, the magnitude of the potential must be accurately measured. Since the potential is developed by the diffusion of relatively few ions across a glass surface, which in itself is a good insulator, the pH electrode has the characteristics of a potential source with a very high internal impedance. Typical values are in excess of 200 MΩ. To prevent the device used to measure this potential from drawing current from the electrode, it must possess an input impedance much higher than that of the pH electrode. (The problem of loading is discussed in Chapter 9.) This requirement is met by use of a potentiometer or a voltage-measuring instrument which employs an electrometer tube or a field-effect transistor in the input stage.

While *in vitro* measurements of pH abound in the life sciences, the

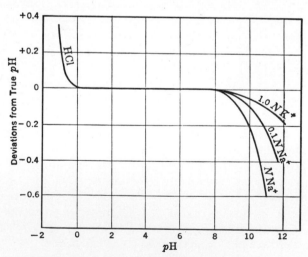

Figure 8-4.   Glass electrode error as a function of solution pH. (From M. Dole, *Theoretical and Experimental Electrochemistry*, McGraw, New York, 1935. By permission.)

continuous recording of pH changes *in vivo* has been carried out less frequently although the number of investigations has increased with the improvement of pH-monitoring equipment. The stability and sensitivity requirements of pH-measuring devices for *in vivo* work can be appreciated by recalling that the range of hydrogen ion concentration compatible with normal cellular function is about one pH unit; therefore, to record continuously pH *in vivo* means that the recording system is never presented with a signal greater than 60 mV. When measuring mammalian arterial blood, the normal pH range is about 7.36 to 7.44, and the signal obtainable is only 5 mV. Accordingly, this amplitude must be adequately displayed by the recording stylus or indicator. If smaller changes within the normal range are to be registered, the recording system must possess a sensitivity and stability in the microvolt range.

One of the earliest to measure pH *in vivo* electrically was McClendon (1915), who passed a platinum gaseous hydrogen, calomel electrode assembly into the stomachs and duodenums of adults and infants to make readings of the pH. Continuous recording of pH was introduced by Gesell and Hertzman (1926). Using a cuvette equipped with a MnO_2 electrode paired with a calomel cell affixed to a continuous aspirating device, they recorded pH changes of arterial and venous blood under a variety of circumstances to investigate the effect of pH on the respiratory center. Voegtlin et al. (1930) introduced the application of the glass electrode for continuously measuring blood pH, using electrodes mounted in a flow-through cuvette. They referred to graphic recording and proved that such an electrode system is insensitive to changes in blood flow. A similar electrode system described by Fruhling and Winterstein (1934) was used to make recordings of the pH of carotid artery blood of dogs. Dubuisson (1937) recorded a pH change of a few tenths of a pH unit within a second after the beginning of contraction of skeletal muscle. Continuous records of pH changes on the surface of the cortices of monkeys were made by Dusser de Barenne et al. (1937). They employed a glass electrode paired with a Ag-AgCl electrode filled with physiological saline to avoid the injurious action of the potassium ion in the calomel electrode.

The technique of prolonged recording of pH in the blood of experimental animals was investigated thoroughly by Nims and his co-workers. In a series of papers (1937) they discussed the construction of electrodes suitable for recording pH in flowing blood and described experiments in which continuous records of pH changes were made for periods up to 8 hr. Elegant records of rhythmic changes of approximately 0.1 pH unit in the anesthetized dog were presented. Marshall and Nims (1937) recorded the blood pH response to a variety of injected substances, and Nims et al.

(1938) showed that by careful adjustment of the respirator, the pH could be maintained at a chosen level in the curarized dog.

Band and Semple (1967) developed a rapidly responding, indwelling arterial glass electrode for the continuous measurement of blood pH. The pH-sensitive cell consisted of a glass electrode and a Ag-AgCl reference electrode, both lying in the lumen of an intra-arterial needle. The outside diameter of the pH-sensitive glass portion of the electrode measured 0.5 to 0.8 mm, the wall thickness 0.0025 to 0.50 mm, and the length 1.5 to 2.0 cm. The 90% response to a change in pH of blood flowing past the electrode at 2 ml/min was 0.5 sec. The two samples of blood used to measure the response time had been equilibrated previously with 4 and 6% CO_2. In a test performed by driving buffers past the electrode *in situ* at high flow rates (10 ml/min), 90% of the response occurred in about 40 msec.

For the most part, the glass electrode is an excellent device for monitoring pH and changes in pH. Some limitations and precautions, however, should be mentioned in connection with its use. The glass electrode exhibits a loss of sensitivity and decreased speed of response after a period of service (i.e., a couple of months). This deterioration may be accelerated, becoming more severe when the electrode is employed in solutions containing proteins. The electrode may be restored repeatedly by etching the glass surface to remove the inactive outer layer. According to Brems (1962), the sensitivity of the glass electrode increases by 0.34%/°C with rising temperature, and the electrical resistance of the glass increases with falling temperature, increasing accordingly the required input impedance of the recording device. Because the active portion of the electrode consists of a thin glass bulb, obvious precautions are required to prevent breakage.

Mattock and Band (1967) have called attention to the limitations of glass electrodes for both pH and cation determinations. In regard to accuracy of measurement, these investigators state:

"It is probably true to say that the accuracy of most pH measurements in terms of interpretative values is relatively poor, and insufficient work has been done to establish how accurate are most of the measurements of cations by electrochemical methods. A good reproducibility or even a good discrimination does not imply good accuracy, since this, if related (as is usual) to an individual ion activity, depends mainly on the validity of the extrathermodynamic assumptions which have to be made in the interpretation of the Nernst equation."

These investigators give the following example showing the degree of difference between accuracy and discrimination which can arise:

"In blood pH measurements it is probably fair to say that a discrimination between samples to within ± 0.004 pH unit ($\equiv \pm 1\%$) is possible, but that accuracy in terms of translation to hydrogen ion activity cannot be any better than ± 0.02 pH unit ($\equiv 4.5\%$). This implies that an operational pH scale for blood can be defined quite closely, without involving interpretation of the pH numbers to beyond a 'notional' activity, but that an absolute activity determination from these numbers can only be uncertain."

8-7. THE pCO₂ ELECTRODE

The pCO₂ electrode was first described by Stow et al. (1957). It consisted of a standard glass pH electrode covered with a rubber membrane permeable to CO_2. Between the glass surface and the membrane was a thin film of water. The solution under test, which contained dissolved CO_2, was presented to the outer surface of the rubber membrane. The film of water equilibrated with the CO_2 in the solution under test by diffusion of CO_2 across the membrane. After equilibration, the pH of the aqueous film was measured by the glass electrode and interpreted in terms of pCO₂ on the basis of the linear relationship between log pCO₂ and pH as described by the Henderson-Hasselbalch equation.

The Stow pCO₂ electrode was improved by Severinghaus and Bradley (1958), who showed both analytically and experimentally that the sensitivity of the electrode could be doubled by including bicarbonate ion in the aqueous medium between the rubber membrane and the glass electrode. These investigators also found that wet Teflon backed with a layer of cellophane 0.002 in. thick was a superior membrane. The optimum aqueous solution consisted of 0.01 M NaHCO₃ and 0.1M NaCl in which the cellophane had been soaked for several hours. In addition to these modifications of Stow's electrode, Severinghaus and Bradley added NaCl to the solution surrounding the silver reference electrode, thus increasing the conductivity of this solution and stabilizing the reference electrode. The resulting modified pCO₂ electrode was twice as sensitive and drifted much less than before. The response time was such that equilibrium was reached in about 2 min after a fourfold rise in CO_2 and in about 4 min after a fourfold fall in CO_2.

Further improvements in stability and response time, achieved by utilization of a flat-plane membrane glass electrode for tissue measurements, were reported by Hertz and Siesjö (1959). The increase in overall stability was also due to the use of a calomel cell (made an integral part of the electrode) instead of the Ag-AgCl reference cell. The response time was reduced to 25 to 30 sec for 90% response by employing a more dilute NaHCO₃ solution (0.0001 N). The use of this dilute solution, however, reduced the sensitivity slightly and introduced an initial rapid drift toward alkalinity, followed later by a slower drift. The use of a 0.001 N solution of

NaHCO₃ appeared to provide a good compromise between drift and response time, although more dilute solutions (even distilled water) were required when rapid response time was the primary consideration. The response times for the electrode at 36°C in saline, equilibrated with different gas mixtures of known CO_2 concentrations, are shown in Fig. 8-5. Because of its unique construction, this electrode could not be used in the horizontal or inverted position.

Severinghaus (1962) reported improvement in both response time and

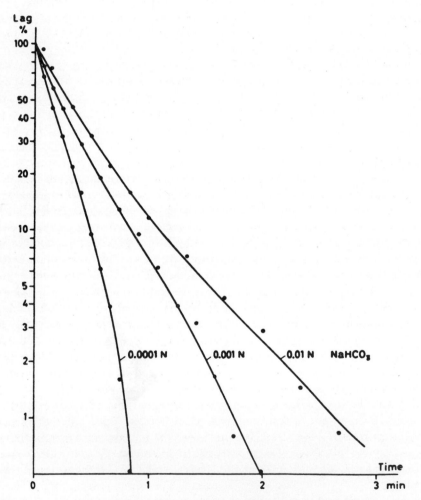

Figure 8-5. The response time of the pCO_2 electrode. [From C. H. Hertz and B. Siesjo, *Acta Physiol. Scand.* **47**:115–123 (1959). By permission.]

linearity of the Severinghaus-Bradley electrode in the low pCO_2 range by replacing the cellophane spacer used to hold the water film on the surface of the glass electrode with very thin nylon mesh from a stocking. Fibers of glass wool or powdered glass wool were also found to constitute good separators. By using a membrane of 3/8-mil Teflon and glass wool for the separator, electrodes with 95% response in 20 sec were constructed. It was discovered that glass wool catalyzed the reaction of CO_2 with water. The response time was found to be almost entirely due to the diffusion rate, which was governed by the membrane thickness and temperature. According to Severinghaus, the response time was reduced further by the addition of hemolyzed blood to the electrolyte. The blood provides carbonic anhydrase activity for 1 or 2 days.

In an effort to reduce the response time further, Reyes and Neville (1967) used 0.5-mil polyethylene as a pCO_2 electrode membrane. No separator or spacing material was placed between the glass surface and the membrane. A commercial preparation of carbonic anhydrase was added to the electrolyte. The response time of this electrode was 6 sec for 90% of a step change from 2 to 5% CO_2.

In commercially available equipment that uses the Astrup method for the determination of blood pCO_2, the same electrode employed for measuring pH directly serves also to determine pCO_2.[1] The procedure makes use of a nomogram shown in Fig. 8-6, the ordinate of which is pCO_2 in mm Hg plotted on a log scale, and the abscissa is pH plotted on a linear scale. Briefly, the method employed is as follows. First, the pH of a small sample of heparinized blood (drawn from a capillary bed such as the lobe of the ear) is measured directly. This is the actual pH value, and it determines a vertical line passing through this point on the pH axis. Next, two other small samples taken at the same as the first are equilibrated under temperature control with two different standard gas mixtures of known pCO_2 60 and 30 mm Hg, for example. The pH of the equilibrated blood samples is then measured directly with the pH electrode. These two values are then plotted on the nomogram (points *A* and *B*, respectively), and a straight line is drawn between them. The intersection of line *A-B* with the vertical line through the actual pH value (point *C*) is projected to the pCO_2 axis, from which the actual pCO_2 is read. This construction also permits reading values of standard bicarbonate, base excess, and buffer base (all in milliequivalents per liter). The basis of this method was reported by Siggaard-Andersen and Engel (1960), and Siggaard-Andersen (1962).

[1] Radiometer Co., Copenhagen, Denmark.

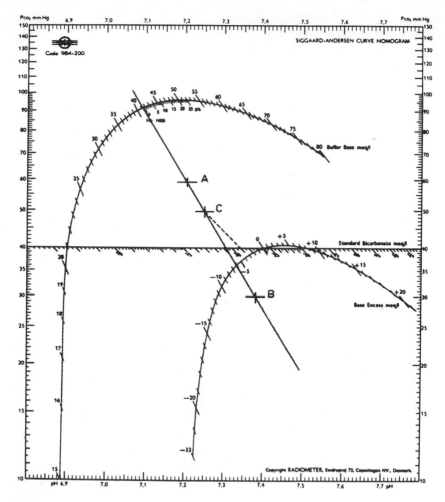

Figure 8-6.   Acid-base nomogram according to Siggaard-Andersen and Engel. (From Radiometer Bulletin 21917E, Copenhagen. By permission.)

8-8.   THE pO₂ (OXYGEN) ELECTRODE

In the study of oxygen concentration levels in biological systems, the oxygen electrode provides a means of measuring the partial pressure of oxygen directly at the point of insertion into the tissue. Localization is limited only by the size of the electrode. This is in contrast to manometric methods, which measure the total oxygen concentration in that portion of a biological system that can be isolated and brought to equilibrium with the oxygen in a manometer. An excellent discussion of the principles and techniques pertaining to the use of the oxygen electrode has been presented by Davies (1962). Davies prefers to call this electrode, which is used to measure dissolved oxygen, an oxygen cathode. This terminology serves to avoid possible confusion with the oxygen electrode as understood in physical chemistry, which operates under equilibrium conditions and possesses a standard potential of +1.229 V relative to the hydrogen electrode. The term oxygen electrode is employed in this book, since it is the designation most often used by workers in the life sciences.

A method for applying the oxygen electrode to measure the partial pressure of dissolved oxygen is diagramed in Fig. 8-7. The oxygen electrode itself is a piece of platinum wire embedded in an insulating glass holder with the end of the wire exposed to the solution under measurement. According to Davies (1962), the principle of operation of the electrode is as follows:

1. When the platinum electrode is made slightly negative (about -0.2 V) with respect to the reference electrode, oxygen reaching the surface of the platinum is reduced electrolytically (i.e., the O$_2$ accepts electrons). The reaction at the cathode is, however, not fully understood.

2. When the platinum is made more negative (-0.6 to -0.9 V), the velocity of the electrolytic reduction is limited by the maximum rate at which O$_2$ can diffuse to the electrode surface and is not affected greatly by the magnitude of the potential difference. In this voltage range it is found that the current flowing is proportional to the oxygen concentration in the body of the solution.

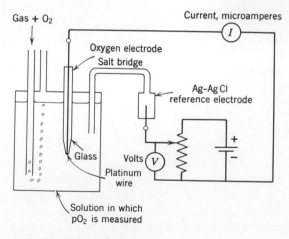

Figure 8-7.   The pO$_2$ electrode.

The shape of the electrode current versus potential relationship is shown in Fig. 8-8a. The electrode is operated in the "plateau" region over which the current shows very little dependence upon the applied voltage. If the potential is held constant (at -0.7 V, e.g.), the current is a linear function of the partial pressure of dissolved oxygen, which is expressed as percent O_2 in Fig. 8-8b.

Although most of the commercially available pO_2 electrodes exhibit a response time of 30 to 60 sec, it is possible to construct electrodes with a very short response time. Figure 8-9 gives the response time of an open-type oxygen electrode to a sudden change in pO_2 as reported by Davies (1962). The 0 to 90% response time of the recording system, including the capacitance of the O_2 electrode and wiring, was determined to be about 25 μsec. The rise time of this particular electrode is seen to be approximately 0.3 msec (300 μsec), which is certainly adequate to monitor continuously localized varying changes in tissue oxygen content.

The oxygen electrode is not free of practical difficulties. The problem known as electrode aging presents itself as a slow reduction in current over time (minutes or hours), even though the O_2 tension of the test medium is maintained at a constant level. Aging requires frequent recalibration of the electrode. The exact cause of aging is not known, but the phenomenon is associated with material attaching itself to the electrode surface. Two measures are often used to combat this problem. First, the electrode is covered with a protective film such as polyethylene, which has the undesirable effect of shielding the electrode from the dissolved O_2, consequently increasing the response time (0 to 90%) to as much as 2.5 min. The second procedure employed to minimize aging is to reverse the flow of current frequently to lower or reverse the accumulation of surface contaminants.

Another problem encountered with the oxygen electrode is created by the presence of the electrode itself. The O_2 diffusion field is maximal in the vicinity of the electrode, causing the concentration of O_2 there to be different from what would exist in the absence of the electrode. This source of error is reduced by constantly rotating or vibrating the electrode or by giving it a special geometrical shape.

Olson et al. (1949) reported an investigation that explored the application of alternating potential techniques to overcome the difficulties attending the use of open, static platinum electrodes. This method employed switching the potential pattern imposed on an electrolytic cell consisting of a platinum electrode of 20-gauge wire about 3 mm long versus a 0.1 M calomel half-cell, both immersed in a 0.1 M KCl solution. Dual cells were used as a means of comparing electrode performance in oxygen and nitrogen-saturated KCl solutions. The applied potential pattern consisted of a square positive pulse followed by an interval during which the applied

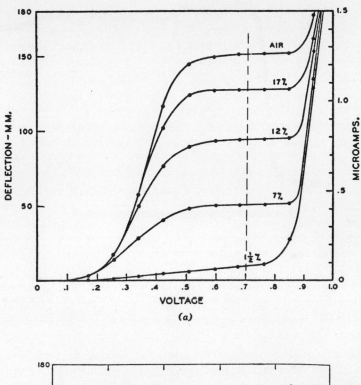

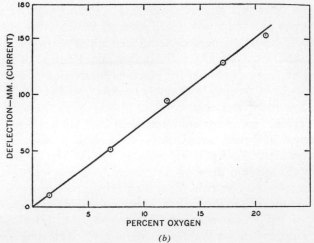

Figure 8-8. (*a*) Current-voltage characteristics of the pO_2 electrode (a). (*b*) Response of pO_2 electrode versus percentage of oxygen; values obtained from (*a*) for polarization voltage of 0.7 V. [From R. A. Olsen, F. S. Brackett, and R. G. Crickard, *J. Gen. Physiol.* **32**:687–703 (1949). By permission.]

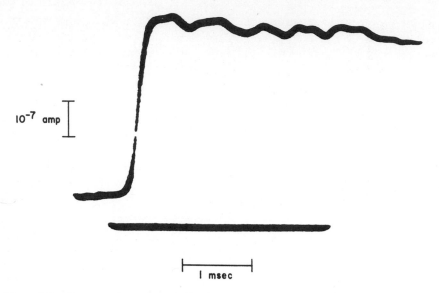

Figure 8-9.   Response time of open-type pO₂ electrode. [From P. W. Davies, *in Physical Techniques in Biological Research,* W. L. Nastuk (ed.), vol. IV, Academic Press, New York, 1962. By permission.]

potential was suddenly reduced to zero by shorting the cell through a resistance. The short was then removed and a square negative pulse applied, after which the short was again induced before application of the positive pulse to begin the next cycle. Observations were made over the range of 30 cycles/sec down to 6 to 12 cycles/min. Because of the time required for stabilization of the oxygen plateau, the maximum rate at which the potential could be switched and stable values of current output obtained was between 5 and 10 cycles/min.

The Clark (1956) type of oxygen electrode (Fig. 8-10) has been employed widely by many biological investigators. It is of single-unit construction with a self-contained Ag-AgCl reference electrode. The entire device is isolated from the solution under measurement by a polythene membrane. This feature allows the electrode to be used for measuring oxygen tension in solutions of poor electrical conductivity or in the gas phase. The stability of response of the Clark electrode depends on the diffusion distance between the platinum surface and the membrane. Care must be exercised to ensure that the membrane is kept taut to maintain the diffusion distance constant.

In physiology the pO₂ electrode has been applied extensively to monitor the partial pressure of oxygen in biological fluids. Among the first to exploit the method were Davies and Brink (1942), who described the construction of a bare platinum electrode paired with a calomel cell polarized with 0.6 V. Using this system they successfully recorded the oxygen tension changes in the arterioles of a cat's brain and in skeletal muscle during contraction. Their paper, which discusses the theory and electrode reactions, as well as many of the practical details of the method, is recommended reading for those wishing to enter the field. Kreuzer et al. (1958) compared the fidelity of the pO₂-electrode method with that of standard chemical procedures.

Two interesting and useful *in vitro* pO₂ electrodes were described by Tobias (1947, 1949). One was built into a hypodermic syringe barrel, and on withdrawal of a blood sample from a vessel into the syringe, the pO₂

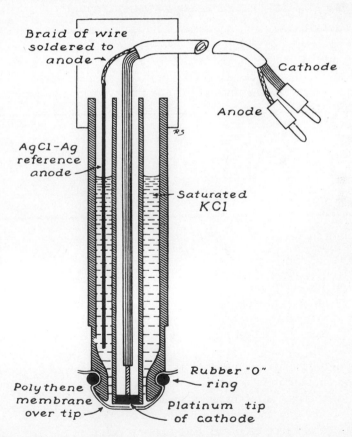

Figure 8-10. The Clark-type pO₂ electrode. [From B. J. Sproule et al., *J. Appl. Physiol.* **11**:365–370 (1957). By permission.]

tension was instantly read on a calibrated galvanometer; the other was built into a hypodermic needle, which Tobias used to measure pO_2 in the eyelid, lip, and vagina.

Detailed descriptions of use of the pO_2 electrode to measure the oxygen tension in the brain of a cat were presented by Davies and Brink (1942). Davies et al. (1943–1944) presented multichannel recordings of the EEG and local oxygen tension changes in experimental animals during convulsions. Using an ingenious occlusion method, Davies et al. (1948) recorded the rate of oxygen consumption on the surface of the cortex of cats before and after electrical stimulation of the brain. Clark (1956) developed a unique electrode assembly for monitoring oxygen tension in heart-lung machines. Clark et al. (1957, 1958) also achieved the remarkable feat of chronically implanting pO_2 electrodes in the brains of cats and he recorded the local oxygen tension over a period of months to years.

The rate of oxygen consumption at synaptic endings of sympathetic ganglia was measured by Bronk et al. (1946), using the occlusion technique. They found that 90 sec elapsed before the oxygen tension dropped to near-zero levels. Posternak et al. (1947), recording in the same region, found that the oxygen consumption was doubled when the ganglia were electrically stimulated at a rate of 15/sec.

In frog and crab nerve fibers, pO_2 microelectrodes were used by Bronk et al. (1947) and Carlson et al. (1948) to record the oxygen consumption during stimulation. They found that oxygen consumption outlasted heat production by as much as 0.5 min.

Regional oxygen tensions have been measured on a variety of other tissues. Davies (1946), who recorded the consumption of oxygen in frog skeletal muscle during and following a single twitch, noted a fall in the oxygen tension during the first half-second and a return to the control level in 2 sec. Oxygen tension measurements have also been recorded by Cater et al. (1957) in the intact lactating mammary gland and in tumors.

For the measurement of pO_2 in solution the oxygen electrode offers several advantages; among them are (a) the current obtained is linearly related to the concentration of oxygen; (b) the electrode can be made small enough to measure concentrations in highly localized areas; (c) when used in vitro, only a small sample of fluid is required; and (d) the measurement requires only seconds as compared to minutes for chemical determination. Electrode configurations have been developed with a response time short enough for continuous recording of transient changes.

Probably the greatest difficulty in the use of the pO_2 electrode is the size of the electrical signal produced. Although provision of a known stable polarizing voltage offers no difficulties, measurement of the current representing the partial pressure of oxygen presents special problems. The current measured by Tobias (1949) was 0.650 μA for a 500-mm Hg oxygen tension. The total range of the indicator used by Davies and Brink (1942) was 0.05 μA for an oxygen tension of 180 mm Hg. The recorder sensitivity employed by Kreuzer et al. (1958) was 0.96 μA, and that described by Clark et al. (1958) produced a full-scale deflection for 0.98 μA. The signal detected by Cater et al. (1957) was 0.01 μA.

8-9. THE COMBINED pO₂ AND pCO₂ ELECTRODE

With care in mechanical design, it is possible to combine the pO_2 and pCO_2 electrode in one assembly. Figure 8-11 shows an arrangement of a pO_2 electrode operating on the Clark principle and a pCO_2 electrode based on the Severinghaus principle, mounted in a temperature-controlled cell to continuously monitor a single stream of fluids or gases.[2] The following performance data are given for this combined electrode.

Characteristic	pCO₂ Electrode	pO₂ Electrode
Response time	1.5 min (38°C)	30–60 sec (38°C)
Volume (minimum)	70 μl (with thermostatted cell)	
Accuracy	1% + error of adjustment	

The practical considerations of the routine use and maintenance of pH,

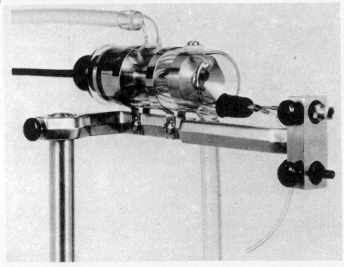

Figure 8-11. The combined pO₂ and pCO₂ electrode. (From Radiometer Catalog, 1967, Copenhagen. By permission.)

---

[2] Radiometer Co., Copenhagen, Denmark.

pO_2, and pCO_2 electrodes in a cardiopulmonary physiology laboratory have been described by Purcell and Rodman (1965). These investigators compared the measurements obtained from these electrodes with those obtained from the classical procedures and emphasized the greater ease, convenience, and simplicity of use provided by the electrodes.

8-10. CATION ELECTRODES

The Nernst equation is the basis of all membrane electrodes, as was pointed out at the beginning of this chapter. Accordingly, the development of specific electrodes for a particular species of ions has logically centered on finding selective membranes that allow the reversible transfer of the desired ions only. Membranes of this type are called permselective membranes, and the desirable characteristics that they should possess were summarized by Sollner (1958) as follows:

"1. The membranes should exhibit an extreme degree of ionic selectivity even at relatively high concentrations, so that the thermodynamically possible maximum of the concentration potential may be approached closely over wide concentration ranges.

"2. The absolute permeability of the membranes for the nonrestricted critical ions should be high, so that all ionic processes across them can occur at a rapid rate; this means the ohmic resistance of the membranes should be low.

"3. The membranes should come readily to equilibrium with electrolytic solutions, so that stable, well-defined states (and potentials) may quickly be established across their thickness, this quality obviously being closely related to the thickness of the membranes and their ohmic resistance.

"4. The membranes should not deteriorate to a significant extent even on prolonged contact with electrolyte solutions.

"5. The membranes should be mechanically satisfactory, i.e., they should be smooth, uniform in thickness over their whole area, and strong enough for the purpose for which they are designed, high mechanical strength being a prerequisite for their successful industrial use.

"6. The preparation of the membranes should be easy and reproducible.

"7. For many scientific purposes the membranes should be of low ion exchange capacity per unit area."

In view of the considerable experience gained over the years in the development and use of the glass electrode for pH measurement, it was certainly to be expected that the possibility of making glass specific for other ions would be investigated. On the basis of the observation by von Lengyel and Blum (1934) that the addition of Al_2O_3 or B_2O_3 to sodium silicate glass caused the glass electrode potential to become strongly dependent on the concentration of several cations besides H^+, Eisenman et al. (1957) and Eisenman (1962) studied the relative cation sensitivities of various glasses as a function of their composition for the purpose of developing an electrode for measuring Na^+ activity in complex mixtures of ions. They constructed glass electrodes from various mixtures of oxides of sodium, aluminum, and silicon, and produced one having 250 times more sensitivity to sodium than potassium at pH = 7.6. They stated that the ultimate limits of specificity were unknown and that in biological fluids containing 0.15 M Na$^+$ or more, the electrode produced a sodium ion voltage with less than 0.2% error in the presence of potassium concentrations up to 30 mM at any pH greater than 5.6. In addition, the electrode was insensitive to calcium, magnesium, ammonia, and lithium ions except when these components were present in unusual concentrations. Although data relating to the rapidity of response were not given, attention was called to the fact that the drift was less than 1.3%/hr. Moreover, the sodium-sensitive electrode could be used with any pH meter and was not poisoned by constituents of serum, cerebrospinal fluid, or brain homogenate, even after it was soaked in these solutions for many hours.

Although the main concern of Eisenman and co-workers was the creation of an electrode for sodium ions, they found that certain mixtures of the oxides resulted in electrodes having a high specificity for potassium. They did not pursue this study further, but certainly this evidence promises a transducer for potassium ion.

Friedman et al. (1959), using a flow-through cuvette-type electrode, recorded continuously the concentration of sodium in the femoral arteries of dogs. They noted that the electrode was flow-sensitive in certain flow ranges, but not in others. Their striking records, made with a direct recorder, illustrate changes of a few milliequivalents per liter in sodium concentration produced by a variety of pressor and depressor drugs.

8-11. ELECTRODES FOR DIVALENT IONS

At least one manufacturer[3] markets a permselective electrode that is sensitive to certain divalent ions. The following material represents a summary of technical information released by this company.

[3] Orion Research, Inc., Cambridge, Mass.

The electrode operation depends on the potential developed across a liquid ion-exchange membrane in which the conducting material is a water-immiscible liquid ion exchanger held by an extremely thin, porous, inert membrane disk. The liquid ion exchanger is a salt of an organophosphoric acid which exhibits a very high specificity for divalent ions. Electrical conductivity between the inner surface of the membrane and the Ag-AgCl reference cell is established by filling the electrode with calcium chloride solution. The calcium ion establishes a stable potential between the calcium chloride solution and the inner surface of the membrane, while the chloride ion provides a stable potential between the reference electrode and the solution. With all junction potentials stabilized, observed changes in potential are produced by changes in the activities of divalent ions in the sample under measurement.

Figure 8-12 compares the conventional glass electrode and the liquid-membrane divalent ion electrode. This electrode has been designed to give almost identical response to calcium and magnesium ions on a molar basis, while providing slightly higher selectivity for Ni^{2+}, Zn^{2+}, Fe^{2+}, and Ca^{2+}. It is slightly less selective for Ba^{2+} and Sr^{2+}. The electrode shows negligible error in the presence of 10^{-2} mole/l sodium or potassium down to 10^{-4} mole/l calcium (or other divalent) ions. The selectivity is tenfold higher for Pb^{2+} than for Ca^{2+}. The electrode detects calcium down to 10^{-5} mole/l. It

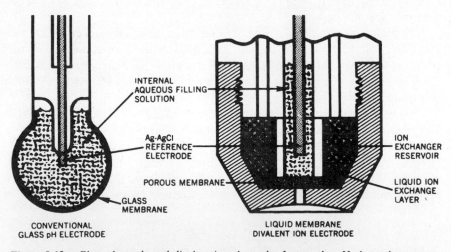

Figure 8-12. Glass electrode and divalent ion electrode. Just as the pH electrode measures hydrogen ion activity, the divalent ion electrode measures divalent activities. In the pH electrode the potential is developed across a glass membrane; in the calcium electrode the membrane is a thin layer of ion exchanger. (From "Divalent Cation Activity Electrode," Orion Research, Inc., Cambridge, Mass., 1966. By permission.)

may be used over a range of pH from 5 to 11 with negligible error resulting from pH changes. The electrode can be employed with any modern expanded-scale pH meter and a conventional calomel reference electrode. It operates over a temperature range of 0 to 50°C and has an electrical resistance of less than 25 MΩ at 25°C. The minimum sample size is less than 5 ml in a 50-ml beaker or 0.3 ml in a special microsample container. Under average operating conditions the minimum useful life of the electrode membrane and ion exchanger is 30 days without replacement.

Ross (1967) reported the development of a simple calcium-selective electrode capable of measuring calcium ion activity in the presence of many common interferring ions. The electrode utilizes a liquid ion-exchanger membrane containing the calcium salt of a disubstituted phosphoric acid and is able to measure free calcium ion activity in the presence of a thousand-fold excess of sodium or potassium ions.

An electrode to measure sulfide ion activity is available commercially, and the following information has been supplied by the manufacturer.[4] This electrode is constructed of unbreakable plastic; because it is a solid-state device, it requires no renewal. No interference is obtained from a wide variety of other anions. The electrode will detect any level of sulfide for which stable standard solutions can be prepared. Its ultimate sensitivity is below 10^{-17} M, and it will follow sulfide activity over the pH range 1 to 12.

8-12.   FLUORIDE ION ELECTRODE

The development of an electrode for measurement of fluoride ion activity has been announced by Frant and Ross (1966). The principle of construction of the electrode is similar to that of a conventional glass pH electrode except that the membrane material is a disk-shaped section of a single-crystal rare earth fluoride, such as LaF_3, NdF_3, or PrF_3. The disk-shaped section (1 cm in diameter, 1 to 2 mm thick) is cemented to the end of a rigid polyvinyl chloride tube filled with a solution containing both fluoride and chloride ions (typically 0.1 M NaF and 0.1 M KCl), and electrical contact is made by inserting a Ag-AgCl electrode into the solution. Electrical connection to the test sample is through a standard saturated calomel cell. Measurements were reproducible to within less than 1 mV.

Because the membrane is permeable only to fluoride ions, the potential developed is given by the Nernst equation. The only significant interference comes from the hydroxide ion, as would be expected on the basis of similarities in charge and ionic radii. The electrode response as a function of pH and fluoride concentration is given in Fig. 8-13.

---

[4] Orion Research, Inc., Cambridge, Mass.

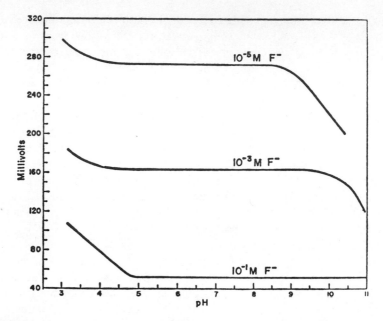

Figure 8-13.   Sensitivity characteristics of the fluoride ion electrode. [From M. S. Frant and J. W. Ross, *Science* **154**:1533–1554 (1966). Copyright 1966 by the American Association for the Advancement of Science. By permission.]

8-13.   CONTINUOUS MONITORING OF BLOOD CHEMISTRY

Gotoh et al. (1966), in a study of cerebral blood flow and metabolism, have reported the simultaneous use of several chemical transducers to monitor venous and arterial blood in more than 80 human subjects. The arrangement of equipment employed by these investigators is illustrated in Fig. 8-14. Arterial and venous blood was passed through similar transparent acrylic cuvettes, which were maintained at body temperature. Transducers mounted in the cuvettes monitored the values of pO_2, pCO_2, pH, Na^+, and K^+ in the circulating heparinized blood. Other physiological data, such as the EEG, ECG, blood pressure, temperature, expired pCO_2, and oxygen saturation, were also recorded. The primary advantage of this system lies in permitting the simultaneous detection of small changes in blood chemistry as rapidly as possible. Gotoh pointed out, however, that the response times of all the chemical transducers are not the same, and therefore the method is not suitable for studies in which time sequences within a second or two are important. The problems encountered with blood clotting were discussed, but the use of an adequate amount of heparin appears to have eliminated these difficulties.

The study of Gotoh and co-workers indicates the possibility of continuous monitoring of blood chemistry for the whole body or specific organs. Besides the surgical techniques required, one of the chief technical limitations of this method at present is the relatively long response time of the chemical transducers.

8-14.   THE LEX-O₂-CON CELL

Hersch (1965) developed a remarkably efficient oxygen fuel cell in which the current delivered reflects the amount of oxygen presented to it. This device contains two especially designed electrodes separated by a thin porous membrane containing only a tiny quantity of electrolyte. When oxygen gas

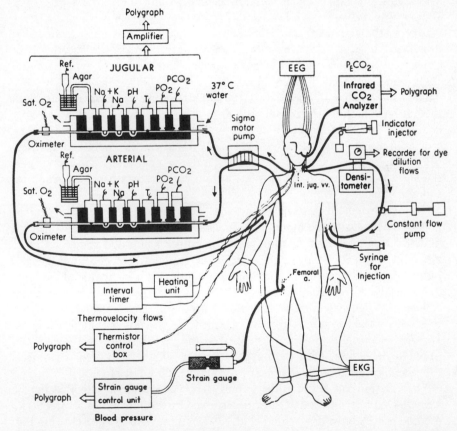

Figure 8-14.   Continuous monitoring of blood chemistry. [From F. Gotoh et al., *Med. Res. Eng.* **5**:15–19 (1966). By permission.]

is admitted to the cell, the oxygen molecules give up their electrons, a voltage is developed and current is delivered. The time integral of the current, therefore, represents the total volume of oxygen admitted to the cell. In reality, all the oxygen molecules passing through the cell are counted because each provides the electrons that appear as current. In fact, the Hersch cell operates on Faraday's law of electrolysis, which states that 96,500 C (A-sec) are required to liberate one chemical equivalent of an element. When applied to the oxygen fuel cell, this means that 8 grams of oxygen provide 96,500 A-sec of current. Stated another way, 1 ml of oxygen at 20°C and 1 atm of pressure provides 287 mA-min of charge.

The Hersch cell has been incorporated into a very practical oxygen analyzer known as the Lex-O_2-Con.[5] This device provides a quantitative indication for the volume of oxygen in the blood sample that is introduced. The reading is expressed in volumes percent, that is, milliliters of O_2 per 100 ml of blood.

The method of using the Hersch cell in the Lex-O_2-Con instrument is illustrated in Fig. 8-15, where the various valves are in the "USE" (i.e., "measure") position. A carrier gas (nitrogen, containing 2% hydrogen and 1% carbon monoxide) is admitted into the gas inlet and passes over a catalyst to remove all traces of oxygen. This oxygen-free carrier gas (with the carbon monoxide) is bubbled into distilled water in the scrubber chamber. The constant bubbling keeps the distilled water circulating. The oxygen-free carrier gas then passes into the Hersch cell and on to a water-filled reservoir, where it escapes. Since there is no oxygen in the carrier gas, the Hersch cell produces no current (although there may be a very small residual current).

The measurement of oxygen in a blood sample is accomplished by filling a 20-μl syringe with the blood to be measured. The blood sample is injected into the scrubber solution through the septum. The blood gradually gives up its oxygen by the partial pressure gradient and because carbon monoxide combines with the hemoglobin, rendering it incapable of carrying oxygen. The carrier gas transports the released oxygen through the Hersch cell, which delivers current that flows until all the electrons have been released by the oxygen. A typical current-time curve is included in Fig. 8-15. An electronic integrator measures the area under the curve and provides a readout when the oxygen current falls to zero. This reading is expressed in terms of the volume of oxygen in 100 ml of blood.

The relationship between the values of oxygen content provided by the Lex-O_2-Con instrument and those determined by the conventional Van Slyke method was examined by Valeri et al. (1972); these data are presented in Fig.

[5] Lexington Instruments, Waltham, Mass. 02154.

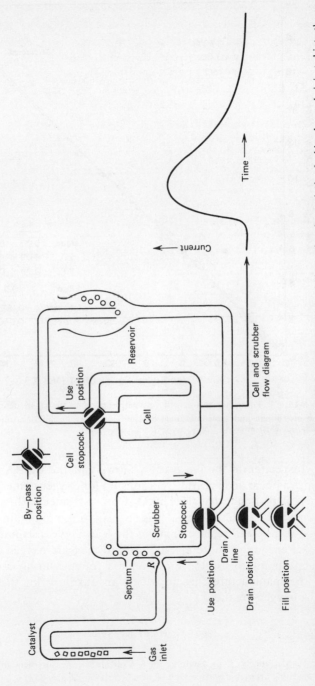

Figure 8-15. The Lex-O$_2$-Con oxygen content analyzer and a current-time record illustrating the analysis of a blood sample injected into the apparatus via the septum. (Courtesy of Lexington Instruments, Waltham, Mass.)

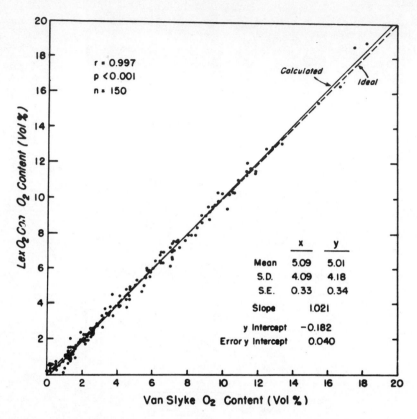

Figure 8-16. Relationship between the oxygen content in blood, as determined by the Lex-O_2-Con instrument and values obtained by the Van Slyke method. [From C. R. Valeri et al., *J. Lab. Clin. Med.* **79**:1035–1040 (1972). By permission.]

8-16. Inspection of the illustration shows that the Lex-O_2-Con instrument provides a linear and accurate relationship for oxygen content.

There is no doubt that the Lex-O_2-Con instrument will see increasing use in biomedical studies. Because it is so easy to use to obtain data of high accuracy, it may well replace many of the Van Slyke instruments. It probably will also encourage more investigators to measure oxygen content and will stimulate many to use the Fick method for measuring cardiac output. In fact, the manufacturer has provided an auxiliary kit that facilitates obtaining oxygen uptake.

REFERENCES

Band, D. M., and S. J. G. Semple. 1967. Continuous measurement of blood pH with an indwelling arterial glass electrode. *J. Appl. Physiol.* **22**:854–857.

Brems, N. 1962. Measurements of pH electrodes and pertinent apparatus. *Acta Anaesthesiol. Scand.* **6**(Suppl. XI):199–206.

Bronk, D. W., F. Brink, C. M. Connelly, F. D. Carlson, and P. W. Davies. 1947. The time course of recovery of oxygen consumption in nerve. *Fed. Proc.* **6**:83–84.

Bronk, D. W., M. A. Larrabee, and P. W. Davies. 1946. The rate of O_2 consumption in localized regions of the nervous system in presynaptic endings in cell bodies. *Fed. Proc.* **5**:11.

Bull, H. B. 1943. *Physical Biochemistry.* Wiley, New York.

Bull, H. B. 1964. *An Introduction to Physical Biochemistry.* F. A. Davies Co., Philadelphia.

Carlson, F. D., F. Brink, and D. W. Bronk. 1948. A method for direct measurement of rate of O_2 utilization by nerve. *Fed. Proc.* **7**:18.

Cater, D. B., A. F. Phillips, and I. A. Silver. 1957a. Apparatus and techniques for the measurement of oxidation-reduction potentials, pH and oxygen tension *in vivo. Proc. Roy. Soc. (London)* **146B**:289–297.

Cater, D. B., A. F. Phillips, and I. A. Silver. 1957b. Induced changes in oxidation-reduction potentials, pH and oxygen tension in the intact lactating mammary gland. *Proc. Roy. Soc. (London)* **146B**:400–415.

Cater, D. B., A. F. Phillips, and I. A. Silver. 1957c. The measurement of oxidation-reduction potentials, pH and oxygen tension in tumors. *Proc. Roy. Soc. (London)* **146B**:382–399.

Clark, L. C. 1956. Monitor and control of blood and tissue oxygen tensions. *Trans. Am. Soc. Intern. Organs* **2**:41–48.

Clark, L. C., and G. Misrahy. 1957. Chronically implanted polarograph electrodes. *Fed. Proc.* **16**:22–23.

Clark, L. C., G. Misrahy, and R. P. Fox. 1958. Chronically implanted polarographic electrodes. *J. Appl. Physiol.* **13**:85–91.

Cooper, R. 1963. Electrodes. *Am. J. EEG Tech.* **3**:91–101.

Davies, P. W. 1946. Rapid bursts of oxygen consumption in stimulated muscle. *Fed. Proc.* **5**:21–22.

Davies, P. W. 1962. In *Physical Techniques in Biological Research.* W. L. Nastuk (ed.). Vol. IV: *Special Methods.* Academic Press, New York.

Davies, P. W., and F. Brink. 1942a. Direct measurement of brain oxygen concentration with platinum electrode. *Fed. Proc.* **1**:19.

Davies, P. W., and F. Brink. 1942b. Microelectrodes for measuring local oxygen tension in animal tissues. *Rev. Sci. Instr.* **130**:524–532.

Davies, P. W., R. G. Grenell, and D. W. Bronk. 1948. The time course of *in vivo* oxygen consumption of cerebral cortex following electrical stimulation. *Fed. Proc.* **7**:25.

Davies, P. W., W. S. McCulloch, and E. Roseman. 1943–1944. Rapid changes in the O_2 tension of cerebral cortex during induced convulsions. *Am. J. Psychiat.* **100**:825–829.

de Bethune, A. J. 1964. Electrode potentials, temperature coefficients. In *Encyclopedia of Electrochemistry.* C. A. Hampel (ed.). Reinhold, New York.

Dole, M. 1935. *Theoretical and Experimental Electrochemistry.* McGraw-Hill, New York.

Dole, M., R. M. Roberts, and C. E. Holley. 1941. The theory of the glass electrode. V. The influence of negative ions. *J. Am. Chem. Soc.* **63**:725–730.

Dubuisson, M. 1937a. A method for recording pH changes of muscle during activity. *J. Physiol.* **90**:47p–48p.

Dubuisson, M. 1937b. pH changes in muscle during and after contraction. *Proc. Soc. Exp. Biol. Med.* **35**:609–611.

Dusser de Barenne, J. C., W. S. McCulloch, and L. F. Nims. 1937. Functional activity and pH of the cerebral cortex. *J. Cell. Comp. Physiol.* **10**:277–289.

Eisenman, G. 1962. Cation selective glass electrodes and their mode of operation. *Biophys. J.* **2**:259–323.

Eisenman, G. 1967. The origin of the glass-electrode potential. In *Glass Electrodes for Hydrogen and Other Cations—Principles and Practice.* G. Eisenman (ed.). Marcel Dekker, New York.

Eisenman, G., D. O. Rudin, and J. U. Casby. 1957. Glass electrode for measuring sodium ion. *Science* **126**:831–834.

Frant, M. S., and J. W. Ross. 1966. Electrode for sensing fluoride-ion activity in solution. *Science* **154**:1553–1554.

Friedman, S. M., J. D. Jamieson, J. A. M. Hinke, and C. L. Friedman. 1959. Drug-induced changes in blood pressure and in blood sodium as measured by glass electrode. *Am. J. Physiol.* **196**:1049–1052.

Fruhling, G., and H. Winterstein. 1934. Registrierung der pH in stromenden Blut. *Arch. Ges. Physiol.* **233**:475–485.

Gesell, R., and A. B. Hertzman. 1926. Regulation of respiration. *Am. J. Physiol.* **78**:206–223.

Glasstone, S. 1946. *The Elements of Physical Chemistry.* D. Van Nostrand, Princeton, N.J.

Gotoh, F., J. S. Meyer, and S. Ebihara. 1966. Continuous recording of human cerebral blood flow and metabolism: methods for electronic monitoring of arterial and venous gases and electrolytes. *Med. Res. Eng.* **5**(2):13–19.

Hersch, P. A. 1965. Method and means for oxygen analysis of gases. U.S. Patent 3,223, 597, December 14.

Hertz, C. H., and B. Siesjö. 1959. A rapid and sensitive electrode for continuous measurement of pCO_2 in liquids and tissue. *Acta Physiol. Scand.* **47**:115–123.

Janz, G. J., and H. Taniguchi. 1953. The silver-silver halide electrodes. *Chem. Rev.* **53**:397–437.

Kolthoff, I. M., and J. J. Lingane. 1955. *Polarography.* Interscience Publishers, New York.

Kreuzer, F., T. R., Watson, and J. M. Ball. 1958. Comparative measurements with a new procedure for measuring the blood oxygen tensions *in vitro. J. Appl. Physiol.* **12**:65–70.

Lengyel, B. von and E. Blum. 1934. The behavior of the glass electrode in connection with its chemical composition. *Trans. Faraday Soc.* **30**:461.

Marshall, C., and L. F. Nims. 1937. Blood pH *in vivo.* 11. Effects of acids, salts, dextrose and adrenalin. *Yale J. Biol. Med.* **10**:561–564.

Mattock, G., and D. M. Band. 1967. Interpretation of pH and cation measurements. In *Glass Electrodes for Hydrogen and Other Cations—Principles and Practice.* G. Eisenman (ed.). Marcel Dekker, New York.

McClendon, J. F. 1915. New hydrogen electrode and rapid method of determining hydrogen ion concentrations. *Am. J. Physiol.* **38**:180–185.

Nims, L. F. 1937. Glass electrodes and apparatus for direct recording of pH *in vivo. Yale J. Biol. Med.* **10**:241–246.

Nims, L. F., and C. Marshall. 1937. Blood pH *in vivo.* 1. Changes due to respiration. *Yale J. Biol. Med.* **10**:445–448.

Nims, L. F., C. Marshall, and H. S. Burr. 1938. The measurement of pH in circulating blood. *Science* **87**:197–198.

Olson, R. A., F. S. Brackett, and R. G. Crickard. 1949. Oxygen tension measurement by a method of time selection using the static platinum electrode with alternating potential. *J. Gen. Physiol.* **32**:681–703.

Orion Research, Inc. 1966. Sulfide ion activity. *Electrode Bulletin.* Cambridge, Mass.

Posternak, J. M., M. A. Larrabee, and D. W. Bronk. 1947. Oxygen requirements of the neurones in sympathetic ganglia. *Fed. Proc.* **6**:182.

Purcell, M. K., and T. Rodman. 1965. Carbon dioxide and oxygen electrodes for arterial blood analysis in a cardiopulmonary physiology laboratory. *Am. J. Med. Electron.* **4**:82–86.

Radiometer, Co. Bulletin 21917E. Copenhagen, Denmark.

Reyes, R. J., and J. R. Neville. 1967. An electrochemical technic for measuring carbon dioxide content of blood. *USAF School Aeros. Med. Tech. Rept.* SAM-TR-67-23.

Ross, J. W. 1967. Calcium-selective electrode with liquid ion exchanger. *Science* **156**:1378–1379.

Severinghaus, J. W. 1962. Electrodes for blood and gas pCO_2, pO_2, and blood pH. *Acta Anaesthesiol. Scand.* **6**(Suppl. IX):207–220.

Severinghaus, J. W., and A. F. Bradley. 1958. Electrodes for blood pO_2 and pCO_2 determination. *J. Appl. Physiol.* **13**:515–520.

Siggaard-Andersen, O. 1962. The pH-log pCO_2 blood acid-base nomogram revised. *Scand. J. Clin. Lab. Invest.* **14**:598–604.

Siggaard-Andersen, O., and K. Engel. 1960. A new acid-base nomogram an improved method for the calculation of the relevant blood acid-base data. *Scand. J. Clin. Lab. Invest.* **12**:177–186.

Sollner, K. 1958. The physical chemistry of ion exchange membranes. *Svensk Kem. Tidsks.* **6–7**:267–295.

Stow, R. W., R. F. Baer, and B. F. Randall. 1957. Rapid measurement of the tension of carbon dioxide in blood. *Arch. Phys. Med. Rehabil.* **38**:646–650.

Tobias, J. M. 1949. Syringe oxygen cathode for measurement of oxygen tension in solution and respiratory gases. *Rev. Sci. Instr.* **20**:519–523.

Tobias, J. M., and R. Holmes. 1947. Observation on the use of the oxygen cathode. *Fed. Proc.* **6**:215.

Valeri, C. R., C. G., Zaroulis, L. Marchionni, and K. J. Path. 1972. A simple method for measuring oxygen content in blood. *J. Lab. Clin. Med.* **79**:1035–1040.

Voegtlin, C., F. F. De Eds, and H, Kahler. 1930. *Public Health Rept. (U.S.)* **45**:2222–2233; also: 1935. *N.I.H. Bull.* 164, Part II, pp. 15–27.

Vogel, J. H. K., R. F. Grover, and S. G. Blount. 1962. Detection of the small intracardiac shunt with the hydrogen electrode: a highly sensitive and simple technique, *Am. Heart J.* **64**:13–21.

9

Electrodes for Bioelectric Events

9-1. INTRODUCTION

In presenting a bioelectric event to an amplifier, a pair of electrodes plays the role of a transducer. As such, the electrodes must transfer the bioelectric event to the amplifier input circuit, which has been designed to accommodate the characteristics of the electrodes. The event, its anatomical location, and the dimensions of the bioelectric generator dictate the type of electrodes to be used, and the electrical characteristics of the electrodes specify the type of amplifier circuit required. When large-area electrodes are employed, the restrictions on input impedance are not too severe, and most vacuum tube and high-input impedance solid-state amplifers suffice. However, when the application calls for small electrodes—and, in particular, microelectrodes, with their inherently high impedance—special high-resistance, low-capacitance, input circuits are needed to transfer the bioelectric event to the amplifying system. Distortionless insertion of the event into the recording apparatus requires, therefore, special consideration of the electrical characteristics of the electrodes and the input impedance of the amplifier.

9-2. THE ELECTRODE–ELECTROLYTE INTERFACE

A truly remarkable variety of electrodes has been used to detect bioelectric events. With the exception of insulated electrodes, which are discussed later, there exists a fundamental component common to all. This component is a metal-electrolyte interface; the metal is the material of the electrode and the electrolyte may be an electrolytic solution or paste such as is used with surface electrodes, or it may be the tissue fluids that come into contact with an electrode inserted below the integument. The electrolyte may also be perspiration that accumulates under a dry electrode applied to skin containing sweat glands.

When a metallic electrode comes into contact with an electrolyte, an ion-electron exchange occurs. There is a tendency for metallic ions to enter into solution and a tendency for ions in the electrolyte to combine with the metallic electrode. Although the details of the reaction may be complex in a given situation, the net result is the existence of a charge distribution at the electrode-electrolyte interface. The spatial arrangement of the charge depends on the manner in which the electrode and electrolyte react. Several types of charge distribution have been proposed. The simplest was conceived by Helmholtz (1879), who postulated that there exists a layer of charge of one sign tightly bound to the electrode and a layer of charge of the opposite sign in the electrolyte. The separation between the two layers of charges (often called the electrical double layer) is of course measured in ionic dimension; Fig. 9-1 diagrams this concept. Parsons (1964) described electrodes in terms of the reactions at the double layer, referring to electrodes in which no net transfer of charge occurs across the metal-electrolyte interface as "perfectly polarized." Those in which unhindered exchange of charge is possible were called "perfectly nonpolarizable." Real electrodes have properties that lie between these idealized limits. MacInnes (1961) stated that the term "electrode polarization" is applied in two ways; first, as just stated and second, as the condition in which the electrode-electrolyte potential is altered by the passage of current.

In a conceptual sense, an electrode-electrolyte interface resembles a voltage source and a capacitor. However, it is well known that current can pass through an electrode-electrolyte interface. Therefore any electrical model for such an interface must include resistance, capacitance, and a potential. Although it is easy to identify these three components, it is by no

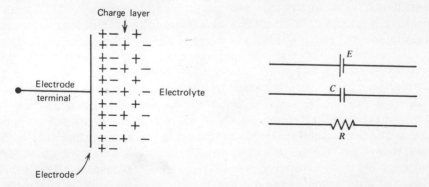

Figure 9-1. The charge distribution at an electrode-electrolyte interface and the three circuit elements (voltage E, capacitance C, and resistance R) that can be used to describe it in terms of an electrical model.

means easy to create an accurate electrical model to include them because their magnitude depends on the electrode metal, its area, the electrolyte, current density, and the frequency of current used for measurement.

9-3. ELECTRODE POTENTIAL

The voltage developed at an electrode-electrolyte interface is designated the half-cell potential. The total voltage between a pair of electrode terminals is therefore the difference in the two half-cell potentials. Since it is impossible to measure the potential developed at a single electrode, an arbitrary standard electrode has been chosen, and electrode potentials are measured with respect to it. The standard electrode is the hydrogen electrode; it consists of a specially prepared platinum surface in contact with a solution of hydrogen ions (of unit activity) and dissolved molecular hydrogen; the activity of the latter is specified by requiring it to be in equilibrium with hydrogen at 1 atm of pressure in the gas phase (Janz and Kelly, 1964).

The potentials of many of the metals used for electrodes are listed in Table 9-1. Inspection of this table indicates that an appreciable voltage can be produced when dissimilar metals are employed. When such electrodes are connected together through the input impedance of the measuring device, a current will flow. The consequences of this situation are discussed later. The table also indicates that a voltaic cell of zero potential will be created if the metals are identical. In practice, even if the same material is used for both electrodes, some potential difference may be measured between the pair. In many instances the presence of a potential would not be objectionable if it were stable. In practice it is not, and its variations constitute a source of artifact.

Many investigators have carried out studies of the stability of electrode potentials; Table 9-2 presents a summary of many of these studies. Forbes (1934) examined the potential difference between amalgamated lead-mercury electrodes in contact with a lead chloride solution, applied to a chamois in contact with the skin. In 10 electrodes, potential differences ranging from 0 to 600 μV were measured. The spontaneous voltage variations ranged between 1.3 and 6.8 μV. A more extensive study was carried out by Greenwald (1936), who measured the potential difference and resistance of pairs of calomel, zinc, and zinc-zinc sulfate electrodes used for recording the electrodermal response. The calomel and zinc electrodes were measured with saline as the electrolyte. The zinc-zinc sulfate electrodes consisted of a zinc plate in contact with a kaolin paste made with zinc sulfate. Between them was a saline solution. The potential difference between the calomel electrodes, before passage of direct current to measure

Table 9-1   Electrode Potentials for Commonly Used Materials in Electrodes* (E^0 values)

Metal and Reaction	Potential ($E^0_{25°C}$) (V)	Temperature Coefficient (mV/°C)
$Al = Al^{3+} + 3e$	-1.662	$+1.375$
$Zn = Zn^{2+} + 2e^-$	-0.7628	$+0.962$
$Zn(Hg) = Zn^{2+} + Hg + 2e^-$	-0.7627	—
$Cr = Cr^{3+} + 3e^-$	-0.744	$+1.339$
$Fe = Fe^{2+} + 2e^-$	-0.4402	$+0.923$
$Cd = Cd^{2+} + 2e^-$	-0.4029	$+0.778$
$Ni = Ni^{2+} + 2e^-$	-0.250	$+0.93$
$Pb = Pb^{2+} + 2e^-$	-0.126	$+0.420$
$Pt(H_2)H^+$	0	—
$Ag + Cl^- = AgCl + e^-$	$+0.2225$†	$+0.213$
$Cu = Cu^{2+} + 2e^-$	$+0.337$	$+0.879$
$Cu = Cu^+ + e$	$+0.521$	$+0.813$
$2 Hg = Hg_2^{2+} + 2e^-$	$+0.788$	—
$Ag = Ag^+ + e^-$	$+0.7991$	-0.129
$Pt = Pt^{2+} + 2e^-$	$+1.2$ approx.	—
$Au = Au^{3+} + 3e^-$	$+1.498$	—
$Au = Au^+ + e^-$	$+1.691$	—

* From A. J. de Bethune, in *Handbook of Electrochemistry*. C. A. Hampel (ed.). Reinhold, New York, 1964.

† MacInnes (1939).

resistance, ranged between 1 to 20 μV and became considerably higher after the dc resistance had been measured. The zinc plates exhibited a potential difference of 450 μV, which quadrupled after the passage of direct current. The potential difference for the zinc-zinc sulfate electrodes was 180 μV, which tripled after the passage of a direct current.

In a similar study Lykken (1959) investigated the potentials developed by many of the electrodes used for the measurement of electrodermal phenomena. He measured the potential difference between pairs of stainless steel, zinc, zinc-mercury, silver, silver-mercury, silver-silver chloride, lead, lead-mercury, and platinum electrodes; in each case the electrolyte was saline. Pairs of zinc and and zinc-mercury in contact with zinc sulfate and saline were also measured. During the first hour of measurement the various electrodes exhibited the following voltages: stainless steel, 10 mV; zinc, 100 mV; zinc-mercury, 82 mV; silver, 94 mV; silver-mercury, 90 mV; silver-silver chloride, 2.5 mV; platinum, 320 mV. For the others listed, the voltage difference was approximately 1 mV. Edelberg and Burch (1962), while conducting galvanic skin response (GSR) studies, reported that

Table 9-2   Fluctuations in Potential Between Electrodes in Electrolytes*

Electrode Metal	Electrolyte Type	Potential Difference Between Electrodes	Reference
PbHg	PbCl₂ in chamois on human skin	0–600 μV (basal) 1.3–6.8 μV (fluctuations)	Ferris (1934) (av. of 10 electrodes)
Calomel	Saline	1–20 μV	Greenwald (1936)
Zn-ZnSO₄	Saline	180 μV	Greenwald (1936)
Zn	Saline	450 μV	Greenwald (1936)
Stainless steel	Saline	10 mV	Lykken (1959)
Zn	Saline	100 mV	Lykken (1959)
ZnHg	Saline	82 mV	Lykken (1959)
Ag	Saline	94 mV	Lykken (1959)
AgHg	Saline	90 mV	Lykken (1959)
Ag–AgCl	Saline	2.5 mV	Lykken (1959)
Pb	Saline	1 mV	Lykken (1959)
PbHg	Saline	1 mV	Lykken (1959)
Pt	Saline	320 mV	Lykken (1959)
Ag, AgCl sponge	ECG paste	0.2 mV 0.07 mV drift in 1 hr	O'Connell et al. (1960)
Ag, AgCl (11-mm disk)	ECG paste	0.47 mV 1.88 mV drift in 1 hr	O'Connell et al. (1960)
Pb (11-mm disk)	ECG paste	4.9 mV 3.70 mV drift in 1 hr	O'Connell et al. (1960)
Zn, ZnCl₂ (11-mm disk)	ECG paste	15.3 mV 11.25 mV drift in 1 hr	O'Connell et al. (1960)

* From L. A. Geddes, *Electrodes and the Measurement of Bioelectric Events*. Wiley, New York, 1972. (By permission.)

stainless steel and aluminum produced high random noise levels. Solder, silver, and copper produced slow wave artifacts. O'Connell et al. (1960) examined the galvanic potentials developed by various electrodes made from silver, lead, and zinc. The highest potential (13 mV) was produced by the zinc-zinc chloride pair and the lowest (0.2 mV) by the silver-silver chloride electrodes affixed to a sponge.

A pair of electrodes made from the same piece of metal, when placed in 0.9% saline and joined through a resistance, will frequently produce a fluctuating "noise" current that often can be eliminated by connecting the electrodes together and allowing them to reach a stable equilibrium with the electrolyte. This technique has been employed by electrophysiologists. A related observation has been that newly prepared electrodes are often noisy when placed in an electrolyte, but with the passage of time the noise decreases. Another method of quieting electrodes is to deposit electrolytically, from a large electrode, a uniform film of material covering both recording electrodes. In this way the minute differences in electrode material are virtually eliminated, and a pair of electrodes having a very small and stable potential difference can be made.

9-3-1. Chlorided Silver Electrodes

The principle just described is frequently applied when silver electrodes are first made. The authors have demonstrated that a new set of cortical electrodes, Fig. 9-23a, (1-mm silver balls) which were scraped to remove surface contaminants, when placed in 0.9% saline and connected to the recording system, produced an unstable random noise signal of several hundred microvolts. Figure 9-2a illustrates the type of record obtained. The noise was diminished by maintaining all of the electrodes positive by about 3 V with respect to a 1 × 2 in. silver plate in the saline for 2 min and reconnecting them to the recording equipment without changing their position in the saline. This process is known as chloriding. The noise record obtained is shown in Fig. 9-2b.

To further demonstrate the phenomenon, the electrodes were scraped to remove the coating, and they became noisy again (Fig. 9-2c). The electroplating current was reapplied, but this time in reverse (electrodes negative by 3 V for 3 min), and much of the electrode noise disappeared (Fig. 9-2d). Finally, the electrodes were most effectively quieted by the simple procedure of chloriding them after the electrolytic cleaning. The polarity was then reversed (electrodes positive), and with a milliammeter in the circuit, the current was turned on and interrupted when it started to fall. After the electrodes were connected to the amplifier, the noise record shown in Fig. 9-2e was obtained. To illustrate that all the noise cannot be attributed to the electrodes, Fig. 9-2f shows the inherent noise level of the amplifying channel under open- and short-circuit conditions.

An ingenious method of stabilizing chlorided silver electrodes while they are in storage was described by Cooper (1956). The method serves to maintain the electrodes short circuited to each other and at the same time keeps them in a chlorided condition. These two actions are brought about by mounting the electrodes with their silver-silver chloride surfaces immersed in a dish of saline in which is mounted a carbon rod projecting out of the solution. At the tip of the carbon rod, Cooper affixed a stainless steel plate to which all the electrode terminals were connected. Thus all electrodes were joined together, and because carbon is slightly electronegative with respect to silver-silver chloride, a small chloriding current was maintained. Therefore during storage, the electrodes were maintained at the same

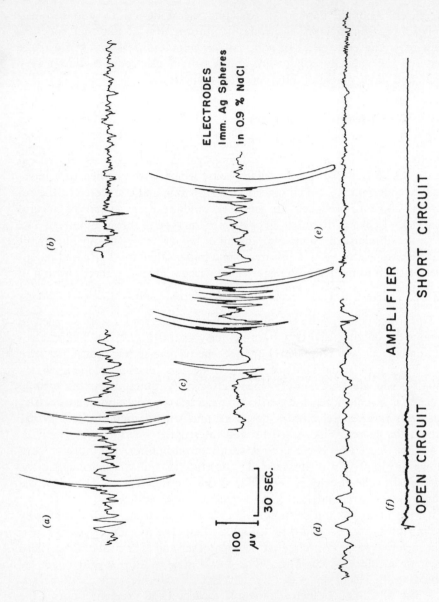

Figure 9-2. Electrode noise.

202

potential to each other and were continuously chlorided. Cooper reported that electrodes treated in this way were adequately stable for use with high-gain dc amplifiers.

Chlorided silver electrodes can be made very stable electrically and, for this reason, enjoy widespread popularity. However, they are not without defects. For example, an electrodeposited chloride coating can be removed easily by abrasion. In addition, silver-silver chloride is photosensitive (i.e., it changes its potential slightly when exposed to light). Therefore, if such electrodes are used with photic stimulation studies, they should be shaded from changing light intensity. Figure 9-3 illustrates the photosensitivity of chlorided silver electrodes.

One of the chief advantages of chloriding a silver electrode is stabilization of the half-cell potential. Initial studies by the authors (1967) have shown that the deposition of a thin layer of silver chloride reduces the low-frequency electrode-electrolyte impedance. If a thick layer is deposited, the impedance at all frequencies is increased. Cole (1962) and the authors (1969) found that a deposit in the range of 500 to 2000 mA-sec/cm² provided the lowest impedance coating. The current density found to be optimum was about 5 mA/cm². For additional data on heavily coated electrodes for electrochemical studies, the report by Janz and Taniguchi (1953) is recommended.

9-3-2.   Stabilization of the Electrode-Electrolyte Interface

Another useful piece of information derives from a consideration of the electrical double layer, namely, the effect of its mechanical disturbance. It

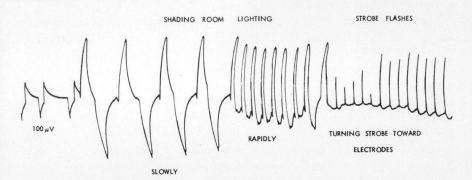

Figure 9-3.   The photosensitivity of a pair of chlorided silver electrodes in 0.9% saline in a lighted room. After the 100 μV calibration, the electrodes were shaded and exposed to light by slowly and rapidly casting a shadow on them by placing the hand above them. Then the light from a flashing stroboscope was directed toward the electrodes to evoke a similar photovoltaic effect due to the action of light on the electrode-electrolyte double layer of charge. [From L. A. Geddes, *Am. J. EEG Technol.* **13**:195–203 1973. By permission.]

has been found that electrodes relatively free of movement artifacts are of the recessed type, in which the electrode-electrolyte interface is removed from direct contact with the subject. Because the double layer is a region of charge gradient which is a source of potential, disturbance of it gives rise to a change in voltage that, although small electrochemically, is often large with respect to the size of the bioelectric events. Movement artifacts produced by disturbance of the electrical double layer are in the frequency range of many of these events; hence filtering techniques can seldom be employed with success. Therefore the electrical stability of an electrode is considerably enhanced by stabilization of the electrode-electrolyte interface. This phenomenon has been demonstrated practically when attempts have been made to measure bioelectric events on moving subjects; for example, Forbes et al. (1921) were perhaps the first to record such measurements when they employed a type of recessed electrode to obtain electrocardiograms and electromyograms on an elephant. When standing, elephants sway from side to side, making it difficult to obtain artifact-free records with plate electrodes. Forbes employed a zinc electrode in the neck of a funnel filled with zinc sulfate. The opening of the funnel was covered with a permeable membrane soaked in saline. Two rubber-gloved assistants held these electrodes against the inner surfaces of the forelimbs of the animal. The electrocardiogram was successfully recorded by a string galvanometer.

In a study of the electrocardiograms of perspiring miners, Atkins (1961) found that the main source of artifacts was contact variations between the electrode metal and the skin. When the electrodes were separated from the skin by a layer of filter paper or gauze soaked with an electrolyte, electrode artifacts virtually disappeared.

Roman and Lamb (1962), using miniature recessed electrodes applied to the skin over each end of the sternum, presented some truly remarkable records of the ECG in which no artifacts were to be observed when the electrodes were tapped or struck or when the subject was jumping or engaged in vigorous activity. These electrodes were employed for monitoring ECG changes in pilots flying in high-performance aircraft. Lucchina and Phipps (1962) similarly demonstrated that their electrodes (Fig 9-15) were free from artifacts when pressure was applied or when the electrodes were displaced. To prove their point, high-quality electrocardiograms were recorded from ambulatory subjects. Similar recessed electrodes have been employed successfully to record the ECG of astronauts, laborers, swimmers, and a variety of other subjects exercising strenuously.

To record the EEG on moving subjects Kado et al. (1964) constructed interesting electrodes in which the metal was tin in contact with a tin chloride solution contained in a small ceramic chamber. Contact between the ceramic chamber and the skin was made via a sponge soaked in physiological saline. Other than removing oil from the scalp, no special precautions were required for the installation of the electrodes. When carefully applied, these electrodes produced remarkably stable EEG recordings in subjects who were moving their heads rapidly.

In summary, the electrical stability of an electrode is related to the stability of the regions of charge gradient. With electrodes in which there is a metal-electrolyte interface, stabilization of the interface prevents the development of variable electrochemical voltages, which have become known as "movement artifacts." With surface electrodes, however, the electrode-electrolyte interface is only one region of charge gradient. Other regions exist between the electrode-electrolyte interface and the skin and underlying tissue fluids. Disturbance of these regions may produce electrochemical voltages of appreciable magnitude. The skin-drilling technique of Shackel (1959), by decreasing the ionic gradient, attenuates movement artifacts produced by disturbance of this region.

The preceding discussion of electrode potentials was presented to alert the reader to the possibility of the presence of voltages of nonphysiological origin. To have confidence in the magnitude of the voltage appearing between the electrode terminals, electrodes should be routinely checked for voltage without the bioelectric event interposed.

Often relatively little attention is given to the large unstable potentials developed when the electrode wires come into contact with electrolytes. Special precautions should be taken after a carefully prepared electrode is joined to the wire connected to the recording apparatus. In the early days of electrocardiography, Pardee (1917) recommended that the connecting wire be riveted to the electrode and the use of solder avoided. Henry (1938) called attention to the fact that if the solder connection joining the electrode to the interconnecting wire became wet with an electrolytic solution, a multimetal electrolytic cell was produced that developed unstable voltages and caused eventual corrosion and breakage of the connection. The simple practice of covering the wire connection at the electrode with a waterproof coating will result not only in a more stable electrode but one that will last longer.

9-4. ELECTRODE IMPEDANCE

In addition to developing a half-cell potential, each electrode exhibits an impedance that is dependent on the nature of the electrical double layer. This impedance is often called the polarization impedance. Through the impedance of both electrodes and the input impedance of the recording apparatus flows a small current derived from the bioelectric event. Because the input impedance of most bioelectric recorders is high, the current is small and the voltage drop caused by the electrode impedance is usually negligible. As pointed out later, however, this situation does not always obtain, and in its absence, besides a loss of amplitude, undesirable waveform distortion of a bioelectric event can occur.

Electrode impedances are complex and can be difficult to measure with high accuracy on living subjects. The term electrode impedance really refers to the impedance at each electrode and does not include the impedance of the biological material between the electrodes. Frequently, however, the term is used to describe the total impedance of the circuit between the electrode terminals. Such an impedance of course includes the impedance at both electrodes and that of the biological material between them. A discussion of the electrical properties of living tissue is presented in Chapter 10.

9-4-1. Electrode Capacitance and Resistance

The presence of a charge distribution at an electrode-electrolyte interface produces not only an electrode potential but also a capacitance. Conceptually, two layers of charge of opposite sign, separated by a distance, constitute a capacitance. The distance between the layers of charge is molecular in dimension; therefore the capacitance per unit area is quite large (Grahame, 1941, 1952). In fact, this is one of the properties that allowed the first electrolytic capacitors to exhibit such large capacitances in relatively small packages.

Measurement of the capacitance, and for that matter the resistance, of a single electrode-electrolyte interface is difficult. The impedances of the electrode-electrolyte interfaces in conductivity cells plagued the early electrochemists who desired to obtain accurate values for the resistivities of electrolytes. Kohlrausch (1897, 1898) reduced the electrode-electrolyte impedance to a negligible value by using platinum-black electrodes, which have a very rough surface, hence large effective area. The large area provides a high capacitance, the reactance of which is negligible at 1000 Hz (the frequency most often used to measure electrolytic resistivity).

Warburg (1899, 1901), a contemporary of Kohlrausch, was one of the first to investigate the components of the electrode-electrolyte interface, and his studies provided a model that equates a single electrode-electrolyte interface to a series resistance and capacitance. It is important to note that the magnitude of each of these components is dependent on electrode type and area (including surface condition), the electrolyte, the frequency, and the current density used to make the measurement. More recently, the Warburg equivalent circuit has been elaborated for conductivity cells by Grahame (1952), Feates et al. (1956), and Robinson and Stokes (1959).

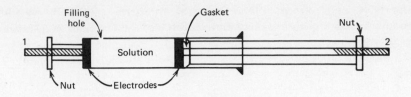

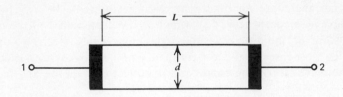

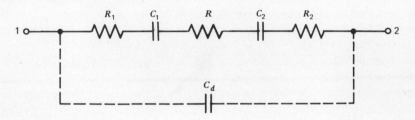

Figure 9-4. The electrolytic conductivity cell and its series-equivalent representation.

To illustrate the difficulty in determing the capacitance and resistance of a single electrode-electrolyte interface, it is merely necessary to set down the expression for the impedance appearing between the two terminals of a pair of electrodes immersed in an electrolyte of resistivity ρ. For convenience, assume that circular electrodes of area A are applied to the ends of a cylinder of electrolyte of length L and diameter d (see Fig. 9-4). The terminal impedance Z_{12} is

$$Z_{12} = Z_1 + \frac{\rho L}{A} + Z_2. \qquad (9\text{-}1)$$

In this expression Z_1 and Z_2 are the impedances of the electrode-electrolyte interfaces at electrodes 1 and 2. Using the series-equivalent (Warburg) model for each electrode-electrolyte interface, the terminal impedance Z_{12} is

$$Z_{12} = R_1 + \frac{1}{j\omega C_1} + \frac{\rho L}{A} + R_2 + \frac{1}{j\omega C_2}. \tag{9-2}$$

In this expression, $R_1 C_1$ and $R_2 C_2$ are the equivalent series resistances and capacitances of the two electrode-electrolyte interfaces. Note that for any given frequency it is possible to use the reactive component of the terminal impedance to obtain the capacitive components (C_1 and C_2), if it is assumed that there are no other capacitances present. In fact there is another capacitive component (C_d), which is the capacitance of the cell itself, consisting of the two electrodes; the intervening electrolyte is the dielectric. In most cases, in the low-frequency region, C_d can be neglected.

Rearranging the foregoing expression to collect the reactive and resistive components provides:

$$Z_{12} = \left(R_1 + \frac{\rho L}{A} + R_2\right) + \frac{1}{j\omega}\left(\frac{1}{C_1} + \frac{1}{C_2}\right). \tag{9-2a}$$

Now if at a single frequency, an impedance bridge (Fig. 9-5) is used to provide the series-equivalent values R_b and C_b, then

$$R_b + \frac{1}{j\omega C_b} = \left(R_1 + \frac{\rho L}{A} + R_2\right) + \frac{1}{j\omega C_1} + \frac{1}{j\omega C_2} \tag{9-3}$$

Equating the resistive and reactive components gives

$$R_b = R_1 + \frac{\rho L}{A} + R_2, \tag{9-4a}$$

$$\frac{1}{C_b} = \frac{1}{C_1} + \frac{1}{C_2}. \tag{9-4b}$$

If it is assumed that the electrode areas are the same, $R_1 = R_2 = R$ and $C_1 = C_2 = C$, where R and C are the equivalent resistance and capacitance of a single electrode-electrolyte interface, then by substitution and rearrangement, the following are obtained:

$$2R = R_b - \frac{\rho L}{A}, \tag{9-5a}$$

$$C = 2C_b. \tag{9-5b}$$

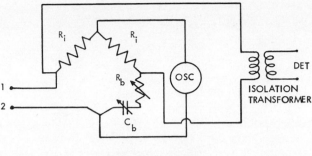

IMPEDANCE BRIDGE

Figure 9-5. Constant-current comparison impedance bridge for measurement of the components of an electrode-electrolyte interface. The value of R_i is chosen to be many times higher than the impedance appearing between the measuring terminals (1, 2). The bridge-balance values (R_b and C_b) are respectively equal to the series-equivalent resistive and capacitive components of the impedance between terminals 1 and 2.

Recalling that R_b and C_b are the series-equivalent bridge-balance values, it can be seen that if there are no other capacitances present, the capacitance of a single electrode-electrolyte interface (at the frequency and current density employed to make the measurement) is twice the bridge-balance capacitance; however, the resistance (R) of a single electrode-electrolyte interface cannot be obtained by this single measurement. The additional information required is indicated by equation 9-5a; namely, the resistivity (ρ) of the electrolyte, the length (L) and area (A) of the cell. Alternatively, if the resistivity is not known, two measurements can be carried out at the same frequency and with the same current (I) density (I/A). Measurements can be repeated with two known values of electrode area (A), which is difficult, or with two different lengths (L) for the conductivity cell; the latter technique is by far the easiest to carry out, and its use is discussed subsequently.

The equivalent series capacitance has been measured in the audiofrequency range for a variety of electrode-electrolyte interfaces using a low current density. Figure 9-6 summarizes the data reported. Inspection of these data reveals that the series-equivalent capacitance decreases with increasing frequency. The magnitude of the capacitance also depends on the surface condition of the electrode. In the illustration, the values for polished metals are the lowest; the values for specially roughened surfaces (e.g., platinum black) are the highest. To obtain the highest capacitance values (curve A) Schwan (1963) sandblasted platinum and then electro-deposited platinum black on this surface. A high electrode-electrolyte capacitance value is, of course, indicative of a low reactive component ($1/2\pi fC$) for the electrode-electrolyte impedance.

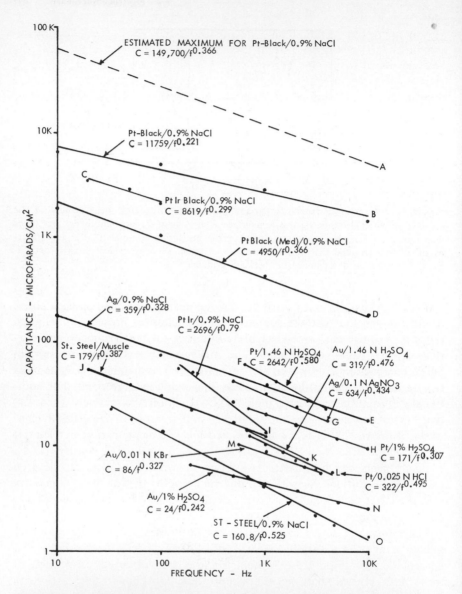

Figure 9-6. Equivalent series capacitance-frequency data for various electrode-electrolyte interfaces. (From L. A. Geddes, *Electrodes and the Measurement of Bioelectric Events,* Wiley, New York, 1972. By permission.)

It is interesting to note that Warburg (1899, 1901) postulated that the capacitance of an electrode-electrolyte interface varies inversely with the square root of frequency; thus $C = Kf^{-0.5}$ where K is a constant depending on the electrode species, electrolyte concentration, and temperature. The capacitance (C) of course should be expressed in $\mu F/cm^2$ with a specified surface and current density. The data in Fig. 9-6 generally support Warburg's hypothesis; however, Fricke (1932) pointed out that the exponent (α) is often less than 0.5. A survey of values calculated from the published literature was presented by Geddes (1972) and showed values for α ranging from 0.22 to 0.79, the majority being slightly less than 0.5.

If it is desired to measure the equivalent resistance of a single electrode-electrolyte interface, the variable-length method (Geddes, 1971, 1973) is the easiest to employ and can be carried out by mounting the electrodes so that the length of electrolytic column can be controlled. The conductivity cell (Fig. 9-4) designed for this purpose uses a disposable syringe with one electrode mounted on the piston and the other on the end of the barrel. An outlet hole in the side at the end permits expulsion of electrolyte to accommodate a decrease in length. With this variable-length conductivity cell, it is only necessary to make measurements at two lengths (L, L') to determine the equivalent resistance and capacitance of a single electrode-electrolyte interface. From the same data, the resistivity of the electrolyte can be determined with high accuracy. The following derivation presents the theory of operation of the variable-length conductivity cell.

Balance condition for length L:

$$R_b + \frac{1}{j\omega C_b} = 2R + \frac{2}{j\omega C} + \frac{\rho L}{A}. \tag{9-3a}$$

Balance condition for a shorter length L':

$$R_b' + \frac{1}{j\omega C_b'} = 2R + \frac{2}{j\omega C} + \frac{\rho L'}{A}. \tag{9-3b}$$

Manipulation of these two expressions to separate R, C, and ρ by equating the resistive and the reactive components gives

$$R = \frac{LR_b' - L'R_b}{2(L - L')} = \frac{LR_b' - L'R_b}{2\Delta L}, \tag{9-6}$$

$$C = \frac{4(C_b C_b')}{(C_b + C_b')} \quad \text{if} \quad C_b' = C_b, \quad \text{then} \quad C = 2C_b, \tag{9-7}$$

$$\rho = \frac{A(R_b - R_b')}{L - L'} = \frac{A\Delta R_b}{\Delta L}. \tag{9-8}$$

Using the variable-length conductivity cell, Geddes (1971, 1973) investigated the validity of the Warburg concept, which states that both the equivalent resistance and the reactance vary inversely as the square root of frequency and that the resistance is approximately equal to the reactance. The data obtained (Fig. 9-7a) indicate that for stainless steel in contact with 0.9% sodium chloride at room temperature both the capacitance and the resistance of a single electrode-electrolyte interface decrease with increasing frequency. Figure 9-7b shows that the reactance of the capacitance $(1/2\pi fC)$ is approximately equal to the resistance.

Perhaps the most remarkable characteristic of the series-equivalent circuit for an electrode-electrolyte interface is the frequency dependence of the values for capacitance and resistance; this condition emphasizes the difficulty of assigning single values for resistance and capacitance. Another interesting relationship is that the ratio of the reactance to the resistance, which is the tangent of the phase angle (ϕ), is approximately unity (i.e., tan

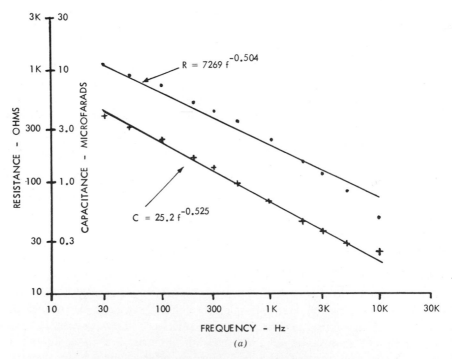

(a)

Figure 9-7.   Stainless steel 0.9% saline electrode-electrolyte interface measured with a current density of 0.025 mA/cm² over a frequency range from 20 Hz to 20 kHz. (a) Series-equivalent resistance (R) and capacitance (C); (b) Series-equivalent resistance (R) and reactance (X = ½πfC). [From Geddes et al., *Med. Biol. Eng.* **9**:511–521 (1970). By permission.]

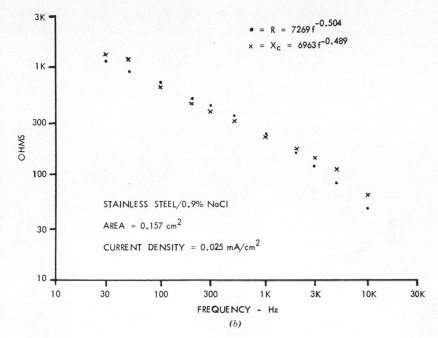

Figure 9-7. (*b*)

$\phi = X/R = 1$). Schwan (1963) reported that the ratio of reactance to resistance for platinum electrodes in contact with saline varied only by a factor of about 2 over a four-decade range of frequency. Figure 9-7*b* supports this statement.

It is important to note that the magnitude of the equivalent resistance and reactance are dependent on current density. Studies by Schwan (1965, 1968), Jaron (1969), and Geddes et al. (1971) have shown that the series-equivalent capacitance increases with increasing current density, the increase being greater in the low-frequency region. The work of Geddes et al. (1971) also revealed that the series-equivalent resistance of an electrode-electrolyte interface decreases with increasing current density, the decrease being largest in the low-frequency region. Because the series-equivalent capacitance increases with increasing current density, the reactance decreases with increasing current density. Since the series-equivalent resistance also decreases with increasing current density the impedance-frequency curves taken at higher current densities will lie below those taken at lower current densities. Figure 9-8 presents this relationship for brass electrodes in contact with 0.6% saline. Note that the high-frequency impedance becomes asymptotic to the resistance of the electrolytic column, revealing that the

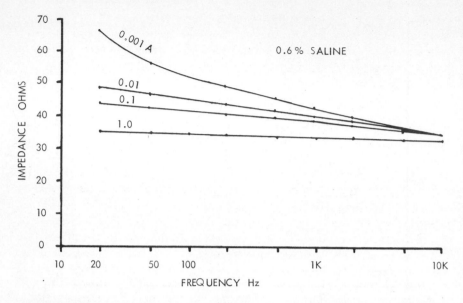

Figure 9-8.   Impedance-frequency characteristics of an electrolytic resistor consisting of two circular brass electrodes (6 cm diameter) separated by a column of 0.6% saline, 15.1 cm long. The numbers on the curves indicate the current levels (in amperes rms) used to measure the impedance-frequency characteristics. [From L. A. Geddes et al., *Med. Biol. Eng.* **11**:747–754 (1973). By permission.]

electrode impedance becomes negligible with respect to this resistance, which is about 32 Ω.

It is noteworthy that as the frequency is decreased, the electrolyte impedance increases for all current densities. However, if the Warburg equivalent (Fig. 9-9a) were totally valid, the impedance would continue to increase to an infinite value as the frequency approaches 0 Hz (i.e., dc). Such a condition does not obtain; instead, the impedance value for each current density becomes finite and there is a relatively constant value for frequencies approaching 0. Thus the Warburg model must be modified by the addition of a parallel resistance R_f (as in Figure 9-9b), which accounts for the faradic (electrochemical) processes that occur at the electrode-electrolyte interface. Electrochemists use the term faradic admittance or resistance to account for this phenomenon.

In summary, a single electrode-electrolyte interface can be modeled by a series resistance and capacitance; the magnitudes of both depend on the type of metal, its area, surface condition, current density, the type of electrolyte, and its concentration. To account for the ability of an electrode-electrolyte interface to pass direct current, it is necessary to add a resistance (R_f) in parallel with the series-equivalent circuit. This resistance accounts for the electrolytic process that can occur at an electrode-electrolyte interface. In addition, an electrode-electrolyte interface exhibits a half-cell potential. Figure 9-9b diagrams this simplified model.

9-4-2. Equivalent Circuit for Electrodes on a Subject

With the admittedly oversimplified model for an electrode-electrolyte interface appearing in Fig. 9-9b, it is possible to create an approximate equivalent circuit that identifies the important components between the terminals of two electrodes applied to living tissue to record a bioelectric event. Figure 9-10a assembles the principal components, including the two electrode-electrolyte interfaces, the conventional model for living tissue (see Chapter 10), and the voltage (E_b) of the bioelectric generator. Inspection of this illustration reveals that there are two sources of capacitance, one due to the electrodes and the other due to the nature of the membranes of the cells that constitute the living tissue. In a practical situation, the physical sizes of the components will govern their impedances; for this reason it is difficult to specify the magnitudes of the reactances and resistances. Nonetheless, a few general statements can be made regarding the impedance-frequency characteristic measured between the electrode terminals 1 and 2.

In the previous discussion, it was shown that the impedance of an electrode-electrolyte interface decreases with increasing frequency. The capacitive nature of the electrical model for living tissue also indicates that its impedance decreases with increasing frequency. Therefore the impedance measured between the terminals of a pair of electrodes applied to living tissue would be high in the low-frequency region, decreasing with increasing frequency, and approaching a relatively constant value when the reactances

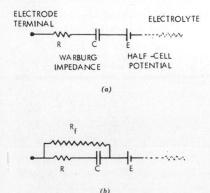

Figure 9-9. Idealized models for an electrode-electrolyte interface. (a) Series-equivalent (Warburg) resistance (R) and capacitance, the magnitudes of which increase with decreasing frequency; E is the half-cell potential. (b) Model including a resistance R_f, which accounts for the electrochemical (dc) impedance of the electrode-electrolyte interface.

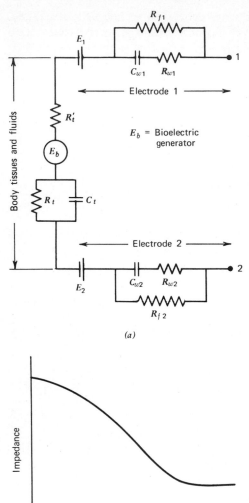

Figure 9-10. (a) Idealized equivalent circuit of electrodes applied to living tissue to record a bioelectric signal (E_b); (b) typical impedance-frequency characteristic measured between electrode terminals (1, 2).

in the circuit become small with respect to their associated resistances. Figure 9-10b illustrates this relationship. In general, with small-area electrodes, the zero-frequency (i.e., dc) impedance will be largely dependent on the electrode area. The frequency at which the impedance starts to decrease will be lower with needle electrodes, when compared with plate or disk electrodes, such as those used for ECG and EEG. With large-area electrodes, the decrease in impedance with increasing frequency usually reflects the decreasing impedance of the living tissues.

It is infrequently recognized that there may be a standing (dc) potential appearing across the electrode terminals in the absence of a bioelectric event. For example, if the two half-cell potentials of the electrodes are unequal, a constant potential will be present whose magnitude and polarity depend on the relative magnitudes of the two half-cell potentials. This standing, or dc-offset potential, is of considerable importance when direct-coupled recording techniques are employed.

9-5. INSULATED ELECTRODES

In remarking earlier that it is possible to detect bioelectric events with electrodes in which there is no electrolytic bridge (i.e., ohmic contact) between the metallic electrodes and the subject, reference was made to the use of electrodes that are completely covered with an insulating material. Such electrodes are, of course, capacitors in which one plate is the elec-trode, the subject is the other "plate" and the dielectric is the insulating covering on the metallic electrode and the dry outer layer of the skin. To obtain an electrode-subject impedance that is as low as possible, every effort is made to attain a high capacitance by using a very thin dielectric having a high dielectric constant. Richardson et al. (1967, 1968) and Lopez and Richardson (1969) described the first insulated electrodes which consisted of an aluminum plate (2.5 × 2.5 cm) that was anodized (i.e., covered with a film of aluminum oxide, which is an insulator). The anodized surface was placed in contact with the subject and on the back of the elec-trode was mounted a field-effect transistor (FET) with the gate connected directly to the insulated electrode. The FET was connected as a source follower. To protect the FET from acquiring a high electrostatic voltage, a high resistance leakage path was provided by using two diodes connected in series opposition.

Wolfson and Neuman (1969) described another insulated electrode consisting of a chip of N-type silicon (6 × 6 mm × 0.3 mm thick) on which was deposited a circular layer of silicon dioxide, 0.2 μ thick and 4.5 mm in diameter. The region beyond the circle and the edge of the chip was insu-lated with a thicker layer of silicon dioxide. The electrode was directly mounted to an ultra-high input impedance amplifier consisting of a metal-oxide semiconductor field-effect transistor (MOSFET) amplifier, arranged as a source follower. A second MOSFET was used as an electronic switch to protect the input transistor from high electrostatic voltages.

There is no doubt that an adequate time constant can be obtained with insulated electrodes to allow recording the ECG (i.e., the product of electrode capacitance and amplifier input resistance is greater than 3 sec). However, attractive as these truly dry electrodes are, certain important practical considerations should be borne in mind. For example, considerable effort is directed toward obtaining a very thin, waterproof, insulating coating. The waterproofing consideration is mentioned because if dry electrodes are placed on human skin, perspiration, which is dilute saline, will soon accumulate perhaps attacking and destroying the dielectric, leading to an ohmic contact with the subject. Also, a thin-film dielectric is easily punctured by stray electrostatic potentials, resulting in the possibility of a conductive contact with the subject. If the dielectric remains intact, a very high input impedance amplifier is required. The magnitude of the input impedance required depends on the time constant desired.

9-6.   TYPES OF SURFACE ELECTRODES

Many types of electrode have been employed to detect bioelectric events. A few of the more familiar types are sketched in Figs. 9-11, 9-13, 9-14, 9-15, 9-17, 9-19, 9-21, 9-22, 9-24, and 9-25. A practical basis for their comparison is the electrode area,[1] and an important characteristic is the impedance measured between the electrode terminals. When large-area electrodes are used, it is customary to measure the dc resistance between the electrode terminals. Direct-current resistance, however, does not by itself describe the electrical circuit constituted by the electrodes and the biological material. To adequately describe this circuit, it becomes necessary to know the resistive and reactive components at all frequencies. In general, the smaller the electrode, the higher the interface impedance. The impedance-frequency characteristics of electrodes of various sizes are discussed in this section.

9-6-1.   Plate and Disk Electrodes

Among the largest recording electrodes are those used for electrocardiography (Fig. 9-11a), consisting of two rectangular (3.5 × 5 cm) or circular (4.75 cm) plates of German silver,[2] nickel-silver, or nickel-plated steel. When these electrodes are applied to a subject with electrode jelly, typical dc resistance values are in the range of 2 to 10 kΩ; the high-frequency impedance amounts to a few hundred ohms. Figure 9-12 illustrates a typical impedance-frequency characteristic for such electrodes.

---

[1] The area referred to here is calculated from the physical dimensions of the electrodes, not the effective area, which in the case of many specially prepared electrodes is much greater.

[2] German silver is an alloy of nickel, copper, and zinc; it contains no silver.

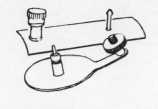   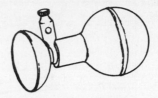

A. METAL PLATES   B. SUCTION ELECTRODE

Figure 9-11. Electrodes for electrocardiography: (*a*) metal plates; (*b*) suction electrode.

In 1910 James and Williams reported that such plate electrodes replaced the more cumbersome immersion (bucket) electrodes traditionally used for recording the ECG. The metal plate electrodes were separated from the subject by cotton or felt pads soaked in concentrated saline. Pardee (1917) indicated that the electrodes used then were 12 × 25 cm, and the saline was described as "strong."[3] The plate electrodes and the electrolytes developed were so practical for electrocardiography that they quickly displaced the immersion electrodes, which had been observed to have serious practical defects that made the taking of an ECG a time-consuming procedure: (*a*) the subject had to remove his boots, (*b*) the subject had to be seated (hence the ECGs of many bedridden patients could not be obtained), and (*c*) spillage of the electrolytes made it difficult to keep the subject insulated from ground.

In electroencephalography, solder pellets a few millimeters in diameter are sometimes applied to the cleaned scalp and contact is established via electrode paste. Small needles inserted subcutaneously are also used. In most studies, however, small silver disks approximately 7 mm in diameter, such as those in Fig. 9-13, are employed. Sometimes the disks are chlorided, and occasionally they are separated from the scalp by a washer of soft felt (Jasper and Carmichael, 1935). Contact with the cleaned scalp in both cases is made by way of an electrolytic paste. In practice, the dc resistance measured between a pair of these electrodes on the scalp varies between 3 and 15 kΩ.

The impedance measured between pairs of the electrodes just described was determined by the authors in the frequency range extending from 0 to 100 kHz. The measurements were made with the same current density at each frequency. Often there were appreciable differences between individual electrodes of the same type. When this occurred, many electrodes were tested and the data averaged. The values plotted in Fig. 9-12 include the impedance of the electrodes and that of the subject between them. In each case dc resistance was measured, using a low-current ohmmeter. Figure 9-

[3] The authors estimate that the concentration of saline was between 5 and 30%.

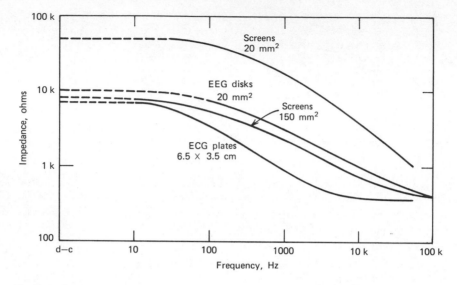

Figure 9-12.   Impedance-frequency characteristics of electrodes applied to human subjects.

12 also presents the impedance-frequency characteristics of several other types of electrodes. In general, for all electrodes the dc resistance is greater than the high-frequency impedance, indicating that if a low-current ohm-meter is used to measure the resistance, the value obtained, although in-dicative of circuit continuity, only approximates the low-frequency impe-dance of the circuit. In the 10- to 100-Hz region, the impedance approxi-mates the dc resistance. Above 100 Hz the impedance decreases progressively, reaching values many times smaller than the magnitude of the dc resistance.

Although the figures given for the impedances of large-surface electrodes can be called typical, considerable variation that is dependent on the quality of application to the subject may be encountered. To demonstrate this point, Schmitt et al. (1961) measured the 60-Hz impedance between standard ECG electrodes on subjects before taking routine electrocardio-

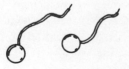

EEG ELECTRODES   Figure 9-13.   EEG scalp electrodes.

grams. Although a median value of 2400 Ω was obtained, even under well-controlled conditions, impedances 40 times this large were encountered. In this investigation, which employed technicians familiar with attaching electrodes to human subjects, impedances as high as 100,000 Ω were occasionally measured.

Although the physical size of the electrode appears to be the property most directly determining its impedance, it is noteworthy that the effective area of the electrode is increased by wetting the skin with electrolytic solutions (e.g., electrode paste or perspiration). Blank and Finesinger (1946) directed attention to the importance of this factor when measuring the resistive component of the galvanic skin reflex. Effective area can also be increased by special treatment of the electrode metal. Electrodeposition of a spongy layer of metal greatly increases the area and reduces the impedance. Use of this technique was described by Marmont (1949), Svaetichin (1951), and Dowben and Rose (1953).

A very useful type of electrode is the suction-cup electrode (Fig. 9-11b), the forerunners of which were described by Roth (1933-1934) and Ungerleider (1939). Such an electrode is extremely practical as an ECG chest electrode and is well suited for attachment to flat surfaces of the body and to regions where the underlying tissue is soft. Although physically large, this electrode has a small area because only the rim is in contact with the skin.

A variant of the plate electrode that permits quick application is contained in a strip of adhesive tape. This electrode (Fig. 9-14) consists of a lightweight metallic screen backed by a pad for electrolytic paste. Measuring approximately 1.5 in. square, it adheres well to the skin and exhibits a relatively low resistance. The adhesive backing holds the electrode in place and retards evaporation of the electrolyte.

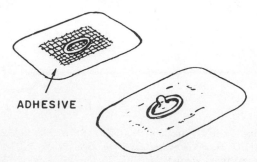

ADHESIVE

Figure 9-14.   Adhesive tape electrode. (Courtesy of Telemedics Dept., Vector Division of United Aircraft Corp., Southampton, Pa.)

9-6-2. The Recessed Electrode

An electrode popular in aerospace studies and patient monitoring, and frequently used on exercising subjects, is the recessed electrode, occasionally referred to as the liquid-junction electrode. In this type (Fig. 9-15) the metal does not contact the subject directly; contact is made via an electrolytic bridge. The principle embodied in the recessed electrode was used

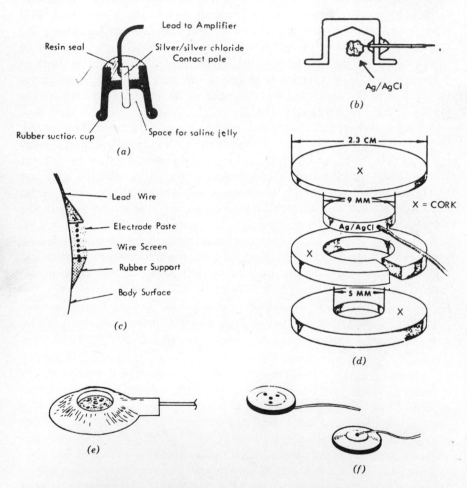

Figure 9-15. Floating or liquid-junction electrodes. (*a*) B. Shackel, *J. Appl. Physiol.* **13:**153–158 (1958); (*b*) D. N. O'Connell et al., *Arch. Gen. Psych.* **3:**252–258 (1960); (*c*) E. Hendler and N. J. Santa Maria, *Aerosp. Med.* **32:**126–133 (1961); (*d*) G. G. Lucchina and C. G. Phipps, *Aerosp. Med.* **33:**722–729 (1962); (*e*) J. Day and M. Lippitt, *Psychophysiology* **1:**174–182 (1964); (*f*) A. Kahn, personal communication, 1964.

by the electrophysiologists of the nineteenth century, when it was customary to employ a metallic electrode in contact with an aqueous solution of one of its salts contained in a porous plug. Surrounding the plug was a saline solution that made contact with the subject. As time passed, the awkwardness of this type of electrode led investigators to contain the salt of the electrode metal in a kaolin plug or paste that adhered to the electrode. Between the kaolin and the subject was a film of saline. Occasionally the saline was omitted, and contact with the subject was made via the salt of the electrode metal. /

The recessed electrode takes many forms. One such electrode was used by Forbes et al. (1921), who employed a fluid-filled funnel containing a zinc rod in the neck; the mouth of the funnel was covered with a permeable membrane soaked in saline. Pairs of these electrodes were applied to elephants to record their electrocardiograms. Baudoin et al. (1938) described a similar electrode consisting of a small rubber cup, which was cemented to the skin. The cup was filled with electrolyte into which a chlorided silver wire dipped. Baudoin et al. used their electrode for a variety of purposes, including recording the EEG.

A modern version of the recessed electrode was described by Haggard and Gerbrands (1947) and Clark and Lacey (1950). Shackel (1958) embodied the principle in an interesting suction-cup electrode consisting of a silver-silver chloride rod mounted centrally in a rubber cup, filled with electrode jelly. This electrode (Fig. 9-15a) was found to have remarkably high electrical stability despite movement of the cup on the skin. The dc resistance between a pair of these electrodes applied to the forearm was 2000 to 7000 Ω.

A similar high-stability recessed electrode, consisting of a silver-silver chloride sponge in a small enclosure resembling a top hat, was described by O'Connell et al. (1960). This electrode, illustrated in Fig. 9-15b, was designed for GSR measurements. A type of recessed electrode that has become popular in aerospace medicine and is now employed extensively for recording bioelectric events on patients and exercising subjects was described by Hendler and Santa Maria (1961). In this electrode (Fig. 9-15c) the metallic conductor is mounted in a flat rubber or plastic washer, which is cemented to the skin by special adhesives.[4, 5] The washer holds the electrode away from the skin, and contact is established via a thick film of electrolytic paste. Choice of the electrode materials and electrolytes depends on the event and the circumstances of measurement. Monel wire screens (Hendler and Santa Maria, 1961), crossed tinned copper wires in a segment

[4] Eastman 910: Eastman Kodak Co., Rochester, N.Y.
[5] Stomaseal: 3M Manufacturing Co., St. Paul, Minn.

of rubber tubing (Rowley et al., 1961), stainless steel screens (Roman and Lamb, 1962; Mason and Likar, 1966), silver disks (Boter et al., 1966), chlorided silver screens and plates (Day and Lippitt, 1964, Fig. 9-15e; Skov and Simons, 1965), and disks of a compressed mixture of silver and silver chloride (Lucchina and Phipps, 1962, 1963, Fig. 9-15d; Kahn, 1964, Fig. 9-15f) have been employed with considerable success. With these electrodes applied to the human thorax, the dc resistance varies with the method of preparing the skin, the type of conducting electrolyte, and the area of the electrodes. In practice dc resistance varying from about 2 to 50 kΩ are typical. Figures 9-12 and 9-16 present the impedance-frequency characteristics of several such electrodes of different areas.

Lucchina's and Kahn's investigations merit special consideration, for they focus attention on important factors relative to the stability of recessed electrodes. Lucchina's (1962) electrode (Fig. 9-15d) consisted of a disk of equal parts of silver and silver chloride made by first grinding and then compressing the mixture under a pressure of 20,000 psi. The disk was then mounted in a cork ring, which held the electrode away from the skin. With a pair of these electrodes applied to the abraded human thorax, the authors reported a dc resistance of 500 to 2000 Ω.

Lucchina and Phipps (1963) made a series of electrodes having different amounts of silver and silver chloride. They measured the voltage difference and resistance between similar electrodes in contact with Graphogel[6] in a test jig and found that reducing the amount of silver chloride decreased the dc resistance but increased the voltage difference. Although they noted that the presence of a minute amount of silver chloride reduced the potential difference between a pair of electrodes, they recommended a 30% silver and 70% silver chloride mixture as the best compromise between voltage difference and resistance.

The electrodes described by Kahn (1964), which are commercially available,[7] are illustrated in Fig. 9-15f. In these electrodes a disk of silver-silver chloride is mounted behind a stiff baffle in which holes have been drilled. Contact between the electrode and the skin is made via electrode jelly that fills the holes. The combination of a stiff baffle and the use of silver-silver chloride results in an electrode of high mechanical and electrical stability with which remarkably clean electrocardiographic records can be obtained from subjects exercising vigorously.

9-6-3.   Multipoint Electrodes

A most interesting type of electrode, which was described by Lewes (1965), is shown in Fig. 9-17. This very practical ECG electrode, now

[6] Tablax Corp., New York, N.Y.
[7] Beckman Instruments, Spinco Division, Palo Alto, Calif.

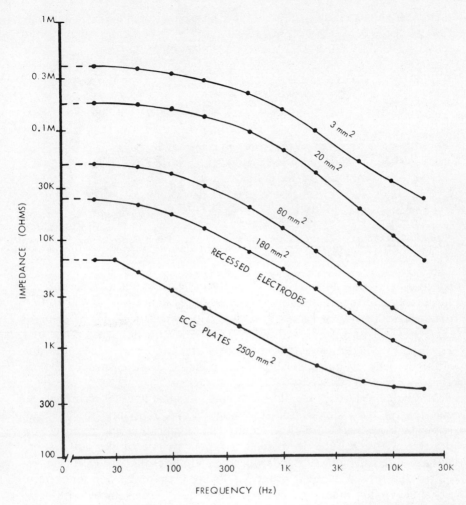

Figure 9-16.   Impedance-frequency characteristics of recessed electrodes of various areas and conventional ECG electrodes applied to the human thorax. [From Geddes and Baker, *Electrocardiol.* **1**:51–56 (1968). By permission.]

designated as the multipoint electrode,[8] consists of a 6 × 5 cm segment of a standard nutmeg grater made of stainless steel or tin-plated soft iron. It is slightly curved to fit over fleshy parts of the body; the abrasive side is placed against the skin. Approximately 1000 fine, active contact points are obtained when the electrode is applied to the skin with a very slight rotary movement that causes the multipoints to penetrate the stratum corneum, the layer responsible for the major part of the skin resistance. When

[8] U.K. Patent Application 52,253/64. Now available from Cardiac Recorders, London, EC1.

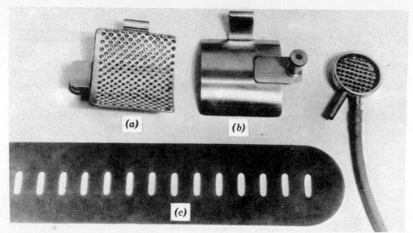

Figure 9-17. Multipoint electrodes: (*a*) limb electrode; (*b*) suction electrode; (*c*) rubber strap. (Courtesy of D. Lewes, Bedford, England.)

penetration occurs, a low-resistance contact is established with the subject. Lewes reported that the multipoint electrode resistance was similar to that obtained with plate electrodes and jelly. The impedance-frequency curves (Fig. 9-18) obtained by Lewes and Hill (1966) over a frequency range of 1 Hz to 1 kHz closely resemble those produced with plate electrodes and electrode jelly. With a smaller 1-in. circular chest electrode, the dc resistance was slightly higher (6 kΩ).

Multipoint electrodes are of special value in some unusual recording circumstances; for example, for screening the ECG in large numbers of human subjects, the short time required for application and removal is a most attractive feature. In a demonstration on one of the authors, installation, recording three standard leads, and removal of the electrodes required only 80 sec. When it is not possible to prepare the skin for conventional electrodes, multipoint electrodes are ideal. For example, with hairy animals, when it is not permissible to remove the hair, coarse multipoint electrodes can be readily employed. Using such electrodes applied directly to the unprepared skin of the horse, Hill (1967) recorded the ECG and impedance respiration. Multipoint electrodes also see useful service in extreme environmental conditions. In situations of low temperature and barometric pressure, it is difficult to store electrode pastes and jellies in their containers. The use of multipoint electrodes eliminates the need for these substances and permits easy recording under field conditions.

9-6-4. Low-Mass Electrodes

When recordings are to be made on subjects experiencing large vibration or acceleration forces, it is important to make the electrodes as small and light as possible/ Thompson and Patterson (1958), Sullivan and Weltman (1961), Roman and Lamb (1962), Lucchina and Phipps (1962), and Simons et al. (1965) have described such electrodes and demonstrated their value. Sullivan and Weltman's electrode weighed 2 mg and consisted of mylar 0.001 in. thick on which was deposited a metallic film. The center was filled with electrode jelly, and Eastman 910 adhesive[9] was employed to cement the electrode to the subject. Remarkably clean electromyograms were obtained on exercising subjects. Thompson's electrodes consisted of small pieces of silvered nylon applied to an area of skin that had been lightly sanded. The electrodes were applied with a special conducting adhesive. Although the electrodes were small and performed remarkably well during vigorous movement, the dc resistance between pairs was in the vicinity of 100,000 Ω, a characteristic that demanded the use of an amplifier with a very high input impedance.

9-6-5. Radio-Transparent Electrodes

Occasionally while a subject is being fluoroscoped or x-rayed, it is desirable to record the electrocardiogram. In many instances the electrodes and the connecting wires are in the x-ray field, consequently obscuring the area of interest. To overcome this problem Castillo and Marriott (1974) developed electrodes that cannot be detected during x-ray visualization. Their electrodes (Fig. 9-19) consist of a foam rubber container (corn plaster) 3 mm thick, saturated with electrode paste. A French vinyl feeding tube (also filled with electrode paste) is connected to the electrode. At the

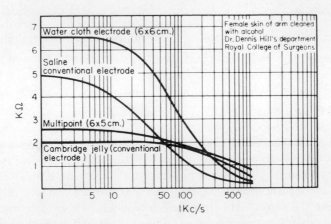

Figure 9-18. Impedance-frequency curves for multipoint and conventional electrodes. (Courtesy of D. Lewes and D. Hill.)

---

[9] Eastman Kodak Co., Rochester, N.Y.

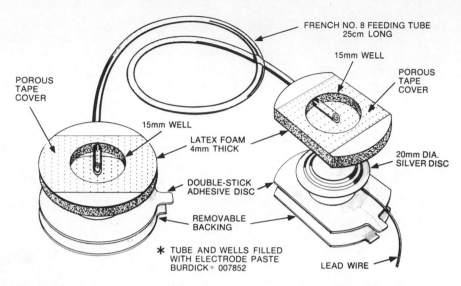

Figure 9-19. Radio-transparent electrodes for electrocardiography [From Castillo and Marriott, *J. Electrocardiol.* 1974, in press. By permission.]

other end of the vinyl tube is a chamber containing electrode paste and a chlorided silver disk, 15 mm in diameter. The wire from the disk is connected to the electrocardiograph. The electrodes are transparent to x-rays because only an electrolytic fluid column is in the x-ray field. Electrode pastes, like tissue fluids, are transparent to x-rays.

Castillo and Marriott reported that the use of vinyl tubes of electrolytic paste adds only 5000 Ω to the electrode impedance. They also stated that these electrodes have been applied to the precordium to record electrocardiograms during 25 cardiac catheterization procedures.

9-6-6.   "Dry" Electrodes

With the increasing availability of solid-state amplifiers with high input impedances, it is becoming recognized that bare conducting surfaces, applied directly to the unprepared skin, can be used as electrodes to detect bioelectric events from human subjects. Such "dry" electrodes seldom remain dry when they are placed on skin that is endowed with sweat glands because perspiration usually accumulates and provides an electrolytic connection with the subject. It is therefore important to recognize that the impedance appearing between the electrode terminals will be high initially and will remain so if no perspiration accumulates to render the stratum corneum (the outer dry layer of the skin) conducting. In fact, if the sweat glands are blocked by drugs (such as atropine) or if the skin is devoid of sweat glands, or in the case of thick, dry skin (as in hypothyroidism), the electrodes may function largely as capacitors and exhibit the characteristics of insulated electrodes (see Section 9-5), which capacitively couple the subject to the recording apparatus.

As just stated, the accumulation of perspiration under dry conducting surfaces, used as electrodes, results in a gradual decrease in the impedance measured between the electrode terminals; Fig. 9-20 documents this fact. The initial value of impedance depends on the type of skin, its thickness, and the area of the electrode. The rate of decrease in impedance is quite variable and depends on a variety of environmental factors and the nature of the subject to whom the electrodes are applied. The following paragraphs provide some quantitative data on these points. In general, there is little change in impedance after about 30 min.

Prior to the availability of high input impedance solid-state amplifiers, studies were undertaken to investigate the practicality of dry electrodes for the long-term recording of bioelectric events. Edelberg (1963) described an efficient dry electrode made by electrodeposition of silver into the layers of the skin. The resistance between a pair of silver depositions was remarkably low, and no electrolytic paste was required; the silver spots were virtually terminals on the subject. The only drawback to these remarkable electrodes is their relatively short life. As time passes, the silver undergoes chemical changes and the spot eventually disappears. Nonetheless, the obvious advantages of these electrodes indicate that investigation of their use will continue.

A most interesting low-mass dry electrode (Fig. 9-21) designed for aerospace research was described by Roman (1966), and technical details were presented by Patten et al. (1966). This electrode, which exhibits many desirable characteristics for human use, can be applied to the skin in only a few minutes. With a pair of these electrodes on the thorax, remarkably clean ECG and impedance respiration recordings can be obtained. To date 500 hr of in-flight and 700 hr of ground recording of the ECG have been logged successfully on Air Force personnel. The electrodes are applied by first rubbing electrode jelly into the skin with a toothbrush and then wiping the skin dry with gauze. Next a film of conducting adhesive[10] is painted or sprayed on the skin, forming a conducting spot about 20 mm in diameter. Then a silver-plated copper wire is placed in the conducting adhesive glue and is captured as drying occurs. When dry, the assembly is coated with insulating cement to cover the electrode (see Fig. 9-21). The impedance of

[10] 43 grams of Duco Household Cement (Dupont S/N 6241), 23 grams of silver powder (Handy and Harman Silflake 135), and 125 cc of acetone.

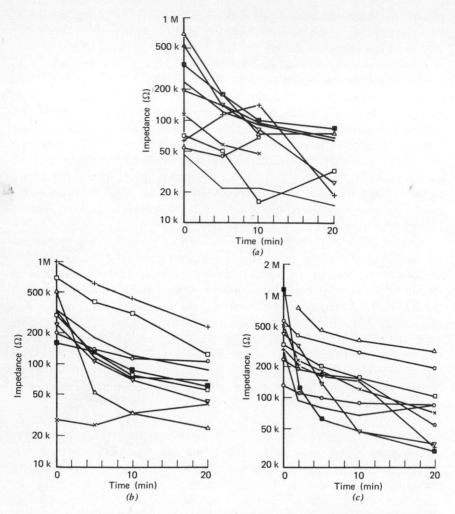

Figure 9-20. Temporal change in impedance encountered with dry electrodes supplied to the right arm and left leg to record the electrocardiogram: (*a*) silver electrodes (3.9 × 6.2 cm); (*b*) stainless steel electrodes (3.9 × 6.2 cm); (*c*) German silver electrodes (3.3 × 5.1 cm). [From Geddes and Valentinuzzi, *Ann. Biomed. Eng.* 1:350–367 (1973). By permission.]

these electrodes is dependent on their area. In the sizes customarily used, the low-frequency impedance is in the range of 50 kΩ, so that an amplifier with an input impedance of 2 MΩ or more is required if distortion-free ECGs are to be recorded.

Lewes (1965) reported that it was possible to obtain electrocardiograms that were indistinguishable from those obtained conventionally, 6 min after applying dry metal electrodes (15 cm²) that were connected to a conventional vacuum tube electrocardiograph. He explained his results by reporting that the accumulation of perspiration lowered the electrode-subject impedance to a level that was adequately low for his instrument. In another study Johnson and Allred (1968) reported using dry silver-screen electrodes connected to a FET differential amplifier (with an input impe-

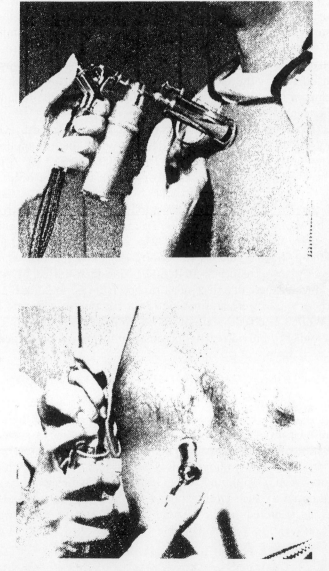

Figure 9-21.   Spray-on electrode. [From *Aerosp. Med.* 37:790–795 (1966). By permission.]

dance of 10^7 Ω and a common-mode rejection ratio of 80 dB.) to record the human electrocardiogram. They measured a range of electrode-subject impedance extending from 20 kΩ to 10 MΩ (for very dry skin). In another study, Bergey et al. (1971) applied bare metal electrodes (2.5 cm diameter) to unprepared human skin to record the electrocardiogram. They made measurements using several different metals and chose stainless steel as the optimum. However, a similar decrease in impedance with time was seen with all metals. After a few minutes the low-frequency impedance with stainless steel electrodes was in the range of 20 to 60 kΩ. In a similar study Geddes et al. (1973) applied dry silver, stainless steel, and German silver ECG electrodes to human skin. The highest initial impedance was about 1 MΩ. With all metals the impedance decreased almost exponentially with time, reaching a range of 50 to 100 kΩ at 30 min; Fig. 9-20 presents a summary of these data.

The electrooculogram (see Chapter 11) has been recorded by Geddes et al. (1973) using dry coin-silver electrodes (1.7 cm diameter) applied bitemporally. The initial impedances ranged from 5100 Ω to 230 kΩ. After about 20 min, the average impedance had dropped by about one order of magnitude.

One of the first practical clinical applications of dry electrodes was described by Wolfe and Reinhold (1973); they employed a dry conducting elastomer $\frac{1}{4}$ in. thick and measuring $2\frac{1}{8} \times \frac{7}{8}$ in. These electrodes were placed in the axillae of humans to acquire the ECG for aural monitoring and telemetery by a frequency-modulated tone transmitted by telephone. The impedance of these dry electrodes ranged from 60 to 2.5 kΩ, averaging 12.7 kΩ; these values were attained within a fraction of a minute after application. Wolfe's electrodes were designed for emergency application by unskilled personnel to provide early diagnostic information on myocardial infarction.

9-7. PRECAUTIONS WITH HIGH-IMPEDANCE ELECTRODES

When high-impedance electrodes are used to measure bioelectric events, special input stages are required.[11] For example, in electrocardiography attention must be given to the averaging resistance networks such as those which constitute the V-terminal (Wilson et al., 1934) or those employed with the various vectorcardiographic lead systems (Schwarzschild et al. 1954). Dower et al. (1959), and King (1964) have challenged the validity of records taken under such circumstances. Although the magnitudes of the distortions encountered in the various situations have not always been critically examined, they are calculable from measured values of electrode

---

[11] See Section 9-14.

impedance and the values of the resistances in the networks to which the electrodes are connected. Rappaport et al. (1949) presented a mathematical analysis of this problem. Schwarzschild's suggestion of using cathode followers ahead of the averaging resistors merits consideration when high-resistance electrodes are to be employed with such resistance networks. Emitter or source follower circuits or unity-gain operational amplifiers will achieve the same end.

When special electrodes are used for electrocardiography, their location is often chosen to minimize artifacts. For example, slight differences in electrode materials, variable contact resistance, and action potentials from contracting muscle masses between the electrodes all produce spurious signals. To obtain ECGs free from muscle artifact, Geddes et al. (1960) developed the MX lead, in which one electrode was placed over the manubrium and the other over the xiphoid process. Standard EEG electrodes (1-cm silver disks), jellied and attached to the skin with adhesive tape, were employed. To attain the same goal Carbery et al. (1960) introduced two electrode placements. In both they used 1-in. stainless steel recessed screen electrodes. In one configuration three electrodes were employed; one was placed over the manubriosternal junction, another over the vertebral column at the lumbrosacral junction, and the third over the vertebral column at the level of the eighth thoracic vertebra. In the other configuration electrodes were placed at the lower margin of the rib cage on the midaxillary lines. The third electrode was placed over the vertebral column at the level of the lumbrosacral junction. In addition they employed a band-pass filter to select only the frequencies of importance in the ECG. They reported that with the first electrode array they obtained satisfactory ECGs on 95% of the subjects tested; the only difficulties were associated with truly hyperasthenic subjects. For the latter group the second electrode array was satisfactory.

Recognizing that ECGs taken on the exercising subject by using limb leads always contain movement artifacts, Mason and Likar (1966) investigated electrode locations on the thorax, which produced records nearly identical with those derived from leads I, II, III. Two electrodes were located on the right and left chest below the clavicles, and the third was on the anterior axillary line halfway between the costal margin and the crest of the ilium.

Rose (1963) reported that if ECG changes are sought which are indicative of the metabolism of the myocardium, such as alterations in the T wave and S-T segment, the location of the electrodes merits special consideration. He found that locating one electrode over the manubrium and the other at the left fifth or sixth interspace at the anterior axillary line produced better results than any of the other possibilities investigated. A similar electrode location was adopted by Gibson et al. (1962) and designated as the T lead by Davis and Thornton (1965). Rose reported that electrodes placed along the sternum, although relatively free from movement artifact, were of little value in indicating ischemic S-T segment shifts.

Thus when taking the ECG with special electrodes placed in nonstandard locations, it is important to examine the type of information to be obtained from the recordings. If only heart rate is desired, the choice of electrodes and their location present no problems. If clinically acceptable records are wanted, it is necessary to compare the results carefully with those obtained with clinically accepted instruments and standard lead configurations. If changes in cardiac metabolism are to be determined, attention to placement is paramount; the location for ECG electrodes which permits recording with a minimum of artifacts is not necessarily the optimum for identification of subtle changes occurring with alterations in the metabolism of cardiac muscle.

9-8. ELECTRODE ELECTROLYTES

When metallic electrodes are placed on the surface of the body, contact is made via electrolytic solutions. If the electrodes are to be left in place for extended periods, evaporation of the solution takes place. To prevent such an occurrence, it is sometimes possible to locate the electrodes in body cavities and use the fluids in these regions as electrolytic conductors; sometimes the cavities can serve as containers for the electrolytes. Although not all the body cavities can be employed in unanesthetized subjects, consideration should be given to using the nose, ear, mouth, axilla, navel, rectum, vagina, and urethra. Often electrodes in these and other areas can be combined with other transducers, such as electrical thermometers or heart-sound pickups. Sometimes the metallic cases of these devices can serve as active, indifferent, or ground electrodes. The fluid in some fluid-coupled pressure transducers makes direct contact with the metallic case of the transducer, which is usually grounded. If this occurs, a ground connection is automatically placed on the subject. Although this may be desirable in many instances, it may constitute a hazard. For example, if the subject comes into contact with the "hot" side of a voltage which is ground-referred, the ground path through the transducer may result in the passage of a sizable current through the subject. In some instances, in which catheter electrodes are employed for measuring blood pressure or for pacemaking and when other devices (such as EEG or ECG instruments) are connected to the subject, there is a real danger of the existence of multicircuit loops in which currents intense enough to precipitate ventricular fibrillation may flow./Reviews of the practical considerations in this area were supplied by Whalen et al. (1964) and Geddes and Baker (1971). Chapter 10 presents a discussion of such electrical hazards.

Electrode jellies and pastes were developed during the early string galvanometer days of electrocardiography when investigators were anxious to eliminate the cumbersome immersion electrodes, which required that the subject be seated with both hands and feet in saline-filled buckets. Study was begun of the behavior of electrodes consisting of sheets of metal wrapped in saline-soaked bandages and applied to the skin, but experience with the immersion electrodes indicated that ECG distortion occurred if the electrode resistance was high. Under these conditions, the string tension had to be reduced to obtain adequate sensitivity, and, as a consequence, the response time of the string was prolonged. Thus to obtain a satisfactory ECG a tight string was required, which meant that the electrode resistance could not exceed a certain value. Large electrodes and strong electrolytes were needed to obtain a low resistance contact with the subject.

James and Williams (1910) were the first to introduce plate electrodes made of German silver. The electrodes were wrapped in saline-soaked gauze and applied to the subject. Cohn (1920) described a more practical electrode of soft lead (22 $\times$ 7 cm) backed by a rubber sheet. The electrode was applied to the skin, which had been rubbed with a saline solution. The ECGs taken with German silver electrodes and lead electrodes were essentially the same as those taken with the immersion electrodes, probably because the resistances in all cases were comparable.

About 1935, when electrode pastes and jellies began to replace the saline-soaked pads, the characteristics of several of the earliest electrode jellies were investigated by Bell et al. (1939). Using lead electrodes (14 $\times$ 5 cm) on human subjects, they measured the dc resistance and 300-Hz impedance with the following substances under the electrodes: (a) 1% saline; (b) a paste of saline, glycerine, water, and pumice; (c) soft green soap; and (d) a recently introduced electrode jelly that contained crushed quartz. They found that when the electrodes were wrapped in gauze, soaked in 1% saline, and applied to the subjects, the dc resistance was highest (3080 Ω). With the other three preparations in direct contact with the electrodes and skin, the resistances were 2010, 2040, and 1100 Ω, respectively. By analyzing their results, Bell and his colleagues quickly found that the presence of an abrasive reduced the resistance considerably. They were able to show that the resistance with green soap was divided by 3 when crushed quartz was added and the mixture rubbed into the skin. They also found that by lightly rubbing the dry skin with glass paper (fine sandpaper), "so that it lost its sheen and white color," and applying the electrolyte, they could obtain very low and extremely stable dc resistance and impedance values. This early observation demonstrated the need for abrasives in electrode pastes and jellies.

A novel method for obtaining a low resistance, which Shackel (1959) described and called the skin-drilling technique, is painless when properly employed. The area of skin where the electrode is to be placed is first cleaned with an antiseptic solution. The region is then abraded with a dental burr in a hand tool. Only the epidermis is eroded and no blood is drawn. The amount of abrasion required depends on the type of skin. Kado (1965) reported that deeply pigmented skin requires more abrasion. In a few seconds, tissue fluid can be seen seeping into the drilled depression. The area is then cleaned with alcohol or acetone. If the skin has been drilled to the proper depth, the subject should feel a slight tingling sensation when the region is cleaned with either of these solutions. The electrode jelly is then applied and the electrode secured.

To test the value of the technique, Shackel compared the resistance values obtained with and without drilling. The drilled sites consistently exhibited values one-fifth to one-tenth of those of undrilled areas. When the electrodes are removed, the drilled site is again cleaned with an antiseptic solution. Lanolin cream is then rubbed in, and the site soon becomes invisible.

A modern reappraisal of traditional electrode jellies for recording the ECG was presented by Lewes (1965), who called attention to the fact that strong electrolytes were essential in the string galvanometer days, when the electrode-subject resistance had to be in the low-kilohm range, but with the advent of electronic instruments with high input impedance the need for a low electrode resistance had disappeared. To prove his point he recorded more than 4000 ECGs with instruments of high input impedance (2 to 4 MΩ), using a remarkable variety of substances as electrode jellies. The recordings made with each substance were compared with those obtained with standard electrode jelly. The substances used were lubricating compounds (K-Y jelly, Lubrifax), culinary compounds (mayonnaise, marrons glacés, French mustard, tomato paste), and toilet preparations (hand cream and tooth paste). All these substances are poor conductors, and all produced ECGs indistinguishable from those taken with standard electrode jelly.

To emphasize his point further, Lewes employed dry polished electrodes (15 cm²) on dry skin and in 6 min obtained entirely satisfactory ECGs indistinguishable from those taken with standard jelly. Examination of the skin under each electrode revealed the presence of a small amount of sweat, which on analysis was found to contain approximately 6 mg of sodium chloride. Additional evidence that strong electrolytes are unnecessary was provided by obtaining entirely satisfactory ECGs within 15 sec after placing a single drop of distilled water under each electrode.

Lewes's studies prove that when instruments of high input impedance are employed to record the ECG, a low electrode-subject resistance is not necessary. His findings, however, relative to the relationship between amplifier input impedance and high-impedance electrodes produced by electrolytic solutions of low ionic content are just beginning to be noticed. For single- or multiple-channel recording with bipolar electrodes, the facts adduced by Lewes are clear. However, King (1964) pointed out that when monopolar recording techniques are employed in which several electrodes are connected through resistors joined to a common point, a high electrode resistance is incompatible with the low value of averaging resistors presently in use (5000 to 300,000 Ω). He further illustrated his point by making recordings with low- and high-resistance electrodes. Although such a condition may obtain when high-resistance electrodes are used in this situation, provision could easily be made to electronically add the voltage from each individual electrode, thereby removing all restrictions on the resistance of electrodes employed in procedures in which averaging techniques are involved.

From studies such as those just reported, it can be seen that two types of electrode preparation are now in use. One has low resistivity and originated in the days when it was necessary to obtain a low-resistance contact with the subject. Such preparations are still used for recording bioelectric events and must be used when electrodes are used to pass current, as in the case of stimulation or defibrillation. The other type of electrode-electrolyte that is available is high in resistivity and resembles skin lotion. Such preparations are suitable for recording bioelectric events with modern equipment which has an adequately high input impedance. Such preparations should never be used with stimulating or defibrillating electrodes. Table 9-3 presents the resistivity values for various electrode-electrolytes.

The electrodes, and electrolytes used with them, must not be considered to be independent from the recording equipment to which the electrodes are connected. Presented elsewhere in this chapter are additional studies relative to the type of distortion encountered when high-impedence electrodes are employed with amplifiers having input impedances that are not high enough.

Although most of the commercially available electrode pastes are satisfactory for recording a variety of bioelectric events, various authors have presented their own recipes. Among these are Jenks and Graybiel (1935), Bell et al. (1939), Marchant and Jones (1940), Thompson and Patterson (1958), Shackel (1958), Lykken (1959), Edelberg and Burch (1962), Asa et al. (1964), and Fascenelli et al. (1966).

Table 9-3 Resistivities of Electrodes-Electrolytes*

Preparation and Supplier	Resistivity[†] (Ω-cm)
Redux Electrode Paste	9.4
Sanborn Div., Hewlett Packard: Waltham, Mass.	
Electrode Cream EC-2	30.0
Grass Instrument Co.: Quincy, Mass.	
Cambridge Electrode Jelly	10.4
Cambridge Instrument Co., Inc.	
Ossining, N.Y.	
Beckman-Offner Paste	5.9
Offner Division, Beckman Instruments Inc.	
Chicago, Ill.	
EKG-Sol	200.0
Burton, Parsons & Co., Washington, D.C.	
Burdick Electrode Jelly	10.0
Burdick Co., Milton, Wis.	
Cardiopan	120.0[‡]
Leichti: Berne, Switzerland	
Cardette Electrode Jelly	313.0[‡]
Newmark Instrument Co.: Croydon, Surrey, England	
Electrode Jelly	118.0[‡]
Smith and Nephew Res. Ltd., Harlow, Essex, England	
Cardioluxe Electrode Jelly	84.0[‡]
Philipps Electrical Ltd., Balham, London	
Electrode Jelly	196.0[‡]
Data Display, Ltd., Liverpool, England	
NASA Flight Paste	13.0
National Aeronautics and Space Administration	
(NASA): Houston, Tex.	
Electrode Cream	82.0[‡]
National Aeronautics and Space Administration	
NASA: Houston, Tex.	
K-Y Lubricating Jelly	323.0[‡]
Johnson & Johnson: Slough, Buckinghamshire, England	
0.9% (physiological) saline solution	70

* From L. A. Geddes, *Electrodes and the Measurement of Bioelectric Events.* Wiley New York, 1972. (By permission.)
† At room temperature.
‡ From Hill and Khandpur, *World Med. Instr.* 7:12–22 (1969) (By permission.)

9-9. TISSUE RESPONSE TO ELECTROLYTES

When recording bioelectric events with surface electrodes, attention should be given to the choice of the metal and electrolyte employed, since each may produce its own physiological effects. The constituents of some electrode pastes can cause allergic reactions, erythema, or discoloration of the skin. Some species of ions stimulate cells; others are toxic. For example, a high concentration of calcium chloride, such as was used in the older electrode jellies and pastes, causes sloughing of the skin. Seelig (1925) showed by subcutaneous injections of calcium chloride that solutions with concentrations greater than 1% produced sloughing.

When recording the GSR, the ionic composition of electrolytes merits special consideration. For example, Edelberg and Burch (1962) conducted a series of ingenious experiments in which the responses at test and control sites were compared; they found that solutions of 1 molar (1.0 M) calcium chloride, ammonium chloride, and potassium sulfate potentiated the GSR by 100 to 300%. Aluminum chloride potentiated by 1000%, and zinc chloride (0.5 M) approximately doubled the response. Very dilute acids, alkalis, and detergents decreased the response. A solution of 0.05 M sodium chloride had negligible effect on the GSR, and Edelberg recommended its use for this purpose. Thus in the routine recording of a bioelectric event from skin surfaces containing sweat glands, what may appear as an artifact may actually be an enhanced GSR. On the other hand, if one is attempting to record the GSR, the electrolyte may enhance or diminish the response. Scarification of the region under the electrode can produce unwanted voltages. Edelberg and Burch (1962) reported that although cuts or skin punctures lower skin resistance, they also reduce the GSR.

9-10. PERCUTANEOUS ELECTRODES

Mooney et al (1974) described a most ingenious method of creating a percutaneous vitreous carbon terminal in human subjects; one part is above the skin, and the other is below; Fig. 9-22 illustrates these devices, which resemble a collar button made of vitreous carbon. Using local anesthesia, the devices can be implanted surgically with the larger part of the collar button below the skin and the smaller part protruding. Healing, without reddening, occurs around the protruding portion in a manner that resembles the skin surrounding the base and sides of finger nails.

Vitreous carbon, which is surprisingly well tolerated by living tissue, is made by firing an organic polymer in an inert atmosphere at about 1800°C. The firing time is adjusted so that all elements other than carbon are eliminated. The resulting hard material is very smooth and retains the

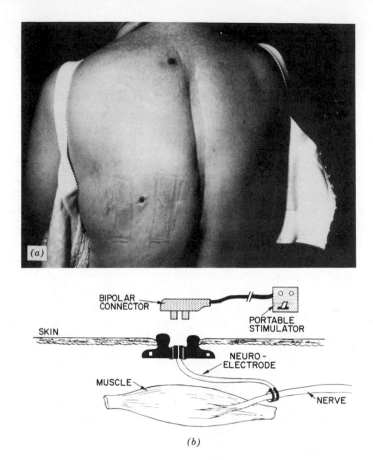

Figure 9-22. (*a*) Vitreous carbon percutaneous implants applied to the human subject; (*b*) implants used as cable connector for electrodes applied to a nerve. [From Mooney et al., *Arch Surg.* **108**:148–153 (1974). By permission.]

shape of the original polymer, except that a shrinkage of about 40% has occurred. The vitreous material can be polished with a diamond polishing compound.

Figure 9-22*a* illustrates a typical percutaneous "collar button" and the appearance of the skin surrounding it 26 months after implantation. Mooney and Hartmann reported implantation of 23 vitreous carbon implants into 11 persons. The implants can be used as cable connectors, as in Figure 9-22*b*, or as stimulating or recording electrodes. They have also been used for skeletal attachment for limb prostheses. Rarely has there been any difficulty with healing or infection. There is no doubt that this remarkable material will be widely used for a variety of purposes.

9-11.   ELECTRODES FOR EXPOSED TISSUE

When the electrical activity of the exposed cortex is recorded, it is customary to employ silver ball electrodes approximately 1mm in diameter, bare or chlorided, and sometimes covered with a small cotton pad. Geddes (1948–1949) described the preparation and use of these electrodes, which are illustrated in Fig. 9-23a. The dc resistance between a pair of these electrodes spaced a few centimeters apart on the human brain is in the 10- to 50-kΩ range.

In some studies it is necessary to employ a pair of what have come to be known as nonpolarizable electrodes. One frequently employed type, illustrated in Fig. 9-23b, is often made from a medicine dropper. A cotton wick is placed in the tapered end, and a cork in the large end holds a chlorided silver wire in contact with the electrolyte in the dropper. These electrodes were described and thoroughly investigated by Burr (1944, 1950). They are frequently used for dc recording because a pair can be made having a voltage difference as small as 10 μV or less. The dc resistance of two cotton wick electrodes in saline is in the 10- to 50-kΩ range. Kahn (1965) described electrodes of this type in which the metal consisted of a compressed mixture of silver and silver chloride. The electrode employed was saline and in some instances plasma. The voltage difference between a saline-filled pair varied between 5 and 10 μV.

A similar type of medicine dropper electrode, developed for total implantation, was described by Rowland (1961). The stem of his electrode measured 15 mm long and 6 mm in diameter, and in it he placed a coiled-coil electrode made from 30-guage silver wire that was in contact with saline. The coiled coil was made by first winding 5 in. of wire around a 20-

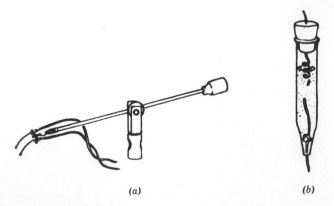

(a)   (b)

Figure 9-23.   Electrodes for exposed tissues: (a) cortical electrodes; (b) wick electrode.

gauge needle and then removing and stretching the coil slightly so that the individual turns did not contact each other. The coil was then wrapped around a needle of the same size and inserted into the stem of the small medicine dropper. This technique permits obtaining a large electrode-electrolyte junctional area in a small space. Rowland reported that the dc resistance range of such electrodes was 30 to 50 kΩ with a potential difference in the millivolt range between pairs. He demonstrated their value in recording six channels of EEG in the cat.

9-12. SUBINTEGUMENTAL ELECTRODES

When it is desired to bring an electrode close to a bioelectric generator, it is often practical to penetrate the skin and advance the electrode through the penetration. Often the electrode is sharp enough to accomplish penetration. Hence a variety of depth and needle electrodes have been described to obtain highly localized extracellular recordings of bioelectric events.

9-12-1. Depth Electrodes

Because electrodes placed on the scalp or cortex detect mainly the electrical activity of the neurons in the superficial layers of the brain, the need has arisen to find a method of detecting the electrical activity of subcortical nerve cells. Two highly successful types of depth electrodes have been developed, one, due to Delgado (1955), (see Figs. 9-24a, 9-24b), the other due to Ray (1966; see Figs. 9-24c, 9-24d). Delgado's electrode consists of a bundle of Teflon-insulated stainless steel wires (0.005 in. in diameter) of differing lengths bonded to a central supporting wire (0.007 in. in diameter) by an insulating varnish. The end of the supporting wire is rounded for ease of insertion into the brain. The ends of the individual wires are staggered 3 mm, and their 1-mm exposed surfaces constitute the individual electrodes. The active area of each electrode is in the vicinity of 0.5 mm². The end of the central supporting wire often serves as an indifferent electrode. The other

Ray's electrode, which is commercially available,[12] consists of a bundle of 18-gauge insulated wires bonded to a length of 24-gauge stainless steel needle tubing with a high-temperature varnish. Each wire is platinum (90%)-iridium (10%) and is 0.0035 in. in diameter; the active electrodes are made by scraping the varnish from the wires at the desired places. The scraped area is then platinized to reduce the tissue-electrode impedance by

[12] Medical Applications Department, Advanced Systems Development Division, IBM, Rochester, Minn.

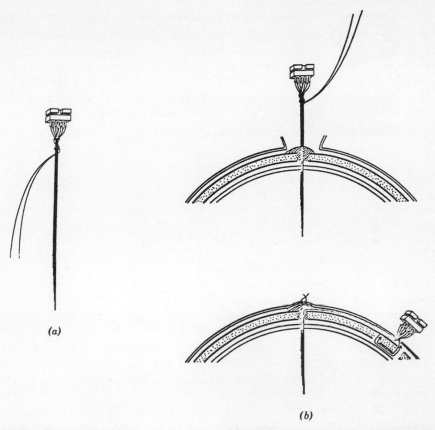

(a)

(b)

Figure 9-24. (a) Delgado's depth electrode; (b) method of insertion. [From J. M. R. Delgado, *EEG Clin. Neurophysiol.* 7:637–644 (1955). By permission.] (c) Ray's depth electrode; (d) method of insertion (now available from Medical Applications Dept. 249, IBM Corp., Rochester, Minn.). [From C. D. Ray, *J. Neurosurg.* 24:911–921 (1966). By permission.]

about one hundred-fold. The contact area employed by Ray was 0.075 × 1.00 mm.

The depth electrodes described by Delgado and Ray have been implanted into the brains of animals and man and left there for prolonged periods to record the electrical activity of subcortical neurones under a variety of normal and abnormal states. Ray reported that the central stainless steel needle that supports the electrodes could be used for the injection of materials into the brain or the passage of a guarded microelectrode. He also stated that his electrodes could serve to measure localized impedance changes; by the application of the proper polarizing voltage, moreover, the electrodes are suitable for the continuous recording of oxygen tension.

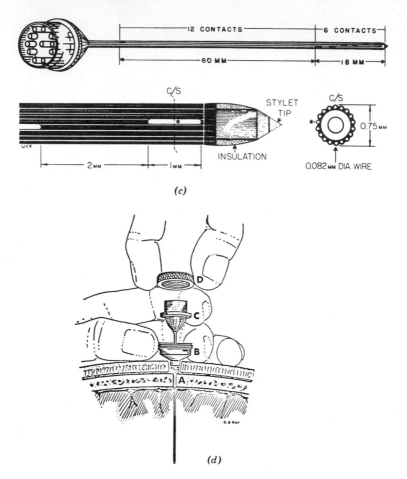

Figure 9-24. (*c*,*d*)

9-12-2. Needle Electrodes

Electromyographers often find it convenient to use a variety of electrodes; some are placed on the skin, whereas others are inserted directly into the muscle being examined. For precise localization, steel needle electrodes are inserted directly into the muscle. Usually the electrodes are coated with an insulating varnish and are bare only at the tip. Frequently one needle electrode is paired with a metallic plate on the surface of the skin. Figure 9-25a illustrates this type of electrode, which was described by Jasper et al. (1945). When the shaft of the needle electrode is coated with insulating varnish, the area of the electrode in contact with active tissue is quite small/ In the case of Jasper's needle electrode, the area was /approximately 0.2 mm²/

/Over the past decade there has arisen the need for EMG electrodes that can be left in place for prolonged periods. To meet this requirement, many interesting electrodes have been developed. The main goals have been ease of insertion, freedom from pain during insertion, mechanical and electrical stability during muscular contraction, minimal interference with muscular movement, and freedom from pain while *in situ.*/Although few types have attained all these goals, some very promising electrodes have been constructed. For example, Basmajian and Stecko (1962) developed a bipolar fine-wire (25-μ in diameter) electrode that is easily inserted and

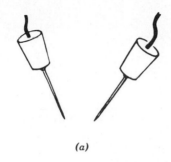

(a)

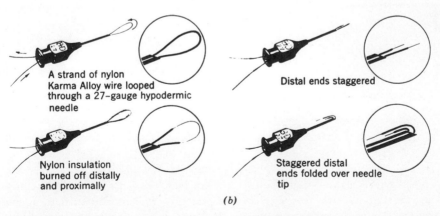

A strand of nylon Karma Alloy wire looped through a 27–gauge hypodermic needle

Distal ends staggered

Nylon insulation burned off distally and proximally

Staggered distal ends folded over needle tip

(b)

Figure 9-25. Electrodes for electromyography. (*a*) Needle electrodes; (*b*) steps in making a bipolar electrode assembly before sterilization. [From Basmajian and Stecko, *J. Appl. Physiol.* **17**:894 (1962). By permission.] (*c*) Scott's electrode. (*d*) Parker's electrode.

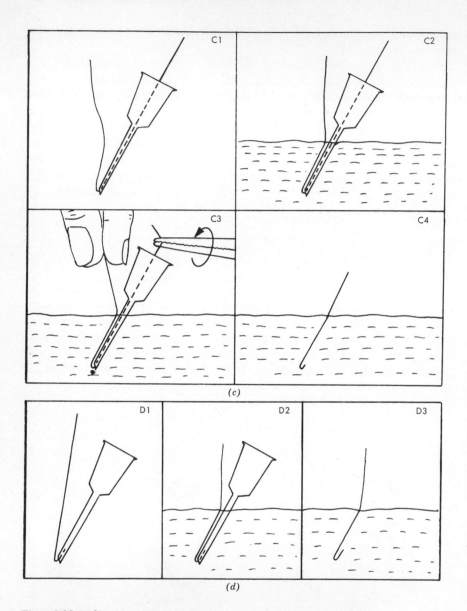

(c)

(d)

Figure 9-25. (*c,d*)

remains well anchored in the muscle./The steps in construction of this electrode are shown in Fig. 9-25b. In the lower right-hand corner of the figure, the electrode is ready for insertion into the muscle by advancing the hypodermic needle. When the depth desired is reached, the needle is withdrawn, leaving the electrode in the muscle. The bent ends serve as hooks to prevent the electrode from coming dislodged.

In a similar fine-wire electrode described by Scott (1965), the insulated wire[13] is passed through the lumen of the needle and bent back to pass along the outside of the needle [Fig. 9-25c(1)]. The hypodermic needle and wire are then inserted to the desired depth in the muscle [Fig. 9-25c(2)]. With the outside wire held firmly, a pair of forceps is applied to the inner wire, and the wire is cut by winding it on the forceps [Fig. 9-25c(3)] so that it contacts the sharp edge of the hypodermic needle. Then the needle is withdrawn, leaving the outer wire in the tissue [Fig. 9-25c(4)]. The active surface of the electrode is approximately the cross-sectional area of the wire.

Another method of inserting fine-wire electrodes was developed by Parker (1966). A short length at the end of a fine wire is bent back upon itself. The bent-back portion is then inserted into the tip of the hypodermic needle [Fig. 9-25d(1)] and the needle and wire are advanced into the muscle [Fig. 9-25d(2)]. At the desired depth the needle is withdrawn, leaving the electrode hooked into the muscle [Fig. 9-25d(3)]. With this technique, monopolar or bipolar electrodes can be installed. The active surface of the electrode is the cross-sectional area of the wire.

The authors have measured the impedance-frequency characteristics of a variety of pairs of stainless steel needle electrodes, similar to those illustrated in Fig. 9-25a. The electrodes were insulated down to the tip, which was left bare. The area of each pair of electrodes was carefully measured before insertion into the left hind limb and right forelimb of an anesthetized dog. After 5 min impedance-frequency curves were determined. The procedure was repeated for each pair of electrodes. Current density was maintained at the same level at each frequency.

The impedance-frequency curves for the various pairs of needle electrodes are presented in Fig. 9-26. Clearly evident at all frequencies is the inverse relationship between electrode area and impedance. Also apparent is a decrease in impedance with increasing frequency. The contours of the impedance-frequency curves of the various electrodes examined are similar to those obtained by Barnett (1937), Offner (1942), Burns (1950), Gray and Svaetichin (1951–1952), Tasaki (1952–1953), Gesteland et al. (1959), Plutchik and Hirsch (1963), and Schwan (1963).

[13] Karma Wire, Driver-Harris Co., Harrison, N.J.

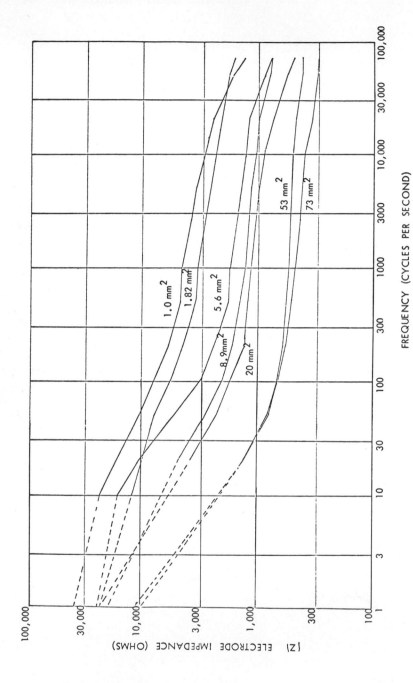

Figure 9-26. Impedance-frequency curves for needle electrodes. [From L. A. Geddes and L. E. Baker, *Med. Biol. Eng.* **4:**439–450 (1966). By permission.]

Occasionally, when it is necessary to record from animals with thick dry hides, the use of plate electrodes is impractical and conventional needle electrodes cannot be easily inserted. To solve this problem, Geddes et al. (1964) developed two types of cutting electrode (Fig. 9-27). These electrodes are made from surgical cutting needles, and their beveled, sharpened shanks permit easy insertion through the hide.

When cutting electrodes are used, movement artifacts can be minimized by inserting the needles in a manner such that the area of the bare metal electrode in contact with the tissues is constant. The safety pin electrode should be inserted through a pinch of skin and fastened. When the pinch is released, the skin will press against the head and spring of the safety pin. The connecting wire is soldered to the brass sleeve, and the sleeve and solder connection are all covered with insulation to prevent their contact with body fluids. To provide strain relief for the solder joint the connecting wire is passed through the coils of the spring and tied. Similarly, with the needle electrode, it is advisable to insulate the soldered portions of the electrode and the part of the shank above the cutting edge and to insert the electrode into the animal far enough so that no bare needle protrudes.

To record the electrical activity of small groups of cells, monopolar and bipolar hypodermic electrodes are often used. Such types, first described by Adrian and Bronk (1929), are shown in Fig. 9-28. The monopolar electrode was made with 36-gauge wire (190 μ diameter), and the bipolar electrode contained two 44-gauge wires (80 μ diameter). These electrodes exhibit dc resistances in the range of tens of kilohms.

9-13.   TISSUE RESPONSE TO IMPLANTED ELECTRODE METALS

In many recording situations electrodes must remain in direct contact with body tissues and fluids for prolonged periods. For example, when electrodes are implanted in muscle and brain tissue to record the bioelectric signals of these structures for periods of months, special consideration must

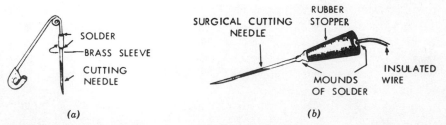

Figure 9-27.   Cutting electrodes: (a) safety pin electrodes; (b) needle electrodes. [From L. A. Geddes et al., *Southwest. Vet.* **18:**56–57 (1964). By permission.]

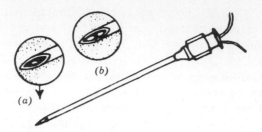

Figure 9-28.   (*a*) Monopolar and (*b*) bipolar hypodermic needle electrodes.

be given to the type of metal employed/There were only a few studies of
the relative toxicity of the various species of metallic ions in the early days
of depth electrode recording in the human brain. Dodge et al. (1955) had
the opportunity to study the tissue response to two electrodes, each
consisting of 6 strands of Formvar-insulated copper wire (97.5 μ diameter),
which had been *in situ* for 6 days. Nineteen months later the brain was
examined histologically. Tissue changes were seen at the points of entry of
the electrodes. Minimal tissue changes were found along the tracks of the
electrodes.

Faced with the problem of recording the electrical activity of structures
deep within the brains of human and animal subjects, Fischer et al. (1957)
studied the response of the brains of cats to 1-cm lengths of 24-gauge wires
left *in situ* for periods up to 4 weeks. The wires employed were of chlorided
silver, bare copper, and stainless steel. Both bare and insulated[14] wires were
employed. After 1 week histological studies showed tissue responses to all
of the materials used. The responses were dependent on the type of metal
employed; the insulating compounds were virtually without tissue response.
Silver and copper wires proved to be the most toxic to brain tissue. After 3
weeks a narrow ring of necrotic tissue surrounded the silver wire/Around
this ring was a circular edematous region 2 mm in diameter./The reaction
to the copper wire at the same time was similar except that an increase in
vascularity had also occurred/The copper wire was encircled by necrotic
tissue and an edematous region. The diameter of the lesion varied between
1.5 and 7 mm./With the stainless steel wire the size of the lesion was determined by the extent of the mechanical trauma produced by its introduction into the brain./Only minimal edema was found/Fischer and his co-
workers concluded therefore that the electrode material of choice for such
studies is stainless steel. /

In another study, carried out by Collias and Manuelidis (1957), bundles
of six stainless steel electrodes (125 μ diameter) were inserted into the

---

[14] Tygon, Formvar, Thermobond M472, and polyethylene.

brains of cats. Describing the histological changes that occurred over periods extending up to 6 months, the investigators found that an orderly sequence of changes took place in the tissue surrounding the electrode track. At the end of 24 hr there was a zone of hemorrhage, necrosis, and edema extending to about 1 mm from the electrode. After 3 days there was less hemorrhage and necrotic debris, and by the seventh day a 0.1-mm layer of capillaries occupied the necrotic zone. By the fifteenth day the capillaries had almost completely replaced the necrotic region, and connective tissue had started to form. After the passage of a month the necrotic debris had disappeared, and a well-defined capsule surrounded the electrode track. Capsule formation was virtually complete after 4 months, at which time a thick, dense capsule completely encircled the electrode.

Robinson and Johnson (1961) carried out studies similar to those just described. Into cat brains they implanted wires (125 μ diameter) of gold, platinum, silver, stainless steel, tantalum, and tungsten, and studied the tissue responses at different times over a period extending to 6 months. Responses similar to those previously described were observed. After about a week the differences betweeen the metals in regard to the reaction produced began to be detectable. Gold and stainless steel evoked the least tissue response; tantalum, platinum, and tungsten produced more. Silver precipitated a vigorous tissue reaction. Encapsulation of all electrodes was evident at 15 days, with thicker capsules around the metals that provoked the greatest tissue response.

The authors hasten to emphasize that these tissue changes were studied in cat brains with electrodes that carried no current. Studies on the responses of other tissues to other electrode materials and on tissue responses to current-carrying electrodes have yet to be made. It is anticipated that the tissue response to current-carrying electrodes will be quite different in view of the many electrolytic reactions that can occur.

9-14. INPUT IMPEDANCE OF THE BIOELECTRIC RECORDER

When recording bioelectric events, it is necessary to make the input impedance of the bioelectric recorder many times larger than the impedance appearing between the electrode terminals. When this technique is employed, only a small current flows through the electrode impedance, and there is a minimal loss of voltage at the electrode-electrolyte interface. However, if the bioelectric recorder has an input impedance that is not high with respect to the impedance of the smallest-area electrode, there can occur a distortion in the waveform of the bioelectric event. Because of the resistive and reactive components of the electrode-electrolyte impedance, the various components of the bioelectric event will not be presented to the bioelectric recorder with the same relative amplitudes they initially posssessed. Moreover, phase distortion accompanies such amplitude-frequency distortion, and the time relations between the various frequency components will be altered. In addition, it is known that the resistive and reactive components of the impedance decrease when high current densities are encountered. If the input impedance of the bioelectric recorder is so low that high current densities result, it is possible for the electrode impedance to become dependent on the amplitude of the bioelectric event. If this occurs small- and large-amplitude signals will be injected differently into the input of the bioelectric recorder. It is thus apparent that the use of an input stage whose impedance is not very high with respect to the electrode-subject impedance virtually guarantees that the bioelectric event will be distorted. A high electrode current density can occur when the electrode area is small (as it is with metal microelectrodes) and a conventional amplifier is employed.

It has already been demonstrated that waveform distortion of clinical significance occurs when high-resistance electrodes are employed with recorders having a low-resistive input impedance. In the early days of electrocardiography, when string galvanometers with their relatively low resistance (5–20 kΩ) were used, Lewis (1915) showed that a normal ECG was distorted when recorded with polarizable platinum electrodes. In such cases attenuated P and T waves and enhanced S waves were obtained. Similarly Pardee (1917), using a string galvanometer and German silver electrodes applied to a bandage soaked in saline, showed that the rectangular wave calibration signal was distorted when the area of each electrode was decreased from 300 to 8 cm². With the smaller electrodes, the calibration signal instead of rising rapidly and exhibiting a flat top, showed a sharp overshoot and an R-C decay to a sustained plateau. On turning off the calibrate signal, there was an undershoot and R-C decay to the baseline. Pardee (1917) observed a similar type of distortion when electrodes were applied to patients with thick, dry skin or when the blood vessels under the electrodes were constricted. The distortion disappeared when an electrolyte was rubbed into the skin. It often disappeared as time passed and the electrolyte penetrated the dry, horny layers of the skin. Although Pardee did not investigate the phenomenon thoroughly, his observations were in agreement with those of previous and later workers, notably Einthoven (1928), who demonstrated that the electrode-subject interface impedance introduced a time constant into the circuit which electrically differentiated the P and T waves.

The practical importance of these facts in recording the ECG was again made evident by Sutter (1944) and Roman and Lamb (1962). These investigators applied small-area electrodes to the chest of a human subject and used them first with an amplifier having a high input impedance to obtain control records. They then lowered the input impedance of the amplifier by connecting different resistances across it. The distortions in the ECG were what would be called clinically significant, consisting of a displacement of the S-T segment and a slight depression in the latter part of the T wave.

Recent studies focusing attention on the relationship between recorder input impedance and electrode impedance were those of Maxwell (1957–1958) and Lewes (1965), mentioned previously. Geddes and Baker investigated the relationship between resistive input impedance and electrode area in recording the ECG (1966) and the EMG (1967). By using electrodes of differing areas and shunting the amplifier input with various resistors (loading), the effect of electrode interface impedance was made to manifest itself.

Figure 9-29, showing a lead II ECG in an anesthetized dog, illustrates the type of distortion encountered when this technique was employed. Stainless steel needle electrodes such as those in 9-25a were employed. The needles were insulated to within 1 mm of the tip. The geometric area in contact with the body tissues and fluids was approximately 1 mm^2. To illustrate the nature of the distortion, a square pulse was inserted in series with the electrodes.

Figure 9-29a shows the control ECG and square pulse recorded with an amplifier having a 4 MΩ resistive input impedance. Figures 9-29b through 9-29e reveal the changes produced by placing resistors of successively lower values across the input of the amplifier. During the various trials the electrodes were not disturbed. In Figs. 9-29a through 9-29d, the recording sensitivity was the same. In Fig. 9-29e the recording sensitivity was doubled for clearer comparison with Fig. 9-29a.

The outstanding changes seen in these records are those expected in a system that is deficient in low-frequency response. Such a situation could be predicted on the basis of the general nature of the impedance-frequency curves of electrodes. With 300 kΩ across the input terminals, there were recognizable P and T wave changes and a noticeable tilt appeared on the square pulse. With 100 kΩ and especially with 30 kΩ across the input terminals, the P and T waves and the square pulse were dramatically changed, all becoming diphasic. As loading was increased, there was a continued loss of overall amplitude, and in Figs. 9-29d and 9-29e the resemblance to the control record was all but lost. In Fig. 9-29e, recorded with twice the amplification, the ECG is vastly different from that in Figs. 9-29a. The outstanding differences are the loss of P and T wave amplitudes and the addition of diphasic components to each. The QRS complex has similarly been changed by exaggeration of the S wave.

The manner in which this type of distortion is related to electrode

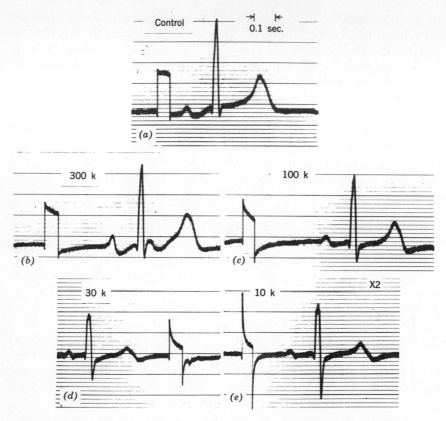

Figure 9-29. Distortion in the ECG produced by lowering input impedance. [From L. A. Geddes and L. E. Baker, *Med. Biol. Eng.* **4**:439–450 (1966). By permission.]

area is shown in Fig. 9-30. In this illustration, ECGs of anesthetized dogs were recorded with various pairs of needle electrodes connected in lead II configuration. The control records, shown along the top of each column, were all obtained with an input impedance of 4.4 MΩ. The changes that occurred as the input impedance of the amplifier was lowered can be appreciated by reading from top to bottom of any column; for example, for the 1-mm² electrodes noticeable distortion occurred when the input impedance was reduced to 100 kΩ. For the 10-mm² electrodes detectable distortion occurred when the input impedance was 20 kΩ. Clearly evident in this illustration is the inverse relationship between distortion, amplifier input impedance, and electrode area.

The relationship between amplifier input impedance and electrode area is not the same for all metals. Cooper (1963) compared the distortions en-

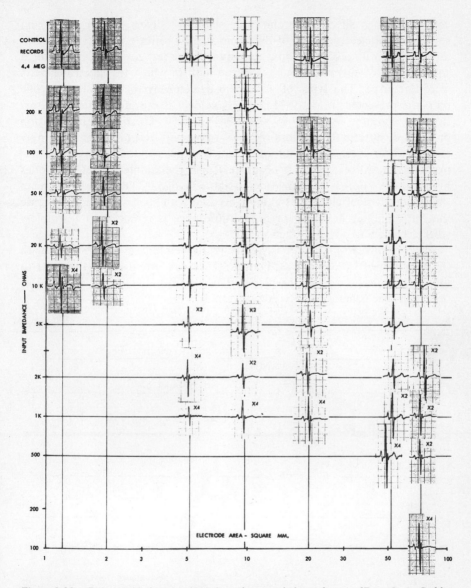

Figure 9-30. Relationship between input impedance and electrode area. [From L. A. Geddes and L. E. Baker, *Med. Biol. Eng.* **4**:439–450 (1966). By permission.]

countered when silver-silver chloride, platinum, silver, copper, gold, and stainless steel electrodes, all of the same area (0.1 mm²), were connected to an amplifier with a 750-kΩ input impedance. The test consisted of passing a square wave of current through a saline bath in which the electrode pairs were immersed. The types of waveform detected by the various electrode pairs are presented in Fig. 9-31. Clearly evident is the same kind of distortion that appeared in Figs. 9-29 and 9-30—namely, electrical differentiation or, stated differently, a loss of low-frequency response. Interestingly enough under these circumstances, the silver-silver chloride electrodes reproduced the waveform most accurately, and the stainless steel electrodes provided the poorest reproduction of the test signal. This does not mean that stainless steel electrodes cannot be used with success; it does indicate that an amplifier having high input impedance is required with stainless steel electrodes of small surface area.

These results, which are consistently reproducible, are in agreement with those described by other investigators. They call attention to the need to use an input stage with an input impedance many times larger than that of the bioelectric generator-electrode system.

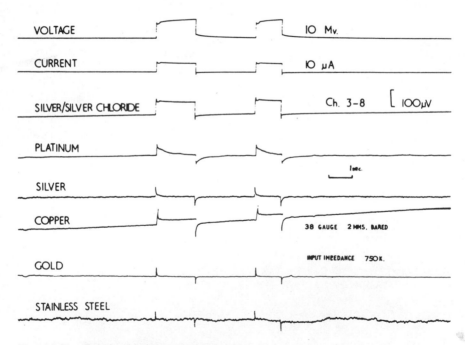

Figure 9-31. Relationship between surface type and constant input impedance for electrodes of various metals. [From R. Cooper, *Am. J. EEG Technol.* **3**:91–101 (1963). By permission.]

The distortion illustrated in Figs. 9-29 through 9-31 is caused primarily by two factors. First, with loading (i.e., the use of an amplifier input circuit in which the input impedance is not high with respect to the electrode-bioelectric generator system) the electrode-electrolyte impedance becomes a dominant part of the input circuit, and the voltage across the input terminals of the bioelectric recorder is less than that under the electrodes. Second, the amount of phase shift is different for the various frequency components of the bioelectric event. With loading, the electrode current density is increased, and the resistive and reactive components of the electrode-electrolyte impedance become nonlinear. Because of this nonlinearity, the magnitude of the electrode impedance becomes a function of the amplitude of the bioelectric event. Thus small- and large-amplitude signals will encounter different impedances. The exact contribution of each of the two sources of distortion is as yet unknown for the various electrodes employed in recording bioelectric events.

Not only does an increase in current density alter the electrode impedance, it also changes the half-cell potential. Even with such a relatively nonpolarizable electrode as the calomel cell, current flow alters the half-cell potential. Rothschild (1938) showed that the maximum current density for this type of electrode was 15 $\mu A/cm^2$ before the half-cell potential was changed. The exact limits of current densities permissible for the various types of electrodes have not as yet been investigated adequately.

9-15. MICROELECTRODES

When it is necessary to investigate the characteristics of the fundamental bioelectric generator (i.e., the single cell), microelectrodes are employed. For an electrode to be classed as a microelectrode, it need only be small enough with respect to the size of the cell in which it is inserted so that penetration by the electrode will not damage the cell.

Electrodes described as micro are of two general types, metallic and nonmetallic. Metallic electrodes consist of a slender needle of a suitable metal sharpened to a fine point or formed by electrolytic etching; nonmetallic electrodes consist of a glass micropipet filled with an electrolyte.

Grundfest and Campbell (1942) reported the method of grinding fine wires to produce 5- to 10-μ points. Grundfest (1950) gave complete details for making 1-μ stainless steel electrodes by electrolytic etching. His technique has become known as "electropointing." Hubel (1957) described a similar method for pointing tungsten wire to obtain electrodes with a tip diameter of 0.4 μ. A most useful and simple automatic electropointing machine for making stainless steel microelectrodes was developed by Mills (1962). With multiple needles mounted radially on a turning rod that dipped them into and out of the etching solution 5 times per minute, the electrodes were pointed to have tip diameters in the range of 1 to 6 μ in 6 hr.

Before use, metal microelectrodes are coated almost to the micro tip with an insulating material that often requires baking in an oven. Guld (1964) described a technique for insulating platinum microelectrodes with a glass covering. When an insulating coating is applied to metal microelectrodes constructed by any of these techniques, it is often difficult to measure the exposed area of the tip, which is rarely if ever covered because of the action of the surface tension of the insulating material. The layer of insulating coating is usually so thin near the tip that microscopic examination frequently fails to uncover the true extent of the insulation, regardless of its color. Under such circumstances the tip area can often be determined by using a method developed by Hubel (1957). A drop of saline is placed on a glass slide and viewed with a microscope. A small wire is then placed in the drop and connected to one pole of a battery; the other pole is connected to the metal microelectrode, which is advanced into the drop and viewed in the microscope. The active area can be estimated by observation of the region from which bubbles are evolved.

As early as 1925 Taylor described the technique of drawing a 35-gauge platinum wire in heated glass tubing. By cutting or breaking the drawn section, an electrode with a tip diameter of less than 1 μ was produced. This method was revived by Svaetichin (1951), who heat-pulled silver solder in a glass tube to produce electrodes with tip diameters of 0.5 to 1 μ. The electrode tip was then covered with electrolytically deposited platinum to lower the electrode resistance. Dowben and Rose (1953) used a mixture of gallium and indium for the metal and heat-pulled the alloy in a glass tube to a tip 2 to 4 μ in diameter; the electrode tip was gold plated to lower the electrical resistance. They pointed out that this particular alloy "wetted" the surface of the glass and produced electrodes having a high degree of uniformity.

It is possible to reduce the impedance of metal microelectrodes by electrolytic processing of the tip. Because some metals, notably platinum and silver, can be laid down in a spongy deposit, electrodeposition of these substances produces a substantial increase in surface area, and a reduction in impedance can be attained without much increase in diameter. A similar technique was described by Marmont (1949), who made an electrode of silver, 13 mm long $\times$ 100 μ in diameter. The electrode was first chlorided, then "developed" by a photographic developer, and the procedure served to decrease the electrode impedance from one-twentieth to one-thirtieth of its "undeveloped" value.

The nonmetallic microelectrode consists of a glass micropipet filled with an electrolyte compatible with the fluid inside the cell being studied. Connection to the electrolyte is made by means of a larger wire inserted into the electrolyte, which fills the stem of the micropipet. The microelectrode thus resembles the larger wick electrode made from a medicine dropper (Fig. 9-23b). There are numerous descriptions of this technique in the literature, and many microelectrode-fabricating machines are available commercially. Reviews of the fabrication techniques have been presented by Kennard (1958), Frank and Becker (1964), and Geddes (1972).

When micropipet electrodes are to be applied to tissue that moves, the tip often breaks. An ingenious solution for this problem was offered by Woodbury and Brady (1956), who introduced the floating micropipet. In their electrode the stem was made of glass tubing 1 to 2 mm in diameter. After filling the micropipet with 3 M KCl, they advanced a thin, flexible tungsten wire into the stem. The friction between the wire and the stem of the micropipet and the fluid surface tension held the micropipet on the wire. The tungsten wire was mounted to a rigid support, and its flexibility permitted the micropipet to follow contracting cardiac muscle.

In the search for precise knowledge of the mechanisms underlying bioelectric phenomena, the microelectrode has made it possible to measure the magnitude of the resting membrane potential and the action potential of an intact single cell and even of separate parts of a cell. Previously, attempts to measure the membrane potential and its excursion relied on killing or damaging the cells under one electrode and placing the other electrode on uninjured cells. This resulted in much ambiguity concerning the conditions at the site of injury. However, with the advent of electrodes small enough to be inserted into single cells without excessive damage, it became possible to measure membrane and action potentials with accuracy and thereby discover the true nature of fundamental bioelectric generators.

When a microelectrode is employed to measure membrane and action potentials, it is located within the cell. The reference (indifferent) electrode is situated outside the cell. The size of an intracellular microelectrode is dictated by the size of the cell and the ability of its enveloping membrane to tolerate penetration by the microelectrode tip. Because single living cells are rarely larger than 0.5 mm (500 μ) and are usually less than one-tenth this size, typical microelectrodes have tip dimensions ranging from 0.5 to 5 μ. When the tip of either a metal or glass micropipet electrode penetrates the cell membrane, the membrane potential suddenly appears between the intracellular and reference electrodes. The electrical circuits in these two situations of measurement will now be analyzed.

9-15-1. Metal Microelectrodes

When a metal microelectrode is advanced into a cell surrounded by other cells or by tissue fluids, as in Fig. 9-32, the potential appearing between terminals connected to the microelectrode and the indifferent electrode is the

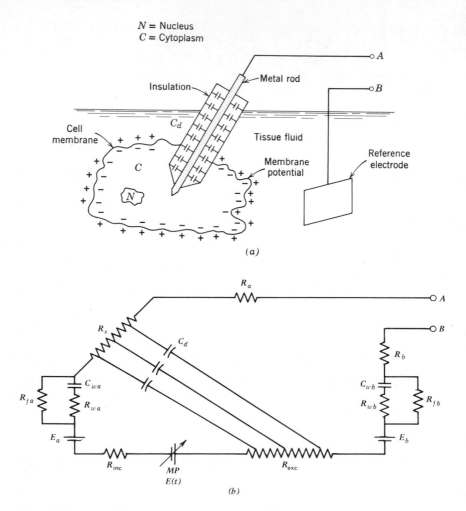

Figure 9-32. Intracelluar metal microelectrode: (*a*) inserted into cell; (*b*) equivalent circuit.

sum of three potentials: the metal-electrolyte potential at the microelec-trode tip which can be designated E_a, the cell membrane potential MP, and the reference electrode-electrolyte potential E_b. When measuring the membrane potential it is assumed that the sum of the first and the third potentials is known and constant.

In addition to the three sources of potential, several impedances are of special importance when action potentials are to be measured. If we neglect the potentials for the moment and trace out the circuit from the active elec-trode terminal A to the terminal of the reference electrode B, we encounter the resistance of the connecting wire R_a (negligible); the resistance R_s of the shaft of the microelectrode (also negligible); the microelectrode tip-intracellular fluid interface impedance constituted by R_{fa}, R_{wa}, C_{wa}; the resistance of the intracellular fluid R_{inc}; the resistance of the extracellular fluid R_{exc}; and the reference electrode-extracellular fluid interface impedance composed of R_{fb}, R_{wb}, C_{wb}. The resistance of the wire connected to the reference electrode R_b is negligible.

In addition to the obvious impedances just identified, there is another of some importance. It is the capacitive reactance of the distributed capacitance C_d between the insulated shaft of the microelectrode and the extracellular fluid. Although the insulated shaft extends into the cell, the capacitance between it and the intracellular fluid can be neglected because the potential difference across it does not change.

An approximate circuit that identifies these components appears in Fig. 9-32b. Although relatively simple in appearance, the circuit cannot be analyzed because the component values cannot be specified. Fortunately the values of some of the components can be neglected, and in many instances it is possible to collect them and synthesize a simple electrical circuit that mimics the electrical behavior of the actual circuit. For example, in comparison to the impedance of the microelectrode tip, the resistance of the shaft of the metal microelectrode R_s can be neglected, as can the resistances of the intracellular and extracellular fluids, R_{inc} and R_{exc}, respectively. Because the area of the reference electrode is many times greater than that of the microelectrode tip, its electrode-electrolyte impedance, composed of R_{fb}, R_{wb}, C_{wb}, can be neglected.

The electrochemical potentials of nonbioelectric origin (E_a, E_b) can be collected to form E', and the equivalent circuit reduces to that in Fig. 9-33. In practice C_d is small and can often be neglected. The impedance of the

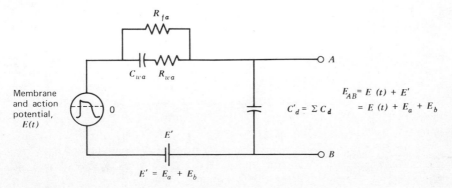

Figure 9-33. Approximate equivalent circuit for a metal microelectrode in a cell.

microelectrode tip, constituted by R_{fa}, R_{wa}, C_{wa}, is inversely dependent on the area of the tip and the frequency. Thus the bioelectric event (i.e., the membrane potential and its excursion) is coupled to the amplifying device by a circuit that has a decreasing impedance with increasing frequency. Figure 9-34 presents typical impedance-frequency characteristics for metal microelectrodes of various areas. The effect of such a circuit on the waveform of an action potential is determined by the input impedance of the amplifier to which it is connected. If the input impedance is not high enough, the low-frequency components of the bioelectric event will be attenuated, as in Figs. 9-29 and 9-30. The relationship between electrode area and input impedance is discussed in Section 9-14.

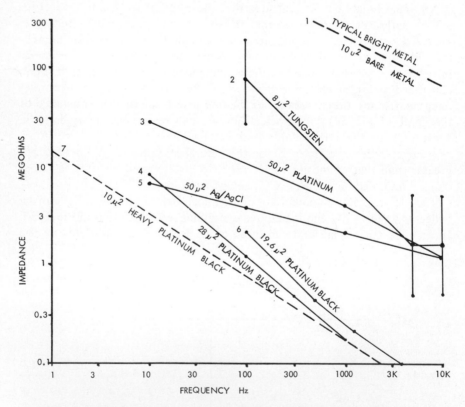

Figure 9-34. Impedance-frequency characteristics of metal microelectrodes. (From L. A. Geddes, *Electrodes and the Measurement of Bioelectric Events*. Wiley, New York, 1972. By permission.)

9-15-2.   The Micropipet

Figure 9-35*a* diagrams a micropipet electrode inserted into a cell for the measurement of the membrane potential. The electrolyte filling the micropipet is frequently 3 M KCl because of its compatibility with the cytoplasm and its low resistivity. The electrode wire in the stem is usually chlorided silver, stainless steel or tungsten. Thus in the circuit between the terminals of the micropipet and the indifferent electrode, there are actually four potentials, as in Fig. 9-35*b*. If we start from terminal A and trace out the circuit, the first potential encountered is E_a, the potential between the electrode metal (A) and the electrolyte filling the micropipet. If the fluid in the cell is different from that in the microelectrode tip, there will be a small potential E_t at the tip. In practice this potential is larger than accountable for on the basis of ionic concentration differences (Nastuk, 1953; del Castillo and Katz, 1955; Adrian, 1956). Next to appear in the circuit is the membrane potential MP, followed by the potential between the indifferent electrode (B) and the extracellular fluid E_b. Thus the potential between the electrode terminals A, B consists of the sum of four potentials: E_a, E_t, MP, and E_b. The variation in MP is designated $E(t)$.

If we now turn to the impedances in traversing the circuit, there are encountered the resistance of the connecting wire R_a, which is negligible; the impedance of the electrode-electrolyte interface in the stem of the micropipet (constituted by R_{fa}, R_{wa}, C_{wa}); the resistance R_t of the electrolyte filling the tip of the micropipet; the resistance of the electrolyte inside the cell R_{inc}; the resistance of the electrolyte outside the cell R_{exc}; the impedance of the reference electrode-electrolyte interface (constituted by R_{fb}, R_{wb}, C_{wb}); and finally the negligible resistance of the wire R_b connecting the reference electrode to terminal B. All these impedances form a series circuit in conjunction with the four potentials previously identified. In addition, a distributed capacitance C_d exists between the fluid in the micropipet and the extracellular fluid. The magnitude of this important capacitance largely determines the response time of the micropipet.

It is possible to assemble the components identified in Fig. 9-35*b* to form an approximate equivalent circuit for the situation in which a micropipet is used to measure the membrane potential. In many measurement situations the relative magnitudes of the various impedances are known, making it possible to simplify the circuit. For example, the resistances of the connecting wires R_a, R_b amount to a fraction of an ohm and can be neglected. In the whole circuit, the resistance of the tip of the micropipet (R_t) is by far the largest, amounting to about 10 to 200 MΩ for typical micropipets filled with 3MKCl (Frank and Becker, 1964). The area of the electrode-elec-

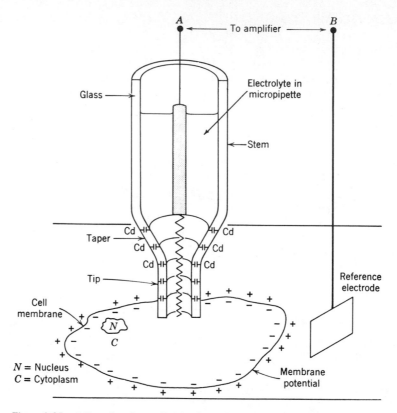

Figure 9-35. Micropipet in a cell: (*a*) schematic; (*b*) equivalent circuit.

trolyte interface in the stem is usually large or can be made large, resulting in the impedance of the circuit composed of R_{fa}, R_{wa}, C_{wa} being negligible with respect to the 10- to 200 MΩ resistance that exists at the tip. Likewise the resistance of the intracellular fluid R_{inc}, the resistance of the extracellular fluid R_{exc}, and the impedance of the reference electrode-electrolyte interface, composed of R_{fb}, R_{wb}, C_{wb}, can be neglected. The distributed capacitance C_d cannot be neglected. Hence with reasonable accuracy the circuit can be reduced to that appearing in Fig. 9-36a. This first simplification shows that the membrane potential *MP* or $E(t)$ is connected to the amplifier input terminals *A, B* via the 10- to 200-MΩ resistance (R_t) of the tip of the micropipet, which is shunted by the distributed capacitance (C_d), amounting to about 0.5 pf per millimeter of tip length. Across the terminals a voltage appears which is the sum of the membrane potential, the potential of the electrode-electrolyte interface in the stem E_a, the tip potential E_t, and the potential of the reference electrode-electrolyte junction E_b.

In many circumstances E_a, E_t, and E_b are stable and can be corrected for in determining the membrane potential. Therefore they can be summed to form E. In addition, the distributed capacitance C_d and tip resistance R_t can be represented as in Fig. 9-34b, where $R_t{}'$ and $C_d{}'$ are the single resistance and capacitance values that approximate the same electrical behavior as R_t with its distributed capacitance C_d.

Inspection of Fig. 9-36b shows that the membrane potential $E(t)$ is coupled to the amplifier terminals A, B via a high series resistance and a moderate shunt capacitance. The effect of this particular combination of circuit elements is to place a limit on the response time of the circuit which

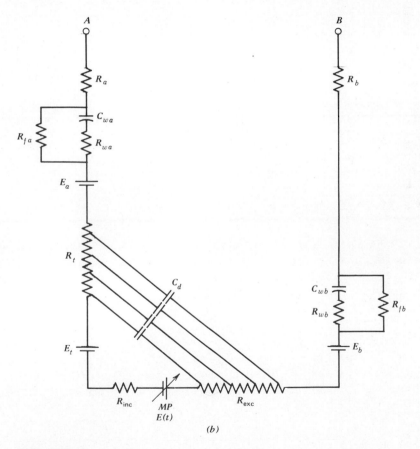

(b)

Figure 9-35. (b)

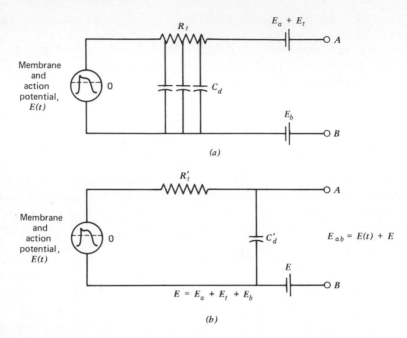

Figure 9-36. Simplified equivalent circuits for a micropipet used to measure membrane and action potentials: (*a*) simplified circuit; (*b*) circuit with lumped parameters.

may limit the faithful presentation of the rapidly changing portions of the action potential to the electrode terminals *A, B*.

9-15-3. Comparison of the Metal Microelectrode and Micropipet Circuits

In summary, the electrical characteristics of metal microelectrodes and of fluid-filled micropipets are quite different. In the former, the metal electrode-electrolyte area is small and accounts for almost all the impedance between the electrode terminals; in the latter, the high impedance is constituted largely by the electrolyte-filled microtip. Both types require the use of an amplifying system having an input impedance many times higher than that of the microelectrode. Failure to use a high enough input impedance causes the metal microelectrode to behave as a high-pass filter. The micropipet behaves as a low-pass filter even when connected to an amplifier with a high input impedance. This limitation can be removed by the use of a "negative input capacity" amplifier. Under the conditions just described, the statement (attributed to Svaetichin by Gesteland et al., 1959) that metal microelectrodes resemble high-pass filters and micropipets resemble low-pass filters is seen to be valid.

One final subtle point must be made regarding the accuracy of the transmembrane potential when measured with a metal microelectrode or a micropipet. First, it is necessary to assume that the input impedance of the measuring apparatus is high enough to ensure that the potential appearing across the terminals of the electrodes is not diminished by connection of the measuring apparatus. In a practical situation the voltage appearing between the microelectrode and reference electrode, when the former is outside the cell, is taken as zero. The actual potential is, of course, the sum of two electrode-electrolyte half-cell potentials and a tip potential when a micropipet is used. The potential at the tip of the metal microelectrode and the micropipet is dependent on the extracellular fluid. When the metal microelectrode or the micropipet tip enters the cell, the sudden change in voltage (from the arbitrary extracellular zero value) is taken as the transmembrane potential. However, there may be a small error associated with use of this technique because when the tips of both the metal microelectrode and the micropipet are in the cell, the potential at the tip is dependent on the composition of intracellular fluid (cytoplasm). Thus the potential revealed when the tip of a metal microelectrode or a micropipet enters a cell is constituted by the transmembrane potential and the difference in potential between that of the tip in contact with extracellular and intracellular fluid. The latter quantity is small and is usually neglected.

9-15-4. Ohmic Noise

Another important characteristic of electrodes derives from the ohmic component of the electrode impedance. All resistors are generators of spurious voltages of all frequencies. This unwanted voltage, called Johnson noise after its discoverer (1928), results from the random motion of the charge carriers in the material making up the conductor. Johnson demonstrated that the actual voltage measured is dependent on the magnitude of the resistance, the absolute temperature, and the bandwidth of the recording system. This voltage varies as the square root of these three quantities, and increasing any or all of them raises the noise voltage displayed by the recording system/For example, Terman (1943) stated that the thermal agitation voltage developed across a 500,000-Ω resistor at 27°C operating into a system with a bandwidth of 0 to 5000 Hz is 6.4 μV rms. Although ohmic noise may not be an important factor when bioelectric recordings are made with large low-resistance electrodes, when the electrode resistance is high, as it is with microelectrodes, and the bandwidth of the recording equipment is wide, resistive noise places a limit on the minimum signal detectable. For this reason it is advisable not to use a bandwidth in excess of that required for faithful reproduction of the waveform under investigation/(see Chapter 13).

9-16. CONCLUSION

Although many penetrating studies of the electrochemistry of electrodes have been made, many factors remain to be investigated before there is an adequate description of the electrical nature of the circuit between a pair of electrodes from which a bioelectric event is recorded. Only when this is accomplished will it be possible to ascribe a proper magnitude to the type of distortion to be expected with the various electrodes and recording systems. The following statement, made by Curtis and Cole in 1938, retains much validity: "Unexplained effects, analogous to polarization impedance are found at metal-electrolyte interfaces, in imperfect dielectrics and internal viscosity of solids, but the equation which describes them all is purely empirical and the use of the term polarization impedance is an admission of our ignorance."

In summary, it is obvious that electrodes can produce their own distortions. To minimize galvanic potentials, the electrodes should be of the same metal, and each should contact the same type of electrolyte. Although a steady electrode potential may not be bothersome, it nonetheless causes current to flow through the input resistance of the bioelectric recorder. Often this is not objectionable, but if electrodes are moved, the resistance of the circuit will alter and will result in a change in current flowing through the input circuit. The use of electrodes with equal half-cell potentials and of a recording apparatus having high input impedance will minimize this type of artifact. Disturbance of the double layer of charge at either electrode will also alter the half-cell potential. Stabilization can be attained by protecting the double layer by moving it away from the source of the movement. This is one of the reasons for the superiority of recessed electrodes. Maintenance of a low current density at the electrode interface will reduce the tendency for the electrode impedance to distort the waveform of a bioelectric event. With large-area electrodes and a bioelectric recorder of high input impedance, the risk of encountering this type of distortion is minimized.

REFERENCES

Adrian, E. D., and D. W. Bronk. 1929. Impulses in motor nerve fibers, Part II. *J. Physiol.* **67**:119–151.

Adrian, R. H. 1956. The effect of internal and external potassium concentration on the membrane potential of frog muscle. *J. Physiol.* **133**:631–658.

Asa, M. M., A. H. Crews, E. L. Rothfield, E. S. Lewis, I. R. Zucker, and A. Berstein. 1964. High fidelity radioelectrocardiography. *Am. J. Cardiol.* **14**:530–532.

Atkins, A. R. 1961. Measuring heart rate of an active athlete. *Electron. Eng.* **33**:457.

Barnett, A. 1937. The basic factors involved in proposed electrical methods for measuring thyroid function. *Western J. Surg. Obstet. Gynec.* **45**:540–554.

Basmajian, J. V. and G. Stecko. 1962. A new bipolar electrode for electromyography. *J. Appl. Physiol.* **17**:849.

Baudoin, A. H. Fischgold, and J. Lerique. 1938. Une nouvelle electrode liquide. *C. R. Soc. Biol.* **127**:1221–1222.

Bell, G. H., J. A. C. Knox, and A. J. Small. 1939. Electrocardiography electrolytes. *Brit. Heart J.* **1**:229–236.

Bergey, G. E., R. D. Squires, and W. C. Sipple. 1971. Electrocardiogram recording with pasteless electrodes. *IEEE Trans. Bio-Med. Eng.* **BME-18**:206–211.

Blank, I. H., and I. G. Finesinger. 1946. Electrical resistance of the skin. *Arch. Neurol. Psychiat.* **54**:544–557.

Boter, J., A. den Hertog, and J. Kuiper. 1966. Disturbance-free skin electrodes for persons during exercise. *Med. Biol. Eng.* **4**:91–95.

Burns, R. C. 1950. Study of skin impedance. *Electronics* **23**:190 and 196.

Burr, H. S. 1944, 1950. In *Medical Physics*. O. Glasser (ed.). Year Book Publishers, Chicago.

Carbery, W. J., W. E. Tolles, and A. H. Freiman. 1960. A system for monitoring the ECG under dynamic conditions. *Aerosp. Med.* **31**:131–137.

Castillo, H., and H. Marriott. 1974. Radio transparent ECG electrodes for use during cardiac catheterization. *Med. Instr.* **8**:116.

del Castillo, J., and B. Katz. 1955. Local activity at a depolarized nerve-muscle junction. *J. Physiol.* **128**:396–411.

Clark, L. C., and R. J. Lacey. 1950. An improved skin electrode. *J. Lab. Clin. Med.* **35**:786–787.

Cohn, A. E. 1920. A new method for use in clinical electrocardiography. *Arch. Intern. Med.* **26**:105–113.

Cole, K. S., and U. Kishimoto. 1962. Platinized silver chloride electrode. *Science* **136**:381–382.

Collias, J. C., and E. E. Manuelidis. 1957. Histopathological changes produced by implanted electrodes in cat brains. *J. Neurosurg.* **14**:302–328.

Cooper, R. 1956. Storage of silver chloride electrodes. *EEG. Clin. Neurophysiol.* **8**:692.

Cooper, R. 1963. Electrodes. *Am. J. EEG Technol.* **3**:91–101.

Curtis, H. J., and K. S. Cole. 1938. Transverse electric impedance of the squid giant axon. *J. Gen. Physiol.* **21**:757–765.

Davis, D. A., and W. E. Thornton. 1965. *Radiotelemetry in Anesthesia and Surgery*. International Anesthesiology Clinics. Little, Brown, Boston, 586 pp.

Day, J., and M. Lippitt. 1964. A long term electrode system for electrocardiography and impedance pneumography. *Psychophysiology* **1**:174–182.

Delgado, J. M. R. 1952. Permanent implantation of multilead electrodes in the brain. *Yale J. Biol. Med.* **24**:351–358.

Delgado, J. M. R. 1955. Evaluation of permanent implantation of electrodes within the brain. *EEG Clin Neurophysiol.* **7**:637–644.

Delgado, J. M. R. 1964. Electrodes for extracellular recording and stimulation. In *Physical Techniques in Biological Research*. W. L. Nastuk (ed.). Academic Press, New York, 460 pp.

Dodge, H. W., C. Petersen, C. W. Sem-Jacobsen, G. P. Sayre, and R. G. Bickford. 1955. The paucity of demonstrable brain damage following intracerebral electrography: Report of a case. *Proc. Staff Meetings Mayo Clinic* **30**:215–221.

Dowben, R. M., and J. E. Rose. 1953. A metal-filled microelectrode. *Science* **118**:22–24.

Dower, G. E., J. A. Osborne, and A. D. Moore. 1959. Measurement of the error in Wilson's central terminal. *Brit. Heart J.* **21**:352–360.

Edelberg, R. 1963. Personal communication.

Edelberg, R., and N. R. Burch. 1962. Skin resistance and galvanic skin response. *Arch. Gen. Psychiat.* **7**:163–169.

Einthoven, W. 1928. Die Aktionsstrome des Herzens. *Handbuch der Normalen und Pathologischen Physiologie.* Julian Springer, Berlin, pp. 758–862.

Fascenelli, F. W., C. Cordova, D. G. Simons, J. Johnson, L. Pratt, and L. E. Lamb. 1966. Biomedical monitoring during dynamic stress testing; 1. *Aerosp. Med:* **37**:911–922.

Feates, F. S., D. J. G. Ives, and J. H. Pryor. 1956. Alternating current bridge for measurement of electrolytic conductance. *J. Electrochem. Soc.* **103**:580–585.

Fischer, G., G. P. Sayre, and R. G. Bickford. 1957. Histologic changes in the cat's brain after introduction of metallic and plastic coated wire used in electroencephalography. *Proc. Staff Meetings Mayo Clinic* **32**:14–22.

Forbes, A., S. Cobb, and McK. Cattell. 1921. An electrocardiogram and an electromyogram in an elephant. *Am. J. Physiol.* **55**:385–389.

Forbes, T. W. 1934. An improved electrode for the measurement of potentials on the human body. *J. Lab. Clin. Med.* **19**:1234–1238.

Frank, K., and M. Becker. 1964. Microelectrodes for recording and stimulation. In *Physical Techniques in Biological Research,* Vol. V, part A. Academic Press, New York and London, 460 pp.

Fricke, H. 1931. The electric conductivity and capacity of disperse systems. *Physics.* **1**:106–115.

Fricke, H. 1932. The theory of electrolyte polarization. *Phil. Mag.* **14**:310–318.

Geddes, L. A. 1948–1949. Cortical electrodes. *EEG Clin. Neurophysiol.* **1**:523. Illustrated on cover of *Sci. Amer.* 1948, **179**, No. 4.

Geddes, L. A. 1972. *Electrodes and the Measurement of Bioelectric Events.* Wiley, New York, 364 pp.

Geddes, L. A. 1973. Measurement of electrolytic resistivity and electrode-electrolyte impedance with a variable-length conductivity cell. *Chem. Instrum.* **4**:157–168.

Geddes, L. A., and L. E. Baker. 1966. The relationship between input impedance and electrode area in recording the ECG. *Med. Electr. Biol. Eng.* **4**:439–450.

Geddes, L. A., and L. E. Baker. 1967. Chlorided silver electrodes. *Med. Res. Eng.* **6**:33–34.

Geddes, L. A., and L. E. Baker. 1971. Response to passage of electric current through the body. *Med. Instr.* **5**:13–18.

Geddes, L. A., L. E. Baker, and McGoodwin. 1967. The relationship between electrode area and amplifier input impedance in recording muscle action potentials. *Med. Biol. Eng.* **5**:561–568.

Geddes, L. A., L. E. Baker, and A. G. Moore. 1969. Optimum electrolytic chloriding of silver electrodes. *Med. Biol. Eng.* **7**:49–56.

Geddes, L. A., J. D. Bourland, G. Wise, and R. Steinberg. 1973. Dry electrodes and holder for electro-oculography. *Med. Biol. Eng.* **11**:69–72.

Geddes, L. A., C. P. Da Costa, and G. Wise. 1971. The impedance of stainless-steel electrodes. *Med. Biol. Eng.* **9**:511–521.

Geddes, L. A., J. D. McCrady, H. E. Hoff, and A. Moore. 1964. Electrodes for large animals. *Southwest. Vet.* **18**:56–57.

Geddes, L. A., M. Partridge, and H. E. Hoff. 1960. An EKG lead for exercising subjects. *J. Appl. Physiol.* **15**:311–312.

Geddes, L. A., J. Rosborough, H. Garner, J. Amend., A. G. Moore, and M. Szabuniewicz. 1970. Obtaining electrocardiograms on animals without skin preparation or penetration. *Vet. Med.* **12**:1163–1168.

Gesteland, R. C., B. Howland, J. Y. Lettvin, and W. H. Pitts. 1959. Comments on microelectrodes. *Proc. IRE* **47**:1856–1862.

Gibson, T. C., W. E. Thornton, W. P. Algary, and E. Craige. 1962. Telecardiography and the use of simple computers. *New Engl. J. Med.* **267**:1218–1224.

Goldstein, A. G., W. Sloboda, and J. B. Jennings. 1962. Spontaneous electrical activity of three types of silver EEG electrodes. *Psychophysiol. Newsl.* **8**:10–16.

Grahame, D. C. 1941. Properties of the electrical double layer at a mercury surface. *J. Am. Chem. Soc.* **63**:1207–1214.

Grahame, D. C. 1952. Mathematical theory of the faradic admittance. *J. Electrochem. Soc.* **99**:370C–385C.

Gray, J. A. G., and G. Svaetichin. 1951–1952. Electrical properties of platinum tipped microelectrodes. *Acta Physiol. Scand.* **24**:278–284.

Greenwald, D. U. 1936. Electrodes used in measuring electrodermal responses. *Am J. Psychol.* **48**:658–662.

Grundfest, H., and B. Campbell. 1942. Origin, conduction and termination of impulses in dorsal spino-cerebellar tracts of cats. *J. Neurophysiol.* **5**:275–294.

Grundfest, H., R. W. Sengstaken, and W. H. Oettinger. 1950. Stainless steel microneedle made by electro-pointing. *Rev. Sci. Instr.*, **21**:360–361.

Guld, C. 1964. A glass-covered platinum microelectrode. *Med. Electr. Biol. Eng.* **2**:317–327.

Haggard, E. A., and R. Gerbrands. 1947. An apparatus for the measurement of continuous changes in palmar skin resistance. *J. Exp. Psychol.* **37**:92–98.

Helmholtz, H. 1879. Studien über electrische Grenzschichten. *Ann. Phys. Chem.* **7**:337–382.

Hendler, E., and L. J. Santa Maria. 1961. Response of subjects to some conditions of a simulated orbital flight pattern. *Aerosp. Med.* **32**:126–133.

Henry, F. 1938. Dependable electrodes for the galvanic skin response. *J. Gen. Psychol.* **18**:209–211.

Hill, D. 1967. In Hales, Marey, and Chauveau, Report on 1966 course "Classical Physiology with Modern Instrumentation." NIH Grant Report HE 05125.

Hubel, D. H. 1957. Tungsten microelectrode for recording from single units. *Science* **125**:549–550.

James, W. B., and H. B. Williams. 1910. The electrocardiogram in clinical medicine. *Am. J. Med. Sci.* **140**:408–421.

Janz, G. J., and F. J. Kelly. 1964. Reference electrodes. In *Encyclopedia of Electrochemistry*. C. A. Hampel (ed.). Reinhold, New York, 1206 pp.

Janz, G. J., and H. Taniguchi. 1953. The silver-silver halide electrodes. *Chem. Rev.* **53**:397–437.

Jasper, H. H., and L. Carmichael. 1935. Electrical potentials from the intact human brain. *Science* **81**:51–53.

Jasper, H. H., R. T. Johnson, and L. A. Geddes. 1945. The RCAMC electromyograph. Canadian Army Med. Rept. C6174.

Jaron, D., S. A. Briller, H. P. Schwan, and D. B. Geselowitz. 1969. Nonlinearity of cardiac pacemaker electrodes. *IEEE Trans. Bio-Med. Eng. BME* **16**:132–138.

Jenks, J. L., and A. Graybiel. 1935. A new simple method of avoiding high resistance and overshooting in taking standardized electrocardiograms. *Am. Heart J.* **10**:683–695.

Johnson, J. B. 1928. Thermal agitation of electricity in conductors. *Phys. Rev.* **32**:97–109.

Johnson, J. B., and J. E. Allred. 1968. High impedance electrocardiogram amplifier-transmitter for use with dry electrodes. Tech. Rept. SAM TR-68-55, 1968. School of Aerospace Medicine, Brooks AFB, Texas.

Kado, R. T. 1965. Personal communication.

Kado, R. T., W. R. Adey, and J. R. Zweizig. 1964. Electrode system for recording EEG from physically active subjects. *Proc. 17th Ann. Conf. Eng. Med. Biol.* Washington, D.C., McGregor and Werner, 129 pp.

Kahn, A. 1964. Fundamentals of biopotentials and their measurement. Biomedical Sciences Instrumentation. 1964. Dallas. *Am. J. Pharm. Educ.* **28**:805–814.

Kahn, A. 1965. Motion artifacts and streaming potentials in relation to biological electrodes. *Digest 6th Int. Conf. Med. Electr. Biol. Eng.,* Tokyo, pp. 562–563.

Kennard, D. W. 1958. Glass microcapillary electrodes. In *Electronic Apparatus for Biological Research.* P.E.K. Donaldson (ed.). Butterworth's, London, Chap. 35.

King, E. E. 1964. Errors in voltage in multichannel ECG recordings using newer electrode materials. *Am. Heart J.* **18**:295–297.

Kohlrausch, F. 1897. Über platinirte Elektroden und Widerstandsbestimmung. *Ann. Phys. Chem.* **60**:315–332.

Kohlrausch, F., and L. Holborn. 1898. *Das Leitvermogen der Elektrolyte.* Teubner, Leipzig, 211 pp.

Lewes, D. 1965a. Electrode jelly in electrocardiography. *Brit. Heart J.* **27**:105–115.

Lewes, D. 1965b. Multipoint electrocardiography without skin preparation. *Lancet* **2**:17–18. U.K. Patent application 52253/64.

Lewes, D., and D. Hill. 1966. Personal communication.

Lewis, T. 1914–1915. Polarisable as against non-polarisable electrodes. *J. Physiol.* **49**:l-lii.

Lopez, A., and P. Richardson. 1969. Capacitive electrocardiographic and bioelectric electrodes. *IEEE Trans. Bio-Med. Eng.* **BME-16**:99.

Lucchina, G. G., and C. G. Phipps. 1962. A vectorcardiographic lead system and physiologic electrode configuration for dynamic readout. *Aerosp. Med.* **33**:722–729.

Lucchina, G. G., and C. G. Phipps. 1963. An improved electrode for physiological recording. *Aerosp. Med.* **34**:230–231.

Lykken, D. T. 1959. Properties of electrodes used in electrodermal measurement. *J. Comp. Physiol. Psychol.* **52**:629–634.

MacInnes, D. A. 1961. *The Principles of Electrochemistry.* Reinhold, New York; Dover, New York, 478 pp.

Marchant, E. W., and E. W. Jones. 1940. The effect of electrodes of different metals on the skin current. *Brit. Heart J.* **2**:97–100.

Marmont, G. 1949. Studies on the axon membrane. *J. Cell. Comp. Physiol.* **34**:351–382.

Mason, R. E., and I. Likar. 1966. A new system of multiple lead electrocardiography. *Am. Heart J.* **71**:196–205.

Maxwell, J. 1957 and 1958. Preparation of the skin for electrocardiography. *Brit. Med. J.* 1957, **2**:942; 1958, **1**:41.

Mills, L. W. 1962. A fast inexpensive method of producing large quantities of metallic microelectrodes. *EEG Clin. Neurophysiol.* **14**:278–279.

Mooney, V., D. B. Hartman, and D. McNeal. 1974. The use of pure carbon for permanent percutaneous electrical connector systems. *Arch. Surg.* **108**:148–153.

Nastuk, W. 1953. The electrical activity of the muscle cell membrane at the neuromuscular junction. *J. Cell. Comp. Physiol.* **42**:249–283.

O'Connell, D. N., and B. Tursky. Special modifications of the silver-silver chloride sponge electrode for skin recording. U.S. Air Force Office of Scientific Research. Contact AF 49 (638)-728, 37 pp.

O'Connell, D. N., B. Tursky, and M. T. Orne. 1960. Electrodes for recording skin potential. *Arch. Gen. Psychiat.* **3**:252–258.

Offner, F. F. 1942. Electrical properties of tissues in shock therapy. *Proc. Soc. Exp. Biol. Med.* **49**:571–575.

Pardee, H. E. B. 1917a. Concerning the electrodes used in electrocardiography. *Am. J. Physiol.* **44**:80–83.

Pardee, H. E. B. 1917b. An error in the electrocardiogram arising in the application of the electrodes. *Arch. Intern. Med.* **20**:161–166.

Parker, T. G. 1966. Personal communication. V. A. Hospital, Houston, Tex.

Parsons, R. 1964. Electrode double layer. In *The Encyclopedia of Electrochemistry*. C. A. Hampel (ed.). Reinhold, New York, 1206 pp.

Patten, C. W., F. B. Ramme, and J. Roman. 1966. Dry electrodes for physiological monitoring. NASA Tech. Note NASA TN D-3414. National Aeronautics and Space Administration, Washington, D.C., 32 pp.

Plutchik, R., and H. R. Hirsch. 1963. Skin impedance and phase angle as a function of frequency and current. *Science* **141**:927–928.

Rappaport, M. B., C. Williams, and P. D. White. 1949. An analysis of the relative accuracies of the Wilson and Goldberger methods for registering unipolar and augmented unipolar electrocardiographic leads. *Am. Heart J.* **37**:892–917.

Ray, C. D. 1966. A new multipurpose human brain probe. *J. Neurosurg.* **24**:911–921.

Richardson, P. C. 1967. The insulated electrode: A pasteless electrocardiographic technique. *Proc. 20th Ann. Conf. Eng. Med. Biol.* **9**:15.7.

Richardson, P. C. 1967. Progress in long-term physiologic sensor development. *Proc. Biomed. Eng. Symp., San Diego.* 39–44.

Richardson, P. C. and F. K. Coombs. 1968. New construction techniques for insulated electrocardiographic electrodes. *Proc. 21st Ann. Conf. Eng. Med. Biol.* **10**:13A.1.

Richardson, P. C., F. K. Coombs, and R. M. Adams. 1968. Some new electrode techniques for long-term physiologic monitoring. *Aerosp. Med.* **39**:745–750.

Robinson, F. R. and M. T. Johnson. 1961. Histopathological studies of tissue reactions to various metals planted in cat brains. ASD Tech. Rept. 61-397, 13 pp. USAF Wright-Patterson AFB, Ohio.

Robinson, R. A., and R. H. Stokes. 1959. In *Electrolyte Solutions,* 2nd ed. Academic Press, New York.

Roman, J. 1966. Flight research program—III. High impedance electrode techniques. *Aerosp. Med.* **37**:790-795.

Roman, J., and L. Lamb. 1962. Electrocardiography in flight. *Aerosp. Med.* **33**:527-544.

Rose, K. D. 1963. Telemetering physiologic data from athletes. *Proc. Int. Telemetering Conf.* **1**:225-241.

Roth, I. 1933-1934. A self-retaining skin contact electrode for chest leads in electrocardiography. *Am. Heart J.* **9**:526-529.

Rothschild, Lord. 1938. The polarization of a calomel electrode. *Proc. Roy. Soc. (London) Ser. B.* **125**:283-290.

Rowland, V. 1961. Simple non-polarizable electrode for chronic implantation. *EEG Clin. Neurophysiol.* **13**:290-291.

Rowley, D. A., S. Glasgov, and P. Stoner. 1961. Fluid electrodes for monitoring the electrocardiogram during activity and for prolonged periods of time. *Am. Heart J.* **62**:263-269.

Schmitt, O. H. M. Okajima, and M. Blaug. 1961. Skin preparation and electrocardiographic lead impedance. *Digest IRE Internat. Conf. Med. Electron.* McGregor and Werner, Washington, D.C., 288 pp.

Schwan, H. P. 1963. Determination of biological impedances. In *Physical Techniques in Biological Research* . W. Nastuk (ed.). Vol. VI, part B. Academic Press, New York and London, 425 pp.

Schwan, H. P. 1968. Electrode polarization impedance and measurements in biological materials. *Ann. N.Y. Acad. Sci.* **148**:191-209.

Schwan, H. P. and J. G. Maczuk. 1965. Electrode polarization impedance: limits of linearity. *Proc. 18th Ann. Conf. Eng. Biol. Med.* McGregor and Werner, Washington, D.C., 270 pp.

Schwarzchild, M. M., I. Hoffman, and M. Kissin. 1954. Errors in unipolar limb leads caused by unbalanced skin resistances, and a device for their elimination. *Am. Heart J.* **48**:235-248.

Scott, R. N. 1965. A method of inserting wire electrodes for electromyography. *IEEE Trans. Bio-Med. Eng.* **BME-12**:46-47.

Seelig, M. C. 1925. Localized gangrene following the hypodermic administration of calcium chloride. *JAMA* **84**:1413-1414.

Shackel, B. 1958. A rubber suction cup surface electrode with high electrical stability. *J. Appl. Physiol.* **13**:153-158.

Shackel, B. 1959. Skin drilling: A method for diminishing galvanic skin potentials. *Am. J. Physiol.* **72**:114-121.

Simons, D. G., W. Prather, and F. K. Coombs. 1965. Personalized telemetry medical monitoring and performance data-gathering for the 1962 SAMMATS fatigue study. SAM-TR-65-17. USAF Brooks AFB, Texas.

Skov, E. R., and D. G. Simons. 1965. EEG electrodes for in-flight monitoring. SAM-TR-65-18. USAF Brooks AFB, Texas.

Sullivan, G. H., and G. Weltman. 1961. A low mass electrode for bioelectric recording. *J. Appl. Physiol.* **16**:939–940.

Sutter, von C. 1944. Ueber die Beeinflussung der Ekg-kurve durch elektrische Eigenschaften der Aufnahmeanordnung. *Cardiologia* **8**:246–262.

Svaetichin, G. 1951. Low resistance microelectrode. *Acta Physiol. Scand.* Suppl. 86, **24**:1–13.

Tasaki, I. 1952–1953. Properties of myelinated fibers in a frog sciatic nerve and in spinal cord as examined with microelectrodes. *Japan. J. Physiol.* **3**:73–94.

Taylor, C. V. 1925. Microelectrodes and micromagnets. *Proc. Soc. Exp. Biol. Med.* **23**:147–150.

Telemedics, Inc. 1961. *Medical Electronics News* **1**(4):9.

Terman, F. E. 1943. *Radio Engineers Handbook,* 1st ed. McGraw-Hill, New York, 1019 pp.

Thompson, N. P., and J. A. Patterson. 1958. Solid salt bridge contact electrodes—System for monitoring the ECG during body movement. Tech. Rept. 58–453. ASTIA Doc. AD215538. April.

Ungerleider, H. E. 1939. A new precordial electrode. *Am. Heart J.* **18**:94.

Warburg, E. 1899. Über das Verhalten sogenannter unpolarisierbarer Elektroden gegen Wechselstrom. *Ann. Phy. Chem.* **67**:493–499.

Warburg, E. 1901. Über die Polarizationscapacität des Platins. *Ann. Phys. (Leipzig).* **6**:125–135.

Weale, R. A. 1951. A new micro-electrode for electrophysiological work. *Nature* **167**:529.

Weinman, J., and Mahler. 1964. An analysis of electrical properties of metal electrodes. *Med. Electr. Biol. Eng.* **2**:299–310.

Whalen, R. E., C. F. Starmer, and H. D. McIntosh. 1964. Electrical hazards associated with cardiac pacemaking. *Ann. N.Y. Acad. Sci.* **111**:922–931.

Wilson, F. N., F. C. Johnson. A. G. Macleod, and P. S. Baker. 1934. Electrocardiograms that represent the potential variations of a single electrode. *Am. Heart J.* **9**:447–458.

Wolfe, A. M., and H. E. Reinhold. 1973. A flexible quick-application ECG electrode system. *Biomedical Electrode Technology.* H. A. Miller and D. C. Harrison (eds.). Academic Press, New York, 447 pp.

Wolfson, R. N., and M. R. Neuman. 1969. Miniature Si-SiO$_2$ insulated electrodes based on semiconductor technology. *Proc. 8th Int. Conf. Med. Biol. Eng. 1969.* Paper No. 14-6. Carl Gorr, Chicago.

Woodbury, J. W., and A. J. Brady. 1956. Intracellular recording from moving tissues with a flexibly mounted ultramicroelectrode *Science* **123**:100–101.

Woodbury, L. A., J. W. Woodbury, and H. Hecht. 1950. Membrane and resting action potentials of single cardiac fibers. *Circulation* **1**:264–265.

10

Detection of Physiological Events by Impedance

10-1. INTRODUCTION

Often it is necessary to measure a physiological event for which there is no specialized transducer. In many circumstances transduction can be carried out by means of the impedance method if the event can be caused to exhibit a change in dimension, dielectric, or conductivity. The elegantly simple technique requires only the application of two or more electrodes, and it has been used successfully for many years to detect a remarkable variety of physiological events. It is extremely practical for phenomena that produce a large change in one or more of the three quantities just mentioned. With the simplest of "transducers"—that is, appropriately placed electrodes—the impedance between them may reflect seasonal variations, blood flow, cardiac activity, respired volume, bladder and kidney volume, uterine contractions, eye movement, nervous activity, muscular contraction, the galvanic skin reflex, the volume of blood cells, clotting, blood pressure, and salivation. In some instances the impedance is dissected into its resistive and reactive components; in others, the total impedance is measured. Often only a change in impedance, with or without resolution into its components, contains information sufficient to describe the physiological event. Many of the techniques that have been employed are presented in this chapter.

The impedance method offers all the advantages of the indirect techniques used in the biomedical sciences, the most important being that in many applications the integument need not be penetrated to make the measurement. Since electrodes are very easy to apply, practicality is an attractive feature of the method. Because a specialized transducer is not required, the same electrodes and the same impedance apparatus often can be used to detect a variety of events in man and animals. In the absence of a

276

transducer, the response time is governed mainly by the event. If the electrodes are small enough, they offer little restraint to the subject and need not modify the phenomenon under study. Unlike many transducers, electrodes are affected little by temperature and barometric pressure changes. This property makes the impedance method practical for monitoring events under changing environmental conditions. In addition, because the usually bothersome galvanic potentials produced when metallic electrodes come into contact with electrolytes are not a part of the signal when the impedance method is employed, the problem of canceling these unwanted voltages is eliminated. A further advantage of the impedance method is obtained through employment of carrier-system techniques, which permit the use of narrow-band amplifiers with consequent enhancement of the signal-to-noise ratio.

The impedance method is subject to the limitations inherent in many indirect techniques. Since frequently the signal is obtained at a distance from the phenomenon, resolution is compromised, and the signal is often difficult to calibrate in true physiological terms. However, uncalibratible signals that directly reflect a physiological event can have considerable value for monitoring changes under a variety of experimentally controlled conditions.

10-2. SAFETY CONSIDERATIONS

When current is passed through living tissue, special consideration must be given to the structures between the electrodes. Muscle (skeletal, cardiac, and smooth), nerve fibers, sensory receptors, glands, and body fluids all form part of the current-carrying circuit. The parameters for electrical stimulation of the irritable tissues in the current path can be found in their strength-duration curves, which are plots of the threshold current required for excitation versus the duration of the single testing stimulus. Figure 10-1 illustrates the general form of the strength-duration curve. Such curves are remarkably similar in form for a wide variety of irritable tissues; the major difference lies in the scale applied to the duration axis.

The threshold current for an infinitely long duration stimulus is designated the rheobase. Although current magnitude is often used to signify stimulus intensity, a better unit might be current density (mA/cm^2). The shortest duration for a stimulus of twice the rheobasic current is called the chronaxie; Figure 10-1 identifies these quantities. The strength-duration curve demonstrates that the shorter the duration of a stimulus, the higher the current required for stimulation. Figure 10-1 also shows that there is a limit to the brevity of a stimulus that will produce excitation, since the strength-duration curve becomes parallel to the current axis for a very

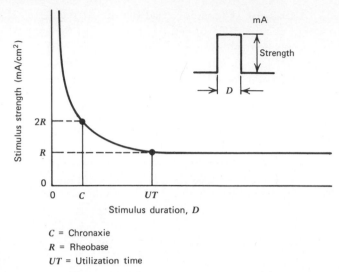

C = Chronaxie
R = Rheobase
UT = Utilization time

Figure 10-1. Typical form for the strength-duration curve of irritable tissue. The values for the stimulus strength (mA/cm²) and duration (D, msec) depend on the type of tissue.

short-duration stimulus; indicating that a stimulus which is shorter in duration will not stimulate, no matter how intense it may be. Although intense stimuli of short duration may not excite irritable tissue, local heating and burning can be produced.

Table 10-1 lists the chronaxie values for a variety of irritable tissues. Interestingly, the tissues in which excitation is propagated slowly have long chronaxie values. The physiological implications of this fact have been discussed extensively by Fredericq (1928) and Davis and Forbes (1936). The various equations that have been developed to describe strength-duration curves are also analyzed in these reports. The strength-duration curve for skeletal muscle is important clinically because it is altered in a characteristic way by denervation and reinnervation.

To minimize or avoid stimulation, pulses having durations many times shorter than the chronaxie must be employed. Sinusoidal current with a frequency of 12,500 Hz could conceivably stimulate the most rapidly recovering tissues, indicating the need to use higher frequencies in the measurement of physiological events by impedance techniques. In practice, frequencies of 20 kHz are usually employed. Although the perception threshold for current is expected to vary widely, depending on the richness of distribution of sensory receptors, the sensation threshold studies carried out to date are in fairly good agreement and reveal the sensitivity to alternating current.

Table 10-1 Chronaxie Values for Irritable Tissues*

Tissue	Time (msec)
Skeletal muscle	
Frog (gastrocnemius)	0.2–0.3
Frog (sartorius)	0.3
Turtle (leg flexors and extensors)	1–2
Man (arm flexors)	0.08–0.16
Man (arm extensors)	0.16–0.32
Man (thigh muscles)	0.10–0.72
Man (facial muscles)	0.24–0.72
Cardiac muscle	
Frog (ventricle)	3
Turtle (ventricle)	9
Dog (ventricle)	2
Man (ventricle)	2
Smooth muscle	
Frog (stomach)	100
Nerve	
Frog (sciatic)	0.3
Man (A fibers)	0.2
Man (vestibular)	14–22
Receptors	
Man (tongue)	1.4–1.8
Man (retinal rods)	1.2–1.8
Man (retinal cones)	2.1–3.0

* Data obtained from Fredericq (1928), Brazier (1951), Hoffman and Cranefield (1960), and Brazier (1951).

The perception of and tolerance to electric current of different frequencies attracted considerable attention at the dawn of the twentieth century when it became necessary to choose a frequency for the distribution of electrical energy. d'Arsonval, of galvanometer fame, showed in 1893 that when current was passed through the human body, no sensation was perceived as the frequency was increased beyond 2500 to 5000 Hz. At much greater frequencies, even with a high intensity, there was no perception of the current. To prove his point in a most dramatic manner, d'Arsonval connected two human subjects (arm to arm) and a 100-W light bulb in series with a high-frequency spark coil that delivered enough current (1 amp) to cause the bulb to burn brilliantly. The subjects through whom the 1-amp, 0.5- to 1-MHz current flowed reported no sensation. In a later study

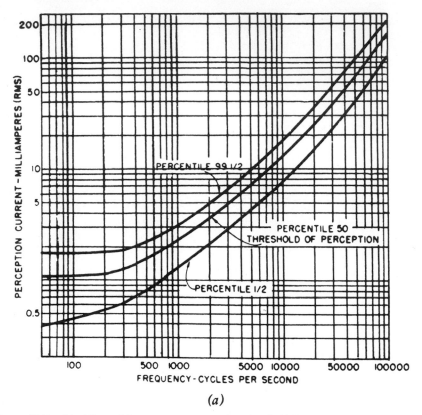

(a)

Figure 10-2. (*a*) Effect of frequency on perception threshold for current, using hand-held electrodes. [From C. F. Dalziel, *IRE Trans. Med. Electron.* **5**:48 (1956). By permission.] (*b*) Threshold of sensation for sinusoidal current applied to neck-abdomen ($\frac{1}{4}$-in. metal ribbon) and transchest (11-mm circular disks) electrodes. [From Geddes and Baker, *J. Assoc. Adv. Med. Instr.* **5**:13–18 (1971). By permission.]

d'Arsonval passed 3 amps through his own body. These demonstrations, of course, paved the way for the use of high-frequency current for heating living tissues and in reality initiated medical diathermy.

When ac generators capable of providing substantial electrical energy with frequencies up to 100,000 Hz became available, further studies were performed to determine the ability of human subjects to perceive and tolerate alternating current. Kennelly and Alexanderson (1910) reported on a series of experiments in which current was passed through subjects via buckets filled with 3% saline into which the hands were immersed. Using the limit of tolerance as the criterion, they plotted graphs of current versus frequency for five subjects. They found that the tolerance to current

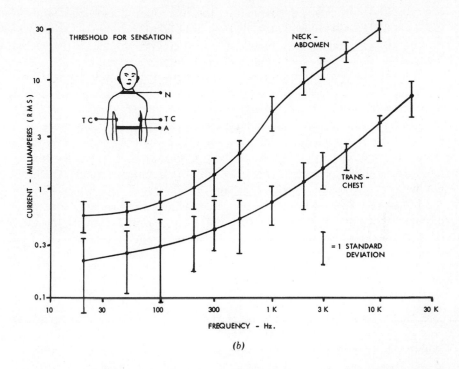

(b)

increased with rising frequency. At 60 Hz the tolerance current varied between 4 and 100 mA. At 11 kHz the tolerance current was 30 mA and at 100 kHz it varied between 450 and 800 mA. Even with these high currents the subjects reported only a slight tingling and a sensation of heat at the wrists.

Dalziel (1956) reported that the tip of the tongue is the most sensitive part of the body and determined the threshold for sensation on 115 subjects as 45 μA for both direct current and 60 Hz alternating current. In another series of experiments he measured the ability of more than 100 male subjects to perceive current flowing in the body through electrodes held in the hands. The threshold for sensation was 5.2 mA for direct current and 1.1 mA for 60-Hz alternating current. Dalziel found that the threshold of sensation for women was two-thirds that of the value for men. In another series of studies using hand-held electrodes, Dalziel measured the threshold for sensation for different frequencies of sinusoidal current. The data he obtained are plotted in Fig. 10-2a.

In a study of the choice of frequency for impedance respiration, Geddes et al. (1962,1969,1971) determined the threshold of sensation for sinusoidal current with electrodes placed on the human thorax. The data obtained (see

Fig. 10-2*b*) are in general agreement with those of Anderson and Munson (1951) and Dalziel (1956); that is, above about 300 Hz the threshold of perception rises as frequency is increased. Both studies emphasize the use of higher frequencies to avoid stimulation of sensory receptors.

Although the perception threshold for current is quite well defined for a particular electrode system and current waveform, it is probably unwise to normalize the sensation current and express it as current density (mA/cm²) to define perception threshold. This point is discussed later when the current level for a painful stimulus is described. For a uniform strip of irritable tissue, current density is likely to be the best quantity to describe a threshold stimulus. However, when stimulating cutaneous areas, which do not have a uniform distribution of sensory receptors and whose various receptors may have different thresholds, it would be surprising indeed to discover that current density is the best normalizing factor. It must be pointed out however that there has been insufficient investigation of this subject.

10-3. PAINFUL STIMULATION

With a given electrode type, when the current is increased to a value above the perception threshold, a variety of different sensations can be encountered depending on the electrode area, location, frequency, and waveform. The variation in sensation probably results from the possibility of stimulating simultaneously touch, pressure, temperature, and pain receptors, and/or their afferent nerve fibers. Despite the many studies carried out in which a variety of current waveforms were applied to electrodes on the surface of human skin, it is difficult to specify the kind of sensation that will be perceived; nonetheless there appears to be some agreement. Using low-frequency sinusoidal current, the sensation under large-area electrodes is often described as buzzing, throbbing, or tingling. Under electrodes of a few square millimeters in area or less, a stinging, burning, or painful sensation is frequently reported.

An interesting sensation, described as a pin prick, can be obtained under a small-area (ca. 0.5 mm) electrode when the voltage is gradually increased; at a critical voltage the pricking sensation is encountered. Mueller et al. (1953) studied this phenomenon using 1200-Hz sinusoidal voltage, which was increased linearly while both voltage and current were recorded. At the point when the pricking sensation was observed, the current was seen to increase markedly, and the impedance under the small-area electrode decreased suddenly. The decrease in impedance was due to a highly localized breakdown of the skin dielectric.

Current levels above the perception threshold are applied to electrode arrays for sensory communication (Gilmer, 1961) and in psychophysiological studies for conditioning. In the latter case, the goal is to achieve a perceptible stimulus that can be controlled in its intensity but is still nonhazardous to the subject. Recent reviews of the studies in these fields was presented by Notermans (1966) and Pfeiffer (1968).

An early study aimed at differentiating between a perceptible (touch) and painful electrical stimulus was reported by Anderson and Munson (1951), who found that the pain threshold for sinusoidal current was about 25 dB above the perception threshold in the frequency range extending from 100 to 10,000 Hz. Gibson (1963), in a preliminary study, discovered that a rectangular pulse lasting 0.5 msec provided the highest ratio of a painful to a touch stimulus. Measurable differences in threshold were found between hairless and hairy skin, the former requiring less current for pain and touch perception. The polarity of the stimulus also affected the perception and pain thresholds. With cathodal stimuli the thresholds were lower, but anodal stimulation produced less reddening under the active (small-area) electrode. In these studies, 11-mm-diameter active electrodes were used.

Having selected the optimum pulse duration (0.5 msec), Gibson conducted two series of experiments in which the number of pulses, with a frequency of 100 Hz, was varied to determine touch and pain sensation thresholds. In the second series, the frequency of the 0.5-msec stimuli was varied, and the thresholds for pain and touch were determined for stimuli consisting of 4 and 20 pulses. Figure 10-3 presents the data obtained, which indicate that the current thresholds for touch and pain, determined with 1 to 20 stimuli (0.5 msec in duration with a frequency of 100 Hz), depend on the site stimulated, the hairless tissues requiring less current for both touch and pain perception. The current required for pain and touch decreases initially with an increasing number of pulses; but a further increase beyond about 4 for hairless tissue and about 10 for hairy tissue decreases the pain and touch thresholds insignificantly.

In the second study, in which 4 and 20 stimuli (each 0.5 msec in duration) were delivered at varying frequencies, it was clearly demonstrated that a frequency of about 100 Hz is generally optimum to evoke pain and touch sensation with the least current. The threshold currents for both sensations were lower with 20 stimuli than with 4. These studies therefore indicate that a stimulation period lasting 0.2 sec using 0.5 msec pulses having a frequency of 100 Hz appears to be optimum for evoking touch and pain sensations. In general the current ratio for pain to touch threshold was found to range between 1.3 and 2.4 for the various body sites.

Numerous other studies have led to a description of the parameters for a painful stimulus. Table 10-2 is a representative compilation. Even though extensive studies such as those of Gibson et al. (1963), Pfeiffer et al. (1971),

Table 10-2　Stimulus Parameters for Pain Sensation

Reference	Stimulus Waveform	Current* (mA)	Electrode size and Location	Remarks
Notermans (1966)	Square wave, 100 Hz; 50% duty cycle, 40 pulses	0.39–0.65 p	Conical, 1 mm radius Dorsum of 2nd finger	Pin-prick pain
Gibson (1963)	Rectangular, 0.5 msec, 100 Hz; 4 to 20 pulses	1.5 p	11 mm diameter active electrode is anode; various sites	Optimum number of stimuli
Gibson (1963)	Rectangular, 0.5 msec, 100 Hz; 20 pulses	1.5 p	11 mm diameter active electrode is anode; various sites.	Optimum frequency for stimulus
Pfeiffer (1971)	Square wave, 50–150 Hz; 50% duty cycle	1–2 p	4 small points on skin of forearm	
Pfeiffer and Stevens (1971)	Rectangular 120 Hz, 3.2 msec	0.8–1.8 p	4 small points on skin of forearm	0.5 sec on, 0.5 sec off
Steinbach and Tursky (1964–1965)	Sine wave, 60 Hz	1.82–10.23 pp	Annular electrode on dorsum of forearm	Applied for 1 sec
Sigel (1953–1954)	Square wave, 10 msec	—	1.5 × 2 in. saline pad on volar upper forearm	Pin-prick sensation with 5 V

Plutchich and Bender (1966)	Square wave, 50 msec	0.7–0.85 p	1 cm diameter on tips of fingers	Applied for 5 sec
Hall et al. (1952)	Sine wave, 60 Hz	4.42–4.67 r	3 × 5 cm electrodes on palm and dorsum of hand	Applied for 0.1 sec
Hawkes and Warm (1960)	Sine wave, 100 Hz 500 1,000 5,000 10,000	1.0 r 1.9 r 2.0 r 5.5 r 10 r	Active electrode on fingertip	
Tursky and Watson (1964)	Sine wave, 60 Hz	1–3 pp 8.5 pp	Concentric electrode (Tursky, 1965) on forearm; inner electrode = 56.4 mm^2; outer = 430 mm^2	Untreated skin; treated skin applied for 0.5 sec
Higgins et al. (1971)	Sine wave, 60 Hz	3.5–4.2	Concentric electrode on left forearm (Tursky, 1965)	In conjunction with another test
Sternbach and Tursky	Sine wave, 60 Hz	6.12–10.23 pp	Concentric electrode (Tursky, 1965) on left forearm	Applied for 1 sec

* p = peak; pp = peak-to-peak, r = rms.

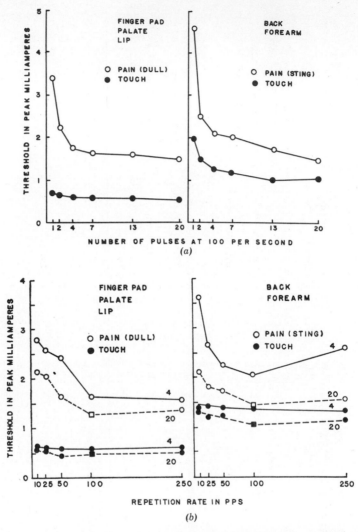

Figure 10-3. Threshold current for touch and pain using an active electrode (11 mm diameter) applied to various areas of the body. (*a*) Values for pain and touch using rectangular pulses (0.5 msec duration; 100 Hz frequency) for different exposure times created by varying the number of stimuli applied. Values for 4 and 20 pulses, each 0.5 msec in duration, for different repetition rates. [From R. H. Gibson, *Proc. 2nd Int. Congr. Technol. Blindness* 2:183–207 (1963). By permission.]

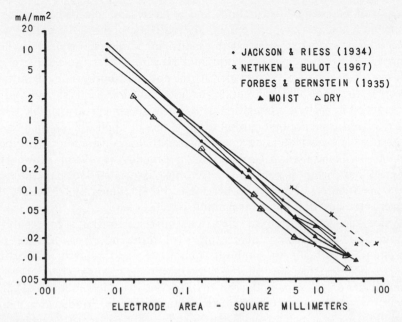

Figure 10-4. Current density (60 Hz rms) versus electrode area for pain sensation. [Data from Jackson and Riess (1934), Forbes and Bernstein (1935), and Netheken and Bulot (1967).]

Tursky and Watson (1964) have been conducted using a variety of wave-forms, the readily available 60-Hz current still seems to be preferred by many investigators; Fig. 10-4 presents the essential data.

There is no agreement on the parameters to be specified to provide a controlled and reproducible pain sensation. For various physical and psychophysiological reasons, a reproducible stimulus intensity is difficult to establish. There have been attempts to normalize a painful sensation by expressing the stimulus in terms of current density, that is, milliamperes per square millimeter of electrode area. Jackson and Riess (1934), Forbes and Bernstein (1935), and Nethken and Bulot (1967) have examined the validity of this procedure. Their data for 60-Hz pain sensation, expressed in milliamperes per square millimeter of electrode area, are plotted versus electrode area in Fig. 10-4. It is quite apparent that the larger the electrode area, the lower the current density for pain sensation. If current density were the correct normalizing factor for specifying pain threshold, a plot of current density versus electrode area would be a straight line parallel to the electrode-area axis. Figure 10-4 shows that such a simple relationship does not exist, probably because sensory receptors are punctate and have a finite density of cutaneous distribution, and a larger-area electrode disproportionately stimulates more receptors; alternatively, perhaps the proportional increase in receptors stimulated results in a disproportionately large increase in perception of the stimulus. However, it is important to emphasize that although current density is not the appropriate quantity to describe the threshold for cutaneous pain, this concept should not be generalized to include stimulation of uniform specimens of irritable tissue, since there is evidence that current density may be applicable in such cases.

Nearly all investigators have emphasized that a constant-current type of circuit should be used, regardless of the stimulus waveform. However, a few feel that current is not the quantity most associated with pain intensity; these investigators (Forbes and Bernstein, 1935; Gilmer, 1937) believe that power is the best descriptor for painful stimuli.

Since the application of electrical current to the skin results in stimulation of a variety of receptors of different types, a pure pain sensation is difficult to establish, quantitate, and reproduce. For this reason, investigators have placed electrodes over regions where there are pain fibers only. Apparently the first to use this technique was Adrian (1919), who placed electrodes on the glans penis and produced a painful sensation using capacitor-pulses of current. More recently Goetzl et al. (1943) and Harris and Blockus (1952) applied stimuli to the tooth pulp to evoke pain. Although the sensation produced in each case was true pain, it has been difficult to standardize and quantitate the pain stimulus, which would be a highly desirable result for studies on the ability of drugs to raise the pain threshold (analgesics). Nonetheless there are devices used to produce painful electrical stimuli, and the name given to the measurement of pain threshold is *algesimetry*. A good account of the difficulties encountered is presented in Beecher's book (1959), which deals with the measurement of subjective responses.

When electrical stimuli are used to produce a painful sensation, it is of paramount importance to consider the safety of the subject. Although any site can be selected for application of the stimuli, it is important to examine all the current pathways to be sure that the heart is not included either directly or indirectly because of the presence of another electrode (e.g., ground) on the subject or a ground fault in the output circuit of the stimulator used to generate the painful stimulus. The safest method of applying painful electrical stimuli places both the active and indifferent electrodes on the same body segment and uses a stimulator with an isolated output circuit. The concentric electrode described by Tursky et al. (1965) offers a practical method of confining the current. The insertion of low-current fuses in series with the output terminals of the stimulator provides additional protection. Adoption of these two safeguards will do much to provide the maximum safety for the subject and make it easier for the investigator to defend his technique to reviewers and critics.

Psychophysiologists who conduct studies on small animals in cages with electrodes on the floor face a particularly difficult problem in delivering a painful stimulation through the animals' feet unless the floor electrodes are kept clean. Fecal matter and urine can initially shortcircuit the electrodes, and dry feces can cover the electrodes with a semiinsulating covering, making it difficult to deliver a controllable painful shock. Alternating current, direct current, and high-voltage pulses have all been used with varying degrees of success. A good review of the techniques was presented by Campbell and Teghtsoonian (1958).

10-4.   THE EFFECTS OF THORACIC CURRENT

When the intensity of current passing through the thorax is increased to a level well above the threshold for cutaneous sensation, contraction of skeletal muscles occurs as a result of direct stimulation of the muscle fibers and/or the motor nerves that innervate them. At about the same level of current, the phrenic and vagus nerves are also stimulated. Stimulation of the phrenic nerves produces tetanic contraction of the diaphragm. Stimulation of the vagus nerves produces the usual spectrum of parasympathetic activity, which includes slowing or arrest of the heart and increased gut motility. In addition, sympathetic nerve fibers are stimulated, yielding effects that oppose the parasympathetic activity; particularly evident is vasoconstriction in many vascular beds. To assign a magnitude for these phenomena, Geddes and Baker (1969) passed current through the thoraxes of dogs ranging in weight from 10 to 18 kg. The dogs were anesthetized with sodium pentobarbital and artificially respired while femoral artery blood pressure was recorded as an indicator of the cardiac activity. Using first the metal-band neck-abdomen electrodes, then transthoracic plate electrodes, the current at each frequency was increased until vagal slowing of the heart was observed. The threshold currents at different frequencies required to obtain vagal slowing in the heart are given in Fig. 10-5.

Figure 10-5 illustrates that in the 10 to 18-kg animal, vagal stimulation is easily achieved with low frequency currents on the order of 50 mA applied either with neck-abdomen or transchest electrodes. Figure 10-5 also shows that the threshold current for vagal stimulation increases with increasing frequency. For example, the threshold current for vagal stimulation with neck-abdomen electrodes at 5 kHz is about 12 times that required at 60 Hz. Similarly with transchest electrodes, the current required to obtain cardiac slowing at 5 kHz is 16 times that required at 60 Hz. Proof that

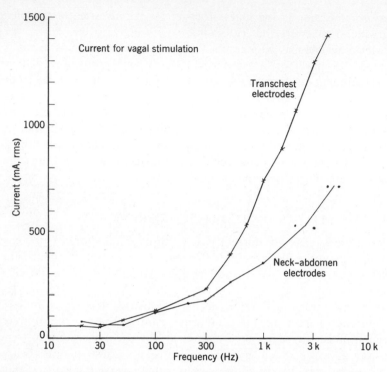

Figure 10-5. Average threshold sinusoidal current for vagal stimulation using transchest and neck-abdomen electrodes applied to dogs weighing 10 to 18 kg. Vagal stimulation was observed by slowing of the heart rate.

slowing of the heart was caused by stimulation of the vagus nerves was verified by the administration of atropine, which blocked the effect. These facts argue strongly in favor of the use of currents high in the kilohertz range for the detection of physiological events by the impedance method, if vagal slowing of the heart is to be avoided.

When thoracic current is further increased, ventricular fibrillation occurs; this is a condition of complete asynchronous contraction and relaxation of all the ventricular fibers, resulting in a loss of cardiac output until defibrillation is achieved. Ventricular fibrillation can result from coronary heart disease, hypoxia of the myocardium, and the use of some drugs. It can be induced by a pacemaker or by other stimuli (e.g., mechanical) falling within the vulnerable period of the ventricles. Once started, fibrillation rarely, if ever, stops spontaneously in man and the larger domestic animals. If it continues for more than 3 min, irreversible damage may occur to the central nervous system, although the heart itself can be resuscitated. In the normal subject, the passage of a relatively low-intensity current of low frequency through the thorax will produce ventricular fibrillation. In particular, ordinary lighting sources are more than sufficient to produce fibrillation; the critical factors are the intensity, pathway, duration of exposure, and frequency of the current. Although it is not desirable to experiment on man to determine the current threshold for fibrillation, studies have been carried out on experimental animals having body weights comparable to the human to identify the dangerous current levels at different frequencies (Ferris et al., 1936; Geddes and Baker, 1969).

In a series of experiments on dogs, the authors determined the threshold current required to produce ventricular fibrillation, using sinusoidal current of different frequencies. Several electrode arrangements were used, and current was passed through the thoraxes of anesthetized animals in which breathing was assisted with a respirator. Blood pressure and the ECG were recorded as indicators of the cardiac function. The procedure consisted of choosing a frequency and increasing the current slowly, while watching the animal's blood pressure and electrocardiogram carefully. A consistent sequence of events occurred with each animal as the current was increased. The first event was strong   contraction of skeletal muscles; this was followed by arrest of spontaneous respiratory movements, vagal slowing of the heart, and initially in most animals there was evacuation of the bladder and bowel. Finally, ventricular fibrillation occurred and blood pressure dropped to a near-zero value. After about 20 sec of fibrillation, the ventricles were defibrillated electrically using high-intensity 60-Hz current applied to transchest electrodes. The procedure was repeated over a frequency range extending from 20 to 3000 Hz. The results (Fig. 10-6) clearly illustrate that as frequency was increased, more current was required to produce ventricular fibrillation. It is particularly important that in the frequency range extending from 20 to 300 Hz, fibrillation was produced in the dog with relatively low currents applied to the electrode arrays. Noteworthy is the fact that the threshold for fibrillation in the region between 20 and 100 Hz is almost independent of frequency. Above 100 Hz the current required to initiate fibrillation is markedly higher, and with all electrode systems the current required to produce ventricular fibrillation increases with increasing frequency. Essentially the same data were obtained by Kouwenhoven et al. (1936), who, using interrupted direct current, found that the threshold current for fibrillation at 1500 Hz was about 10 times that at 60 Hz. Much earlier, Prevost and Battelli (1900) discovered that the threshold voltage for fibrillation at 2000 Hz was 10 times that for 200 Hz. This evidence strongly recommends the choice of frequencies high in the kilohertz region for the measurement of physiological events by the impedance method to avoid the risk of ventricular fibrillation.

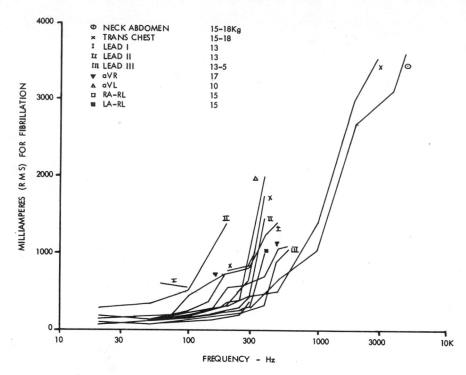

Figure 10-6. Threshold sinusoidal current for precipitation of ventricular fibrillation in the dog using various electrode locations. Ventricular fibrillation was precipitated by gradually increasing the current while monitoring the electrocardiogram and blood pressure.

The magnitude of thoracic current necessary for the precipitation of fibrillation at any frequency is related to the size of the subject. Since the low-frequency threshold current for fibrillation is adequately described by the current required at 60 Hz, the effect of body size in relation to fibrillation threshold can be studied at this frequency. Ferris et al. (1936) carried out the first quantitative studies of this type, using guinea pigs, rabbits, cats, dogs, pigs, sheep, and calves. The authors also carried out similar studies. All these data are plotted in Fig. 10-7 for the various species and electrode locations; the duration of current flow for the studies was 5 sec.

Figure 10-7 clearly shows that the threshold 60-Hz current required for the precipitation of ventricular fibrillation is dependent on the weight of the subject and the location of the electrodes. The straight lines describing these relationships were calculated by the least-squares method from the data. It is interesting to note the difference in threshold currents for the electrode positions employed. The values required for the precipitation of

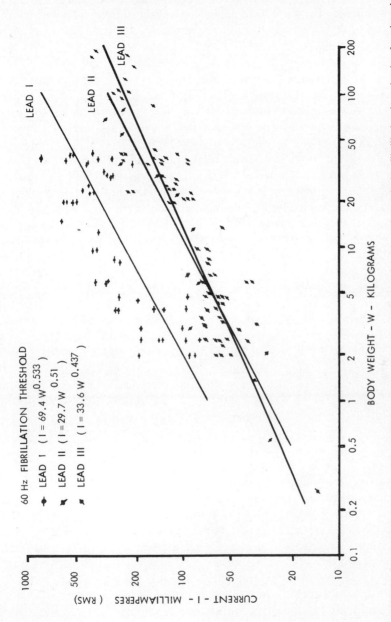

Figure 10-7. Threshold 60-Hz current (applied for 5 sec) required for the precipitation of ventricular fibrillation in animals of various body weights. (Lead I = right to left fore limb; lead II = right fore limb-left hind limb and lead III = left fore limb-left hind limb.) [Redrawn from Geddes et al., *IEEE Trans. Bio-Med. Eng.* **BME-20**:465–468 (1973).]

293

ventricular fibrillation with electrodes on the forelimbs (lead I) are about three times those required when the current is applied between the fore and hind limbs (leads II and III). In general the 60-Hz current required for the precipitation of ventricular fibrillation varies approximately as the square root of body weight.

Particularly important in this illustration is the value of 60-Hz current required to precipitate ventricular fibrillation in the 70-kg animal (which approximates the weight of an adult man). From Fig. 10-7 it would appear that 215 mA rms of 60-Hz current flowing for 5 sec through the left arm-left leg circuit (lead III) will fibrillate the ventricles if species differences are disregarded. Only a slightly higher current (260 mA) is required between the right forelimb and left hind limb (lead II), but a much higher current (670 mA) is required when applied across the forelimbs (lead I). Dalziel (1956) estimated that a 60-Hz thoracic current of between 100 and 275 mA would in all likelihood produce ventricular fibrillation in man.

It was stated earlier that in addition to frequency, electrode location, and body weight, the duration of exposure to current affected the threshold value for the precipitation of ventricular fibrillation. A study of the significance of this factor was carried out by Geddes et al. (1973). Figure 10-8 illustrates the manner in which the threshold current for the precipitation of ventricular fibrillation increases with a decrease in the duration of exposure to 60-Hz current. The data for lead III (left forelimb to left hind limb) were chosen for presentation because the current required with lead III was the lowest of the three limb leads. The illustration also shows that for a given body weight, the amount of current required to induce ventricular fibrillation increases with decreasing duration of exposure. For a duration of exposure in excess of about one second, the threshold current for the precipitation of ventricular fibrillation decreases very little.

The most dangerous situation for the precipitation of ventricular fibrillation exists when a catheter is placed in the right or left ventricle. Mechanical stimulation of the myocardium by the catheter tip as the heart beats can cause extrasystoles and tachycardia, which can lead to ventricular fibrillation. However, when the catheter is filled with an electrolyte (e.g., saline or blood), or when a catheter electrode (for temporary cardiac pacemaking) is in a ventricle, the opportunity arises for current to gain access to the ventricular myocardium. In such a circumstance, a very small current can precipitate ventricular fibrillation. To provide quantitative data on this point, the authors (1971) carried out studies using anesthetized dogs (10–15 kg) with standard saline-filled catheters in the right and left ventricles, placed there by passage down the jugular vein and right carotid artery.

To guarantee that the catheters remained in contact with the endocardium, a small negative pressure was applied to hold the ventricular wall

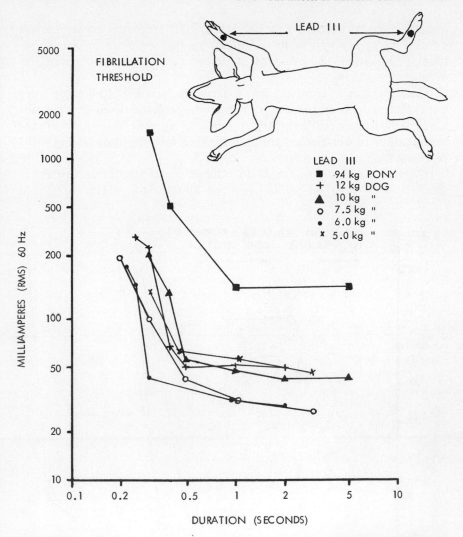

Figure 10-8. Threshold 60-Hz current required to precipitate ventricular fibrillation when period of exposure is varied. [From Geddes et al., *IEEE Trans. Bio-Med. Engng.* **BME-20**:465–468 (1973). By permission.]

against the tip of the catheter. Sinusoidal current was applied for 5 sec between the catheter fitting and a left leg electrode. Blood pressure and lead III electrocardiogram were recorded, and the threshold current for fibrillation was determined in a frequency range extending from 30 to 350 Hz. The ventricular fibrillation threshold current levels appear in Fig. 10-9, which indicates that the lowest current for fibrillation occurs in the frequency range between 30 and 100 Hz. In this frequency region current values ranging from 50 to 400 μA (rms) applied for 5 sec produced ventricular fibrillation. These findings are in agreement with those reported by Whalen et al. (1964).

It is important to recall that the current levels in Fig. 10-8 apply when the catheter tip is in contact with the endocardium. Even a slight displacement of the catheter tip raises the current required for the precipitation of ventricular fibrillation. Therefore the data in Fig. 10-9 represent the worst-case situation.

In a practical circumstance, it is a voltage source that causes current to flow. To shed light on the implications of the data in Fig. 10-9, it is

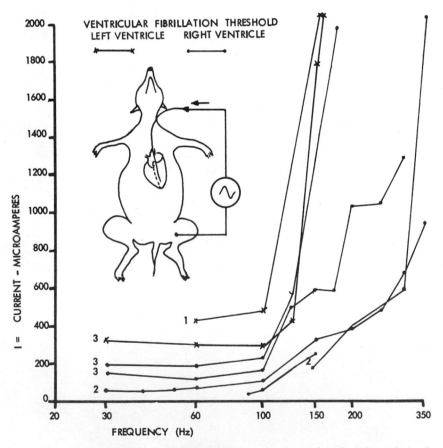

Figure 10-9. Threshold 60-Hz current applied for 5 sec for the precipitation of ventricular fibrillation with catheters in the right and left ventricles. [From L. A. Geddes and L. E. Baker, Response to passage of electric current through the body. J.A.A.M.I. 1971, **5**(1):13–18.]

necessary to consider two distinct situations; one in which a catheter-electrode is placed in a ventricle and the other in which a saline-filled catheter is placed in the same location. In the first case, the electrode impedance amounts to about 500 Ω, at 60 Hz; therefore a voltage of 2.5 mV (rms) would cause 50 μA (rms) of 60 Hz current to flow and precipitate ventricular fibrillation. With saline- and blood-filled catheters the situation is entirely different, as was clearly pointed out by Monsees and McQuarrie (1971). Using resistivity values of 70 and 150 Ω-cm for physiological saline and blood, respectively, the resistance of standard cardiac catheters can be calculated. For example, an 8F catheter has an internal diameter of 1.42 mm; for a 100 cm length, the resistances when filled with saline and blood are 0.44 and 0.95 MΩ, respectively. The voltages necessary to cause 50 μA (rms) to flow in these catheters, to precipitate ventricular fibrillation when the tips are in contact with the endocardium, are 22 and 47.5 V (rms), respectively. The two cardiac catheter situations described indicate that special precautions must be taken to prevent cardiac catheters from carrying 60-Hz current.

Repetitive pulses are not used at present for the measurement of physiological events. However they could be, and certain precautions must be observed if this technique is to be used safely. The chronaxie of mammalian myocardium has been found to be around 2 msec (Brooks et al., 1955). Slowly repetitive stimuli of this duration evoke single ectopic contractions, but there is a real danger of ventricular fibrillation if the repetition rate is increased or if a single stimulus of high intensity falls in the early phase of the relatively refractory period (the "vulnerable period" of the myocardium). To eliminate any possibility of such potentially lethal stimulation, pulses of low intensity and extremely short duration are mandatory.

In summary, the data in Figs. 10-2 (sensation threshold), 10-5 (vagal stimulation threshold), and 10-6 through 10-9 (threshold current at different frequencies for ventricular fibrillation) all demonstrate that when the impedance method is used to measure physiological events, it is wise to choose a frequency in the range above 20 kHz. Frequencies lower than 5 kHz are particularly hazardous if substantial current flows, since ventricular fibrillation may result. The use of higher frequencies not only provides the protection sought in the avoidance of tissue stimulation but permits the safe use of currents of a magnitude that could be dangerous if the frequency were lower. Since in many cases physiological events produce relatively small impedance changes, it is desirable to use as large a current as is safe to obtain the largest electrical signal per unit of physiological event. A safe high-frequency current is one that does not stimulate irritable tissue and does not cause local tissue heating which, of course, alters cell function and local blood supply.

10-5. LEGAL ELECTROCUTION

In view of the hazardous current thresholds just described, it is of interest to consider the values that have been used for the legal execution of convicted criminals. Much has been written on this subject, and an excellent account of the circumstances surrounding the first legal executions, starting in 1890, was presented by MacDonald (1892) who also reported the pathological findings on the first seven electrocutions. More recently, Bernstein (1973) described the heated controversy between Edison and Westinghouse on the subject of death by electric current. It will be recalled that Edison strongly advocated the use of direct current because of its high safety and Westinghouse championed alternating current because it could be transmitted efficiently over large distances, using high voltage which, with a transformer, could be reduced to any convenient voltage at the receiving end of the transmission line.

In the first legal executions, about 1500 to 1700 V were applied to wetted sponge electrodes applied to the head and sacrum. About 2 to 7 A of 60-Hz current flowed, the current being applied initially for 20 sec and reapplied shortly thereafter. In many installations, direct current was used with equal success. The pathological findings associated with death from electric current have been reported by Spitzka and Radash (1912), Jex-Blake (1913), Jaffe (1928), Langworthy (1930), Hassin (1933), Pritchard (1934), and Alexander (1938). These reports indicate that there is virtually complete thermal destruction of the central nervous system in legal electrocution; brain temperatures as high as 140°F have been measured. Ventricular fibrillation has also been reported. There is general agreement that in legal execution, consciousness is lost instantly and death is due to thermal destruction of the central nervous system.

10-6. CURRENT DENSITY DISTRIBUTION

When current is applied to living tissue, the spatial manner in which current is distributed is virtually unknown because of differing resistivities of tissues and fluids and because of their particular arrangement between the current-injecting electrodes. Except for a few simple cases, it is this situation that limits estimation of the calibratability of many physiological events detected by impedance. Moreover, there is no simple method for accurate measurement of current density distribution in anisotropic tissue. The insertion of a voltage-measuring probe provides a voltage that is dependent on the current density and the resistivity of the material surrounding the probe. Knowledge of the resistivity allows calculation of the current density, provided introduction of the probe does not alter the current distribution. It must also be recognized that living tissue has different electrical properties in different directions; therefore accurate specification of the local current density requires knowledge of the resistivity and voltage gradient along three axes. The practical measurement of these quantities is by no means easy. Those who desire to explore this difficult but important problem are directed to the reviews presented by the authors (1969, 1970, 1971).

Although measurement of current density distribution is a formidable task, an estimate of current distribution can be made by knowing the resistivity values of various body tissues and fluids. Reviews of the extensive literature on this subject have been presented by Schwan (1963) and Geddes and Baker (1967). Although many biological specimens have been measured, some of the values appearing in the literature were determined without due regard to electrode polarization errors. Table 10-3 lists representative resistivity values. It is important to note that dead tissue exhibits a lower resistivity than living tissue.

With alternating current of the frequencies and intensities (nonstimu-

Table 10-3   Resistivities of Biological Specimens*

Specimen	Resistivity† (Ω-cm)	Species
Blood	150‡	Human
Plasma	63	Mammals
Cerebrospinal fluid	65	Human
Bile	60	Cow-pig
Urine	30	Cow-pig
Cardiac muscle (R)	750	Dog
Skeletal muscle (T)	1600	Dog
Skeletal muscle (L)	300	Dog
Lung	1275	Mammals
Kidney	370	Mammals
Liver	820	Dog
Spleen	885	Dog
Brain (R)	580	Mammals
Fat	2500	Mammals

* From L. A. Geddes and L. E. Baker, *Med. Biol. Eng.* **5**; 271–293 (1967).

† Average values for body temperature and the low-frequency region (<1 MHz). R = random orientation; T = transverse current; L = longitudinal current.

‡ Magnitude depends on packed-cell volume (see Section 10-22).

lating and nonheating) used to measure physiological events, there appear to be no detectable alterations in cell function due to current flow. The effect of current density on body tissues and fluids has not been adequately investigated. Most body fluids are not simple electrolytes but are suspensions of cells and large molecules. The extent to which these fluid components are modified by current awaits investigation. One study by Poppindiek (1964), pertinent to the techniques in which blood flow is measured by impedance change, showed that no detectable change occurred in canine blood when it sustained a current density of 0.5 A/cm^2 for 3 hr. Studies on the nonthermal effects of current flow on other biological tissues and fluids will undoubtedly be carried out. There are virtually no data on the impedance offered by living tissue to the high current densities such as used in ventricular defibrillation.

10-7.   ELECTRODE SYSTEMS

When the impedance technique is used to measure a physiological event, one of two methods is generally employed. With both, the physiological event is placed between the measuring electrodes in such a way that the event alters the current density distribution between the electrodes, thus manifesting itself as a change in impedance. In one method, the electrodes are in direct contact with the preparation, and a relatively low impedance circuit is formed; in the other, they are insulated from the subject, and a relatively high impedance capacitive circuit results.

Bipolar and tetrapolar electrode systems are currently employed to derive a signal from a physiological event by means of the impedance technique. With the bipolar arrangement two types of circuitry are employed; with the tetrapolar system, only one circuit configuration is needed. All circuits require a source of alternating current and an amplifier having an input impedance that is high with respect to the impedance between the electrode terminals. The impedance signal is recovered by use of a detector, which may be a null indicator, a high-impedance voltmeter, or a phase-sensitive circuit.

In many instances the physiological event changes the impedance by a small amount, and only the change contains the useful information. Under this circumstance, the voltage reflecting the change in impedance is amplified and displayed, without dissection into resistive and reactive components. If separation of these components is desirable, phase-sensitive detecting systems are necessary.

Although the circuits to be described are those most frequently employed, in some cases in which movement has been converted into corresponding changes in capacitance, the variation in capacitance has been employed to frequency modulate a carrier. On a few occasions a direct voltage was applied to the electrodes and the physiological event altered the conductivity and/or capacitance of the circuit, thereby modulating the direct current.

10-8. IMPEDANCE–MEASURING CIRCUITS

10-8-1. Bridge Circuit

When two electrodes are employed, the impedance bridge circuit diagrammed in Fig. 10-10 can be used. In such an arrangement, the oscillator voltage E is applied to two opposite corners of the bridge and the detector is connected to the other two. When the ratio arms Z_1, Z_2 are resistors of equal value, the impedance bridge becomes a comparison bridge. The balancing arm RC may consist of parallel resistance and capacitance decade units which are adjusted to balance the bridge for the basal (Z_0) impedance between the electrode terminals. At balance, the value of the balance arm gives the equivalent parallel resistive and reactive components of the tissue-electrode circuit. If R and C are placed in series and the bridge is balanced, the new values for R and C give the equivalent series circuit between the electrode terminals. These equivalents are valid only for the frequency employed. With most bridges the impedance is measured in terms of a parallel or a series equivalent, but not both. Often it is desirable to transform one equivalent into the other; for example, if in a given case R_s and C_s are the series resistance and capacitance at a particular frequency f, the parallel equivalents R_p and C_p at the same frequency are given by the following:

is equivalent to

$$R_p = \frac{1 + (2\pi f C_s R_s)^2}{4\pi^2 f^2 C_s^2 R_s}, \qquad R_p = R_s + \frac{X_s^2}{R_s},$$

$$C_p = \frac{C_s}{1 + (2\pi f C_s R_s)^2}, \qquad X_p = X_s + \frac{R_s^2}{X_s}.$$

Frequently it is desirable to carry out the reverse process, that is, to express a series circuit in terms of a parallel one. Rearrangement of the expressions

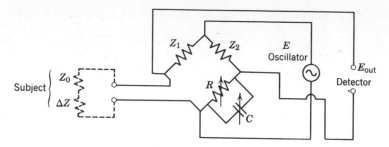

Figure 10-10. Impedance bridge.

just given provides the following relationships:

$$R_s = \frac{R_p}{1 + (2\pi f C_p R_p)^2}, \qquad C_s = C_p \left[1 + \frac{1}{(2\pi f R_p C_p)^2}\right].$$

With the bridge circuit, the changes in impedance reflecting the physiological event produce a varying output voltage (E_{out}) which, after amplification and rectification, is displayed to produce a record related to changes in the physiological event. It must be emphasized that an output is obtained if there is a change in either the resistive or the reactive component or in both. If it is desired to examine the magnitude of each component individually, a phase-sensitive detector is required.

If the bridge is operated at the balance point and without the use of a phase-sensitive detector, an output voltage is obtained if the impedance being measured increases or decreases. Under this operating condition, direction indication is lost. However, if after the bridge has been initially balanced, it is then unbalanced slightly by the addition of a small resistance in series with the impedance being measured, the output voltage from the bridge will increase and decrease in accordance with corresponding changes in the impedance being measured. The amount of resistance added is dictated by the maximum change in impedance required to drive the bridge toward the balance point.

Precautions must be taken in using the bridge circuit to avoid having the size of the output voltage become dependent on the magnitude of Z_0, the basal impedance. For the same ΔZ if Z_0 is small, more current will flow through Z_1 and Z_0, and the output (ΔE_{out}) will be large. This sensitivity dependence on Z_0 can be eliminated by making Z_1 much greater than $Z_0 + \Delta Z$, which allows the bridge to have the properties of the constant-current circuit, which is described next.

10-8-2. Constant-Current Circuit

The constant-current bipolar electrode system is depicted in Fig. 10-11. Current from the oscillator is fed symmetrically to the electrodes through two resistances R, R, which are high in value with respect to the total impedance $(Z_0 + \Delta Z)$ between the electrodes. With this circuit configuration the current through the subject is determined by these resistances (R, R) and the oscillator voltage (E), and it is relatively independent of the electrode-subject impedance $(Z_0 + \Delta Z)$. The detector is connected across the electrodes, and the voltage present is a function of the basal impedance between the electrodes Z_0 and any change ΔZ due to the physiological event. It can easily be shown that the voltage across the electrodes is given by

$$E_{out} = \frac{E(Z_0 + \Delta Z)}{2R + Z_0 + \Delta Z}.$$

If R is made much greater than Z_0 and ΔZ is much less than Z_0, then

$$E_{out} \doteqdot \frac{E(Z_0 + \Delta Z)}{2R},$$

$$\doteqdot \frac{EZ_0}{2R} + \frac{E\Delta Z}{2R}.$$

Rectification of these signals after amplification yields a large constant signal $(EZ_0/2R)$ plus a smaller one $(E\Delta Z/2R)$ proportional to the impedance change due to the physiological event. The larger signal, reflecting the basal impedance of the electrode-subject circuit, is often eliminated from the output by blocking this dc component with a capacitance or by canceling it with an opposing voltage.

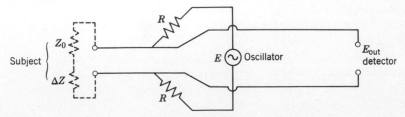

Figure 10-11. Symmetrical constant-current circuit. (For simplicity the constant-current circuit is illustrated by an oscillator and two resistances R, R, which are much larger than $Z_0 + \Delta Z$.)

10-8-3.   Tetrapolar Circuit

The third method for monitoring impedance changes employs four electrodes (see Fig. 10-12). In this tetrapolar circuit the oscillator voltage (E) is fed to the current electrodes I_1, I_2, which are farthest apart on the preparation. Usually a constant-current generator is employed as the current source. Between the current electrodes are the potential-measuring electrodes M_1, M_2, which receive a voltage determined by the current density distribution in the preparation. Amplification and rectification of this voltage (E_{out}) yield a signal related to the "basal" tissue impedance between the potential-measuring electrodes and any changes associated with the physiological event.

10-8-4.   Comparison of Circuits

Each of the three circuits (bridge, constant-current, and tetrapolar) has unique characteristics that are ideal for some applications and less suitable for others. Of the three, the bridge circuit has been the most commonly employed. The wide range of impedance that can be measured is an attractive feature of this configuration. With appropriate components it can be employed to detect the changes in capacitive reactance either when the electrodes do not touch the subject or when they are in direct contact with the preparation. Calibration of the balance arm RC permits derivation of an equivalent circuit for the preparation between the electrodes at the frequency employed. A comparison of the magnitude of the oscillator and detector voltages and the phase angle between them permits dissection of the output signal into its reactive and resistive components.

One of the difficulties with the bridge circuit relates to isolation of the detector and oscillator circuits above ground potential. If both the oscillator and the subject are to be grounded, as by grounding their common point, the detector circuit must be lifted above ground by an appropriate isolating device. Practically, this requires the use of a special low-capacitance transformer.

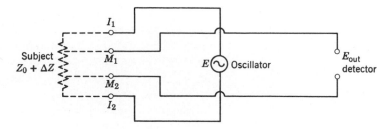

Figure 10-12.   Tetrapolar circuit.

Another drawback to the bridge circuit involves its adaptation for physiological recording. If the impedance of the arm (Z_1) in Fig. 10-10 is not high with respect to the impedance of the tissue, the magnitude of the output signal produced by ΔZ will be dependent on the basal level of impedance (Z_0) between the electrode terminals. This situation arises when the amount of current flowing through the preparation is determined both by Z_1 and by the impedance between the electrode terminals. Should the latter change the current will also change, and the magnitude of the voltage produced by the physiological event will depend on the value of Z_0. This undesirable feature of the bridge circuit can be minimized by a calibration technique in which a resistor of known value is switched into the circuit in series with the preparation. One method of obtaining an output that is not dependent on the electrode-subject impedance is to make the arm of the bridge adjacent to the subject (Z_1) high in resistance with respect to the impedance between the electrode terminals. Under these conditions the bridge circuit takes on the characteristics of the constant-current circuit. For a truly constant-current circuit, however, Z_1 must be controlled by a feedback circuit arranged so that the current through the subject is maintained at a constant value despite any change in Z_0.

The bridge circuit may be employed to measure the impedance between electrodes which are being used simultaneously to record bioelectric events if the oscillator and the detector are isolated from each other and ground and if the impedance of the arm of the bridge adjacent to the subject (Z_1) is made high as previously described. When the oscillator voltage is low and its frequency is beyond the frequency spectrum of bioelectric events, only simple filtering is required in the bioelectric recorder to eliminate the oscillator voltage.

Many of the practical inconveniences of the bridge circuit can be eliminated by use of the symmetrical constant-current circuit shown in Fig. 10-11. In essence, this circuit resembles that of the familiar shunt-type ohmmeter. With the constant-current circuit, the oscillator voltage is applied to the electrodes through two series resistors, a thousand or more times the nominal impedance between the electrode terminals. In this circumstance the impedance of the electrodes and the biological material will not determine the current flowing through the preparation. Although the level of impedance between the electrode terminals will determine the size of the static signal presented to the detector, the same change in impedance, reflecting the physiological event, will always produce the same amplitude signal. The use of a relatively high source voltage and two resistors R, R to obtain the constant-current characteristic is a simple, practical technique. A more sophisticated method uses a low-voltage operational amplifier, connected to provide a constant-current output. Although the use of such a device guarantees constant-current operation, the associated circuitry makes it difficult to obtain isolation from ground; thus the symmetry and low capacitance to ground, characteristically obtained with ordinary resistors, is lost. However, the use of high value resistors requires the availability of a substantial voltage for the oscillator.

Another feature of practical value in the physiological application of the constant-current circuit is the few controls needed for its operation. If direct-coupled recording is required, only one control is needed to adjust the bucking voltage necessary to eliminate the large signal produced by the basal impedance between the electrode terminals. A second control can regulate the amplitude of the display.

A less attractive feature of the constant-current circuit is its limited ability to measure events over a large range of impedance. With a wide range of basal impedance, the amplifier and demodulator are presented with a wide range of voltage on which are superimposed the smaller changes due to the physiological event. This calls for an amplifier having a high input impedance and a wide dynamic range to guarantee linearity of reproduction. For this reason the constant-current circuit is most conveniently employed to detect physiological events when the impedance between the electrode terminals is low, that is, when there is direct electrolytic contact between the tissue and the electrodes.

The constant-current circuit in Fig. 10-11 constitutes a symmetrical system. A requisite that often presents practical difficulties is isolation of the oscillator and detector from each other and from ground. When proper isolation and symmetry are achieved, no change in operation will occur if either or neither side of the input is grounded. This feature permits connecting the circuit to electrodes that are connected to other devices for the measurement of bioelectric events.

When resistors are employed to obtain the constant-current characteristic, a prime requisite is high stability in oscillator voltage. Small variations in amplitude, such as noise or ripple, will appear with the output signal. When direct-coupled recording is employed, the stability requirements for the oscillator can be lessened by deriving the bucking voltage in the output circuit from the oscillator voltage.

With the constant-current circuit it is also possible to employ a detector that will permit dissection of the impedance into its resistive and reactive components. In most applications this is unnecessary. With the circuit in Fig. 10-11 a change in either capacitive reactance or resistance, or both, will alter the output of the system. If only the change in impedance, without its dissection, reflects the physiological event, the constant-current circuit, with its few controls and its freedom from the influence of basal electrode-subject impedance, is unusually practical for the measurement of a variety of physiological events.

The tetrapolar arrangement (Fig. 10-12) is popular among those who measure thoracic and peripheral pulses by impedance plethysmography. It was originally developed by Bouty (1884) to eliminate electrode polarization errors in the measurement of the specific resistance of electrolytes. Nyboer (1944, 1959) and Bagno (1959) have presented good accounts of the physiological application of this circuit. Because the current is admitted to the subject by electrodes that are distant from the measuring electrodes, with a homogeneously conducting medium there exists the possibility for a more uniform distribution of current density in the preparation between the measuring electrodes, despite a relatively large asymmetry in current density distribution in the vicinity of the current electrodes (see Figs. 10-37a and 10-37b). Inasmuch as variations in current density distribution are reflected at the surface of a volume conductor as changes in potential, one could expect artifact produced by movement of the current electrodes to be reduced when recording from potential electrodes located in a region in which the current density distribution remains more nearly uniform.

With a high-impedance detecting system, the voltage appearing across the potential-measuring electrodes M_1, M_2 (Fig. 10-12) is independent of their impedance. If the output impedance of the oscillator is made high with respect to the impedance between the current electrodes I_1, I_2, the constant-current feature is achieved. When this condition is satisfied, accurate measurements can be made of potential changes occurring between the potential electrodes, which reflect changes in the internal current density distribution.

In practice, the equipment used with the tetrapolar arrangement need not require more than three controls, two for balance and one for amplitude. It is possible to employ a phase-sensitive detector to dissect the impedance change into its resistive and reactive components. The tetrapolar method, when applied to the measurement of the resistivity of homogeneously conducting materials in an electrolytic cell, permits the creation of a uniform current density distribution between the potential electrodes. Therefore, resistivity measurements can be made without electrode polarization impedance errors. However, when the tetrapolar circuit is applied in the measurement of physiological events, uniform current density distribution is not likely to exist because of the differing resistivities of biological material and the relationship between the size of the electrodes and the extent of the volume conductor. Although a proper measurement of resistivity cannot be made under such circumstances, the tetrapolar circuit is useful in determining physiological events by impedance change. The primary disadvantage of the method is the requirement of four rather than two electrodes on the subject or preparation.

When any of the circuits just described is used to measure the impedance between the electrode terminals, and such impedance is not dissected into its reactive and resistive components, it is not at all times clear which component contains the information related to the physiological event. When low frequencies are employed the impedance may be strongly reactive; with high frequencies the equivalent circuits are mainly resistive. Many investigations must still be carried out to discover whether in a particular case, the resistive or the reactive component contains the more meaningful data.

10-8-5. Guard-Electrode Technique

When the conducting property of a specimen is measured with electrodes that are small with respect to its size, the current spreads beyond the elec-trodes as in Fig. 10-13*a*. This situation, which often exists when physio-

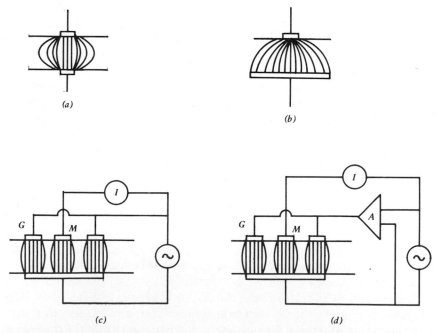

Figure 10-13.   Current spread in a conductor and the use of a concentric guard electrode (*G*) to achieve uniform current density distribution. (*a*) Current spread in a conductor with similar electrodes. (*b*) Current spread with different sized electrodes. (*c*) Current spread with guard electrode maintained at same potential as measuring electrode (*M*). (*d*) Guard electrode driven by a unity-gain amplifier (*A*).

logical events are measured by impedance, plagued the early physicists seeking an accurate value for the resistivity of a material. Current spread also occurs when a small electrode is used in conjunction with a large electrode, as in Fig. 10-13b. To achieve a uniform current density distribution under an electrode, a guard-ring electrode is applied. Figure 10-13b shows that the current distribution with small and large electrodes applied to a conducting specimen extends well beyond both electrodes. To obtain a uniform current density distribution under the smaller electrode, a concentric guard electrode is placed around the smaller electrode, and the potential of the guard electrode is maintained at the potential of the smaller electrode used for current measurement (see Fig. 10-13c). Note that this technique prevents current spread from the smaller electrode connected to the current meter and achieves a more uniform current density distribution in the specimen. The current flowing in the guard electrode is not measured; it merely aids in providing a uniform current density distribution around the main current path in the specimen. The modern method of applying a guard electrode employs an operational amplifier of unity gain to drive the guard electrode; the technique is illustrated in Fig. 10-13d.

The guard-electrode technique is sometimes applied when the constant-voltage system is used to measure impedance or impedance change. Graham (1965) reported its use in the measurement of respiration in the human with a chest-to-back electrode arrangement operated at 50 kHz. Without the guard applied, the basal impedance was 400 Ω, which increased to 404 Ω with inspiration. When the electrode on the back was guarded, the basal impedance was 8000 Ω (the increase presumably due to forcing more current through aerated lung), and the same inspiratory volume increased the impedance by 80 Ω. In this application, which measured the ventilation of one lung, a 20-fold respiratory impedance change was obtained by using the guard-electrode technique. In a similar study Cooley and Longini (1968) chose the guard-electrode technique to detect respiration in man and the dog. Application of the guard increased the measured basal transthoracic impedance. The ratio of the change in respiratory transthoracic resistance using the guard-electrode technique to that with simple bipolar electrodes varied with the size of the guarding electrode; ratios ranging from 39 to 67.5 were obtained.

Lifshitz and Klemm (1966) and Lifshitz (1970) applied guard electrodes to each of a bipolar pair of electrodes on the head to detect pulsatile cerebral blood flow by the method known as rheoencephalography (see Section 10-14-8). The basal impedance and the pulsatile changes were compared with and without the guard electrode, using the constant-voltage method with frequencies ranging from 25 kHz to 2 MHz. The average ratio of the basal impedance with guarded electrodes to that with unguarded electrodes was 3.39. When the amplitude of the pulsatile impedance with guarded electrodes was compared with that of unguarded electrodes, it was found that use of the guard electrodes more than doubled the size of the desired pulsatile impedance change.

Severinghaus (1971) reported the use of a single electrode, guarded by four driven segments, applied to the chest to detect pulmonary edema in humans using 100-kHz current. In the following year Severinghaus et al. (1972) added four additional potential-sensing electrodes between the driven four-quadrant electrodes and the central measuring electrode to improve penetration of the current into the thorax. With this system, which mainly measured the impedance of the region below the guarded electrode, apparent lung resistivity was measured. Only a small decrease in resistivity was found to accompany a relatively large increase in intrathoracic fluid. However, the respiratory impedance change amounted to 63 Ω/l in an adult human. This high impedance coefficient is consistent with the values obtained by others who have used guarded electrodes to detect respiration.

From the foregoing, it can be seen that use of the guard-electrode technique can confine the current flow. In the biological application, however, the anisotropic nature of biological tissue indicates the need for caution in attempting to direct the current flow by the use of guarded electrodes.

10-8-6.   Electrodeless Impedance Measurements

By the use of electromagnetic induction, it is possible to measure the resistivity of a conducting substance without the application of electrodes; this technique is used quite extensively in geophysical exploration. The first to apply this method to obtain signals reflecting respiration and pulsatile blood flow were Tarjan and McFee (1968, 1970), who employed three identical, rigidly mounted coaxial coils separated by a distance approximately equal to their radii. The central coil was energized with 100-kHz current and the two outer coils were connected in series opposition, as in Fig. 10-14. The arrangement therefore constitutes a differential transformer. With the three-coil assembly well removed from conducting materials, amplitude and phase adjustments were made to obtain the smallest possible unbalance signal from the coils connected in series opposition.

When such a balanced three-coil assembly is brought near conducting material, a current is induced in it. The magnitude of the current is proportional to the conductivity. The induced current produces a magnetic field of its own, which alters the voltage induced in one or both of the two pickup coils. With fixed geometry, the unbalance voltage can be detected and

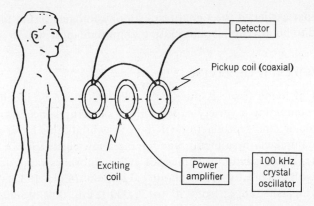

Figure 10-14. The electrodeless method of measuring impedance and impedance change using electromagnetic induction. [From Tarjan and McFee, *Ann. N.Y. Acad. Sci.* **170**:462–475 (1970). By permission.]

processed to provide a measure of the conductance of the material and any variations it experiences.

Tarjan and McFee (1968, 1970) detected respiration in the human by mounting the coil assembly a short distance from the thorax. By carefully placing the axis of the coil assembly over the heart, and requesting that the subject hold his breath at full inspiration, recordings strikingly similar to ventricular volume changes were obtained. With the assembly placed near the head, the investigators recorded pulsatile changes reflecting cerebral blood flow. In this application, they were even able to detect metallic tooth fillings.

The electrodeless method for detecting impedance changes exhibits some interesting characteristics. For many reasons, the elimination of electrodes provides great practicality and allows nonstressful measurements to be made. Magnetic fields penetrate readily into biological tissue, and subintegumental events can be detected more easily than by the use of surface electrodes. However with electromagnetic induction, the magnitudes of the signals provided by physiological events are small, and they decrease with increasing distance from the coil assembly; thus care must be exercised to obtain the optimum placement of the coil assembly which constitutes the transducer. If artifacts are to be avoided, no movement of the subject (with respect to the coil assembly) must occur. It is also important to prevent the induced currents from attaining a magnitude sufficient to stimulate irritable tissue or to cause heating. Finally, as with all other impedance-measuring techniques, it is difficult to calibrate the signal obtained in terms of the magnitude of the physiological event. Nonetheless, as pointed out earlier, if the signal tracks a physiological event faithfully, it can be used to obtain timing and relative-amplitude information.

10-9. IMPEDANCE OF LIVING TISSUE

The unit of living tissue is the single cell, which can be idealized as an electrolyte containing a variety of subcellular structures, necessary for metabolism, repair, and reproduction (if the cell exhibits this latter property), enveloped completely by a membrane having a low electrical leakage in the resting state. The capacitance values for cell membranes range from 0.1 to $3 \, \mu F/cm^2$ with a typical value of about $1.0 \, \mu F/cm^2$ (Cole, 1933). The resistivity of cytoplasm ranges from 10 to 30,000 Ω-cm; 300 to 400 Ω-cm are typical values for mammalian cells (Cole, 1933). Biological tissue consists of an aggregation of cells of differing shapes bonded together and surrounded by tissue fluids which are electrolytes. Therefore, current passing through a specimen of living tissue can pass around the cells by way of the environmental fluid (Fig. 10-15a) if the current is dc or varies slowly (low frequency). If the frequency is high enough, the reactance of the capacitance of the cell membranes will be small and current will flow through the cytoplasm as well as the environmental fluid (Fig. 10-15b). Therefore the low-frequency impedance is high and the high-frequency impedance is low, as idealized in Fig. 10-15c. The transition from the high to low value is characteristic for the type of tissue and reflects the capacitive nature of cell membranes. This characteristic feature of living tissue, recognized by Philippson (1920), led to the concept of equivalent circuits. The circuit at the right in Fig. 10-16a is frequently used to describe the passive electrical behavior of biological specimens. In the measurement of the impedance-frequency characteristics of tissue, precautions must be taken to avoid stimulation of the tissue and to assure awareness of errors introduced by the impedance of the electrode-tissue interface, which increases with decreasing frequency. The latter phenomenon makes it difficult to obtain accurate low-frequency impedance and dc resistance measurements with a bipolar electrode system.

To display the electrical properties of tissue specimens in a more informative manner, Cole (1929, 1933) employed the impedance-locus method used earlier by Carter (1925) to describe the impedance and phase angle of two-terminal networks containing resistances and reactances. With this method the series-equivalent reactance is plotted against resistance. For the idealized circuit on the right in Fig. 10-16a, the impedance-locus plot consists of a semicircle of radius $R_m/2$ on the resistance axis with its center located at $R_s + R_m/2$ units from the origin (Fig. 10-16b). The line joining the origin to a point on the semicircle is the impedance (Z_f) at the

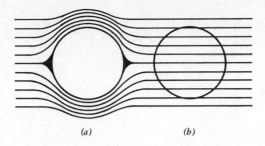

(a)   (b)

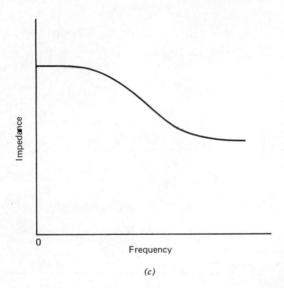

(c)

Figure 10-15. Pathways for (a) low-frequency current and (b) high-frequency current for a cell in an electrolyte; (c) the resulting idealized impedance-frequency characteristic.

frequency (f). Increasing the frequency moves the point f in a counter-clockwise direction on the semicircle. The angle (θ) made by the impedance vector with the resistance (horizontal) axis is the phase angle between the voltage and current measured at the terminals of the network. In the capacitive circuit shown, the current leads the voltage under steady-state, sinusoidal conditions.

When the impedance-locus method is used to display the impedance-frequency characteristics of a biological specimen, the pattern obtained is slightly different from that in Fig. 10-16b. Typical impedance-frequency and phase-frequency characteristics for a single frog egg suspended in an electrolyte are shown in Fig. 10-17; Fig. 10-18 is the impedance-locus plot

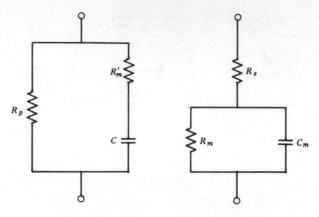

(a) Idealized equivalent circuits for living tissue

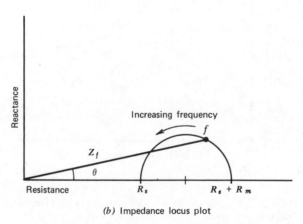

(b) Impedance locus plot

Figure 10-16. (a) Idealized equivalent circuits for living tissue; (b) the impedance-frequency characteristic for living tissue represented by the impedance locus (reactance versus resistance). Z_f is the impedance at frequency f and θ is the phase angle.

for the same specimen. Recalling that the resistivity of electrolytes is constant over a considerable frequency range, it is interesting to note that the circuit measured between the electrode terminals exhibits capacitive reactance (due to the cell membrane). The center of the semicircle in the impedance-locus plot lies slightly below the resistance axis because the cell membrane is not an ideal capacitor. A line between the point where the arc of the semicircle crosses the resistance axis and the center of the circle makes an angle α with a perpendicular line through the center of the circle.

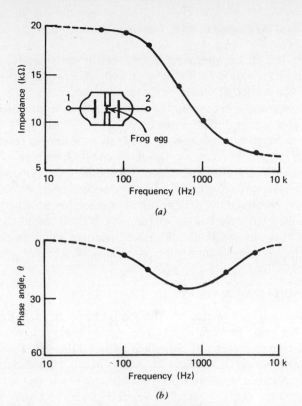

(a)

(b)

Figure 10-17. (*a*) Impedance-frequency characteristic of a single frog egg in an electrolyte; (*b*) phase-frequency characteristic. [Redrawn from Cole, K. S. and R. M. Guttman, *J. Gen. Physiol.* **25**:765–775, (1942).]

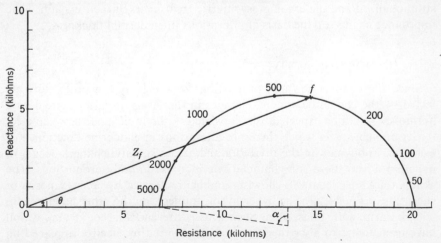

Figure 10-18. Impedance-locus plot for a single frog egg suspended in an electrolyte. [Redrawn from Cole, K. S. and R. M. Guttman, *J. Gen. Physiol.* **25**:765–775, (1942).]

This angle is the membrane phase angle. If the cell membrane were a perfect insulator, α would be 90°, the tangent of α would be infinity, and the center of the semicircle would be on the resistance axis.

An alternate and quicker method of collecting data from which the impedance-locus plot can be obtained was described by Teorell (1947). With this method, a low-frequency square-wave generator, of known resistive output impedance, applies current to the biological specimen. By careful measurement of the waveform of voltage across the specimen and of the current in the circuit, it is possible to obtain the necessary data to plot the impedance locus. Although the data require considerable time to process, the method has the attractive feature of tracking a fairly rapid change in the components of tissue impedance. To date little use has been made of this technique, which is quite common in circuit analysis.

10-10. SEASONAL VARIATIONS IN IMPEDANCE

The conducting properties of the body have been found to vary throughout the year. For example, Crile et al. (1922) discovered that the resistivity of excised samples of biological material depended on the time of the year during which they were removed. Barnett (1940) noted that the 11.16-kHz impedance measured between electrodes on the upper arms of 20 normal subjects varied cyclically over the period of a year. During the winter months the impedance was stable in the vicinity of 100 Ω; it increased from 140 to 250 Ω during the summer, an increase of 40 to 150%. There also occurred a 1- to 4-degree increase in phase angle during the summer. Similar changes were exhibited by the majority of 50 patients institutionalized and undergoing psychiatric treatment. Barnett explained the impedance change on the basis of alterations in epidermal thickness.

10-11. ENDOCRINE ACTIVITY

Since the composition and proportions of the body are profoundly affected by the endocrine system, changes in the levels of various circulating hormones would be expected to be revealed in the impedance between electrodes on subjects in which there are alterations in endocrine function. For example, in diseases of the thyroid gland, gross somatic changes occur. In hypothyroidism there is a characteristic increase in body proportions. The skin is thick, dry, coarse, yellowish, and characterized by heavy deposits of subcutaneous material. The hyperthyroid subject, on the other hand, is thin with a warm, soft, moist skin. Such gross differences in body composition have been found to alter the impedance measured by electrodes placed on the surface of the body.

Brazier (1935) presented two most provocative papers showing that in the intact human the phase angle[1] is directly related to thyroid function. In normal subjects, with both arms immersed up to the elbows in saline solutions serving as electrodes, she measured the impedance and phase angle at 20 kHZ and noted a difference in the phase angle between males and females. In 150 women with thyrotoxicosis she found that the phase angle was directly related to the metabolic rate and was independent of meals, muscular exercise, and the effect of autonomic drugs. Less correlation was found for hypothyroidism, but there was a measurable change when treatment of such subjects with thyroid-stimulating drugs or thyroid extract was begun.

Response to Brazier's paper was almost immediate. Horton and Van Ravenswaay (1935) reexamined the data; they called attention to the fact that the ratio of reactance to resistance was the tangent of the phase angle but stated that for the small angles encountered, the two were nearly equal. By strategically locating electrodes they were able to measure the impedance of the superficial and deep layers of the arms separately. However, they were unable to establish a distinct correlation with thyroid function.

Barnett (1937) thoroughly investigated the problem and was able to obtain impedance values for the skin and deep tissue layers. The phase angle for normal skin was 71.5 degrees, and for deep tissue layers 5 to 10 degrees. He found that the important quantity was not the phase angle, which was almost constant, but the impedance value. He plotted the skin impedance for normal, hyperthyroid, and hypothyroid individuals in a range of frequencies extending from below 100 Hz to above 40 kHz. The three curves (Fig. 10-19) were significantly different, the curve for the hypothyroid subjects (3) lying above that for the normal (1) and the curve for the hyperthyroid (2) lying below. Choosing 11.15 kHz, Barnett studied 458 cases and showed that a plot of basal metabolic rate (BMR) versus the reciprocal of the impedance (Fig. 10-20) correlated almost 80%. A BMR of -2% was equivalent to 109.7 Ω, and a range of 84 to 135 Ω represented a BMR spread of $+10$ to -13%.

Although the impedance method uncovers changes in the conducting properties of the body which are related to thyroid function, in comparison to other thyroid tests, it is not an adequately sensitive indicator for clinical use.

In the studies of impedance associated with thyroid dysfunction, small changes in impedance in the human were observed to be related to age and sex (Brazier, 1935). The impedance changes reflecting estrogenic activity in

[1] Brazier used the tangent of the phase angle and the phase angle in radians interchangeably because the two were nearly identical at the frequency employed.

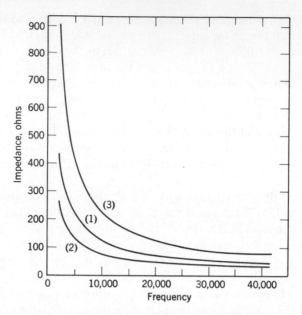

Figure 10-19. Skin impedance versus frequency for normal (curve 1), hyperthyroid (curve 2), and hypothyroid (curve 3) subjects. [Redrawn from A. Barnett, *West. J. Surg. Obstetr. Gynecol.* **45** (October 1937.)]

the white rat were reinvestigated by Farzaneh (1953). Using approximately 100 animals and measuring the 15-kHz impedance between the limbs, at estrous he observed a decrease in impedance of 20% and an increase in phase angle of approximately 5 degrees. In ovariectomized animals, the phase angle remained constant but the impedance varied slightly. Farzaneh also observed that thyroid activity altered the impedance. Much more remains to be investigated to discover the cause of the impedance changes that accompany changes in the level of estrogenic hormones in the circulation.

10-12.   BODY FLUID SHIFTS

By considering the whole body as an electrolytic conductor, it is possible to use a change in impedance of the body, or part of it, as an indicator of volume change. This consideration is the basis of impedance plethysmography, which is concerned mainly with pulsatile changes in impedance and their relation to pulsatile blood flow. These applications are discussed elsewhere in this chapter. However, the basal impedance values for the whole body and for the thorax have been used to indicate blood loss and the accumulation of fluid. These two applications are now described.

10-12-1. Blood Volume Changes

Underwood and Gowing (1965) reported that the impedance between widely spaced electrodes on experimental animals reflected blood volume. In their studies on dogs and cats, they used a bipolar electrode arrangement; one electrode was placed on the sternal notch and the other in the lumbar region. A 10-kHz square wave of current was employed, and the impedance change was measured as blood was withdrawn from the animals. A 10% change in blood volume was found to produce a 1.5-Ω change in resistance.

The authors have verified these observations, using a tetrapolar electrode arrangement applied to dogs. The current electrodes were placed on the right forelimb and left hind limb, and the potential electrodes on the left forelimb and right hind limb. A 50-kHz constant-current system was used. Withdrawal of blood increased the impedance; the addition of blood decreased it. A coefficient of 0.16% change in resistance for a 1% change in blood volume was obtained. A nearly linear relationship was observed for a +30% change in blood volume (calculated on the basis of blood

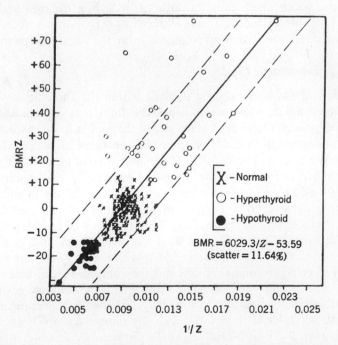

Figure 10-20. The relationship between the reciprocal of impedance (1/Z) at 11.15 kHz and basal metabolism rate (BMR) for normal, hyperthyroid, and hypothyroid subjects. [From A. Barnett, *West. J. Surg. Obstetr. Gynecol.* **45** (October 1937).]

constituting 7% of body weight). The addition of isotonic saline, which has a lower resistivity than blood, produced larger changes in impedance.

Attempting to identify the individual extracellular and intracellular fluid volume changes, Salansky and Utrata (1972), using rabbits and guinea pigs, characterized the impedance measured between the hind limbs by the circuit appearing in Fig. 10-16a. They represented the extracellular fluid compartment by R_p and the intracellular current pathway by the series circuit (R_M' C). The magnitudes of the components of each of these two current pathways were determined by making impedance measurements at 1 and 800 kHz. Using a variety of maneuvers, blood and body fluid volume changes were induced, and their effect on the intracellular and extracellular equivalent circuits was examined. The investigators found that changes in extracellular fluid volume primarily affected the value of R_p.

Despite the attractiveness of the method of using total body impedance to identify blood loss or infusion, the impedance change obtained is small. Underwood and Gowing used bipolar electrodes that required an extremely stable electrode-subject impedance. The tetrapolar electrode system is more appropriate for such measurements because it eliminates errors due to the impedance of the measuring electrodes. The method described by Salansky and Utrata, which offers some promise of dissecting the measured impedance change into extracellular and intracellular components, is interesting and will no doubt see further investigation using the tetrapolar method.

10-12-2. Intrathoracic Fluid

Detection of the accumulation of fluid within the thoracic cavity is of considerable clinical importance. Since the fluid that accumulates is an electrolyte, attempts have been made to use changes in basal thoracic impedance to quantitate the accumulation or disappearance of such fluid.

Van DeWater et al. (1970, 1971, 1972) and Dove et al. (1971) employed the tetrapolar method used in thoracic impedance cardiography (see Section 10-14-5) to measure changes in pleural fluid volume in human subjects. Both groups found that aspiration of pleural fluid increased the basal 100-kHz thoracic impedance slightly. Typical values of impedance change were in the range of 0.001 Ω/ml of fluid aspirated. Pomerantz et al. (1969, 1970) measured 100-kHz impedance changes in the dog and man using the tetrapolar electrode technique. In the dog they obtained a decrease in impedance of about 0.006 Ω/ml of saline infused into the thoracic cavity. In a human subject with pleural effusion, they obtained an increase in impedance of 0.005 Ω/ml of fluid withdrawn. In a similar study Berman et al. (1971) measured the 100-kHz tetrapolar impedance change in dogs in response to hemorrhage, shock, and the intravascular infusion of saline.

Small changes in impedance accompanied hemorrhage and shock and they obtained a decrease in impedance of 0.012 Ω/ml of saline infused into the vascular system. Luepker et al. (1973) obtained similar results using dogs. Severinghaus et al. (1971, 1972) used a four-quadrant guarded electrode applied to the thoraxes of dogs to measure the 100-kHz change in lung impedance in response to saline infusion. A decrease in impedance amounting to 1% was produced by a 4% increase in lung water.

Although the impedance method can detect a change in thoracic fluid volume, a relatively large volume change is required to produce a reliable impedance change. In the dog and man the magnitude of the impedance change is in the vicinity of ten milliohms per milliliter of fluid volume change. With a stable tetrapolar constant-current instrument and mechanically stable potential-measuring electrodes the method can be used to monitor changes in intrathoracic fluid volume; however, it cannot distinguish between the presence of intravascular and extravascular fluid. Moreover, the resting expiratory level must be stable to permit interpretation of the impedance change as a change in thoracic fluid. Within these constraints, the noninvasive nature of the tetrapolar impedance technique may be of clinical value for monitoring thoracic fluid shifts if the measuring electrodes can be retained in the same plane for prolonged periods (or replaced in exactly the same locations) and if respiratory impedance changes do not obscure measurement of the basal impedance.

10-13.   RESPIRATION

Mention was made in Chapter 4 (Section 4-2) of the studies by Atzler and Lehmann and Fenning, who employed the capacitance change principle to detect respiration. Other investigations have been carried out in which the impedance changes between two or four electrodes in direct contact with the chest wall have been employed to detect respiration. A good review of the circuits used in these studies was presented by Pacella (1966).

While recording cardiac impedance pulses with electrodes on the thorax, Nyboer (1944) noted variations in the baseline impedance which correlated with a simultaneously recorded spirogram. Schaefer et al. (1949) developed an impedance system for recording respiration in animals and man, using electrodes inserted subcutaneously in the chest wall. That such transthoracic impedance changes were related to the volume of air moved was demonstrated by Goldensohn and Zablow (1959), who passed a 10-kHz constant current between electrodes on the wrists and detected the respiratory signal from similar electrodes placed farther up on each arm. Geddes et al. (1962) described a two-electrode constant-current system in which respiration was detected by measuring the 50-kHz impedance changes appearing between electrodes placed on the surface of the chest of animals and man. A high correlation between impedance change and volume of air breathed has been demonstrated by Goldensohn and Zablow (1959), Geddes et al. (1962), Robbins and Marko (1962), Hanish (1962), Allison (1962), Allison et al. (1964), McCally et al. (1963), Kubicek et al. (1963–1964), Ax et al. (1964), Baker et al. (1965–1966), Pallett and Scopes (1965), and Hamilton et al. (1965).

Figure 10-21 is a typical three-channel record of an electrocardiogram, an impedance pneumogram, and a spirogram in the human subject made with electrodes at the level of the xiphoid process and along the midaxillary lines. While the recording was being made, the subject was asked to vary his depth of respiration. The impedance and ECG recordings were made from the same pair of electrodes (Geddes et al., 1962). The excursions of the spirometer were detected by coupling a low-torque potentiometer to the pulley suspending the bell (Chapter 2, Section 2-4). Using the same impedance pneumograph, the authors have recorded respiration from horses, dogs, monkeys, cats, rabbits, rats, mice, alligators, frogs, and a camel. The magnitude of the impedance change encountered with respiration depends on body size and the location of the electrodes.

Throughout the years there has been some discussion concerning the importance of frequency for measurement of the respiratory impedance change. Apart from safety considerations previously discussed, which call for the use of a high-frequency current to avoid tissue stimulation, there appears to be no particular advantage to the choice of one frequency over another. This fact is illustrated by Fig. 10-22a which shows the impedance change in a human subject produced by a vital capacity maneuver. It is noted that the change in transthoracic from full inspiration to maximum expiration is practically the same in the frequency range of 50 to 600 kHz.

Figure 10-22b presents a continuous impedance-frequency plot obtained on a dog using a variable-frequency constant-current generator connected to transthoracic electrodes placed along the midaxillary lines at the level of the xiphoid process. The animal was connected to a constant-volume respirator to maintain a constant tidal volume. In the frequency range extending from 10 Hz to 100 kHz, the impedance change for a constant respiratory volume is essentially the same. The decrease in basal (resting-expiratory level) impedance reflects both the decrease in electrode-subject impedance and the reactive nature of the cells that constitute the thorax of the animal.

The relationship between impedance change (ΔZ) and volume of air (ΔV) moved is approximately linear under most circumstances. For the human, the coefficient $\Delta Z / \Delta V$ depends on the size of the subject and the location of the electrodes. In the studies carried out by Baker (1965), who used

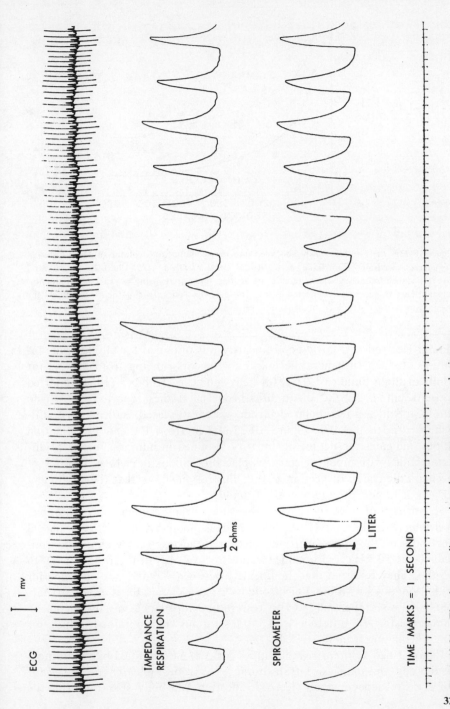

ECG

1 mv

IMPEDANCE
RESPIRATION

2 ohms

SPIROMETER

1 LITER

TIME MARKS = 1 SECOND

Figure 10-21. The electrocardiogram, impedance pneumogram and spirogram.

323

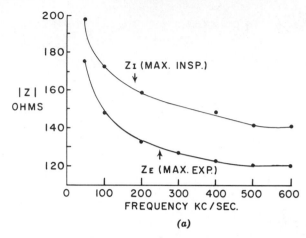

Figure 10-22. (*a*) The relationship between impedance change and volume of air at different frequencies. [Redrawn from Baker et al., *Am. J. Med. Electron.* **4**:75 (1965). By permission.] (*b*) Impedance-frequency characteristic of a dog measured using a variable-frequency, constant-current generator connected to transthoracic electrodes. During the measurement the animal was respired with a constant-volume respirator.

bipolar electrodes, a fairly good linearity was obtained for all electrode locations studied. In general he found coefficients ranging from 6.0 Ω/l for adults of slight build to 1.0 Ω/l for heavy subjects. Kubicek (1964) reported a coefficient of 1.2 Ω/l of air breathed. The studies reported by Allison (1962), in which a tetrapolar electrode system was used, indicated a coefficient of 0.3 to 0.4 Ω/l. Figure 10-23, taken from Baker's investigation (1966), indicates the degree of linearity obtained in human subjects of differing builds with bipolar electrodes placed on midaxillary lines at different levels on the chest. Inspection of this illustration shows that the coefficient $\Delta Z/\Delta V$ is largest for adults of slight build.

A variety of electrode locations have been studied. For example, Weltman and Ukkestad (1969), like Goldensohn and Zablow (1959), placed electrodes on the upper arms and measured the respiratory changes in impedance at 50 kHz and obtained values for $\Delta Z/\Delta V$ in the range of 0.6 to 2.5 Ω/l. They reported that the linearity between ΔZ and ΔV was superior to that obtained with other electrode locations. Khalafalla et al. (1970) carried out low-frequency (280-Hz) respiratory-impedance measurements on humans using 14 different lead configurations and obtained values for $\Delta Z/\Delta V$ ranging from 0.1 to 1.31 Ω/l.

Figure 10-24 summarizes the values for $\Delta Z/\Delta V$ obtained by the authors on the dog and man using transthoracic electrodes. Clearly the values for $\Delta Z/\Delta V$ are dependent on electrode location and body size; however, the

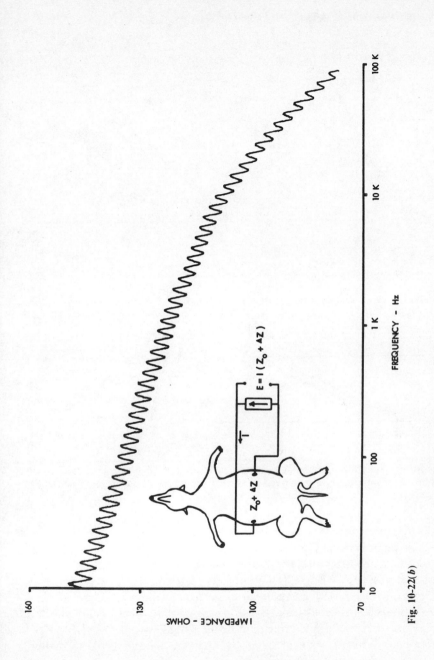

Fig. 10-22(b)

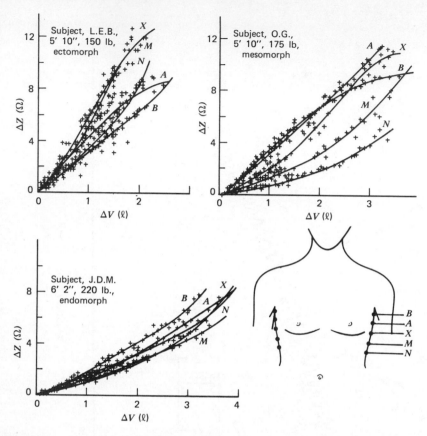

Figure 10-23. Transthoracic impedance changes (ΔZ) versus respired volume (ΔV) measured with bipolar electrodes applied to subjects of light, medium, and heavy builds. [From Baker and Geddes, *Med. Biol. Eng.* **4**:374 (1966). By permission.]

data in this illustration do not reveal the linearity of the $\Delta Z/\Delta V$ relationship. This point is demonstrated by Fig. 10-23, which shows the linearity of the impedance change with the volume of air inspired by subjects of differing somatotypes. With tall thin subjects (ectomorphs), the largest amplitude is obtained with transthoracic electrodes at the level of the xiphoid process. However, the best linearity is obtained with electrodes higher on the chest near the axilla, the price paid being a smaller value for $\Delta Z/\Delta V$.

With endomorphs (corpulent subjects), all values for $\Delta Z/\Delta V$ are smaller, and the best linearity is obtained with electrodes near the axilla, as is the case with the mesomorph. Similar observations have been reported by Kubicek et al. (1964), Hamilton et al. (1965), and Logic et al. (1967).

Valentinuzzi et al. (1971) conducted a study of the impedance change per liter of air inspired ($\Delta Z/\Delta V$) in subjects of widely differing body weights, using transthoracic electrodes placed to obtain the maximum value for $\Delta Z/\Delta V$. Their data (Fig. 10-25) reveal an inverse relationship between the maximum value for the impedance coefficient in ohms per liter and body weight. This almost hyperbolic relationship ($\Delta Z/\Delta V = 453/W^{1.08}$, where W is the body weight in kilograms) has been called the law of impedance pneumography. An approximate relationship for the maximum value of the

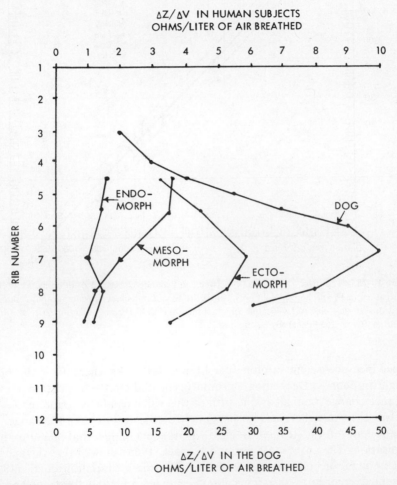

Figure 10-24. The relationship between the maximum impedance coefficient ($\Delta Z/\Delta V$ $\Omega/\text{l.}$) and electrode location in subjects of differing body types. Note the general inverse relationship between impedance coefficient and body proportions and the influence of electrode location. [From Valentinuzzi et al., *Med. Biol. Eng.* **9**:157–163 (1971). By permission.]

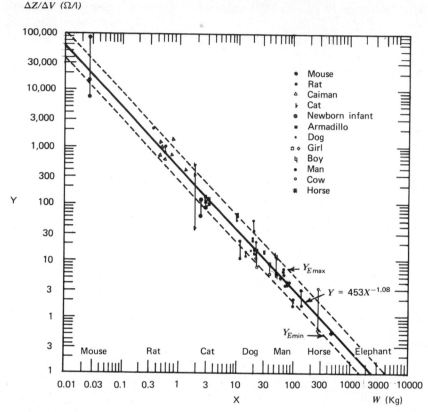

$\Delta Z/\Delta V$ (Ω/l)

Figure 10-25. The inverse relationship between impedance change (ΔZ) in ohms per liter of air breathed (ΔV) and body weight (W), called the law of impedance pneumography, obtained with transthoracic electrodes located for maximum $\Delta Z/\Delta V$. [From Valentinuzzi et al., *Med. Biol. Eng.* **9**:157–163 (1971). By permission.]

impedance coefficient in ohms per liter is $1000/W$, where W is the body weight in pounds. Depending on somatotype and electrode location, an impedance change as small as one-fifth of this value can be encountered.

Over the years there has arisen some discussion regarding the capacitive component of the transthoracic impedance change that accompanies respiration. The authors (Baker and Geddes, 1965) showed that the capacitance change accompanying respiration is small. Hamilton et al. (1965) presented recordings showing volume change (ΔV) and the transthoracic resistance (ΔR) and capacitance (ΔC) change during respiration in the human subject. The ΔR and ΔC recordings tracked volume change equally well. A penetrating quantitative study of the relative importance of ΔR and

ΔC was carried out by Pasquali (1967), who employed transthoracic electrodes ranging in size from 1 to 64 cm² applied to the human thorax, measuring the components of the thoracic impedance and their change at 100 kHz. From an extensive series of measurements, Pasquali concluded that although the percentile changes in resistance and capacitance were approximately equal, the capacitance change contributed negligibly to the transthoracic impedance change because the reactance change was small compared with the resistance change accompanying respiration. In a similar study Cooley and Longini (1968) concluded that the respiratory impedance change was mainly resistive.

Use of the guarded-electrode technique (see-Section 10-8-5) has been applied to obtain signal enhancement in the detection of the respiratory-impedance change. Graham (1965) reported a 20-fold increase in impedance change by using the guarded-electrode method. Similarly Cooley and Longini (1968) reported ratios ranging from 39 to 67.5. In both cases, along with this signal enhancement, guarding produced an increase in basal (resting expiratory level) impedance. In a study directed toward detecting intrathoracic fluid accumulation by measurement of lung resistivity, Severinghaus et al. (1972) used a guarded electrode paired with an unguarded one applied to the human thorax. The measuring electrode was guarded by four driven segments arranged around the central measuring electrode. The potentials used to drive each of the four segments were obtained from four small electrodes located between the measuring and guarding electrodes. Although only a small impedance change was accompanied by an alteration in intrathoracic fluid volume, the respiratory impedance change was large, amounting to 63 Ω/l. No comparisons were made using unguarded electrodes.

It is clear that guarding produces a significant enhancement in respiratory impedance change. However, more studies must be carried out to determine the optimum size and location for guarded electrodes. Whether there is a somatotype factor (see Fig. 10-24) and an electrode-location factor (see Fig. 10-23) remains to be investigated.

Ever since it was found that an increase in transthoracic impedance accompanied respiration, there has been speculation regarding the factors that contribute to the respiratory impedance change. The matter is unsettled because measurements of current density distribution have not been carried out to determine the pathways of the current injected by thoracic electrodes. Some investigators believe that a respiratory redistribution of blood in the pulmonary vascular circuit contributes importantly to the inspiratory impedance increase; this theory has been countered on many occasions. Others believe that despite the small fraction of injected current traversing the lungs, the increase in lung resistivity with inspiration is the major contributor to the impedance change. Baker (1966), using dogs, found that approximately 80% of the injected current traversed the posterior thoracic path and 5% passed through the anterior path. Approximately 10% of the current flowed through the liver and diaphragm, and 5% flowed through lung tissue. Many investigators believe that dimensional changes of the thorax and/or redistribution of its contents underlie the impedance change. At this time, it is difficult to assign the degree of contribution made by each factor associated with the respiratory-impedance signal.

Practicality is probably the most attractive feature of the impedance method for measurement of respiration. Nothing is simpler than affixing electrodes to a subject and connecting them to the recording equipment. Since the impedance change is related to the volume of air moved, the method can be calibrated. Although calibration requires the use of a spirometer or other volume-measuring instrument, the calibrating device can be removed and respiratory volumes measured without obstructing the air stream. Another attractive feature of the method is availability of the electrocardiogram from the same pair of electrodes.

Perhaps the most unattractive feature of the measurement of respiration by impedance is the need to calibrate each subject with a volume-measuring device. No single calibration factor can be specified for each species or subject. However, once a calibration value has been obtained on a subject for electrodes in a given location, this factor remains fairly constant.

As with any physiological event that is measured with electrodes, movement causes a variation in impedance and produces unwanted signals. Therefore precautions must be taken to avoid this complication.

10-14. BLOOD FLOW

When the impedance change technique is applied to the determination of blood flow, three methods are available. With the first, cardiac output (liters per minute) is determined by applying the dilution technique. With the second, stroke volume, that is, the systolic discharge from the left ventricle, is determined by measurement of the impedance change between electrodes placed on or in the heart. In the third method, which employs electrodes that encompass a segment of the body, attempts are made to calibrate the pulsatile impedance signal in terms of blood flow in the field between the electrodes. The various applications of each of these methods will be described.

10-14-1. Cardiac Output, Dilution Method

One of the earliest studies to determine cardiac output employed the impedance method. By measuring transarterial impedance in dogs and by intravenously injecting 1.5% saline, Stewart (1897, 1921) was able to identify the time of arrival and the passage of the blood containing the injected saline. He accomplished this by using a simple impedance bridge, one arm of which was the transarterial impedance. The alternating current for the bridge was derived from an inductorium. The detector was a telephone receiver. Passage of the hyperconducting blood unbalanced the bridge and directed the investigators to collect blood at that moment for future determination of its salinity. Cardiac output was determined by use of the dilution formula. Continuous recording of the change in conductivity of the blood as it passed an arterial detector was accomplished by Romm (1924) and Gross and Mittermaier (1926). In both studies the conductivity curve was not calibrated because the information sought was circulation time. These two studies paved the way for Wigger's (1944) investigations, which employed a flow-through conductivity cell inserted in a femoral artery. Using the original Stewart constant-injection method, Wiggers obtained in anesthetized dogs cardiac output values that were in good agreement with those measured by other observers. White (1947) refined the method by devising two types of hypodermic needle electrodes, which were inserted directly into an artery. As the injected saline passed the electrodes, the intra-arterial impedance at 70 kHz was continuously recorded on an oscilloscope. Despite certain practical difficulties, he obtained cardiac outputs differing between -12 and $+22\%$ from the values obtained by the Fick method.

When sodium chloride is employed as the injected material, some is lost from the vascular tree. Since this naturally affects the limit of accuracy attainable, the exact amount lost has been the subject of much debate which has caused the accuracy of the saline method to be questioned. Chinard (1962) stated that 5% of intravenously injected saline is lost in passing through the lungs. Saline is also removed from the circulation via the kidneys and capillaries. That the loss in one trip from vein to artery must be small can be deduced from studies in which the saline method has been checked against the Fick and dye-dilution methods. These studies, which were reviewed by Smith et al. (1967), indicate that the saline method gives values within approximately $\pm 5\%$ of those obtained with the dye-dilution and Fick methods.

To eliminate loss of the conducting material injected, Goodwin and Saperstein (1957) used autogenous plasma instead of saline. Blood from an artery was aspirated at a constant rate through a conductivity cell operated at 2500 Hz for conductivity measurements. In a series of 24 dogs Goodwin and Saperstein compared the conductivity method and the Evans blue technique and obtained remarkably similar results. The difference in the mean values was 0.3%.

When sodium chloride is used as the indicator to determine cardiac output, the transducer is a conductivity cell through which arterial blood is caused to flow. The dilution curve, which results from the venous injection of hypertonic saline (e.g., 5%) is obtained by continuously recording the impedance of arterial blood measured between the electrode terminals of the conductivity cell, as in Fig. 10-26. As with all indicator-dilution curves, which result from the rapid venous injection of the indicator, calibration is achieved by preparing blood samples with known amounts of indicator. These samples are then passed through the transducer, and the deflections obtained are recorded. However, when sodium chloride is used as the indicator, it is possible to calibrate the transducer electrically by short-circuiting a resistance in series with the conductivity cell, provided two requirements are satisfied. The first requirement is that a constant-current system be used to record the impedance change exhibited by the conductivity cell as the diluted hypertonic saline-blood mixture passes through.

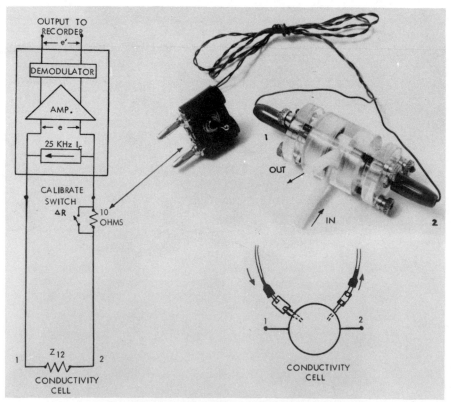

Figure 10-26. Flow-through conductivity cell in which the electrolyte takes a spiral flow pathway, and constant-current impedance-recording equipment used with it to record dilution curves for the measurement of blood flow.

The second requirement relates to the establishment of an equivalent concentration for the deflection on the recording obtained by short-circuiting the calibrating resistor in series with the conductivity cell.

The first requirement—namely, the use of a constant-current source—is easily satisfied. A constant-current source is essential to obtain the same voltage change across the conductivity cell for the same change in blood resistivity ($\Delta\rho$), irrespective of the magnitude of the impedance of the blood within the conductivity cell. If a constant-current source is not available, a constant-voltage source can be converted to a constant-current source by placing a resistor in series with it and the conductivity cell. The value of the series resistance should be about 100 or more times larger than the basal impedance of the conductivity cell when blood is flowing through it.

The change in concentration (ΔC) of sodium chloride in the blood, which is equivalent to the resistance change (ΔR) produced when the calibrating resistor is short-circuited, can be established by knowing the manner in which the resistivity of blood decreases by the addition of sodium chloride. The following derivation presents the underlying theory.

Figure 10-27 diagrams a cylindrical column of blood of diameter d, cross-sectional area A, and length L which is the separation between the electrodes within the cell. The conducting properties of the circuit measured between the electrode terminals 1 and 2 are described by the impedance of the entire circuit. At a single frequency the impedance of an electrode-electrolyte interface can be represented equally well by a series or a parallel combination of resistance and capacitance; for simplicity, the series-equivalent has been shown.

The impedance (Z_{12}) between electrode terminals 1 and 2 consists of three parts: the impedance of the blood-electrode interface at electrode 1 (Z_1), the impedance (resistance) R_B of the cylindrical column of blood between electrodes 1 and 2, and the impedance of the blood-electrode interface at electrode 2 (Z_2); therefore,

$$Z_{12} = Z_1 + R_B + Z_2.$$

If the electrodes are of the same metal and have equal areas, their impedances are equal; therefore $Z_1 = Z_2 = Z$ and $Z_{12} = 2Z + R_B$; and since $R_B = \rho L/A$, $Z_{12} = 2Z + \rho L/A$.

To determine the manner by which the impedance (Z_{12}) between the electrode terminals varies with a change in the resistivity (ρ) of the intervening electrolyte (blood), it is merely necessary to differentiate with respect to concentration (C); therefore,

$$\frac{dZ_{12}}{dC} = \frac{2\,dZ}{dC} + \left(\frac{L}{A}\right)\frac{d\rho}{dC}.$$

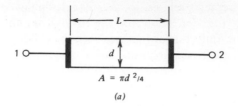

$$A = \pi d^2/4$$

(a)

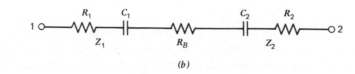

(b)

Figure 10-27. (a) Conductivity cell of length L and diameter d and (b) equivalent circuit in which Z_1 and Z_2 are the impedances of the electrode-electrolyte interface and R_B is the resistance of the intervening biological fluid; $R_B = \rho L/A$ when ρ is the resistivity of the fluid.

In a study on the impedance of stainless steel electrodes, the authors (1972) found that the change in electrode impedance due to increasing electrolyte (saline) concentration from 0.6 to 5% was small with respect to the change in impedance measured between the terminals of the conductivity cell when dilution curves are obtained. Therefore the foregoing expression reduces to

$$\frac{dZ_{12}}{dC} \doteq \frac{L}{A}\left(\frac{d\rho}{dC}\right).$$

This expression indicates that the change in impedance measured between the electrode terminals is independent of the impedance of the electrodes and does not depend on the resistance of the blood column. Hence the factors that establish the baseline of the impedance recording are unimportant. Because the dilution curve is measured only from the baseline, the recorded amplitude is a function of the geometry of the conductivity cell (L/A) and the manner in which the resistivity of the blood changes with added sodium chloride $(d\rho/dC)$. Therefore, to calibrate a conductivity cell electrically, it is necessary to know the dimensions of the cell (L/A) and the manner in which the resistivity of a blood sample is reduced with the addition of sodium chloride. The resistivity of blood is, of course, a function of packed-cell volume and temperature.

To equate the change in impedance ΔZ_{12} (produced by short-circuiting the calibrating resistor ΔR) to a change in concentration of sodium chloride in blood, one simply rearranges the previous expression and substitutes ΔR for ΔZ_{12} and ΔC for dC. Performing this manipulation yields

$$\Delta C = \frac{\Delta R}{d\rho/dC} \left(\frac{A}{L}\right).$$

This expression shows that it is necessary to know the dimensions of the conductivity cell (A/L) and the manner in which the resistivity of blood is decreased $(d\rho)$ by an increase in its concentration of sodium chloride (dC). The former is easily measured, the latter $(d\rho/dC)$ requires that resistivity measurements be made on blood samples to which known amounts of sodium chloride have been added.

Measurements were made at 37°C on blood samples from several species to reveal the nature of the dependence of the resistivity on the amount of added sodium chloride and packed-cell volume (H). Samples of the desired H in the range of 0 to 70% were prepared by centrifuging the blood and adding the desired volume of cells. To each of these samples, known amounts of sodium chloride were added and the concentration was calculated by dividing the weight of the sodium chloride, in grams, added by the volume of the blood sample, in liters. Resistivity measurements were made with a variable-length conductivity cell (Geddes, 1973), which was surrounded by a temperature-controlled water jacket (37°C); the assembly was mounted on an agitator to prevent the blood cells from settling while measurements were being made. The conductivity cell was connected to a constant-current 25-kHz impedance measuring instrument. A typical resistivity versus saline concentration curve obtained for a canine blood sample appears in Fig. 10-28. This figure shows that the reduction in resistivity produced by the addition of sodium chloride to a blood sample depends on its packed cell volume (H), the value for $d\rho/dC$ being large for the high packed-cell volumes.

While recording dilution curves, the concentration of sodium chloride in the blood rarely increases by more than 1.0 g/l; therefore the slopes $(\Delta\rho/\Delta C)$ of the resistivity versus added sodium chloride were calculated in this region for the data obtained from each of the dogs over a range of H extending from 0 to 70%. The blood samples were centrifuged and different plasma-cell mixtures were prepared to determine a wide range of values, illustrating the manner in which the change in resistivity with added sodium chloride $(\Delta\rho/\Delta C)$ depends on H; Fig. 10-29 presents this relationship. This curve, which represents the best fit using an exponential, permits calculation of the change in concentration (ΔC) which is indicated by the recorder deflection obtained by short-circuiting a resistance (ΔR) placed in series with the conductivity cell.

In the measurement of cardiac output, to obtain high accuracy when

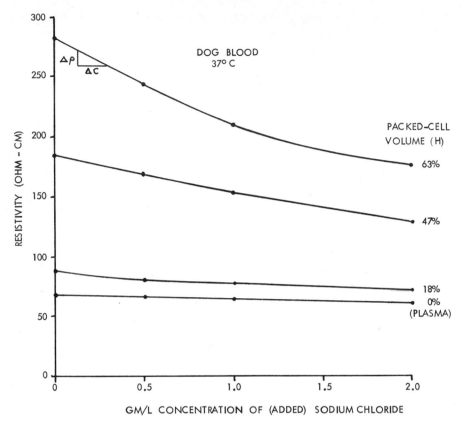

Figure 10-28. The manner in which the resistivity of blood decreases with increasing sodium chloride content. [From Geddes et al., *Cardiovasc. Res. Center Bull.* **10**:91–106 (1972). By permission.]

calibrating a conductivity cell by using a resistor to simulate a change in resistivity of the electrolyte within the cell, it is necessary to attain a uniform current density distribution in the electrolyte. This is particularly important when the electrolyte contains a suspension of particles having a resistivity and density different from the electrolyte that supports them, which occurs when whole blood is the electrolyte and its resistivity is reduced by the addition of sodium and chloride ions. Accordingly, an investigation was carried out on a variety of types of conductivity cells to determine the best method of obtaining a uniform current density distribution within the electrolyte. Cells with annular electrodes across the flow stream and along it were constructed and evaluated. All such cells produced large-amplitude pulsations in conductivity when arterial blood was caused to flow through them because in flowing blood, the cells concentrate in the axial stream and plasma is concentrated in the peripheral stream. Since plasma has a much lower resistivity than packed cells (Geddes and Baker, 1967), the current in such conductivity cells is carried mainly by the plasma and as flow-velocity changes with each heart beat, there is a pulsatile reorientation of red blood cells that modulates the current density distribution. With conductivity cells of this design, which have frequently been used by those who employed the saline-conductivity method, the pulsatile oscillations have amounted to between 5 to 20% of the amplitude of the dilution curve. To eliminate them, electrical filtering has often been used with the risk of distorting the dilution curve. To minimize pulsatile changes in resistivity, a new style of conductivity cell (Fig. 10-26) was developed in which blood enters and leaves tangentially with a flow that is parallel to the electrode surfaces. The cell is cylindrical, and the electrodes are at opposite ends of the cylinder. Blood enters tangentially at one electrode, swirls around and along the cylindrical cell, and leaves tangentially at the opposite side of the other electrode. When this type of cell is placed in an arteriovenous shunt, the pulsatile oscillations in conductivity are small with respect to the amplitude of the dilution curve. No electrical filtering is necessary, which guarantees that the form of the dilution curve is faithfully reproduced.

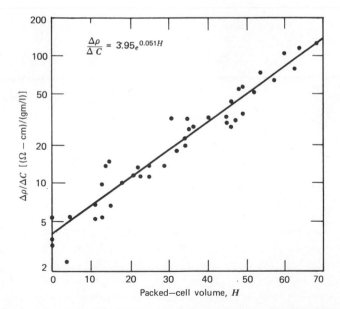

Figure 10-29. The relationship between $\Delta\rho/\Delta C$ and packed-cell volume (H) for canine blood. [From Geddes et al., *Cardiovasc. Res. Center Bull.* **10**:91–106 (1972). By permission.]

A very convenient method of obtaining a large number of measurements of cardiac output without blood loss is depicted in Fig. 10-30. The conductivity cell is placed in an arteriovenous shunt in a subject in which blood clotting is retarded by the use of an anticoagulant. Thus the subject's blood pressure maintains a constant flow of blood through the conductivity cell.

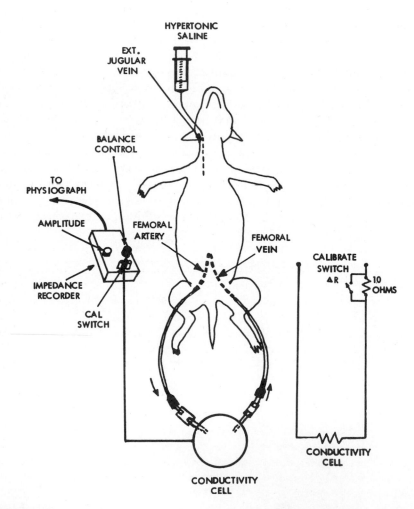

Figure 10-30. Arrangement employed to obtain multiple dilution curves without blood loss. The conductivity cell is placed in an arteriovenous shunt and the indicator (sodium chloride solution) is injected into a large central vein (or the right atrium or ventricle). The dilution curve is obtained by continuously recording the impedance appearing between the terminals of the conductivity cell. Electrical calibration of the conductivity cell is achieved by short-circuiting a calibrating resistor (ΔR) in series with the conductivity cell.

The amount of flow can be controlled by choice of the diameter and length of the tubing used.

To obtain a dilution curve for the determination of cardiac output, a known volume of hypertonic (e.g., 3 to 5%) sodium chloride is injected into a large central vein (e.g., the jugular). The saline mixes with the central circulation and a diluted blood-sodium chloride sample passes through the conductivity cell and a continuous recording of the impedance between its terminals produces the dilution curve (see Fig. 10.31) which was obtained from a dog by injecting 2 ml of 5% NaCl, which is an injection of 0.1 gram of NaCl.

To calculate cardiac output from the dilution curve, it is necessary to establish the concentration-equivalent for the calibrating resistor; the value given in Fig. 10-30 is 10 Ω. The conductivity cell (Fig. 10-26) used to obtain the dilution curve had a cross-sectional area (A) of 1 cm² and a length (L) of 1 cm; therefore $A/L = 1.00$. A centrifuged sample of the animal's arterial blood showed that the packed-cell volume (H) was 50%; therefore the value for $\Delta\rho/\Delta\rho C$ from Fig. 10-29 is 50.1. The concentration equivalent (ΔC) for the amplitude obtained when the 10-Ω calibrating resistor (ΔR) was short-circuited is

$$\Delta C = \frac{\Delta R}{\Delta\rho/\Delta C}\left(\frac{A}{L}\right) = \frac{10}{50.1} \times 1.0 = 0.199 \text{ gram NaCl per liter of blood.}$$

To process the dilution curve, the artifact caused by recirculation of the indicator must be eliminated. Kinsman et al. (1929) developed the technique for accomplishing this goal by replotting the downslope of the dilution curve on semilogarithmic paper, as in Fig. 10-32. The portion of the downslope that is exponential becomes a straight line. Extrapolation of this linear segment on the semilog plot to a concentration corresponding to 1% of the maximum height ($C_{max}/100$) of the dilution curve permits obtaining concentration values at different times during recirculation and allows completion of the exponential downslope of the dilution curve. From Fig. 10-32 the time for the 1% maximum concentration value was 32 sec. By measuring the area under the corrected dilution curve and dividing it by its base length (which corresponds to 32 sec), a mean height is obtained which is converted to a mean concentration ($\bar{c}$) by simple proportion as shown in Fig. 10-31. Cardiac output (CO l/min) can now be calculated by using the standard expression:

$$CO = \frac{60 \times \text{mg of indicator injected}}{\text{mean concentration} \times \text{duration of dilution curve}}$$

$$= \frac{60 \times 0.1}{0.087 \times 32} = 2.16 \text{ l/min}$$

At present, cardiac output values determined by the electrical calibration method are being compared with those obtained using the dye-dilution and Fick methods. In a preliminary study by the authors (1972), the values obtained by the saline method agreed well with those obtained with the dye technique (correlation coefficient 0.813) and with the Fick method (correlation coefficient 0.94). In the former case, the saline values averaged 10.7% high; in the latter, the values were about 1% low. Subsequent studies (Geddes et al., 1974) indicate that the electrically calibrated saline indicator method will overestimate cardiac output by about 10%.

The data reported here were obtained with a flow-through conductivity cell placed in an arteriovenous bypass as shown in Fig. 10-30. This technique does not require the withdrawal of blood through the cell to inscribe the dilution curve; it also eliminates the need for thermostatically controlling the temperature of the conductivity cell. The price paid is the need to use an anticoagulant to prevent the blood from clotting. Maintenance of the conductivity cell at body temperature and at the same time allowing use of the withdrawal technique, which requires only a minimal amount of anticoagulant, can be achieved by using a conductivity cell mounted within a catheter (see Fig. 10-33). The conductivity cell consists of two annular electrodes located within the lumen of the catheter. With the catheter in a major artery, withdrawal of blood by a motor-driven syringe will allow

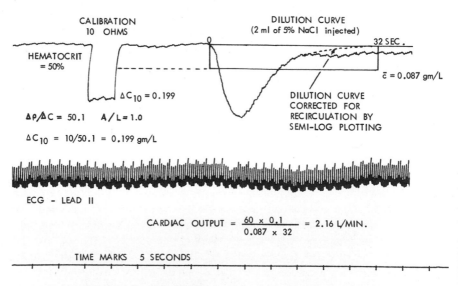

Figure 10-31.   Dilution curve obtained by injecting 2 ml of 5% NaCl solution into the right atrium. The conductivity cell was placed in an arteriovenous shunt as shown in Fig. 10-30. The conductivity cell had an area (A) to length (L) ratio of 1.0.

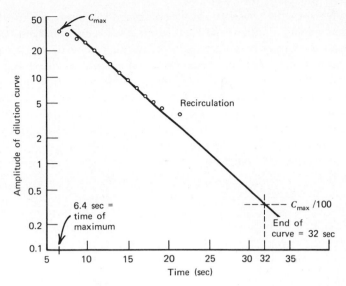

Figure 10-32. Semilog plot of the downslope of the dilution curve in Fig. 10-31. Note that the portion of the downslope of the dilution curve that is exponential is linear in the semilog plot. Extrapolation of the line joining the points forming the straight line allows the acquisition of values for the dilution curve during recirculation. In practice, extrapolation is carried out to find a time corresponding to 1% of the maximum height of the dilution curve. In this example the end of the dilution curve was found to occur at 32 sec and the amplitudes between 15 sec (when recirculation became apparent) and 32 sec (the end of the curve) were used to complete the dilution curve in Fig. 10-31.

inscription of the dilution curve by withdrawal of a very small amount of blood into the catheter, since the electrodes are so close to the bloodstream. The electrical calibration technique can also be applied if a value for A/L, the ratio of electrode area divided by length (effective electrode separation) is known. This ratio can be obtained by measurement of the difference in the series equivalent high-frequency resistance $(R_1 - R_2)$ of two samples of saline having known resistivity $(\rho_1 - \rho_2)$ values; that is,

$$A/L = (\rho_1 - \rho_2)/(R_1 - R_2).$$

Although use of sodium chloride as an indicator has been criticized because the substance is diffusible (Chinard et al., 1962), it offers genuine practical advantages, not the least of which are its low toxicity and high repeatability (because it is rapidly cleared from the circulation). This feature, of course, admits the possibility of overestimating the values obtained for cardiac output. Thus one is faced with the choice of high accuracy with the restriction of taking only a few dilution curves (because of indicator buildup) versus a slight overestimation of cardiac output with the freedom to obtain multiple determinations with considerably less indicator buildup. Elimination of the need to mix calibrating solutions when the electrical calibration method is used with sodium chloride makes the use of this indicator even more attractive. The only price paid for this feature is the availability of $\Delta\rho/\Delta C$ data for the blood of the species employed and withdrawing a small sample of blood for the determination of its packed-cell volume (H). Table 10-4 presents the available data for $\Delta\rho/\Delta C$ for various species.

10-14-2. Ventricular Emptying

The fractional emptying of the left ventricle in the dog was determined by Holt (1956–1962) and Holt and Allensworth (1957) using a modification of the sodium chloride indicator-dilution technique. By injecting a known amount of hypertonic sodium chloride into the left ventricle and continuously recording conductivity in the aorta, it was possible to calculate the volume of the left ventricle and the amount discharged per beat (stroke volume). Elegant as this technique is, it depends on the assumption that perfect mixing occurs in the left ventricle. That this is not always the case was shown by Irisawa et al. (1960).

The mathematical expression for the aortic concentration of a material

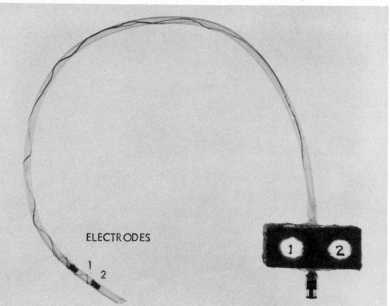

Figure 10-33. Conductivity cell contained within a transparent arterial catheter; 1 and 2 are annular electrodes contained within the catheter.

Table 10-4 Electrical Calibration Data ($\Delta\rho/\Delta C$) for Conductivity Cells;* Used with Saline Indicator Method for Measuring Cardiac Output

Species	$\Delta\rho/\Delta C$† [Ω-cm/(gram)(l)]	Correlation Coefficient
Dog	$3.95e^{0.051H}$	0.970
Sheep	$4.15e^{0.041H}$	0.958
Camel	$3.975e^{0.0354H}$	0.984

* See page 339 for a discussion of the electrical calibration technique. For additional values for $\Delta\rho/\Delta C$, see Geddes et al., *Med. Biol. Eng.* 1975 (In press).
† 37°C.

injected into the left ventricle can be derived if two assumptions are made. The first is that the weight (m grams) of the material injected into the left ventricle is contained in a volume, which is small with respect to the diastolic volume of the ventricle (V ml); the second is that uniform mixing takes place in the ventricle. The injection is made as quickly as possible just before systolic ejection. Then, if uniform mixing has occurred, and the stroke volume (v ml) remains constant for each beat, the aortic concentration (C mg/ml) will decrease in a stepwise fashion. For the first beat the aortic concentration will be m/V grams/ml. The number of grams ejected is mv/V, and the number remaining in the ventricle is $m - mv/V$ or $m(1 - v/V)$ grams. The ventricle then fills, and the diastolic volume is again V ml, into which this weight of material is diluted. The aortic concentration for the second beat is then $(1 - v/V)m/V$. The process continues to be repeated, and the general expression for the aortic concentration for the nth beat becomes

$$C_n = \frac{m}{V}\left(1 - \frac{v}{V}\right)^{n-1}.$$

Figure 10-34 illustrates the concentration as the injected material is cleared from the left ventricle for stroke volumes v equal to 40, 50, and 60% of the diastolic volume V. Thus from calibrated records of these data, ventricular diastolic volume and stroke volume can be calculated. Cardiac output can also be determined by multiplying the stroke volume v by heart rate.

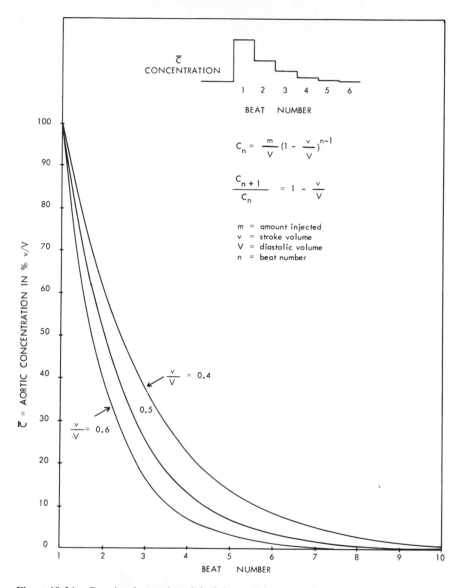

Figure 10-34. Fractional emptying of the left ventricle.

10-14-3. Stroke Volume by Direct Impedance Cardiography

Rappoport and Ray (1927) recorded the impedance changes in a tortoise heart as it was kept beating *in vitro*. The heart, suspended in a beaker of saline, constituted one electrode; the other was placed nearby in the solution. The investigators noted a change in impedance of 10% with each heart beat. Rushmer et al. (1953) affixed electrodes to the interior walls of the right and left ventricles of dogs. In one animal they placed electrodes at the apex and the base of the right and left ventricles. They recorded a decrease in impedance during diastole and an increase during systole. Although the recordings resembled those made with cardiometers, their studies on models and animals led them to believe that the method contained variables which were difficult to quantitate, and they abandoned the technique in favor of others which appeared more promising at that time. Mello-Sobrinho (1963) and Geddes et al. (1965, 1966) reinvestigated the value of the method, using electrodes (insulated except at the tip) inserted into the left ventricle at the base and the apex of canine hearts. Accordingly, the cardiac chambers functioned as conductivity cells of varying dimensions; the impedance decreased with filling and increased with emptying. Since the resistivity of cardiac muscle is approximately five times that of blood, the current is largely confined to the ventricle. Figure 10-35 is a typical record of the 80-kHz impedance changes recorded with this technique.

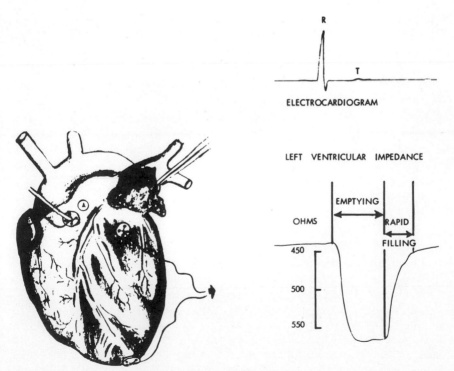

Figure 10-35. Left ventricular impedance cardiogram in the dog. [From Geddes et al., *Cardiovasc. Res. Center Bull.* **4**(4)118-130 (1966). By permission.]

By injecting or withdrawing from the ventricle known amounts of blood with the outlet and inlet valves closed, it is possible to calibrate the impedance change in terms of volume. In preliminary studies with this method calibration factors of 3 to 10 Ω/ml were obtained for the left ventricles of 10-kg dogs. At present, dynamic calibration factors are being derived by recording impedance changes and simultaneously determining the cardiac output by means of the direct Fick method. Initial studies have yielded calibration factors slightly less than those determined by the injection and withdrawal method.

This technique is very easy to apply to lower animals. Figure 10-36 illustrates the filling and emptying of a frog heart with two pin electrodes passed through the apex and the base of the ventricle. The ventricular electrogram was obtained from the same electrodes.

10-14-4.   Pulsatile Blood Flow by Impedance Plethysmography

The use of the impedance change technique for recording peripheral volume pulses was first described by Mann (1937). In a few years there appeared numerous papers on the subject, and the technique soon became known as impedance plethysmography. Pioneering in this field were Nyboer (1943, 1944, 1950, 1959), Brook and Cooper (1957), Polzer et al. (1960), and Polzer and Schuhfried (1961). Nyboer became the advocate of the tetrapolar electrode method, whereas most of the other investigators cited employed two-electrode systems. Although the literature shows that the impedance change is mainly resistive at the frequencies presently employed (20–100 kHz), Mann (1953) demonstrated the existence of a reactive component at 10 kHz, when the impedance was measured between electrodes on each forearm. With either the two- or the four-electrode system it is easy to obtain impedance changes strikingly similar to those recorded with capsule plethysmographs. The real difficulty lies in the lack of accurate methods to relate the impedance change to a volume change.

The basis for impedance plethysmography as applied to body segments is the decrease in impedance when a volume of blood is introduced between the measuring electrodes. The expression most frequently employed to relate the measured impedance change to the volume change can be derived by assuming that there is a homogeneous conducting material and a uniform current density distribution between the measuring electrodes. Obviously these requirements are never satisfied in practical situations, and to minimize some of the resulting errors, current is introduced to the specimen by widely spaced electrodes. The current distribution between electrodes placed on homogeneous conducting cylinders of differing lengths can be seen in Figs. 10-37a and 10-37b. Note that in both cases there is the same

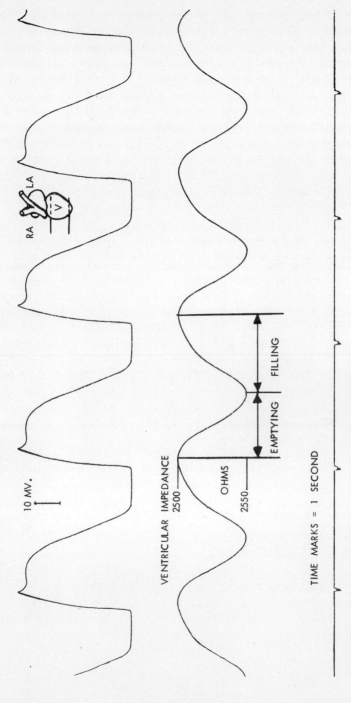

Figure 10-36. Frog ventricular electrogram and impedance cardiogram.

347

distortion of the lines of equal current at each electrode, but in the central region a–a' (Fig. 10-37b) the current distribution is more uniform.

To illustrate how a volume change can be identified by a resistance change, we remove the conducting cylinder a–a' and place electrodes over its ends. For a length L, area A_0, and resistivity ρ, the resistance is $R_0 = \rho L / A_0$. Consider now the addition of a volume ΔV of conducting material to the segment without producing a change in length. The cross-sectional area will increase uniformly to A_1, and the resistance measured between the electrode covering the ends will be $R_1 = \rho L / A_1$. The difference in resistance reflects the volume change; therefore:

$$\Delta R = R_1 - R_0 = \frac{\rho L}{A_1} - \frac{\rho L}{A_0} = \rho L \left(\frac{1}{A_1} - \frac{1}{A_0} \right),$$

but

$$V_0 = L A_0 \quad \text{and} \quad V_1 = L A_1.$$

Substituting,

$$\Delta R = \rho L \left(\frac{L}{V_1} - \frac{L}{V_0} \right)$$

$$= \rho L^2 \left(\frac{V_0 - V_1}{V_1 V_0} \right) = - \frac{\rho L^2 (V_1 - V_0)}{V_1 V_0}.$$

If V_1 is not appreciably larger than V_0 (i.e., the volume added, $\Delta V = V_1 - V_0$, is small), then:

$$\Delta R = - \left(\frac{\rho L^2}{V_0^2} \right) \Delta V.$$

Thus it can be seen that an increase in the volume of conducting material of resistivity ρ will be accompanied by a decrease in resistance appearing between electrodes separated by a distance L. Sometimes, instead of calculating the volume V_0 between the electrodes, the basal impedance value is used. This can be inserted into the formula by multiplying the expression $R_0 = \rho L / A_0$ by L/L to obtain $R_0 = \rho L^2 / V_0$. Substitution of this relationship in the foregoing equation gives

$$\Delta R = - \left(\frac{R_0^2}{\rho L^2} \right) \Delta V,$$

or by rearranging,

$$\Delta V = - \left(\frac{\rho L^2}{R_0^2} \right) \Delta R.$$

It is important to recall that this expression was derived assuming a uni-

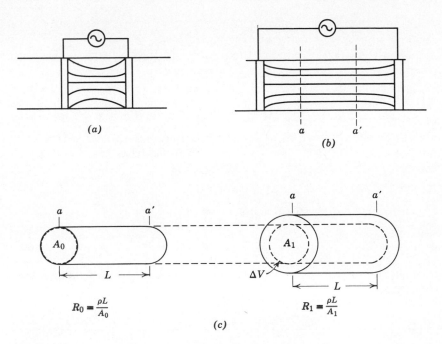

Figure 10-37. Simplified basis for impedance plethysmography: (*a*) current distribution with closely spaced electrodes; (*b*) current distribution with widely spaced electrodes; (*c*) the result of adding a volume ΔV to the conducting cylinder a–a'. $R_1 - R_0 = \Delta R = -(\rho L^2 / V_0^2)\Delta V$.

form current density distribution through a homogeneous conductor of uniform cross-sectional area. In the physiological application, this situation is almost never attained because when pulsatile blood flow measurements are made with the impedance method, the applied current is carried by at least two parallel conducting paths, tissue and blood. Although the resistivity of the latter is easy to measure, that of the former is not because it consists of a variety of tissues, each having a characteristic value of resistivity. For this reason it is useful to perform an analysis of a two-compartment model to derive an expression for the change in blood volume that is reflected by a change in the impedance appearing between the potential-measuring electrodes (a–a' in Fig. 10-37b). It will be shown that by making fairly reasonable assumptions, the two-compartment model reduces to the one-compartment model just described.

Consider the two-compartment model illustrated in Fig. 10-38 in which A_t and A_b are the cross-sectional areas of the tissues and blood respectively, and L is the spacing between the potential-measuring electrodes a, b. The resistivities of tissue and blood are ρ_t and ρ_b. Now the resistance R_{ab}

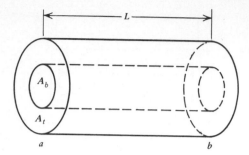

Figure 10-38. Two-compartment model for a body segment in which A_t represents its area occupied by tissue and A_b represents the area occupied by blood; $R_t = \rho_t L/A_t$ and $R_b = \rho_b L/A_b$, when R_t and R_b are the resistances of the tissue and blood paths, ρ_t and ρ_b are the tissue and blood resistivities, respectively, and L is the spacing of the potential-measuring electrodes.

appearing between electrodes a, b is given by

$$\frac{1}{R_{ab}} = \frac{1}{R_t} + \frac{1}{R_b},$$

where R_t and R_b are the resistances of the tissue and blood paths respectively. Accordingly

$$R_t = \frac{\rho_t L}{A_t} \quad \text{and} \quad R_b = \frac{\rho_b L}{A_b}.$$

Substitution of these relationships and manipulation gives

$$R_{ab} = \frac{\rho_t \rho_b L}{\rho_b A_t + \rho_t A_b}.$$

Now it is assumed that when an increment of blood (ΔV_b) enters the region between the potential-measuring electrodes, the tissue area (A_t) remains essentially the same; or stated another way, the change in area of the segment results from a small increase in the area of the blood conductor (A_b). Accepting this fairly reasonable physiological assumption permits derivation of an expression for the change in resistance appearing between the potential-measuring electrodes (a, b) when blood enters the region between them.

Recalling that length multiplied by area is equal to volume, it is possible to multiply the right-hand side of the preceding expression by L/L and substitute for the volume of tissue ($V_t = A_t L$) and blood ($V_b = A_b L$) to obtain the following:

$$R_{ab} = \frac{\rho_t \rho_b L^2}{\rho_b V_t + \rho_t V_b}.$$

To obtain a value for the change in resistance due to the entry of blood into the segment, it is merely necessary to differentiate R_{ab} with respect to V_b. Performing this operation, and recalling that V_t is assumed to be constant, gives

$$dR_{ab} = - \left(\frac{\rho_b \rho_t^2 L^2}{(\rho_t V_b + \rho_b V_t)^2} \right) dV_b.$$

By remembering that $V_t = LA_t$ and $V_b = LA_b$, it is possible to make these substitutions and rearrange the expression to obtain a relationship that links the change in blood volume dV_b with the change in resistance dR_{ab}; carrying out this manipulation gives

$$dV_b = - \frac{(\rho_b A_t + \rho_t A_b)^2}{\rho_t^2 \rho_b} dR_{ab}.$$

Although this expression permits calculation using a two-compartment model, it is practically impossible to determine the areas occupied by tissue (A_t) and blood (A_b). It is, however, convenient to use the basal resistance (R_{ab}) as a measure of their magnitudes. Therefore, as shown previously

$$\rho_b A_t + \rho_t A_b = \frac{\rho_t \rho_b L}{R_{ab}} .$$

When this relationship is substituted into the expression for dV_b, the following is obtained:

$$dV_b = - \rho_b \left(\frac{L}{R_{ab}} \right)^2 dR_{ab}.$$

Note that this expression is the same as that derived for the change in resistance in a single blood cylinder when a volume of blood is added to it. In its application it is important to recall the basic assumptions: (1) the cross-sectional area of the tissue mass remained constant, (2) the area of the blood conductor increased with entry of a volume of blood in the region between the potential-measuring electrodes, and (3) the length L was constant.

If it is assumed that impedance (Z) may be substituted for resistance (R), the expression for the blood volume change (ΔV) can be rewritten as

$$\Delta V = - \left(\frac{\rho L^2}{Z_0^2} \right) \Delta Z,$$

where ρ = resistivity of the blood,
  L = distance (cm) between the potential-measuring electrodes,
  Z_0 = basal impedance of the thorax measured at end diastole,
  ΔZ = change in impedance attributable to the stroke volume in the absence of arterial runoff.

The negative sign merely signifies that the entry of blood produces a decrease in impedance between the potential-measuring electrodes.

When this simple expression is put to practical use to calculate the volume of blood (ΔV) entering the body segment between the potential-measuring electrodes, both physiological and physical factors come into play, thereby making it difficult to determine ΔV accurately. It is important to note that the peak-to-peak amplitude of the pulsatile impedance change ($\Delta Z'$ in Fig. 10-39) is a measure of the difference between blood flow into and out of the body segment between the potential-measuring electrodes. Since ΔZ is supposed to measure the volume change produced only by the inflow of blood into the body segment, some means is required to estimate what this change would be in the absence of arterial runoff. Development of a suitable method is particularly difficult in the case of thoracic impedance cardiography. Despite differences between the ideal and practical situations, the impedance method is useful and very convenient in estimating the change in blood volume of a body segment during each beat of the heart.

10-14-5. Thoracic Impedance Cardiography

If electrodes are placed to encompass the thorax, impedance changes reflecting cardiac activity are recordable with ease. Bipolar and tetrapolar electrode arrangements have been placed on the arms, on either side of the thorax, on the back, and around the neck and chest at the level of the diaphragm. Clear cardiac impedance pulses can be recorded with any of these electrode configurations. Figure 10-40 illustrates the type of recording made with the tetrapolar electrode array applied to a human subject. The electrocardiogram, made from the same pair of electrodes, is presented to identify the location of the impedance pulse in the cardiac cycle.

A number of investigators have studied the thoracic impedance cardio-

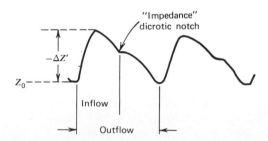

Figure 10-39. Typical pulsatile impedance change ($\Delta Z'$) due to the inflow minus outflow of blood in the region between the potential-measuring electrodes; Z_0 is the basal impedance, and the decrease in impedance ($\Delta Z'$) appears as an upward deflection in the recording. The inflow period shown on the impedance record may not be the same as the true period of ventricular ejection.

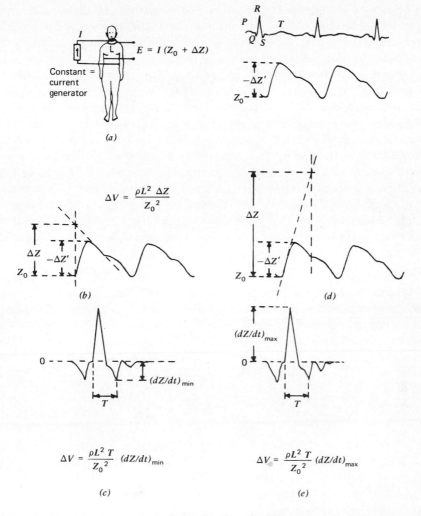

Figure 10-40. (a) A typical thoracic impedance cardiogram; to the left is the conventional electrode arrangement. A decrease in impedance ($-\Delta Z'$) is shown by an upward deflection in the recording. (b) The backslope extrapolation technique used to obtain the impedance change (ΔZ), which reflects the total volume of blood entering the region between the potential-measuring electrodes. Electronic differentiation of the impedance pulse ($\Delta Z'$) provides a means of recording continuously the slope of the impedance pulse (c), and its use to obtain ΔZ, which is equal to $T(dz/dt)_{min}$. (d) The forward extrapolation technique for obtaining ΔZ. The steepest slope $(dZ/dt)_{max}$ is obtained by electrical differentiation (e), and ΔZ is equal to $T(dZ/dt)_{max}$.

gram, hoping to calibrate it in terms of the systolic discharge from the heart. Probably the earliest were Atzler and Lehmann (1932) and Atzler (1933, 1935), who placed electrodes in front of and behind the thorax and detected ultrahigh-frequency impedance changes synchronous with cardiac activity. Because their circuit was mainly capacitive, they called the method "Dielektrographie." Later Nyboer et al. (1940) described precordial impedance changes that also reflected cardiac activity. Probably in an attempt to standardize electrode placement, Holzer et al. (1945) measured the 14-kHz cardiac impedance pulses appearing between electrodes placed on the arms and legs. Their study examined the impedance pulses in human subjects in health and disease, measuring impedance changes by means of the standard electrocardiographic lead configurations. They called their method "Rheokardiographie."

Improving the capacitive method of Atzler and Lehmann, Whitehorn and Pearl (1949) employed a 10.7-MHz current and were able to record impedance pulses with high fidelity, stating:

"Values for stroke volumes, cardiac output and cardiac indices calculated from such records, on the basis of preliminary calibration of the instrument by introduction of known volumes of saline between the plates, fall within the range of accepted normal values, but conclusions as to the validity of the method are not yet possible."

Mann (1953), using his 10-kHz capacigraph, which recorded only the capacitance changes between single electrodes placed on each forearm, believed that these changes were due mainly to blood volume changes within the thorax, although he admitted the presence of smaller changes in the arms. Zajic et al. (1954), using 270 kHz applied to one electrode on the neck and another either in the pelvic area or on the thighs, observed changes in the impedance pulse with manuevers which were known to change stroke volume. In one study Nyboer (1959) presented records called "radiocardiograms," taken at several levels on the precordium with his tetrapolar electrode system.

At present, the use of thoracic impedance cardiography is being actively investigated because it is virtually the only noninvasive method available to estimate stroke volume (the volume of blood ejected with each heart beat). Figure 10-40 illustrates the methods used to obtain human thoracic impedance cardiograms from a tetrapolar electrode system employing a constant-current sinusoidal generator; at present a frequency in the range of 20 to 100 kHz is employed. To indicate its temporal relation to the cardiac cycle, the electrocardiogram has been included.

Nyboer, one of the pioneers in the use of electrical impedance to measure blood volume changes, developed what is now called the backslope or end-systolic extrapolation technique (1959) to obtain a value for the impedance change (ΔZ) that reflects the entry of blood between the potential-measuring electrodes when no outflow occurs. Allison and Nyboer (1965) verified the accuracy of the method using an hydraulic model.

Referring to Fig. 10-40b, just beyond the peak of the impedance pulse ($\Delta Z'$) the physiological conditions are such that inflow to the thoracic segment between the potential-measuring electrodes (L cm apart) is minimum and outflow is maximum. Therefore it is fairly reasonable to assume that backward extrapolation of the steepest part of the postpeak impedance curve to a vertical line erected at the beginning of the pulse (which signals the beginning of ventricular ejection) would provide an impedance change (ΔZ) that corresponds to the inflow if no outflow existed. Therefore the stroke volume (ΔV) entering the segment can be calculated by using the expression given previously, namely:

$$\Delta V = \frac{\rho L^2}{Z_0^2} (\Delta Z).$$

In this expression, ρ is the resistivity of the blood (Ω-cm) for the packed-cell volume that exists, and Z_0 is the basal thoracic impedance between the potential-measuring electrodes which are L cm apart.

Because graphical extrapolation involves visual estimation of the steepest part of the immediate postpeak impedance curve, it is often more convenient to employ electronic differentiation to identify this slope and use a simple mathematical expression to derive the impedance change (ΔZ) that reflects volume inflow without outflow. Figure 10-40c illustrates application of the derivative to the impedance pulse (dZ/dt) to obtain the approximate ejection time (T). Thus the slope (dZ/dt)$_{min}$, multiplied by the ejection time (T) gives a corrected value for the impedance change (ΔZ) without outflow, that is,

$$\Delta Z = T(dZ/dt)_{min}.$$

Entering ΔZ into the expression just given allows calculation of the approximate stroke volume. Cardiac output is equal to stroke volume multiplied by heart rate.

The correction method developed by Kubicek et al. (1966) assumes that at the beginning of inflow to the interelectrode segment, outflow is minimal and inflow is maximal. Therefore forward extrapolation of the steepest part of the impedance pulse, if continued to the end of the ejection period (T), which is often taken as the dicrotic notch in the impedance record (see Fig. 10-40d) would provide an impedance change (ΔZ) that is corrected for outflow. Entry of this value into the expression presented previously provides an approximate value for stroke volume (ΔV). Often the impedance dicrotic notch is not prominent, and the onset of the second heart sound is used to identify the end of the ejection period. However, use of the electrical differentiation technique permits determination of the approximate ejection period (T) without the aid of the phonocardiogram; details of this technique are now presented.

The lack of precision associated with the forward extrapolation technique can be eliminated by recording the derivative of the impedance pulse. The maximum value of the derivative $(dZ/dt)_{max}$, when multiplied by the ejection time T, as identified in Fig. 10-40e, provides a value for ΔZ that is corrected for outflow; that is,

$$\Delta Z = T(dZ/dt)_{max}$$

Entry of ΔZ into this expression along with appropriate values for the resistivity of the subject's blood (ρ Ω-cm at body temperature), L the distance (cm) between the potential-measuring electrodes, and the basal impedance (Z_0), provides a reasonably accurate value for stroke volume (ΔV). Cardiac output is equal to stroke volume multiplied by heart rate.

Another method for determining ΔZ was presented by Kinnen (1965, 1970), who proposed use of the mean intercept. With his technique a value for ΔZ is obtained by carrying out the backward slope extrapolation (see Fig. 10-40b); then a value for ΔZ is obtained by use of the forward-slope method, as in Fig. 10-40d. The value ΔZ most representative of true inflow is taken as the mean of these two ΔZ values.

It is quite clear that the methods described yield different values for ΔZ, the impedance change representing inflow with no outflow. The verification studies conducted to date partly reflect the different techniques used to validate the value for stroke volume and cardiac output. Several investigators have compared the data obtained using the thoracic impedance cardiogram with those obtained using the indicator-dilution, Fick and flowmeter methods in man and animals; Table 10-5 summarizes the results.

A quick inspection of Table 10-5 indicates that the impedance method by and large overestimates cardiac output and stroke volume. The reason for the variability in the correlation has not been identified; however, the lack of agreement cannot be blamed entirely on the impedance method, which is an instantaneous method. When compared with average methods (Fick and indicator), moreoever, the impedance method requires that the stroke volume be absolutely constant while the comparison is being made. Physiologically, this situation is difficult to achieve. In the case of the flowmeter comparisons, blood flow in the ascending aorta is only about 95% of the cardiac output; 5% is delivered to the coronary arteries. In addition, accurate calibration of blood flowmeters is extremely difficult.

The correlative studies described above related the magnitude of the corrected (ΔZ) thoracic impedance change to stroke volume. Dissection of the impedance change into its reactive and resistive components was reported by Namon and Gollan (1970). Using four 2.5 × 2.5 cm electrodes applied to the midline of the canine thorax, the 37-kHz resistive and reactive components of the pulsatile impedance change were recorded separately over a wide range of stroke volumes. The investigators found that the magnitude of the reactive component varied between 25 and 100% of the amplitude of the resistive component. In correlation studies, it was discovered that the amplitude of the reactance pulse correlated better with stroke volume (as measured by the indicator-dilution method) than did the amplitude of the pulsatile change in resistance. No data were given on values for stroke volume obtained from the reactive or resistive impedance pulses.

Namon and Gollan also recorded resistive and reactive thoracic impedance pulses on man. They learned that the best results were obtained when the two current-injecting electrodes were placed on the back over the spine. No correlation data were presented in their initial study.

Although it is too soon to evaluate the method of recording the reactive thoracic impedance pulses, two observations made by Gollan and Namon merit attention. The first has already been mentioned—namely the overall amplitude of the pulsatile reactance change exhibited a higher correlation with stroke volume. The second relates to a reduced sensitivity to artifact. For example, light tapping of the electrodes did not produce artifacts in the reactance recording. There is no doubt that the future will see additional studies of the reactive component of the thoracic impedance cardiogram. It is not obvious now, however, what technique will be used to calibrate a recorded reactance change in terms of stroke volume.

Many of the required values for the resistivities of blood samples at body temperature (see Section 10-22) are available (Geddes and Baker, 1968; Geddes et al.,1972, 1973) for entry into the various stroke volume equations; however, the best method for correcting the recorded amplitude ($\Delta Z'$) to obtain a value for ΔZ that reflects only inflow is by no means settled.

Investigations have been undertaken to identify the phenomena underlying the thoracic cardiac impedance pulse. Bonjer et al. (1952), in a series of ingenious experiments that consisted of wrapping first the heart and then the lungs in rubber sheeting and perfusing each with a stroke pump, concluded that the thoracic impedance changes were due mainly to perfusion of the pulmonary vascular circuit by the output from the right ventricle and that only a small component was due to direct volume changes of the heart. By the injection of hypertonic saline into the left and then the right ventricles of dogs during diastole, L. E. Geddes and Baker (1972) showed that the thoracic impedance change contained unequal

Table 10-5 Thoracic Impedance Cardiography Correlations*

Cardiac output relationship (l/min) $Z(CO) = A(CO) + B$	Correlation Coefficient	Standard Error of Estimate	Subjects	Reference Method for $A(CO) + B$	ΔZ Processing Method	Principal Investigator and Year	Remarks
$0.942(CO) + 0.007$	0.959	0.026	Dogs	Fick	Backslope	Allison (1966)	14–42 kg body weight
$1.124(CO) - 0.097$	0.976	0.107	Dogs	Cardio-green	Backslope	Allison (1966)	14–42 kg body weight
$1.18(CO)$	—	—	Human	Cardio-green	Max derivative	Kubicek (1966)	Resting and postexercise
$0.86(CO) + 2.93$	0.680	2.33	Human	Dye	Forward slope	Harley (1967)	24 cardiac patients
$0.73(CO) + 4.91$	0.579	2.34	Human	Radioisotope	Max derivative	Judy (1969)	
$0.71(CO) + 2.06$	0.83	—	Human	Cardio-green	Max derivative	Smith (1970)	Adults—tilt table
$0.90(CO) + 0.62$	0.94	—	Human	Cardio-green	Max derivative	Smith (1970)	Adults—tilt table
$0.8(CO)$ to $1.2(CO)$	0.95	—	Human	Fick	Double slope	Kinnen (1970)	25 patients
$0.8(CO)$ to $1.2(CO)$	0.84	—	Human	Fick	Double slope	Kinnen (1970)	67 patients
$0.8(CO) \oplus 4.3(CO)$	0.58	—	Human	Radioisotope	Max derivative	Baker (1971)	17 normal adults
$1.0(CO) + 0.52$	0.68	1.63	Human	Cardio-green	Max derivative	Baker (1971)	10 normal adults
$0.96(CO) + 0.56$	0.66	1.54	Human	Cardio-green	Max derivative	Baker (1971)	21 normal adults
$1.43(CO) + 1.08$	0.923	0.593	Human	Cardio-green	Max derivative	Van De Water (1971)	One subject
ca. $1.055(CO)$	—	—	Human	Cardio-green	Max derivative	Lababidi (1971)	Children (cardiac patients)
$0.91(CO) + 0.218$	0.92	—	Dogs	EM flowmeter	Max derivative	Baker (1971)	Aortic blood flow

Stroke-volume
relationship (ml),
$Z(SV) = P(SV) + Q$

Relationship	P	Q	Subject		Reference	Description
$1.42(SV) + 3.5$	0.94	—	Human	Press. gradient	Max derivative	Bache (1969)	Cardiac patient
$1.42(SV) - 5.8$	0.96	—	Human	Press. gradient	Max derivative	Bache (1969)	Cardiac patient
$0.93(SV) + 2.0$	0.91	—	Human	Press. gradient	Max derivative	Bache (1969)	Cardiac patient
$0.44(SV) + 5.3$	0.58	—	Human	Press. gradient	Max derivative	Bache (1969)	Cardiac patient
$1.37(SV) + 12.4$	0.62	—	Human	Press. gradient	Max derivative	Bache (1969)	Cardiac patient
$0.65(SV) - 1.0$	0.78	—	Human	Press. gradient	Max derivative	Bache (1969)	Cardiac patient
$0.77(SV) + 0.4$	0.68	—	Human	Press. gradient	Max derivative	Bache (1969)	Cardiac patient
$1.53(SV) - 5.5$	0.87	—	Human	Press. gradient	Max derivative	Bache (1969)	Cardiac patient
$0.92(SV) + 2.3$	0.94	1.9	Dogs	EM flowmeter	Max derivative	Kubicek (1970)	Aortic blood flow
$0.90(SV) + 15.2$	0.87	—	Human	Cardio-green	Max derivative	Smith (1970)	Head up (8 subjects)
$1.01(SV) + 0.82$	0.96	—	Human	Cardio-green	Max derivative	Smith (1970)	Head up (8 subjects)

* Complete agreement would be indicated by $Z(CO) = 1.00 (CO) + 0.00$ or $Z(SV) = 1.00(SV) + 0.00$.

contributions from the left and right ventricles. They also demonstrated that when the saline was injected into the ventricles during diastole there was virtually no thoracic impedance change, clearly showing that the thoracic impedance cardiogram indicates systolic discharge.

The impedance method does not always provide a highly accurate value for stroke volume and cardiac output, but it does track changes in these quantities quite well; hence the impedance method has value for monitoring subjects. The matter of correlation in subjects with cardiac defects is now under investigation and although the stroke volume values appear to be in error, the recordings are quite characteristic of the type of defect. This fact alone may add to the value of the impedance cardiogram in cardiac diagnosis.

10-14-6.   Impedance Plethysmography of the Extremities

A reduction in blood flow to the extremities occurs in many types of cardiovascular disease. Accordingly, to assist in the diagnosis of peripheral vascular diseases and in evaluating the effect of therapeutic measures, considerable effort has been directed toward the development of quantitative methods to measure peripheral blood flow. The only accurate method available (venous-occlusion plethysmography) is cumbersome to apply, and clinicians have almost abandoned it. The impedance method, however, is much easier to use and therefore offers attractive clinical possibilities. It has not seen extensive use because of difficulties in relating the impedance change, which is measured in ohms, to units of blood flow, namely, milliliters per minute. Excellent accounts of this history and development of the impedance method are to be found in Nyboer's two monographs (1959, 1970).

Before describing impedance plethysmography of the extremities, the method that it may ultimately replace—namely, venous-occlusion plethysmography—must be understood because it provides a reasonably accurate measure of blood flow into an extremity. Most important, this technique will undoubtedly be used to verify the accuracy of the data obtained by impedance plethysmography.

The principle of the venous-occlusion plethysmographic technique was described by Brodie (1905). Figure 10-41 shows application of the pneumatic method to the finger and arm. (Water-filled systems have also been employed.) When applied to the finger (Fig. 10-41a), a hollow capsule is placed around a digit and sealed to it with any convenient thick paste (a disposable syringe barrel makes a convenient plethysmograph). The air in the chamber is connected to a sensitive pressure transducer, which in turn is connected to a graphic recorder. Also connected to the pneumatic system is

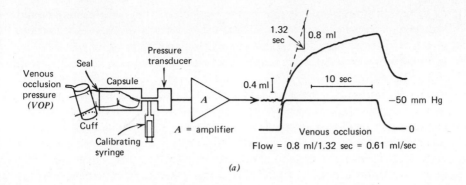

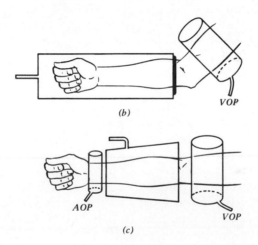

Figure 10-41. Application of venous-occlusion plethysmography to measure blood flow in the digit (a), forearm and hand (b), and forearm only (c). The method consists of measuring the rate of swelling of the member when venous outflow is arrested by quickly inflating a cuff to venous occluding pressure (VOP), usually about 50 mm Hg. To measure flow in the forearm only, inflow and outflow to the hand are arrested by inflating cuff to above arterial occluding pressure (AOP).

a small syringe, which is used to inject a known volume of air for calibration purposes. Just central to the capsule, an inflatable cuff is wrapped around the finger. The cuff is later employed to occlude venous outflow from the digit.

To measure digital blood flow, the apparatus is set up as in Fig. 10-41a. Because of the pulsatile expansion of the digit, small oscillations in pressure are recordable from the air surrounding the finger. When a determination of blood flow is to be made, the venous-occlusion cuff is suddenly inflated to about 50 mm Hg, a pressure above venous and below arterial diastolic pressure. When this is done, arterial inflow starts to swell the digit, and the pressure in the capsule increases—at first, linearly with each heart beat, as in Fig. 10-41a. While the capsule pressure continues to increase, the linear rise gives way to an exponential rise because venous blood pressure increases and the net pressure driving blood (arteriovenous) becomes less with each heart beat. A second reason for the exponential nature of the pressure rise relates to the nonlinear pressure-volume characteristic of the vascular bed. A continued application of the occluding pressure will result in venous pressure overcoming the pressure in the occluding cuff, and venous outflow will be reestablished. However, the measurement is not continued until this point is reached; the occluding pressure is reduced long before the plateau in capsule pressure is attained.

The blood flow per unit time into the digit is calculated by drawing a tangent to the capsule pressure curve where it departs from the baseline at the onset of venous occlusion. This slope of this tangent is converted to volume by recording capsule pressure while injecting a known volume of air while the finger is still inside. A time calibration is also placed on the record. Sample calculations for digital volume flow appear in Fig. 10-41a.

Figure 10-41 also shows how venous occlusion plethysmography is applied to the hand and forearm (Fig. 10-41b) and to the forearm only (Fig. 10-41c). In the latter case blood flow into the hand is arrested by inflating a cuff to well above arterial systolic pressure (arterial occluding pressure, AOP). The same technique is applied to measure blood flow in the lower extremities. Excellent descriptions of the pneumatic and hydraulic techniques have been presented by Burch (1944), Wise (1944), Abramson (1944), and Wolstenholme and Freeman (1954).

When electrodes are applied to the finger within a closed chamber, as in Fig. 10-42, the pulsatile impedance change is strikingly similar to the pulsatile pressure change in the air within the chamber. This fact has been well documented with bipolar and tetrapolar electrode systems; an example of the latter from Nyboer's studies (1970) is illustrated in Fig. 10-42. Therefore, it would seem that the two recordings reflect the same event, and it ought to be a straightforward task to verify the volume flow obtained by use of the impedance method with that determined by venous-occlusion plethysmography. However such an investigation is very difficult to carry out because of the considerable artifact that the venous-occlusion technique imposes on the impedance method, as pointed out by Van der Berg and Alberts (1954), who applied it to the digits. One such study was performed successfully by Young et al. (1967), who modeled a dog hind limb as a truncated cone (between the potential-measuring electrodes) and used a

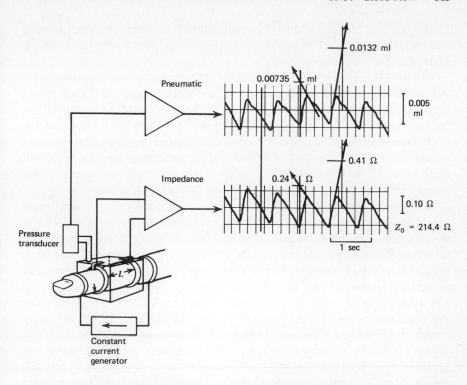

Heart Rate = 75/min; Volume of Digit = 14.5 ml; Length, L = 3.1 cm

	Flow (ml/heart beat)	
Extrapolation Technique	Pneumatic	Impedance
Backward	0.00735	0.00753
Forward	0.0132	0.0128
	Flow [ml/(min)/(100 ml of digit)]	
Backward	3.80	3.89
Forward	6.83	6.62

Figure 10-42. Pneumatic and impedance plethysmography of the digit.

slightly different impedance expression: $\Delta Z/Z_0$ = 1.6 $\Delta V/V$, where ΔZ is the decrease in impedance when a volume ΔV entered the hind limb with a basal impedance Z_0 and volume V. An electromagnetic blood flowmeter probe was applied centrally to the femoral artery to examine the correlation of the flow calculated by the impedance method with that actually entering the member. Collateral circulation was virtually eliminated by ligating the middle sacral artery.

The results obtained by Young et al., who made measurements on 5 dogs, showed that the venous-occlusion impedance plethysmographic data obtained (using their formula) were 1.2% above the values for blood flow (ml/min as measured with the electromagnetic flowmeter). A plot of the impedance flow (Z_f) versus electromagnetic flowmeter (E_f) measurements provided the relationship $Z_f = 0.98\ E_f + 3.9$ ml with a correlation coefficient of 0.98, thereby indicating that venous-occlusion impedance plethysmography can provide quantitative blood flow data in an extremity.

When impedance plethysmography is applied to determine peripheral blood flow, the venous-occlusion method is almost never used, principally because it is so cumbersome. In addition, there is no agreement on the best technique for converting the recorded impedance change to the volume of blood that flows through the body segment between the potential-measuring electrodes. At present, the extrapolation techniques shown in Fig. 10-40 offer the most promise if the venous-occlusion technique is to be avoided. To the best of knowledge of the authors, there have been no studies that compare segmental blood flow determined by nonocclusive impedance plethysmography with values obtained using a member-encircling capsule in conjunction with the venous-occlusion technique. Certainly the results of such a study would provide extremely valuable information. While anticipating the fruits of such work, it is of some interest to apply the graphical extrapolation techniques to both the pneumatic (pressure) and impedance recordings (Fig. 10-42) to examine the correlation between the blood flows predicted by the two different nonocclusive techniques.

The end-systolic (backslope) graphical construction has been applied to both the pneumatic and impedance recordings illustrated in Fig. 10-42. The volume of blood entering the region within the finger-surrounding capsule amounts to 0.00735 ml per heart beat for the pneumatic recording. For the impedance recording, the basal impedance (Z_0) between the potential-measuring electrodes 3.1 cm apart and at the edges of the capsule is 214.4 Ω, and the extrapolated value for the impedance change (ΔZ) is 0.24 Ω. Using a typical value of 150 Ω-cm for the resistivity of blood, the predicted volume entering the body segment is

$$\Delta V = \frac{\rho L^2}{Z_0^2} \Delta Z = \frac{150 \times 3.1^2}{214.4^2} \times 0.24 = 0.00753\ \text{ml}.$$

The forward extrapolation technique has been applied to both the pneumatic and impedance recordings appearing in Fig. 10-42. The pneumatic recording indicates a flow of 0.0132 ml per heart beat. The extrapolated impedance change (ΔZ) amounts to 0.41 Ω and using the same values for L and Z_0, the volume obtained by the impedance method is

$$\Delta V = \frac{\rho L^2}{Z_0^2} \Delta Z = \frac{150 \times 3.1^2}{214.4^2} \times 0.41 = 0.0128 \text{ ml}.$$

It is customary to normalize the values for blood flow in terms of flow in milliliters per minute per 100 milliliters of tissue; therefore, the four values for digital flow have been calculated for a heart rate of 75 beats/min and a digital volume of 14.5 ml and are shown in Fig. 10-42. Table 10-6 indicates that these values compare reasonably well with digital blood flow obtained by venous-occlusion plethysmography using a member-encircling capsule. The agreement may be purely fortuitous, however, because the extrapolation techniques for the impedance pulse, as applied to the digit, have not been verified by flow determinations obtained by other methods.

Since the amplitude of the impedance pulse is lowered dramatically by any reduction in the lumen of the arterial supply, the impedance method offers an excellent noninvasive method for estimating the patency of the large arteries supplying the arm and leg. Applications of the impedance method to the arm and leg are illustrated in Fig. 10-43. Comparisons between the right and left sides often provide qualitative information on the symmetry of blood supply to the members. In addition, with the increase in vessel replacement by surgery, impedance plethysmography of the members offers a convenient means of estimating the patency of a vascular prosthesis. Figure 10-43 presents typical recordings obtained from the arms and legs of human subjects.

Table 10-6   Segmental Blood Flow in Man*

Body Segment	Flow [ml/min/100 ml of segment]		
	Normal	Maximum	Minimum
Finger	15–40	90	0.2
Hand	6 (0.5–16.5)	22	2.5 (0.3–4.7)
Forearm	2.9 (0.4–7.3)	12.6 (3.7–25.4)	0.7 (0.5–1.0)
Leg	1.4 (0.8–2.6)	3.6	1.2 (0.4–1.5)
Calf	1.4 (0.4–2.4)	—	—
Foot	2.7 (0.5–7.8)	18.1 (11–34)	—

* Data from *Handbook of Circulation*, D. S. Dittmer (ed.). Aerospace Medical Laboratory, Wright Air Development Center, USAF Wright-Patterson AFB, Ohio, 1959.

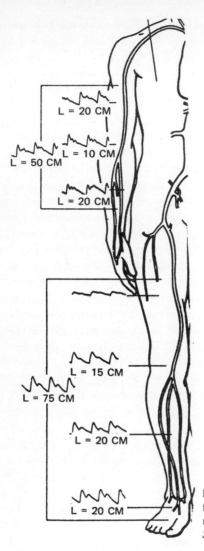

Figure 10-43. Impedance pulses obtained with different electrode separations applied to the extremities. [Redrawn from R. Allison, *J. Am. Geriatr. Soc.* **17**:685–693 (1969).]

L = 20 CM
L = 10 CM
L = 50 CM
L = 20 CM
L = 15 CM
L = 75 CM
L = 20 CM
L = 20 CM

10-14-7.   Impedance Phlebography

Venous occlusion by a blood clot in the limbs is difficult to detect, and there is a real danger of the clot becoming dislodged and passing through the right heart into the pulmonary vascular circuit, occluding blood flow to alveoli, where oxygen is taken up and carbon dioxide is released. Accordingly, any technique that offers promise of identifying venous clots is of considerable interest to the clinician. Wheeler et al. (1972), Gazzaniga et al. (1972,1973), Dmochowski et al. (1972), Deuvaert et al. (1973), and Steer et al. (1973) employed the impedance method to assess the venous drainage rate. Wheeler et al. (1972) designated the method "impedance phlebography." With this technique, basal impedance of a segment of an extremity (arm or leg) is measured, then venous outflow is occluded. A decrease in impedance occurs due to swelling of the member. On release of the venous occlusion, the segmental impedance increases, and its rate identifies the ability of the venous system to drain the segment. If the major veins are obstructed by a blood clot, the initial volume increase (indicated by a decrease in impedance) is smaller than in the normal subject. On release of the venous occlusion, the rate of volume decrease (indicated by an increase in impedance) is smaller.

The clinical value of this method is still under investigation. One of the variables that needs standardization is the method for achieving venous occlusion. The original technique for venous occlusion required the subject to take a deep and sustained inspiration to occlude venous outflow from the legs. Since this technique gave variable results, use of the Valsalva maneuver was adopted; however, this technique produces a considerable change in heart rate and blood pressure and therefore introduces new variables. The technique that shows the most promise employs a pneumatic (blood pressure) cuff around the extremity. To occlude venous outflow, the pressure is rapidly increased to about 40 mm Hg, a value above venous pressure but well below arterial pressure. A recording of basal impedance and the changes it experiences during and after occlusion should provide a record that will allow clinical evaluation of the method to identify venous obstruction in the extremities.

Even though the impedance changes encountered are small and are on the order of 0.2 to 0.5% of the basal impedance, it has been possible to identify venous occlusion using the method. A variant of the technique employs a simultaneous comparison of the recordings obtained from homologous body segments. The initial results presented by Gazzaniga et al. (1972) using this method are extremely promising.

10-14-8. Rheoencephalography (REG)

Measurement of cerebral blood flow is extremely difficult because the conventional pneumatic and hydraulic plethysmographic techniques, which employ a member-encircling chamber, cannot be employed. The only reliable method of determining the amount of blood that flows through the brain per minute was described by Kety and Schmidt (1945,1948). With this technique, the subject inhales nitrous oxide (N_2O, 15%) and exhales to the atmosphere for a period of 10 min, the time necessary for cerebral venous blood to reach equilibration with the tension of N_2O in brain tissue. During the 10-min period, 5 paired samples of arterial and jugular-vein blood are drawn and graphs are plotted of the arterial and venous blood concentrations of N_2O. From these data and using the dilution formula, cerebral blood flow per 100 grams of brain tissue can be calculated. Typically in man the flow amounts to about 55 ml/min per 100 grams of brain tissue.

Clearly measurement of cerebral blood flow is difficult, and any noninvasive, nonhazardous method for obtaining information on cerebral circulation is extremely attractive to the neurologist, the neurosurgeon, and the vascular surgeon. Probably for this reason Polzer and Schuhfried (1950) investigated the value of the impedance method to estimate cerebral blood flow. They placed a pair of electrodes on the head of a patient having an occlusion of one carotid artery and measured the 20-kHz pulsatile impedance changes, first on one side of the head and then on the other. On the affected side the height of the pulsatile impedance change was diminished, thereby indicating a possible relationship with cerebral blood flow. Since that time, numerous studies have been carried out; one book has been published (Jenkner, 1962), and three international symposia have been held on the subject (Martin and Lechner, 1963; Lechner et al., 1969; Markovich, 1970). Review papers have been presented by Lifshitz (1963), Geddes (1964), McHenry (1965), Perez-Borja and Meyer (1964), and Hadijev (1972). Although not all these reviews are laudatory of the method, there is considerable interest in the potential of rheoencephalography, and several instruments are available commercially. There is undeniable evidence that useful qualitative information regarding cerebral perfusion can be obtained by rheoencephalography, but there is no agreement on the optimum electrode placement or instrumentation technique. Therefore the results obtained must be evaluated in view of the type of recording technique employed.

A typical bipolar recording of the REG from a normal subject appears in Fig. 10-44. The electrodes were arrayed as shown, forehead to mastoid, and the impedance changes were measured at 70 kHz using about 1 mA (rms). The first and fifth channels show the EEG; the second and fourth display the REG. The EEG and REG recordings were made from the same pair of electrodes. Lead II ECG was included as a temporal reference.

In this record, it is observed that the REGs from the right and the left sides are slightly different in waveform; this is a fairly common finding in normal subjects. Markovich (1965) reported a 17% difference in area under pulses recorded from the right and left sides of the head is within normal limits. The pulse transmission time from the heart to the head is evident from the relationship between the R wave of the ECG and the onset of the impedance pulse. This interval is often described as the appearance time. It

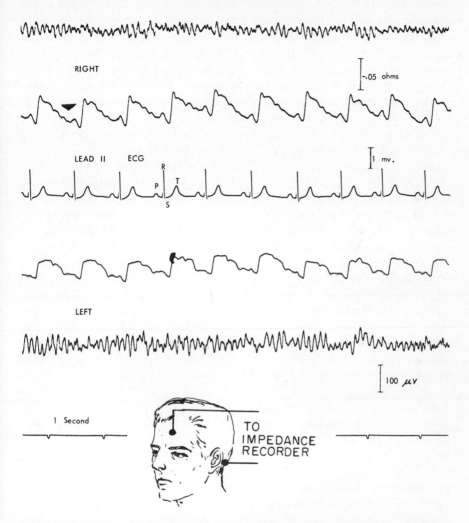

(A decrease in impedance is shown upward.)

RIGHT

-.05 ohms

LEAD II   ECG

1 mv.

LEFT

100 μv

1 Second

TO
IMPEDANCE
RECORDER

Figure 10-44.   Rheoencephalogram (channels 2 and 4) and the electroencephalogram (channels 1 and 5) obtained from the same pairs of electrodes. The ECG (lead II) is included to illustrate the temporal locations of the REG in the cardiac cycle. A decrease in impedance is shown upward.

is customary to measure the peak amplitude (usually 20–200 mΩ) and the rate of rise of the impedance pulse (ohms per second). Often the time from the onset to the peak is also measured. It is hoped that alterations in these quantities will be found to accompany cerebrovascular disease.

As previously stated, the type of rheoencephalographic recording obtained is not unrelated to the type of circuit and the size and location of the electrodes applied to the subject's head. Since it has not been possible to quantitate recordings in terms of blood flow, recourse is made to comparison of the waveforms obtained from homologous areas of the head; an asymmetry usually indicates a difference in vascular supply. Therefore, two or more channels of data are usually recorded simultaneously, although serial single-channel recordings were made from homologous areas in the first studies by Polzer and Schuhfried (1950).

Figure 10-45a illustrates the method employed when two separate instruments, each with its own current source, are used to compare the pulsatile impedance changes on two sides of the head. This technique has been designated REG I by Martin and Lechner (1963). The early studies employed impedance-bridge circuits (which often had the characteristics of a constant-voltage conductance-measuring system). To guarantee that cranial current of the same intensity flows on each side of the head, the constant-current circuit should be used; however, the frequency of the current in each of the two channels must differ from that in the other, and the amplifier demodulator (AD) for one channel must be sensitive only to current of its own frequency. Thus each channel must incorporate a constant source of alternating current and a narrow-band filter to select its own frequency of alternating current. Since the pulsatile impedance signal is very small, only the impedance change (ΔZ) is recorded; the basal impedance of the head (Z_0) is rejected by the use of capacitive coupling after demodulation. Usually a time constant in excess of 2 sec is employed. However, if it is desired to display the pulsatile impedance on a baseline that represents the basal impedance (Z_0) of the head, a biasing signal derived from the current source is applied to the amplifier demodulator. Lechner et al. (1966) advocated recording the basal and pulsatile impedance, calling the record the "total rheoencephalogram."

With the method known as REG I, the same electrodes are used for current injection and potential measurement. Near the electrodes, the current density is highest; consequently impedance changes in these regions are more easily detected than are changes deep within the brain. This defect is attenuated by the two methods designated REG II and monopolar REG.

Probably because clinicians desire to obtain information about the circulation in many areas of the brain, Lechner and Rodler (1961,1966) advocated the use of a single current source for multichannel rheoencephalography; their method is illustrated in Fig. 10-45b. The technique of recording was designated REG II by Martin and Lechner (1963). With this system, a sine wave generator applies a constant current to the head through electrodes placed on the forehead and occiput. The pulsatile im-

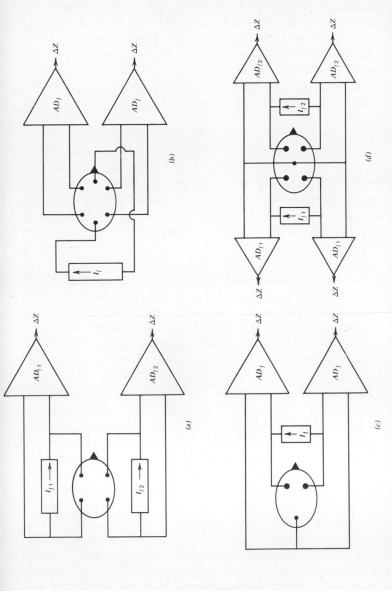

Figure 10-45. Rheoencephalography techniques. (*a*) Bipolar (rheoencephalography I) recording of the rheoencephalogram in which the same electrodes are used for current injection and signal measurement. Multichannel use requires that the amplifier demodulators (AD) detect only the frequency of its current generator. (*b*) Multichannel (rheoencephalography II) employing a single current source (I_{f_1}) and multiple recording channels, each with the same electrical characteristics. [Lechner and Rodler (1961), 66.] (*c*) Monopolar rheoencephalography, employing large-area current-injecting electrodes (to obtain a low current density), which allows use of one current electrode and a single potential-measuring electrode. [Markovich and Namon (1965).] (*d*) Monopolar rheoencephalography employing large-area, current-injecting electrodes and two current sources to permit recording impedance pulses from four regions of the head. [Namon and Markovich (1970).]

371

pedance changes are detected by pairs of potential-measuring electrodes placed on the head as in Fig. 10-45b. As many pairs of potential-measuring electrodes as desired can be applied; therefore their size (and impedance) is unimportant when an amplifier demodulator with a high input impedance is employed. An important practical attribute is that all the amplifier demodulators are identical and sensitive only to the frequency of the applied alternating current. Separation of the current and potential electrodes ensures a more symmetrical and uniform current distribution; therefore, differences in circulation between cerebral hemispheres should be optimally displayed.

Markovich and Namon (1965) and Namon and Markovich (1966,1970) pointed out that in the measurement of impedance the area of the electrodes used to apply current affects dramatically the amplitude of the measured impedance pulse. After documenting this fact, they recommended that the current electrodes should be no less than 6 cm in diameter (to obtain a low current density under them). These investigators detected pulsatile impedance changes using one current electrode paired with another potential-sensing electrode placed at any convenient location. Figure 10-45c illustrates the monopolar recording technique applied to detect the frontal-to-occipital impedance changes on the left and right sides of the head. Figure 10-45d illustrates the monopolar technique used to compare the vertex-frontal and vertex occipital impedance pulses. With this arrangement four different circulatory regions may be examined.

Lifshitz and Klemm (1966) and Lifshitz (1970) applied the guard-electrode technique to obtain a deeper and more uniform penetration of the current into brain tissue. They compared the basal and pulsatile impedance changes measured over a frequency range extending from 25 kHz to 2 MHz using unguarded and guarded electrodes applied to the heads of human subjects. They found that guarding more than trebled the basal impedance and more than doubled the pulsatile impedance change. This observation indicates that in all probability use of the guarding technique forced more current to pass through the skull than when unguarded bipolar (current-injecting and current-measuring) electrodes are used. If so, this technique merits further study.

There is no agreement regarding the frequency of choice for any of the rheoencephalographic techniques just described. The first consideration, of course, is safety for the subject; this dictates that a frequency above 20 kHz be used to minimize the risk of stimulating cutaneous receptors. A second consideration relates to the peculiar arrangement of conducting tissues between scalp electrodes and the brain. For current to gain access to the brain by means of scalp electrodes, it must traverse the scalp and the skull, entering the brain through the cerebrospinal fluid. The resistivity of the scalp is much lower than that of the bony cranium, and the cerebrospinal fluid has a resistivity even lower than that of blood (Radvan-Ziemnowicz et al., 1964). Thus low-frequency current can easily pass between the electrodes through scalp tissue, and only a small fraction will pass through the high-resistivity calvarium to enter the brain. If the frequency is high enough, the reactance of the path constituted by the scalp-calvarium and brain substance will be low, and current will gain easier access to the brain. Hence it ought to be possible to identify an empirically determined frequency that is high enough to secure current penetration into the brain to detect its pulsatile changes accompanying blood flow.

Two investigations have concerned themselves with the importance of the frequency of the current used for rheoencephalography. In a study by Gougerot and Marstal (1965), REG recordings were made in the frequency range extending from 400 to 8000 Hz. They concluded that there was no optimum frequency within this range. In a study that encompassed a much wider frequency range, Lifshitz and Klemm (1966) and Lifshitz (1970) found that increasing the frequency from 25 kHz to 2 MHz decreased the basal impedance and increased pulsatile impedance changes for both unguarded and guarded electrodes. Practical difficulties attributed to stray capacitance made it impractical to use frequencies above 500 kHz. Lifshitz therefore recommended a frequency of 120 kHz as a practical compromise, since the increase in size of the pulsatile impedance change above this frequency was small.

Although it is well known that the pulsatile impedance change detected by scalp electrodes is a reflection of pulsatile blood flow, there is no agreement on the relative contributions of the extracranial and intracranial circulations. However the relative contributions of each can be demonstrated by the simple technique of placing a tight band caudal to the electrodes to cut off the extracranial blood flow. When this is done, there is a significant reduction in pulsatile amplitude with some electrode arrays and circuits; with others, in particular the REG II system, the reduction in amplitude is less, indicating deeper penetration of the current and better detection of intracranial circulation.

In evaluating the etiology of the cardiac-synchronous pulsatile impedance change, it must be remembered that the cerebral circulation is contained within a rigid container, the skull, and the simple plethysmographic model, which assumes that the pulsatile amplitude reflects member swelling and a temporal difference between inflow and outflow, may not be totally applicable. Nonetheless, an increase in blood volume between the measuring electrodes reduces the impedance. Lechner et al. (1965) proposed that the well-known reduction in blood resistivity with increasing blood-flow velocity (see Section 10-22) contributes to the pulsatile impedance change. Certain maneuvers, known to alter cerebral blood flow, can be applied to reveal the types of relationship between the REG and blood flow. The first and foremost of these is occlusion of a carotid artery (by manual compression). This maneuver usually reduces the amplitude of the pulsatile impedance change on the side of the occlusion. However, the cerebral circulation is derived from four main vessels that eventually join at the circle of Willis at the base of the brain. Occlusion of one of these vessels does not totally deprive that side of the brain of circulation. Nonetheless, the result of transient occlusion of a carotid (or vertebral) artery may provide useful information regarding the possible contribution of the vessel which was occluded.

Other maneuvers that decrease brain perfusion also reveal themselves in the REG, although not always in a desirable manner. For example, venous compression or the performance of a Valsalva maneuver occludes venous outflow (and reduces brain perfusion) and usually increases the amplitude of the REG. Most important, body position, which also affects the resistance to venous outflow, influences the REG amplitude. In the head-up position the REG is smaller than it is when the body is horizontal. With the head-down position, the REG amplitude is increased. In describing an REG, therefore, it is important to specify the position of the subject. It may be that useful clinical information can be derived from the REG changes that occur in response to body-position changes.

Another maneuver that reduces brain perfusion is hyperventilation, which reduces arterial pCO_2, thereby producing cerebral vasoconstriction. The expected reduction in the amplitude and decrease in steepness of the ascending limb of the REG is not always manifest with all recording methods. On the other hand, the inhalation of 5 to 7% CO_2 for 5 to 10 min increases the amplitude and slope of the REG (Hadijev, 1972).

Another important factor determining the amplitude of the REG is heart rate. An increase in heart rate decreases the amplitude; a decrease in rate increases the amplitude. Therefore, heart rate should be specified when measuring the components of the REG. The REG changes in response to an increase in heart rate have not been investigated extensively.

There are clearly identifiable changes in the REG following the administration of drugs; an excellent account of these has been presented by Hadijev (1972), who stated that nicotinic acid increases the rising phase of the REG pulse. Nitroglycerin increases the amplitude of the REG.

The clinical value of the various rheoencephalographic methods has not been established. Progress is slow because there are so many different techniques in use. Hadijev's review (1972) describes the clinical evaluations established to date. The really attractive feature of the REG is its noninvasive and painless nature. A second attribute is its continuous recording aspect and ability to indicate immediate changes in response to stimuli (carotid and jugular occlusion, hyperventilation, etc.). Although there is no method available at present for converting the pulsatile impedance change to pulsatile flow, the potential for correlating REG changes with cerebrovascular disease exists and, with the passage of time, the useful correlations will be established. Its use as a safe screening technique may well be its most valuable contribution.

10-15.   BLADDER VOLUME

Bipolar and tetrapolar electrode systems have been used to measure the volume changes accompanying filling and emptying of the urinary bladder. Talibi et al. (1970) employed the tetrapolar electrode system to measure the impedance of the canine bladder containing different volumes of saline. In this study the impedance appearing between the potential electrodes applied to the bladder was represented by a parallel resistance (R_2) capacitance (C_1) circuit in series with a resistance (R_1) as identified in Fig. 10-46b, which shows the method they employed and the data obtained. Their results indicate that the values for R_2 or C_1 could be used as quantities reflecting bladder volume.

A different method of measuring the volume of the canine urinary bladder was described by Waltz et al. (1971). The bladder was surgically exposed and two ring electrodes were applied to the bladder wall; then the incision was closed. Current from the ring electrodes flowed through the bladder contents and the surrounding tissues and body fluids. As the bladder filled, the ring electrodes moved farther apart in the conducting medium of the body, and the resistance measured between the electrode terminals increased. The interelectrode resistance change controlled the frequency of a resistance-capacity oscillator, which in turn was used to indicate bladder volume. Figures 10-46d and 10-46e illustrate the method employed and the relationship between bladder volume, interelectrode resistance, and frequency as a dog bladder was filled with saline and emptied.

Denniston and Baker (1975) developed a novel method of recording bladder emptying with body-surface electrodes applied to the dog. A constant-current (100-kHz) tetrapolar system was employed with one of the current-injecting band-electrodes placed just above the xiphoid process and the other wrapped around both hind limbs (see Fig. 10-46f). Two disk electrodes were used to measure the potential; one was placed midline on the abdomen over the umbilicus and the other over the pubis. The bladder was catherized and urine that was collected earlier was infused while impedance was being recorded. The relationship between impedance change and urine volume indicated by Fig. 10-46f is 0.017 Ω/ml of urine.

The method is elegantly simple and appears to be the only noninvasive method for recording bladder emptying. The impedance-volume coefficient is high because urine has the lowest resistivity of all biological fluids. There is no reason to believe that the technique will not work in human applications, and it may be attractive in some clinical situations. With low intensity current at 100 kHz, the method is obviously nonhazardous.

The methods just described for measuring bladder volume by impedance provide a practical nonobstructive method for studying the bladder reflex. As yet only limited use has been made of these techniques.

10-16. KIDNEY VOLUME

Variations in the impedance between electrodes encompassing the kidney were described by Lofgren (1951). He found that when a solution of dextran was forced into the rat kidney a decrease in the 2-and the 200-kHz impedance occurred. He then proceeded to employ the method to study the change in kidney volume in response to injections of drugs.

10-17. UTERINE CONTRACTIONS

Kornmesser and Nyboer (1962) developed an interesting noninvasive method of recording uterine contractions during labor in the pregnant human female. The method employed is sketched in Fig. 10-47. Four silver electrodes (10-cent coins) were mounted in a band that maintained the electrodes against the abdomen in the position shown in Fig. 10-47a. A low-intensity current (100 kHz) was admitted by the two outer electrodes (I_1, I_2), and the voltage that is proportional to the impedance between the potential-measuring electrodes (E_1, E_2) was continuously recorded after amplification and demodulation.

The record of the impedance change between the two potential-measuring electrodes was called an impedance hysterogram (IHG) by the authors. A typical example of uterine contractions from a pregnant human female appears in Fig. 10-47b, along with the electrohysterogram (EHG), which is a recording of the slow changes in potential detected by electrodes on the abdomen (Larks, 1960).

On the basis of clinical observations, Kornmesser and Nyboer suggested that the recorded impedance changes were related to mechanical displacement of the uterus during contraction. Such a suggestion is not

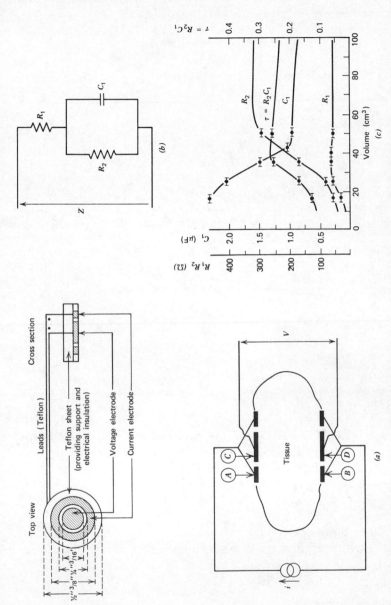

Figure 10-46. The measurement of urinary bladder volume using concentric (tetrapolar) electrodes. (*a*) The electrode system and its application to the bladder; (*b*) the equivalent circuit between the potential-measuring electrodes; (*c*) the manner in which the components of the equivalent circuit vary with bladder volume when saline is injected and withdrawn. [From M. A. Talibi, et al., *Brit. J. Urol.* **42**:56–65 (1970). By permission.] (*d*) The measurement of urinary bladder volume by impedance: electrodes applied to the outer surface of the bladder of a 50-kg dog; the interelectrode impedance is used to control the frequency of a resistance-capacity oscillator. (*e*) The impedance and frequency values for various bladder volumes with saline in the bladder. [Redrawn from Waltz et al., *IEEE Trans. Bio-Med. Eng.* **BME-18**:42–46 (1971).] (*f*) Bladder emptying in the dog. (Courtesy of J. C. Denniston and L. E. Baker.)

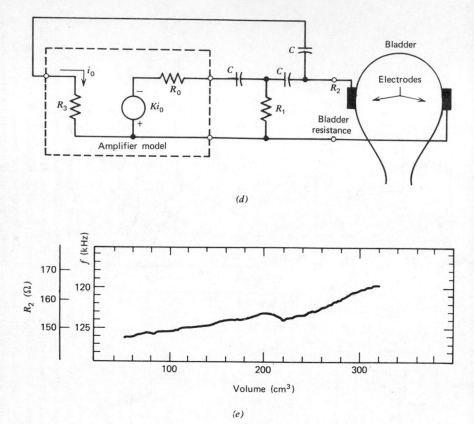

(d)

(e)

Figure 10-46(*d,e*)

without good foundation because during contraction the uterine contents (fetus and amniotic fluid) were displaced in a direction away from the potential-measuring electrodes. Amniotic fluid and urine have the lowest resistivities of all biological fluids (Geddes and Baker, 1967), and it is not surprising that displacement of this highly conducting mass is detectable with abdominal electrodes.

Impedance hysterography would appear to be a safe practical method for recording the frequency of uterine contractions with properly placed electrodes, but little use has been made of this technique.

10-18.   EYE MOVEMENTS

The position of the eye and the characteristic movements it executes are often factors of interest. Records of these events, called electrooculograms

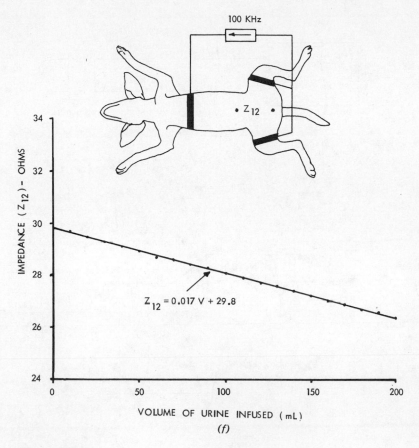

Figure 10-46(*f*)

(EOG), are described in Chapter 11. Two methods have been employed to measure eye position. In one technique, pairs of electrodes either above and below or at the inner and outer canthus of one eye detect a position-dependent component of the corneoretinal potential. The other method requires that the eye be placed in a strong magnetic field, and the voltage induced in coils embedded in a contact lens, or affixed to the sclera, are used to obtain the position-indicating signal. With this technique Robinson (1963) detected signals corresponding to vertical, lateral, and rolling movements of the eye. Fuchs and Robinson (1966) mounted a three-turn search coil to the sclera of a monkey eye and detected signals proportional to vertical and horizontal components of eye movement.

Each of the methods has its advantages and difficulties. The potential-detecting method provides a small signal which is often accompanied by

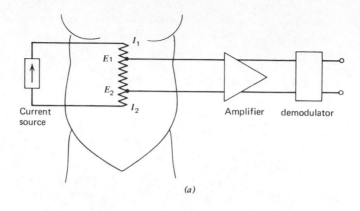

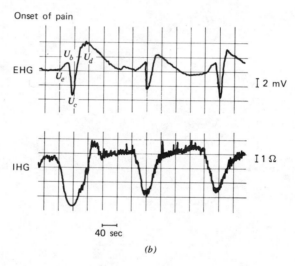

Figure 10-47. Arrangement of equipment for recording uterine contractions by impedance change, a record of which is called the impedance hysterogram (IHG). Also shown is the electrohysterogram (EHG), the voltage change that accompanies uterine contractions, detectable with electrodes placed on the abdomen. [From J. Nyboer, and J. G. Kornmesser, *Harper Hosp. Bull.* **20**:248–261 (1962). By permission.]

muscle action potentials and electrode potentials. Furthermore, Byford (1962) has reported that for horizontal eye movement there is a lack of agreement between this voltage signal and one measured by optical tracking of the eye. The more difficult method of using search coils offers high precision but requires restraint of the head, exacting techniques for fabrication of the coils, as well as complex equipment.

Sullivan and Weltman (1963) have shown that eye movements can be recorded by using the impedance method. Geddes et al. (1965) verified their observations on man and the horse. Because a signal free from electrode potentials and muscle potentials can be obtained with open or closed eyes, the technique has some attractive features. To illustrate the type of signal obtained, a pair of electrodes was placed above and below one eye of a human subject. The electrodes were connected to a direct-coupled impedance recorder and to a high-gain preamplifier to permit recording the electrooculogram along with the impedance oculogram. The upper tracing of the record obtained (Fig. 10-48) shows the impedance oculogram (ZOG); the lower, the EOG. The subject was instructed to gaze from one object to another, both in a vertical plane. In the center of the record he was told to clench his jaw. The EOG record illustrates the muscle-action potentials which are absent from the impedance tracing.

Figure 10-49 is an impedance oculogram made on a horse during the induction of anesthesia. In this and many other species there are conspicuous oscillatory eye movements during light anesthesia. The figures on the record indicate the frequency of the eye movements in oscillations per minute. Although the phenomenon is somewhat dependent on the type of anesthetic employed, many veterinarians use eyeball movements to indicate the depth of anesthesia. A record of them can serve as a means of identifying the depth of anesthesia while graphic recordings of other events are being made.

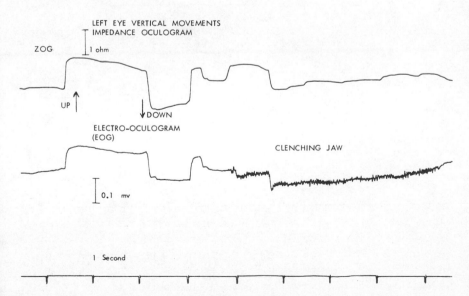

Figure 10-48. Impedance oculogram and electrooculogram from same electrodes.

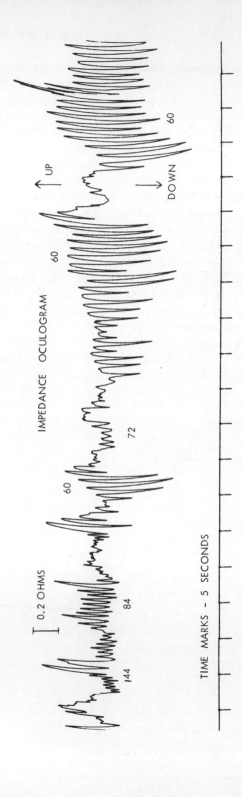

Figure 10-49. Impedance oculogram in the horse. [From Geddes, *Southwest. Vet.* **19:**23–25 (1965). By permission.]

382

Sullivan and Weltman (1963) described a nearly linear relationship between impedance change and eye position in the vertical plane. The authors have verified these observations. When the impedance method is employed to detect horizontal eye movements, the size of the signal and the linearity appear to be less. No studies have been conducted to determine the optimum location of two pairs of electrodes for obtaining purely orthogonal signals, nor have any investigations been carried out to identify the origin of the impedance change. Presumably impedance changes are due to changes in current distribution resulting from movement of the eyeball, which consists of materials of a resistivity differing from that of the surrounding tissue.

Unassociated with eye position, pulsatile impedance changes have been recorded from canine and human eyes by Bishop and Nyboer (1962). Whether these changes can be related to blood flow has not been investigated.

10-19. NERVOUS ACTIVITY

Certainly the most famous of all the impedance-change recordings is that presented by Cole and Curtis (1939), who showed (Fig. 10-50) that accompanying the action potential of nerve, there is a transient decrease in transmembrane impedance. This impedance change led directly to investigations of the ion fluxes that underlie genesis of the action potential. Impedance changes associated with the activity of cerebral neurons have been recorded with extracellular electrodes. For example, Adey et al. (1962) recorded impedance changes in dendritic layers deep within the brain using 30 μV applied to coaxial electrodes, which measured the impedance change at 1000 Hz. They found that with the electrodes in the hippocampal area of cats, arousal decreased the resistive component of the impedance by 1 to 2%. On the other hand, sleep, and anesthesia produced by pentobarbital, increased the impedance by as much as 6%. In addition to these baseline shifts rhythmic oscillations in impedance occurred in a frequency range extending from 0 to 20 Hz. More recently Kado and Adey (1965) reported dissection of the impedance changes into resistive and reactive components. While recording impedance in the amygdala, hippocampus, and midbrain reticular formation in the cat, they observed that brief alerting stimuli decreased the resistance and increased the capacitance measured between electrodes in these regions. These interesting impedance changes await correlation with other parameters of nervous activity.

The impedance changes accompanying anoxia of the brain and spinal cord of cats have been demonstrated by Van Harreveld and Biersteker

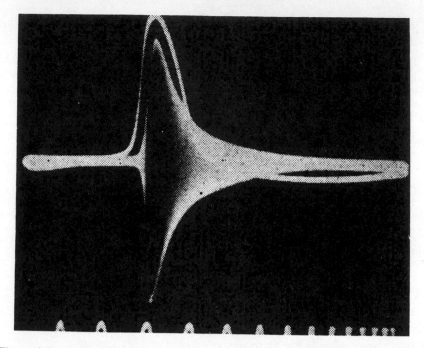

Figure 10-50. Action potential of the squid giant axon and the impedance change (10 kHz) that accompanies it, as signaled by an unbalance of the impedance bridge. Time marks 1.0 msec. [From Cole and Curtis, *J. Gen. Physiol.* **22:**649–670 (1939). By permission.]

(1963). By clamping blood vessels and causing cats to breathe nitrogen, they produced tissue anoxia that in both cases resulted in an increase of impedance amounting to 16 to 25%. Such changes were completely reproducible and reversible. Their significance at the cellular level awaits explanation.

An early study by Grant (1923) appeared to indicate some promise of applying the impedance method for locating brain tumors. Using a thin bipolar probe electrode connected to an impedance bridge, he found that as the probe was advanced into the brain, the impedance was constant until the tumor was encountered. When glioma tissue surrounded the electrodes, the impedance decreased by one-half to one-third.

10-20. MUSCULAR CONTRACTION

The contraction of the three types of muscle—cardiac, skeletal, and smooth—can easily be recorded by the impedance method.

10-20-1.   Cardiac Muscle

The isometric contraction of cardiac muscle has been demonstrated to produce an impedance change. Rosenbleuth and del Pozo (1943) measured this change between electrodes inserted into a tortoise ventricle, which was prevented from shortening. An impedance change of approximately 10%, which appeared coincident with contraction and outlasted it, was measured. The precise relationship of this impedance change to the action potential awaits further investigation.

10-20-2.   Skeletal Muscle

In many studies it is necessary to obtain a signal that indicates the contraction of skeletal muscle without measuring force. Traditionally the electromyogram has been chosen as an indicator of muscular contraction. Although this signal is related (but not proportional) to muscular contraction, in some instances it cannot be conveniently employed. Another method, described by Geddes (1966), consists of using a caliper myograph to measure the amount of lateral force development at the belly of the muscle. Frequently this method is not practical. When it is not possible to measure tension directly or to use the EMG or the caliper myograph, it may be advisable to investigate application of the impedance method to derive a signal related to muscular contraction.

The position of the tongue was transduced to an electrical signal by Petrovick and Brumlik (1961–1962) via the impedance method. With the tongue acting as one plate of a capacitor and the other plate embedded in a denture, movements of the tongue during speech were recorded. This technique may offer promise for speech therapy studies. The same authors employed the method to detect the muscular tremor in Parkinson's disease.

Dubuisson (1933) employed the impedance method to indicate muscular contraction by measuring the impedance between electrodes directly on the surface of an exposed frog gastrocnemius muscle. A record of the decreasing impedance accompanying contraction, made with needle-electrodes passed through the ends of the muscle, is shown in Fig. 10-51 (Geddes and Hoff, 1963). With this particular electrode arrangement, contraction moves the electrodes closer together and increases the cross-sectional area of muscle between them. Both factors contribute to a reduction in impedance. Electrodes placed across the belly of the muscle do not give a reliable impedance change with contraction.

The authors have detected the contraction of skeletal muscles in human subjects by measuring the impedance change between electrodes placed on the skin above the muscle. This change was used to control a solenoid valve and to operate an artificial muscle affixed to an orthosis.

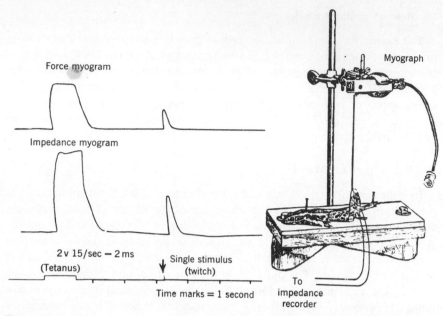

Figure 10-51. Frog muscle myogram and impedance myogram. (From Geddes and Hoff, *Proceedings of the San Diego Symposium for Biomedical Engineers,* 1963, p. 119. By permission.)

To illustrate the type of signal obtainable with the contraction of skeletal muscle in man, two pairs of electrodes were placed on the skin over the biceps muscle. One pair was placed over the origin and insertion; the other across the belly of the muscle. Impedance changes were recorded at 50 kHz while the subject contracted the muscle voluntarily. The records obtained are given in Fig. 10-52. With the electrodes placed along the muscle, a standing subject lifted and lowered a 5-lb weight from a position of full extension of the elbow through an angle of approximately 90 degrees. The EMG and impedance changes were recorded from the same electrodes. In the lower part of the record, below the time line, are the recordings obtained from electrodes over the belly of the muscle. In the first portion of the record the weight was clamped, resulting in isometric contraction of the muscle. Just past the middle of the record, the weight was released and the muscle contracted isotonically.

When the impedance method is employed to record the contraction of skeletal muscle, great care must be exercised in placing the electrodes and in interpreting the records. The impedance change is not necessarily proportional to the force or the amount of shortening. The electrodes measure only the impedance between them, which during muscular contraction may

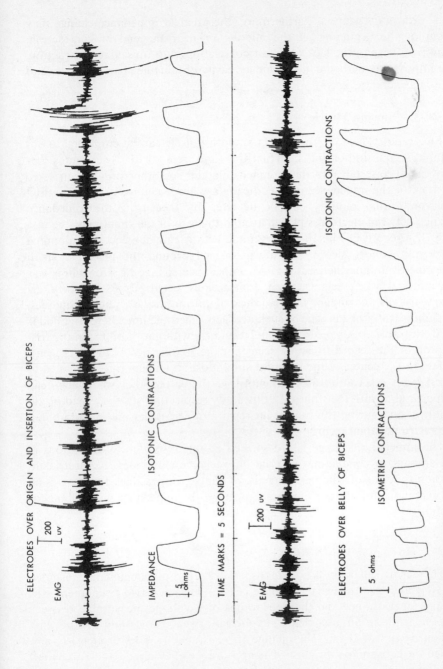

ELECTRODES OVER ORIGIN AND INSERTION OF BICEPS

EMG

$\left[\begin{array}{c}200 \\ uv\end{array}\right.$

IMPEDANCE   ISOTONIC CONTRACTIONS

$\left[\begin{array}{c}5 \\ ohms\end{array}\right.$

TIME MARKS = 5 SECONDS

ELECTRODES OVER BELLY OF BICEPS

EMG

$\left[\begin{array}{c}200 \ uv\end{array}\right.$

ISOTONIC CONTRACTIONS

ISOMETRIC CONTRACTIONS

$\left[\begin{array}{c}5 \ ohms\end{array}\right.$

Figure 10-52. Impedance myograms and the EMG.

387

vary with many factors. Furthermore, the greatest impedance change may occur at the beginning, at the middle, or near the end of contraction. However, despite the lack of direct correlation with muscular contraction, the impedance method can provide an easily obtainable signal indicative of muscular activity.

10-20-3. Smooth Muscle

Electrodes placed on, in, or over smooth muscle can be employed to obtain a signal indicating contractions and relaxation. Electrodes appropriately inserted into the stomach, bladder, or other organs can serve to monitor the impedance change during a volume change or deformation. Gastrointestinal motility can be detected by measuring the impedance change between electrodes placed around the wall of the small intestine of a dog. The record in Fig. 10-53 was made with a pair of electrodes mounted in a split rubber sleeve, which was placed around the proximal small intestine of an anesthetized dog. An impedance change of a few ohms was encountered when segmentation contractions occurred. Respiratory artifacts usually accompany the recording of gut motility by other techniques; to demonstrate the absence of such artifacts when the impedance method is used, respiration was recorded simultaneously with gut motility. In the first portion of the record it can be seen that the frequencies of the two events differ. In the center of the record a small dose of epinephrine was given to arrest both respiration and gut motility; thereafter, the two phenomena reappeared at different times. In this study respiration started ahead of gut motility, and during this period no respiratory artifacts are identifiable in the gastrointestinal recording.

The impedance change just described is obviously due to alterations in the amount of conducting material between the electrodes. Accurate calibration in terms of volume change is, of course, impossible; however, as an indirect indicator of gastrointestinal motility, the impedance method may be useful.

10-21. GALVANIC SKIN REFLEX

The terms galvanic skin response (GSR) [or psychogalvanic response (PGR)] and electrodermal response (EDR) designate two phenomena: the change in resistance and the appearance of a voltage measurable between one electrode in an area richly supplied by sweat glands and another in a region devoid of them. The change in resistance (the Féré effect) is now called the exosomatic response. The appearance of a voltage (the Tarchanoff phenomenon) is now termed the endosomatic response (see Chapter 11).

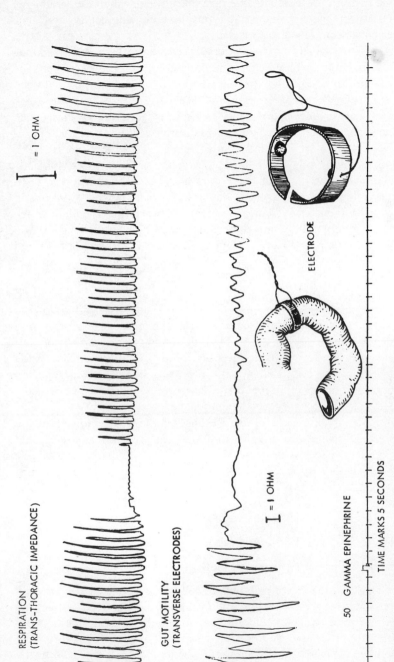

RESPIRATION
(TRANS-THORACIC IMPEDANCE)

$I = 1$ OHM

GUT MOTILITY
(TRANSVERSE ELECTRODES)

$I = 1$ OHM

ELECTRODE

50   GAMMA EPINEPHRINE

TIME MARKS 5 SECONDS

Figure 10-53.   Gastrointestinal motility detected by impedance change.

389

Both events appear in response to an emotional stimulus and reflect a change in the activity of the autonomic nervous system. Frequently, only the resistance change component is recorded.

Although direct current is usually employed to measure the resistance change, it is possible to observe the phenomenon by using the impedance method. The limiting frequency for its detection by impedance has not been established. McLendon and Hemingway (1930) observed that the GSR measured by dc resistance change was 45 times larger than the impedance change measured at 1.5 MHz. The two measurements were carried out simultaneously on human subjects. Using frequencies as high as 10 kHz, Forbes and Landis (1935) were able to detect the GSR in a few subjects. They pointed out, however, that there were gross individual differences. In some subjects the upper frequency was 1 kHz. Both Forbes (1936) and Montagu (1958) found a good correspondence between the potential change (endosomatic signal) and the impedance change in the low frequency region below 100 Hz. Nichols and Daroge (1955), Tolles and Carberry (1959), and Taylor (1962) called attention to the advantages of using alternating current in minimizing electrode polarization problems in detecting the GSR. Nichols and Daroge employed 60 Hz, Tolles and Carberry used 5 Hz, and Taylor used 65 Hz. Nichols and Daroge stated that the amplitude of the GSR decreased with increasing frequency and that there is little response with frequencies above 1 kHz. At 60 Hz they found the response to be half that which is measured when using direct current. A similar decrease in the amplitude of the impedance change with increasing frequency was reported by Yokota and Fujimori (1962). More research must be carried out to correlate the effect of frequency on the impedance change with the resistive and voltaic components of the GSR. Because of the low frequency of the GSR signal, high-gain direct-coupled amplifiers are traditionally used, and drift has frequently been a problem. If the exosomatic component of the GSR can be adequately measured with alternating current, carrier amplifiers can be used to provide high stability and a high signal-to-noise ratio.

10-22.   THE RESISTIVITY OF BLOOD

10-22-1.   The Volume of Cells in a Sample

Blood is a suspension of red cells, white cells, and platelets in plasma, an electrolyte containing a myriad of other dissolved and suspended substances. The percentage of cells in a blood sample is called the packed-cell volume (H). Because the red cells are by far the most numerous, their percentage, which is called the hematocrit, is very nearly equal to the packed-cell volume, except in certain disease states. Blood cells themselves contain electrolytes surrounded by an insulating membrane; therefore the resistivity of a blood sample is dependent on its packed cell volume (H). Blood is an electrolyte, and its resistivity is dependent on temperature. Moreover, because of the capacitive nature of the cell membranes, the resistivity is dependent on the frequency of measurement.

Maxwell (1873, 1904) developed an expression for the resistivity of a suspension of spheres of known resistivity in an electrolyte of known resistivity. Fricke (1925), by including a form factor (f), extended the Maxwell expression to allow its application to suspensions of nonspherical particles. The Maxwell-Fricke expression for the resistivity ρ of a suspension of blood cells in plasma of resistivity ρ_p with a packed-cell volume of $H\%$ is

$$\rho = \rho_p \frac{1 + (f - 1)H/100}{1 - H/100}$$

The form factor (f) for spheres is 1.5. It has been shown by Cole et al. (1969) that the Maxwell-Fricke expression is valid over a considerable range for a suspension of particles of various shapes, including rods. Figure 10-54 plots the foregoing expression for various form factors (f). For convenience, the ratio of ρ/ρ_p is plotted versus packed-cell volume (H). It will

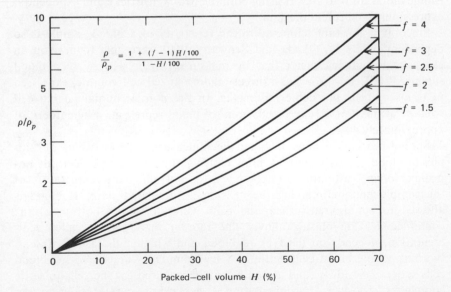

Figure 10-54. The Maxwell-Fricke expression for the resistivity of a blood sample (ρ) in terms of plasma resistivity (ρ_p) and a form factor (f) and packed-cell volume (H).

be of interest to compare the shapes of these curves and those obtained by measurement of blood samples.

Because a semilogarithmic plot of resistivity versus packed-cell volume is nearly linear, an exponential representation of the form $\rho = Ae^{\alpha H/100}$, where A and α have values for the type of blood and H is the packed-cell volume, can be employed. Note that the Maxwell-Fricke expression predicts an infinite value for the resistivity of a sample of packed cells ($H = 100\%$); the exponential representation predicts a finite value for packed cells. Since a H above 80 is usually incompatible with life, either expression can be used to represent the relationship between resistivity and H. Ease of calculation of course favors the Maxwell-Fricke expression; however, a form factor must be chosen for its use. The exponential representation is easier to derive from measured data using the least-squares method, and it does not require selection or determination of the form factor.

Values for the resistivities of blood samples have been presented in reviews by Schwan (1963) and Geddes and Baker (1967). However resistivity data for body temperature are not common. At present, values for body temperature (37°C) are available for human blood at 1 kHz (Rosenthal and Tobias, 1948), and for dog blood at 100 kHz (Kinnen et al., 1964) and at 25 kHz (Geddes and Sadler, 1973). The values obtained in these studies are presented in Table 10-7. Figure 10-55 shows the type of relationship for canine blood for 0 to 70% H using both the Maxwell-Fricke and exponential expressions to represent the data.

Since at a constant temperature the resistivity of a blood sample is so dependent on its H, Okada and Schwan (1960) were able to develop an electrical hematocrit meter that by measuring the resistivity of a blood sample of 0.02 ml, provided a direct reading in red cell volume, expressed in terms of cells per cubic millimeter. In the normal human, a red cell concentration of 5×10^6 red cells/mm³ of blood represents a hematocrit of approximately 40%.

Special precautions must be taken when measuring the resistivity of samples of blood. Apart from preventing clotting and eliminating electrode impedance errors, attention must be given to controlling the temperature of the sample and maintaining the cells in a suspended state. If blood is allowed to stand undisturbed, the cells will fall to the bottom of the container, leaving plasma above. The rate of this process, called sedimentation, depends on the type of blood and whether disease is present. Normal equine blood cells settle in a few minutes, whereas bovine blood cells settle very slowly, and a month may be required for the cells to settle completely. The rate of sedimentation is increased in certain diseases, and "sed rate" has been used as a diagnostic measurement.

Sedimentation rate has been measured by resistivity change by Nelson and Wilkinson (1972). The conductivity cell, which contained multiple

Table 10-7   Resistivity of Blood at Body Temperature

Species	Maxwell-Fricke Expression	Exponential Expression	Frequency (kHz)	Reference
Human		$62.9e^{0.0195H}$	1	Rosenthal and Tobias (1948)
Human	$\dfrac{58.0(1 + 0.75H/100)}{(1 - H/100)}$	$53.2e^{0.022H}$	25	Geddes and Sadler (1973)
Canine		$56.6e^{0.022H}$	100	Kinnen et al. (1964)
Canine	$\dfrac{58.6(1 + 1.25H)}{(1 - H/100)}$	$53.7e^{0.025H}$	25	Geddes and Sadler (1973)
Bovine	$\dfrac{58.3(1 + 0.5H/100)}{(1 - H/100)}$	$54.2e^{0.020H}$	25	Geddes and Sadler (1973)
Equine	$\dfrac{61.5(1 + H/100)}{(1 - H/100)}$	$57.0e^{0.024H}$	25	Geddes and Sadler (1973)
Sheep		$55.6e^{0.020H}$	25	Geddes and Sadler (1973)
Camel		$56.4e^{0.0162H}$	25	Geddes and Sadler (1973)

platinum electrodes, measured 1 × 0.3 cm by 10.3 cm in height. The resistivity change showed a characteristic pattern with time as the cells settled. Attractive as this method appears, the authors pointed out that the optimum cell design had not been achieved.

Mention was made earlier of the importance of temperature control in resistivity measurement. Blood, like most electrolytes, exhibits a negative temperature coefficient of resistivity amounting to about 2%/°C.

10-22-2.   Blood Clotting by Resistivity Measurement

Impedance changes have been shown to accompany the clotting of blood. Rosenthal and Tobias (1948) measured such changes at 1 kHz in a thermostatistically controlled chamber in which a blood sample was placed. They noted an increase in resistivity after 5 min as the blood clot was forming. Blood samples treated with anticoagulants exhibited no such changes within a 1-hr period. The investigators noted the absence, with this technique, of the changes in clotting time that occur with motion of the blood. Henstell (1949) continued these studies, using 60 Hz with particular

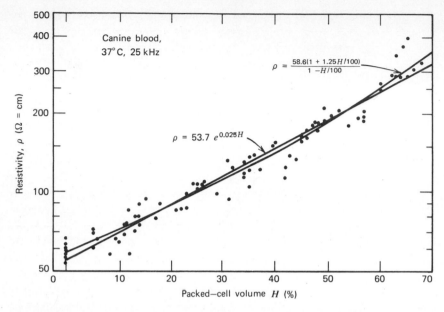

Figure 10-55. The specific resistance of canine blood at 37°C and 25 kHz versus packed-cell volume (H) represented by the Maxwell-Fricke relationship (using a form factor of 2.25) and the exponential expression. [From Geddes and Sadler, *IEEE Trans. Bio.-Med. Eng.* **BME-11**:336–339 (1973). By permission.]

interest in the configuration of the electrodes. He found a circular loop with a horizontal crossbar to be the optimum shape. Using these electrodes he plotted impedance versus time curves over a 48-hr period. He reported that with his electrodes the normal clot resistance for adult white males is 311 ±44.4 Ω and for adult white females 179 ±33.5 Ω. The impedance clotting time was found to be 10.3 ±1.0 min for normal males and 9.5 ±0.94 min for normal females. He also noted changes in the impedance-clotting relationship in diseases of the blood.

An interesting conductivity cell for measuring coagulation time and clot retraction was described by Haley and Stolarsky (1951). Their conductivity cell contained a needle and plate electrode and accommodated 0.8 ml of blood. Impedance-time measurements were made at 10 kHz and at room temperature. The typical recording showed four transition points, and the second coincided with the occurrence of fibrin formation (verified by visual observation). The third transition correlated with clot formation, and the fourth with clot retraction. The largest change in impedance accompanied clot retraction; only small changes were associated with fibrin and clot formation.

A different approach to determine clotting time was taken by Richardson and Bishop (1957). The blood was contained in a tube fitted with two rod electrodes, and the assembly was placed on a platform that oscillated ±45 degrees from the horizontal, six times per minute. A record of the 60-Hz impedance change showed a sharp transition at the time that the clot was formed.

Mungall et al. (1961) continued studies of the impedance changes in clotting blood. Using 100 kHz and a thermostatically controlled conductivity cell, they recorded resistive and reactive changes in blood over a 100-min period. Their records, made on normal subjects and patients with blood disorders, revealed several transitional points that await clarification.

In using impedance to detect blood clotting, attention must be directed toward other factors that produce impedance change. Paramount among these are temperature and sedimentation rate. The design of a blood-containing cell must be such that no impedance change is produced by these two factors. Although temperature control is easily achieved, special care must be devoted to proper design of the electrodes to eliminate errors due to sedimentation. An interesting solution to both problems was presented by Ur (1970), who designed a differential system employing two conductivity cells; in one a sample of untreated blood was placed, and in the other was placed a sample of the same blood, to which an anticoagulant had been added. The two cells formed two arms of an impedance bridge. With the passage of time, a characteristic difference in impedance was obtained which allowed determination of clotting time.

10-22-3.   Blood Velocity by Resistivity Measurement

The resistivity of an unsedimented blood sample depends on temperature, packed-cell volume, frequency, and type of blood. Since the resistivity of packed cells (ca. 500 Ω-cm) is so much higher than plasma (ca. 70 Ω-cm), any situation that can cause an increased fraction of the measuring current to flow through the plasma will decrease the resistivity of the sample. Consistent with this fact, it has been found that imparting flow to a blood sample results in a redistribution of cells and plasma and a reduction in resistivity. This effect has been reported by Sigman et al. (1937), Velick and Gorin (1940), Coulter and Pappenheimer (1949), Molnar et al. (1953), Moskalenko and Naumenko (1959), and Liebman and Cosenza (1962). All these studies have shown that the decrease in resistivity is related to velocity of flow, the reduction decreasing linearly as the blood starts to move; then the decrease becomes less with increasing velocity, and soon there is no further decrease in resistivity. This work has also demonstrated that the magnitude of the reduction in resistivity dends on the percentage of cells; plasma alone exhibits no reduction in resistivity with increasing velocity. The study by Pappenheimer and Coulter showed that with increasing flow velocity, the cells tend to accumulate in the axial stream which is surrounded by a plasma sheath that preferentially carries the current. In pulsatile flow there is not only a pulsatile variation in axial concentration of cells, but their orientation varies; hence quite large amplitude variations in resistivity can be measured by pulsatile flow through a rigid conductivity cell.

Even though the resistivity versus flow velocity relationship is nonlinear, it has been used to record blood flow. Sugano and Oda (1960) measured flow-dependent impedance changes with perivascular electrodes and also with electrodes thrust into vessels. They obtained excellent recordings but admitted that flow calibration was difficult. Liebman and Cosenza measured blood flow velocity in teeth using a miniature tetrapolar electrode array implanted into canine teeth.

Although a decrease in impedance can be recorded which reflects flow velocity, calibration is difficult. The few impedance-flow calibrations made to date indicate a considerable nonlinearity between these two quantities. However, the practical applicability of the method cannot be denied.

In explosive decompression studies, the tiny bubbles that appear in the venous system were recorded by Leverett (1962), using the impedance method. The impedance of blood flowing in a vein was measured by electrodes placed outside the vessel. The passage of air bubbles altered the impedance considerably, giving a semiquantitative indication of their presence.

10-23. BLOOD PRESSURE IN MICROVESSELS

A very interesting application of the impedance method to measure blood pressure in tiny vessels is due to Wiederhelm and Rushmer (1964), who employed a micropipet (0.5 to 5 μ in diameter) as the sensor. It was filled with 2 M saline and connected to an electrical actuator that could apply pressure to the saline. The saline in the pipet and the blood in a tiny blood vessel of frog mesentery constituted an electrical resistance, the value of which depended on the position of the saline-blood interface in the micro tip. The micropipet-animal resistance constituted one arm of a 1000-Hz impedance bridge. The detector consisted of an amplifier connected to the actuator. The bridge was then balanced and set to hunt for a fixed position of the meniscus. The current driving the actuator, which constantly rebalanced the bridge, was proportional to the blood pressure. The system exhibited a response time of .35 msec to a step function of pressure. The remarkably clean and faithful records revealed a blood pressure of 20/15 mm Hg in the microcirculation of the frog mesentry.

10-24. SALIVATION

An increase in the impedance of the canine submaxillary salivary gland accompanying secretion was noted by Bronk and Gesell (1926). Nervous stimulation and drug-induced salivation produced an impedance change of slightly more than 10% just before the appearance of saliva.

10-25. CONCLUSION

The flexibility of the impedance method to detect a wide variety of physiological events is its chief attribute. Its chief drawback is the difficulty encountered in calibrating the impedance in true physiological terms. At present many studies are underway to establish the relationship between impedance values and physiological events. In many, the signals are being dissected into their resistive and reactive components, with a view to determining which component contains the more meaningful information. It is too soon, however, to draw conclusions regarding the true value of the impedance method for the measurement of physiological events.

In conclusion, a word of caution is addressed to those who will investigate the use of impedance or impedance changes as a means of transduction. In every study adequate care must be exercised to guarantee that the change in impedance measured between the electrodes is due to the physiological event investigated and is not an artifact caused by changes in impedance at the electrode-electrolyte-tissue interface. In addition, the safety of the subject must be borne in mind.

REFERENCES

Abramson, D. L. 1944. *Vascular Responses in the Extremities of Man in Health and Disease.* University of Chicago Press, Chicago.

Adey, W. R., R. T. Kado, and J. Didio. 1962. Impedance measurements in brain tissue using microvolt signals. *Exp. Neurol.* 5:47–60.

Adrian, E. D. 1919. The response to human sensory nerves to currents of short duration. *J. Physiol.* 53:70–85.

Alexander, L. 1938. Electrical injuries to the central nervous system. *Med. Clin. N. Am.* 22:663–688.

Allison, R. D. 1962. Volumetric dynamics of respiration as measured by electrical impedance. Ph.D. thesis, Wayne University, Detroit, Mich.

Allison, R. D. 1966. Arterial-venous volume gradients as predictive indices of vascular dynamics. *Instrumentation Methods for Predictive Medicine.* T. B. Weber and J. Poyer (eds.). Instrumentation Society of America, 215 pp.

Allison, R. D. 1966. Stroke volume, cardiac output and impedance measurements. *Proc. Ann. Conf. Eng. Med. Biol.* paper 8.5.

Allison, R. D., E. L. Holmes, and J. Nyboer. 1964. Volumetric dynamics of respiration as measured by electrical impedance plethysmography. *J. Appl. Physiol.* **19**:166-173.

Allison, R. D., and J. Nyboer. 1965. The electrical plethysomography determination of pulse volume and flow in ionic circulatory systems. *New Istanbul. Center Clin. Sci.* **7**:281-306.

Anderson, A. B., and W. A. Munson. 1951. Electrical excitation of nerves in the skin at audiofrequencies. *J. Acoust. Soc. Am.* **23**:155-159.

d'Arsonval, A. 1893a. Action physiologique des courants alternatifs à grande fréquence. *Arch. Physiol. Norm. Pathol.* **5**:401-408; 789-790.

d'Arsonval, A. 1893b. Influence de la fréquencies sur les effets physiologiques des courants alternatifs. *Comptes Rendus.* **116**:630-633.

Atzler, E. 1933. Neues Verfahren zur Funktionsbeurteilung des Herzens. *Deut. Med. Wochenschr.* **59**:1347-1349.

Atzler, E. 1935. Dielektrographie. *Hand. Biolog. Arbeitsmethod.* **5**:1073-1084.

Atzler, E. and G. Lehmann. 1932. Über ein neues Verfahren zur Darstellung der Herztätigkeit (Dielektrographie). *Arbeitsphysiologie* **5**:636-680.

Ax, A. F., R., Andreski, R. Courter, C. DiGiovanni, S. Herman, D. Lucas, and W. Orrick. 1964. Measurement of respiration by telemeter impedance strain gauge and spirometer. *Proc. ISA 2nd Nat. Biomed. Sci. Instr. Symp.* pp. 1-12.

Bache, R. J., A. Harley, and J. C. Greenfield. 1969. Evaluation of thoracic impedance plethysmography as an indicator of stroke volume in man. *Am. J. Med. Sci.* **258**:100-113.

Bagno, S. 1959. Impedance measurements of living tissue. *Electronics* **32**:62-63.

Baker, L. E. 1962. Impedance spirometry. SWIRECO Conference, Houston, Texas, April.

Baker, L. E., and L. A. Geddes. 1965. Quantitative evaluation of impedance spirometry in man. *Am. J. Med. Electr.* **4**:73-77.

Baker, L. E., and L. A. Geddes. 1966. Transthoracic current paths in impedance spirometry. *Proc. Symp. Biomed. Eng.* Marquette University, Milwaukee, **1**:181-186.

Baker, L. E., and L. A. Geddes. 1970. The measurement of current density distribution in biological materials. *Proc. 2nd Int. Symp. Electrother. Sleep Electroanesth. Graz, Austria. Excerpta Med.* **11**:3-11.

Baker, L. E., and L. A. Geddes. 1971. Factors affecting the measurement of current density distribution in living tissue. *Neuroelectric Research.* D. V. Reynolds and A. E. Sjoberg, (eds.). Charles C Thomas, Springfield, Ill.

Baker, L. E., L. A. Geddes, and H. E. Hoff. 1966. A comparison of linear and non-linear characterizations of impedance spirometry. *Med. Biol. Eng.* **4**:371-379.

Baker, L. E., L. A. Geddes, H. E. Hoff, and C. J. Chaput. 1966. Physiological factors underlying transthoracic impedance variations in respiration. *J. Appl. Physiol.* **21**:1491-1499.

Baker, L. E., W. V. Judy, L. E. Geddes, F. M. Langley, and D. W. Hill. 1971. The measurement of cardiac output by means of electrical impedance. *Cardiovasc. Res. Center Bull.* **9**:135-145.

Barnett, A. 1937. The basic factors involved in proposed electrical methods for measuring thyroid function (parts I–IV). *West. J. Surg. Obstet. Gynecol.* **45**:322-326, 380-387, 540-554, 612-623.

Barnett, A. 1938. The phase angle of the normal human skin. *J. Physiol.* **93**:349-366.

Barnett, A. 1940. Seasonal variations in the epidermal impedance of human skin. *Am. J. Physiol.* **129**:306-307.

Beecher, H. 1959. *Measurement of Subjective Responses.* Oxford University Press, New York.

Berman, I. R., W. L. Sehertz, E. B. Jenkens, and H. V. Hufnagel. 1971. Transthoracic electrical impedance as a guide to intravascular overload. *Arch. Surg.* 102:61–64.

Bernstein, T. 1973. A grand success. *IEEE Spectrum* 10:54–58.

Bishop, S., and J. Nyboer. 1962. Electrical impedance plethysmography of canine and human eyes. *Harper Hosp. Bull.* 20:142–151.

Bonjer, F. H., J. van der Berg, and M. N. J. Dirken. 1952. The origin of the variations of body impedance occurring during the cardiac cycle. *Circulation* 1:415–420.

Bouty, E. 1884. Sur la conductibilité électrique de dissolutions salines très étendues. *J. Phys.* 2:325–355.

Brazier, M. A. B. 1935. The impedance angle test for thyrotoxicosis. *West. J. Surg. Obstetr. Gynecol.* 43:429–441, 514–527.

Brazier, M. A. B. 1960. *The Electrical Activity of the Nervous System.* Macmillan, New York, 273 pp.

Brodie, T. G., and A. E. Russell. 1905. On the determination of the rate of blood flow through an organ. *J. Physiol.* 33:XLVII–XLVIII.

Bronk, D. W., and G. Gesell. 1926. Electrical conductivity, electrical potential and hydrogen ion concentration measurements on the submaxillary gland of the dog recorded with continuous photographic methods. *Am. J. Physiol.* 77:570–589.

Brook, D. L. and P. Cooper. 1957. The impedance plethysmograph—Its clinical application. *Surgery* 42:1061–1070.

Brooks, C. McC., B. F. Hoffman, E. E. Suckling, and O. Orias. 1955. *Excitability of the Heart.* Grune & Stratton, New York, 373 pp.

Burch, G. E. 1944. Sensitive portable plethysmograph. In *Methods in Medical Research,* vol. I. V. R. Potter (ed.) Year Book Publishers, Chicago.

Burns, R. C. 1950. Study of skin impedance. *Electronics* 23:190–196.

Byford, G. H. 1962a. Non-linear relations between the corneo-retinal potential and horizontal eye movements. *J. Physiol.* 168:14P–15P.

Byford, G. H. 1962b. A sensitive contact lens photoelectric eye movement recorder. *IRE Trans. Bio-Med. Elect.* 4:236–243.

Campbell, B. A., and R. Teghtsoonian. 1958. Electrical and behavioral effects of different types of shock stimuli on the rat. *J. Comp. Physiol. Psychol.* 51:185–192.

Carter, C. W. 1925. Graphic representation of the impedance of networks containing resistances and two reactances. *Bell Syst. Tech. J.* 4:387–400.

Chinard, F. P., T. Enns, and M. F. Nolan. 1962. Indicator-dilution studies with "diffusible" indicators. *Circ. Res.* 10:473–490.

Cole, K. S. 1929. Electric impedance of suspensions of spheres. *J. Gen. Physiol.* 12:29–36.

Cole, K. S. 1933. Electrical conductance of biological systems. *Cold Spring Harbor Symp. Quant. Biol.* 1:107–116.

Cole, K. S. 1968. *Membranes, Ions and Impulses.* University of California Press, Berkeley and Los Angeles.

Cole, K. S., and H. J. Curtis. 1939. Electric impedance of the squid giant axon during activity. *J. Gen. Physiol.* 22:649–670.

Cole, K. S., and R. M. Guttman. 1942. Electric impedance of the frog egg. *J. Gen. Physiol.* 25:765–775.

Cole, K. S., C. L. Li, and A. E. Bak. 1969. Electrical analogues for tissues. *Exp. Neurol.* **24**:459–473.

Cooley, W. L., and R. C. Longini. 1968. A new design for an impedance pneumograph. *J. Appl. Physiol.* **25**:429–432.

Coulter, N., and J. R. Pappenheimer. 1949. Development of turbulence in flowing blood. *Am. J. Physiol.* **159**:401–408.

Crile, G. W., H. R. Hosmer, and A. F. Rowland. 1922. The electrical conductivity of animal tissues under normal and pathological conditions. *Am. J. Physiol.* **60**:59–106.

Dalziel, C. F. 1956. Effects of electric shock on man. *IRE Trans. Med. Electron.* **PGME-5**:44–62.

Davis, H., and A. Forbes. 1936. Chronaxie. *Physiol. Rev.* **16**:407–441.

Denniston, J. C. and L. E. Baker. 1975. Measurement of urinary bladder emptying using electrical impedance. *Med. Biol. Eng.* **13**:305–306.

Deuvaert, F. E., J. R. Dmochowsky, and N. P. Couch. 1973. Positional factors in venous impedance plethysmography. *Arch. Surg.* **106**:43–55.

Dmochowski, J. R., D. F. Adams, and N. P. Couch. 1972. Impedance measurements in the diagnosis of deep venous thrombosis. *Arch. Surg.* **104**:170–173.

Dove, G. B., B. E. Mount, and J. M. Van De Water. 1971. Bioelectric impedance-clinical applications. *J. Am. Assoc. Adv. Med. Instr.* **5**:111.

Dove, G. B., J. M. Van De Water, and R. W. Horst, 1971. The application of impedance to the intensive care patient. *Proc. San Diego Symp. Biomed. Eng.* **10**:161–166.

Dubuisson, M. 1933. Recherches sur les modifications que surviennent dans la conducibilité électrique du muscle au cours de la contraction. *Arch. Intern. Physiol.* **37**:35–57.

Farzaneh, T. 1953. Endocrine factors influencing impedance and impedance angle. Ph.D. thesis, Ohio State University, 124 pp.

Fenning, C. 1936–1937. A new method for recording physiological activities. I. *J. Lab. Clin. Med.* **22**:1279–1280.

Fenning, C., and B. E. Bonnar. 1936–1937. A new method for recording physiological activities, II. *J. Lab. Clin. Med.* **22**:1280–1284.

Fenning, C., and B. E. Bonnar. 1939. Additional recordings with the oscillato-capacitograph. *J. Lab. Clin. Med.* **25**:175–179.

Ferris, L. P., B. G. King, P. W. Spence, and H. B. Williams. 1936. Effect of electric shock on the heart. *Elect. Eng.* **85**:498–515.

Forbes, T. W. 1936. Skin potential and impedance response. *Am. J. Physiol.* **117**:189–199.

Forbes, T. W., and A. L. Bernstein. 1935. The standardization of sixty-cycle electric shock for practical use in psychological experimentation. *J. Gen. Psychol.* **12**:436–442.

Forbes, T. W., and C. Landis. 1935. The limiting AC frequency for the exhibition of the galvanic skin (psychogalvanic) response. *J. Gen. Psychol.* **13**:188–193.

Fredericq, H. 1928. Chronaxie. *Physiol. Rev.* **8**:501–544.

Fricke, H. 1924. A mathematical treatment of the electrical conductivity of colloids and cell suspensions. *J. Gen. Physiol.* **6**:375–384.

Fricke, H. 1925. A mathematical treatment of the electric conductivity and capacity of disperse systems. *Phys. Rev.* (Ser. 2), **24**:575–587.

Fuchs, A. F., and D. A. Robinson. 1966. A method for measuring horizontal and vertical eye movement chronically in the monkey. *J. Appl. Physiol.* **21**:1068–1070.

Gazzaniga, A. B., R. H. Bartlett, and J. B. Shobe. 1973. Bilateral impedance rheography in deep venous thrombosis. *Arch. Surg.* **106**:835–837.

Gazzaniga, A. B., A. F. Pacela, R. H. Bartlett, and T. R. Geraghty. 1972. Bilateral impedance rheography in the diagnosis of deep vein thrombosis of the legs. *Arch. Surg.* **104**:515–519.

Geddes, L. A. 1962. Recording respiration and the EKG with common electrodes. *Aerosp. Med.* **33**:791–793.

Geddes, L. A. 1973. Measurement of electrolytic resistivity and electrode-electrolyte impedance with a variable-length conductivity cell. *Chem. Instr.* **4**:157–168.

Geddes, L. A., and L. E. Baker. 1967. The specific resistance of biological material—A compendium of data for the biomedical engineer and physiologist. *Med. Biol. Eng.* **5**:271–293.

Geddes, L. A. and L. E. Baker. 1969. Hazards in the use of low frequencies for the measurement of physiological events by impedance. *Med. Biol. Eng.* **7**:289–296.

Geddes, L. A. and L. E. Baker. 1971. Response to the passage of electric current through the body. *J. Assoc. Adv. Med. Instr.* **5**:13–18.

Geddes, L. E., and L. E. Baker. 1972. Thoracic impedance changes following saline ejection into right and left ventricles. *J. Appl. Physiol.* **33**:278–281.

Geddes, L. A., P. Cabler, A. G. Moore, J. Rosborough, and W. A. Tacker, 1973. Threshold 60-Hz current required for ventricular fibrillation in subjects of various body weights. *IEEE Trans. Bio-Med. Eng.* **BME-20**:465–468.

Geddes, L. A., and C. P. DaCosta. 1973. The specific resistance of canine blood at body temperature. *IEEE Trans. Bio-Med. Eng.* **BME-20**(1):51–53.

Geddes, L. A., C. P. DaCosta, and L. E. Baker. 1972. Electrical calibration of the saline-conductivity method for cardiac output. *Cardiovasc. Res. Center. Bull.* **10**(3):91–106.

Geddes, L. A., C. P. DaCosta, and G. Wise. 1971. The impedance of stainless-steel electrodes. *Med. Biol. Eng.* **9**:511–521.

Geddes, L. A. and H. E. Hoff. 1963. The measurement of physiological events by impedance change. *Proc. San Diego Symp. Bio-Med. Eng.* **3**:115–122. La Jolla, Calif. See also *Am. J. Med. Electron. 1964*, **3**:16–27.

Geddes, L. A. and H. E. Hoff. 1965. Continuous measurement of stroke volume of the left and right ventricles by impedance. International Conference on Medical Electronics and Biological Engineering, Tokyo, 1965. *Japan. Heart J.* **7**:556–565.

Geddes, L. A., H. E. Hoff, C. W. Hall, and H. D. Millar. 1964. Rheoencephalography. *Cardiovas. Res. Center Bull.* **2**:112–121.

Geddes, L. A., H. E. Hoff, D. M. Hickman, and A. G. Moore. 1962. The impedance pneumograph. *Aerosp. Med.* **33**:28–33.

Geddes, L. A., and H. E. Hoff, Marey, and Chauveau. 1962. Annual Report, NIH Grant HTS 5125—*Classical Physiology with Modern Instrumentation*. The Heart Institute, National Institute of Health, 53 pp.

Geddes, L. A., H. E. Hoff, A. Mello, and C. Palmer. 1966. Continuous measurement of ventricular stroke volume by electrical impedance. *Cardiovas. Res. Center Bull.* **4**:118–130.

Geddes, L. A., H. E. Hoff, A. Moore, and M. Hinds. 1966. An electrical caliper myograph. *Am. J. Pharm. Ed.* **30**:209–211.

Geddes, L. A., J. D. McCrady, and H. E. Hoff. 1965. The impedance nystagmogram—A record of the level of anesthesia in the horse. *Southwest. Vet.* **19**:23–25.

Geddes, L. A., E. Peery, and R. Steinberg. 1974. Cardiac output using an electrically calibrated flow-through conductivity cell. *J. Appl. Physiol.* **37**:972–977.

Geddes, L. A. and C. Sadler. 1973. The specific resistance of blood at body temperature. *Med. Biol. Eng.* **11**:336–339.

Gibson, R. H. 1963. Requirements for the use of electrical stimulation of the skin. *Proc. Int. Congr. Technol. Blindness* **2**:183–207.

Gilmer, B. von H. 1937. The sensitivity of the finger to alternating electrical current. *Am. J. Psychol.* **49**:444–449.

Gilmer, B. von H. 1961. Toward cutaneous electropulse communication. *J. Physiol.* **52**:211–222.

Goetzl, F. R., D. Y. Burrill, and A. C. Ivy. 1943. A critical analysis of algesimetric methods with suggestions for a useful procedure. *Quart. Bull. Northwestern Univ.* **17**:280–291.

Goldensohn, E. S., and L. Zablow. 1959. And electrical impedance spirometer. *J. Appl. Physiol.* **14**:463–464.

Goodwin, R. S., and L. A. Saperstein. 1957. Measurement of the cardiac output in dogs by a conductivity method after a single intravenous injection of autogenous plasma. *Circ. Res.* **5**:531–538.

Gougerot, L., and N. Marstal. 1965. Quelques remarques sur la fréquence utilizée en rheoencephalographie. *First Symposium on New Developments. Rheoencephalographia.* F. Martin and H. Lechner, (eds.). Verlag Wiener Medizinischen Akademie, Vienna, 298 pp.

Graham, M. 1965. Guard ring use in physiological measurements. *IEEE Trans. Bio-Med. Eng.* **BME-12**:197–198.

Grant, F. C. 1923. Localization of brain tumors. *JAMA* **8**:2168–2169.

Gross, R. E., and R. Mittermaier. 1926. Untersuchungen über das Minutenvolumen des Herzen. *Arch. Ges. Physiol.* **212**:136–149.

Hadijev, D. 1972. Impedance methods for investigation of cerebral circulation. *Progr. Brain Res.* **35**:25–85. Elsevier, New York.

Haley, T. J., and F. Stolarsky. 1951. Changes in electrolytic resistance of blood following coagulation and clot retraction. *J. Appl. Physiol.* **4**:46–52.

Hamilton, L. H., J. D. Beard, and R. C. Kory. 1965. Impedance measurement of tidal volume and ventilation. *J. Appl. Physiol.* **20**:565–568.

Hanish, H. 1962. Telemetry of respiration and the electrocardiogram from the same pair of electrodes. *15th Annual Conference on Engineering, Biology, and Medicine.* Carl Gorr, Chicago, 66 pp.

Harley, A., and J. C. Greenfield. 1968. Determination of cardiac output in man by means of impedance plethysmography. *Aerosp. Med.* **39**:248–252.

Harns, S., and L. E. Blockus. 1952. The reliability and validity of tooth-pulp algesimetry. *J. Pharm. Exp. Therap.* **104**:135–148.

Harris, S. C. and L. E. Blockus. 1952. The reliability and validity of tooth-pulp algesimetry. *J. Pharmacol.* **104**:135–148.

Hassin, G. B. 1933. Changes in the brain in legal electrocution. *Arch. Neurol. Psychiat.* **30**:1046–1060.

Hawkes, G. R., and J. S. Warm. 1960. The sensory range of electrical stimulation of the skin. *Am. J. Psychol.* **73**:485–487.

Henstell, H. H. 1949. Electrolytic resistance of the blood clot. *Am. J. Physiol.* **158**:367–387.

Higgins, J. D., B. Tursky, and G. E. Schwartz. 1971. Shock-elicited pain and its reduction by concurrent tactile stimulation. *Science* **172**:866–867.

Hill, H. E., H. G. Flanary, C. H. Kornetsky, and A. Winkler. 1952. Relationship of electrically induced pain to the amperage and wattage of the shock. *J. Clin. Invest.* **31**:464–472.

Hoffmann, B. F., and P. F. Cranefield. 1960. *Electrophysiology of the Heart.* McGraw-Hill, New York, 323 pp.

Holt, J. P. 1956. Estimation of the residual volume of the ventricle of the dog's heart by two indicator dilution techniques. *Circ. Res.* **4**:187–195.

Holt, J. P. 1962. Left ventricular function in mammals of greatly different size. *Circ. Res.* **10**:798–806.

Holt, J. P. and J. Allensworth. 1957. Estimation of the residual volume of the right ventricle of the dog's heart. *Circ. Res.* **5**:323–326.

Holzer, W., K. Polzer, and A. Marko. 1945. *RKG, Rheokardiographie.* Wilhelm Maudrich, Vienna, 46 pp.

Horton, J. W., and A. C. Van Ravenswaay. 1935. Electrical impedance of the human body. *J. Franklin Inst.* **20**:557–572.

Irisawa, H., M. F. Wilson, and R. F. Rushmer. 1960. Left ventricle as a mixing chamber. *Circ. Res.* **8**:183–187.

Jackson, T. A., and B. F. Riess. 1934. Electric shock with different size electrodes. *J. Gen. Psychol.* **45**:262–266.

Jaffe, R. H., 1928. Electropathology. *Arch. Pathol.* **5**:837–870.

Jenkner, F. L. 1959. Rheoencephalography. *Confinia Neurol.* **19**:1–20.

Jenkner, F. L. 1962. *Rheoencephalography.* Charles. C. Thomas, Springfield, Ill. 81 pp.

Jex-Blake, A. J. 1913. Death by electric currents and by lightning. **1**:425–430, 492–498, 548–552, 601–603.

Judy, W. V., F. M. Langley, K. D. McCowen, D. M. Stennett, L. E. Baker, and P. C. Johnson. 1969. Comparative evaluation of the thoracic impedance and isotope dilution methods for measuring cardiac output. *Aerosp. Med.* **40**:532–536.

Kado, R., W. R. Adey. 1965. Method for the measurement of impedance changes in brain tissue. *Digest 6th International Congress on Medical, Electronic, and Biological Engineering,* Okamura Publ. Co., Tokyo, 638 pp.

Kado, R., W. R. Adey, and D. O. Walter. 1966. Regional specificity of impedance characteristics of cortical and subcortical structures evaluated in hyperapnea and hypothermia. Abstracts of Papers, XXIII Int. Cong. of Physiological Sci. Tokyo, 549 pp.

Kennelly, A. E., and E. F. W. Alexanderson. 1910. The physiological tolerance of alternating-current strengths up to frequencies of 100 kilocycles per second. *Electron World* **50**:154–156.

Kety, S. S., and C. F. Schmidt. 1945. The determination of cerebral blood flow in man by the use of nitrous oxide in low concentrations. *Am. J. Physiol.* **143**:53–66.

Kety, S. S., and C. F. Schmidt. 1948. The nitrous oxide method for the quantitative determination of cerebral blood flow in man: Theory, procedure and normal values. *J. Clin. Invest.* **27**:476–483.

Khalafalla, A. S., S. P. Stackhouse, and O. H. Schmitt. 1970. Thoracic impedance gradient with respect to breathing. *IEEE Trans. Bio. -Med. Eng.* **BME-17**:191–198.

Kinnen, E. 1965. Estimation of pulmonary blood flow with an electrical impedance plethysmograph. School of Aerospace Medicine, Tech. Rept. SAM TR-65-81.

Kinnen, E. 1970. Cardiac output from transthoracic impedance variations. *Ann. N.Y. Acad. Sci.* **170**:747–756.

Kinnen, E., and C. Duff. 1970. Cardiac output from transthoracic impedance records using discriminant analysis. *J. Am. Assoc. Adv. Med. Instr.* **4**:73–78.

Kinnen, E., and Kubicek, W. 1963. Thoracic cage impedance measurements. Impedance product system. School of Aerospace Medicine, Tech. Rept. SAM TDR-63-69.

Kinnen, E., W. Kubicek, P. Hill, and G. Turton. 1964. Thoracic cage independance measurements. Tech. Documentary Rept. SAM-TDR-64-5. USAF School of Aerospace Medicine, 14 pp.

Kinnen, E., W. Kubicek, and R. Patterson. 1964. Thoracic cage measurements. Impedance plethysmographic determination of cardiac output. School of Aerospace Medicine, Tech. Rept. TDR-64-15.

Kinnen, E., W. Kubicek, and D. Witsoe. 1964. Thoracic cage impedance measurements. Impedance plethysmographic determination of cardiac output. School of Aerospace Medicine, Tech. Rept. TDR-64-23.

Kinsman, J. M., J. W. Moore, and W. F. Hamilton. 1929. Studies on the circulation I. Injection method: Physical and mathematical considerations. *Am. J. Physiol.* **89**:322–330.

Kirk, S., Y. Hukushima, S. Kitamura, and A. Ito. 1971. Transthoracic electrical impedance variations associated with respiration. *J. Appl. Physiol.* **30**:820–826.

Kornmesser, J. G., and J. Nyboer. 1962. Electrical and dynamic changes in uterine activity during labor. *Harper Hosp. Bull.* **20**:248–261.

Kouwenhoven, N. B., and D. R. Hooker. 1936. Electric shock; effects of frequency. *Elect. Eng.* **55**:384–386.

Kris, C. 1960. *Vision: Electro-oculography. Medical Physics,* Vol. 3. Year Book Publishers, Chicago, 754 pp.

Kubicek, W. G., A. H. L. From, R. P. Patterson, D. A. Witsoe, A. Castenda, R. C. Lilleki, and R. Ersek. 1970. Impedance cardiography as a noninvasive means to monitor cardiac function. *J. Assoc. Adv. Med. Instr.* **4**:79–84.

Kubicek. W. G., J. N. Kamegis, R. P. Patterson, D. A. Witsoe, and R. H. Mattson. 1966. Development and evaluation of an impedance cardiac output system. *Aerosp. Med.* **37**:1208–1212.

Kubicek, W., E. Kinnen, and A. Edin. 1963. Thoracic cage impedance measurements. School of Aerospace Medicine, Tech. Rept. TDR-63-41.

Kubicek, W. G., E. Kinnen, and A. Edin. 1964. Calibration of an impedance pneumograph. *J. Appl. Physiol.* **19**:557–560.

Kubicek, W. G., D. A. Witsoe, and R. P. Patterson. 1967–1968. Development and evaluation of an impedance cardiographic system to measure cardiac output and other cardiac parameters. NASA Report NAS 9-4500. NASA Manned Spacecraft Center, Houston. Tex.

Lababidi, Z., D. A. Ehmke, R. E. Durnin, P. E. Leaveston, and R. M. Lauer. 1971. Evaluation of impedance cardiac output in children. *Pediatrics* **47**:870–879.

Langworthy, O. R. 1930. Abnormalities in the central nervous system by electrical injuries. *J. Exp. Med.* **51**:943–968.

Larks, S. 1960. *Electrohysterography*. Charles C. Thomas, Springfield, Ill., 123 pp.

Lechner, H., N. Geyer, E. Lugarese, F. Martin, K. Lifshitz, and S. Mardovich. 1969. Rheoencephalography and plethysomographic methods. (*Proc. 2nd Int. Symp. Graz, Austria, April 19–22, 1967*). Excerpta Medica Foundation, Amsterdam, 239 pp.

Lechner, H., N. Geyer, and H. Rodler. 1966. Die Funktion-rheographie. *Wein. Med. Wochenschn.* **116:**391 400.

Lechner, H., and H. Rodler. 1961. Ein neue Method zur Registrierung intracranelier Kreislauf Veränderungen. *Elektromed.* **6:**75.

Lechner, H., H. Rodler, and N. Geyer. 1965. Theoretical aspects of the nature of the rheoencephalogram. *First Symposium on New Developments. Rheoencephalographia.* F. Martin and H. Lechner (eds.). Verlag Wiener Medizinischen Akademie, Vienna, 208 pp.

Lechner, H., H. Rodler, and N. Geyer. 1966. The technical development of field rheography. *Proc. Eur. Symp. Med. Electron., World Med. Electr.* 150 153.

Leverett, S. 1962. Personal communication. School of Aerospace Medicine, Brooks AFB, Texas.

Liebman, R. M., J. Pearl, and J. Bagno. 1962–63. Electrical conductance properties of blood in motion. *Phys. Biol. Med.* **7:**177–194.

Liebman, R. M., and F. Cozenza. 1962–1963. Study of blood flow in the dental pulp by an electrical impedance technique. *Phys. Biol. Med.* **7:**167–176.

Lifshitz, K. 1963a. Rheoencephalography: I. Review of the technique. *J. Nerv. Mental Disease* **136:**288.

Lifshitz, K. 1963b. Rheoencephalography: II. Survey of clinical applications. *J. Nerv. Mental Disease* **137:**285.

Lifshitz, K. 1970. Electrical impedance cephalography; electrode guarding and analog study. *Ann. N.Y. Acad. Sci.* **170:**532–549.

Lifshitz, K., and K. Klemm. 1966. The use of electrode guarding in rheoencephalography. *Proc. 19th Ann. Conf. Eng. Med. Biol.* **8:**39.

Lofgren, B. 1951. The electrical impedance of a complex tissue and its relation to changes in volume and fluid distribution. *Acta Physiol. Scand. Suppl. 81,* **23:**1–51.

Logic, J. L., M. G. Maksud, and L. H. Hamilton. 1967. Factors affecting transthoracic impedance signals used to measure breathing. *J. Appl. Physiol.* **22:**362 364.

Luepker, R. V., J. R. Michael, and J. R. Warbasse. 1973. Transthoracic electrical impedance: Quantitative evaluation of non-invasive measure of fluid volume. *Am. Heart J.* **85:**83 93.

MacDonald, C. F. 1892. The infliction of the death penalty by means of electricity. *Trans. Med. Soc. State N.Y.* 400 427.

Mann, H. 1937. Study of the peripheral circulation by means of an alternating current bridge. *Proc. Soc. Exp. Biol. Med.* **36:**670 673.

Mann, H. 1953. The capacigraph. *Trans. Am. Coll. Cardiol.* **3:**162–175.

Markovich, S. E., and R. Naman. 1965. Theory and facts concerning rheoencephalography. *Trans. 4th Conf. Cerebrovasc. Dis. 1964.* Grune & Stratton, New York, pp. 68–86.

Martin, F., and H. Lechner. 1963. *Rheoencephalographia Wien,* Verlag Wiener Medizenschen Akademie, Vienna.

Martin, F., and H. Lechner. 1965. Rheoencephalography. *First Symposium on New Developments in the Field of Rheoencephalography.* Geneva, 1963. Verlag Wiener Medizenschen Akademie, Vienna, 298 pp.

Maxwell, J. C. 1904. *A Treatise on Electricity and Magnetism.* 3rd Ed. Clarendon Press, Oxford, England. 506 pp. (1st Ed. 1873)

McCally, M., G. W. Barnard, K. E. Robins, and A. Marko. 1963. Observations with an electrical impedance respirometer. *Am. J. Med. Electron.* 2:322–327.

McHenry, L. C. 1965. Rheoencephalography. *Neurology* 15:507–517.

McLendon, J. F., and A. Hemingway. 1930. The psychogalvanic reflex as related to the polarization-capacity of the skin. *Am. J. Physiol.* 94:77–83.

Mello-Sobrinho, A. 1963. Impedance plethysmography of the canine ventricles. M. S. thesis, Baylor University College of Medicine. Houston, Tex. 85 pp.

Molnar, G. W., J. Nyboer, R. L. Levine. 1953. The effects of temperature and flow on the specific resistance of human venous blood. U.S. Army Med. Res. Lab., Fort Knox, Ky., Rept. 127.

Montagu, J. D. 1958. The psychogalvanic reflex. *J. Neurol. Neurosurg. Psychiat.* 21:119–128.

Monsees, L. R., and D. G. McQuarrie. 1971. Is an intravascular catheter a conductor? *Med. Electron. Data* 12:26–27.

Moskalenko, Y. E., and A. I. Naumenko. 1959. Movement of the blood and changes in its electrical conductivity. *Bull. Exp. Biol. Med.* 47:211–215.

Mueller, E. E., R. Loeffel, and S. Mead. 1953. Skin impedance in relation to pain threshold testing by electrical means. *J. Appl. Physiol.* 5:746–752.

Mungall, A. G., D. Morris, and W. S. Martin. 1961. Measurement of the dielectric properties of blood. *IRE Trans. Bio-Med. Electron.* BME-8:109–111.

Namon, R., and F. Gollan. 1970. The cardiac electrical impedance pulse. *Ann. N.Y. Acad. Sci.* 170:733–746.

Namon, R., and S. Markovich. 1966. Monopolar rheoencephalography. *EEG Cli. Neurophysiol.* 22:272–273.

Namon, R., and S. Markovich. 1970. Monopolar rheoencephalography. *Ann. N.Y. Acad. Sci.* 170:652–660.

Nelson, C. V., and A. F. Wilkinson. 1972. Electronic measurement of sedimentation rate. *J. Maine Med. Assoc.* 63:160.

Nethken, R. P., and M. A. Bulot. 1967. Threshold of electrical signal on the upper human arm. *Trans. Reg. 3 IEEE Meeting.*

Nichols, R. C., and T. Daroge. 1955. An electric circuit for the measurement of the galvanic skin response. *Am. J. Psychol.* 68:455–461.

Notermans, S. L. H. 1966. Measurement of the pain threshold determined by electrical stimulation and its clinical application. *Neurology* 16:1071–1086.

Nyboer, J. 1944. Electrical impedance plethysmography, O. Glasser. *Medical Physics,* Vol. 1. Year Book Publishers, Chicago, 744 pp.

Nyboer, J. 1950. Electrical impedance plethysmography. *Circulation* 2:811–87.

Nyboer, J. 1959. *Electrical Impedance Plethysmography.* Charles C. Thomas, Springfield, Ill., 243 pp.

Nyboer, J. 1965. Tetrapolar electrical resistive impedance measurements as indices of vascular, cardiac and respiratory volume changes. *Proc. Eur. Symp. Med. Electron,* Part 2. Brighton, England.

Nyboer, J. 1970. *Electrical Impedance Plethysmography,* 2nd ed. Charles C. Thomas, Springfield, Ill.

Nyboer, J., S. Bagno, A. Barnett, and R. H. Halsey. 1940. Radiocardiograms. *J. Clin. Invest.* **19**:773.

Nyboer, J., S. Bagno, and L. F. Nims. 1943. The impedance plethysmograph, an electrical volume recorder. *Off. Sci. Res. Dev.* Comm. on Aviation Med. Rep. 149, 12 pp.

Okada, R. H., and H. P. Schwan. 1960. An electrical method to determine hematocrits. *IRE Trans. Med. Electron.* **ME-7**:188–192.

Pacella, A. F. 1966. Impedance pneumography—A survey of instrumentation techniques. *Med. Biol. Eng.* **4**:1–15.

Pallett, J. E. and J. W. Scopes. 1965. Recording respirations in newborn babies by measuring impedance of the chest. *Med. Biol. Eng.* **3**:161–168.

Pasquali, E. 1967. Problems in impedance pneumography. Electrical characteristics of skin and lung tissue. *Med. Biol. Eng.* **5**:249–258.

Patterson, R., W. G. Kubicek, E. Kinnen, G. Noren, and D. Witsoe. 1964. Development of an electrical impedance plethysmograph system to monitor cardiac output. *Proc. 1st Ann. Rocky Mt. Conf. Biomed. Eng.,* Colorado Springs, Colo. pp. 56–71.

Perez-Borja, C., and J. S. Meyer. 1964. A critical evaluation of rheoencephalography in control subjects and in proven cases of cerebrovascular disease. *J. Neurol. Neurosurg. Psychiat.* **27**:66–72.

Petrovick, M. S., and J. Brumlik. 1961–1962. Clinical measurements of biological vibrations in normal and disease states. Symposium on Recent Developments in Research Methods and Instrumentation, National Institutes of Health, October 9–12, 1961. *15th Annual Conference on Engineering in Medicine and Biology.* Carl Gorr, Chicago, 66 pp.

Pfeiffer, E. A. 1968. Electrical stimulation of sensory nerves with skin electrodes for research, diagnosis, communication and behavioral conditioning: A survey. *Med. Biol. Eng.* **6**:637–651.

Pfeiffer, E. A., and D. S. Stevens. 1971. Problems in electro-aversive shock in behavior therapy. In *Neuroelectric Research.* D. V. Reynolds and A. E. Sjoberg (eds.) Charles C. Thomas, Springfield, Ill.

Plutchick, R., and H. R. Hirsch. 1963. Skin impedance and phase angle as a function of frequency and current. *Science* **141**:927–928.

Polzer, K., and F. Schuhfried. 1950. Rheographische Untersuchungen am Schädel. *Z. Nervenheilke.* **3**:295–298.

Polzer, K., and F. Schuhfried. 1961. Application of rheography in vascular disease. *Spec. Issue., J. Oester. Krank-Ztg.* **8–9**:5.

Polzer, K., F. Schuhfried, and H. Heeger. 1960. Rheography. *Brit. Heart J.* **22**:140–148.

Pomerantz, M., R. Baumgartner, J. Lauridson, and B. Eiseman. 1969. Transthoracic electrical impedance for the early detection of pulmonary edema. *Surgery* **66**:260–268.

Pomerantz, M., F. Delgado, and B. E. Eiseman. 1970. Clinical evaluation of transthoracic electrical impedance as a guide to intrathoracic fluid volumes. *Ann. Surg.* **171**:686–694.

Poppendiek, H. E., G. L. Hody, N. D. Greene, J. L. Glass, and J. E. Hayes. 1964. *In vivo* study of the effects of alternating currents on some properties of blood in dogs. *Phys. Med. Biol.* **9**:215–217.

Powers, S. R., C. Schaffer, A. Boba, and Y. Nakamura. 1958. Physical and biologic factors in impedance plethysmography. *Surgery* **44**:53–61.

Prevost, J. L. and F. Battelli. 1900. Influence du nombre des periodes sur les effets mortels des courants alternatifs. *J. Physiol. Path. Gen.* **2**:755–766.

Pritchard, E. A. 1934. Changes in the nervous system due to electrocution. *Lancet* **1**:1163–1167.

Radvan-Ziemnowicz, S. A., J. C. McWilliams, and W. E. Kucharski. 1964. Conductivity versus frequency in human and feline cerebrospinal fluid. *Proc. 17th Ann. Conf. Eng. Med. Biol.* MacGregor & Werner; Washington, D.C., 108 pp.

Rappoport, D., and G. B. Ray. 1927. Changes of electrical conductivity in the beating tortoise ventricle. *Am. J. Physiol.* **80**:126–139.

Richardson, A. W., and J. C. Bishop. 1957. A new accurate and reliable method to record blood coagulation times using an AC bridge principle. *J. Am. Pharm. Assoc.* **46**:553–555.

Robbins, K. C., and A. Marko. 1962. An improved method of measuring respiration rate. *15th Annual Conference on Engineering in Medicine and Biology.* Carl Gorr, Chicago, 66 pp.

Robinson, D. A. 1963. A method of measuring eye movements using a scleral search coil in a magnetic field. *IEEE Trans. Biomed. Eng.* **BME-10**:137–145.

Romm, S. O. 1924. Zur Bestimmungsmethode der Umlaufzeit des Blutes im Kreislauf. *Arch. Ges. Physiol.* **202**:14–24.

Rosenbleuth, A., and E. G. del Pozo. 1943. The changes of impedance of the turtle ventricular muscle during contraction. *Am. J. Physiol.* **139**:514–519.

Rosenthal, R. L., and C. W. Tobias. 1948. Measurement of the electric resistance of human blood use in coagulation studies and cell volume determination. *J. Lab. Clin. Med.* **33**:1110–1122.

Rushmer, R. F., T. K. Crystal, C. Wagner, and R. Ellis. 1953. Intracardiac plethysmography. *Am. J. Physiol.* **174**:171–174.

Salansky, I., and F. Utrata. 1972. Electrical tissue impedance of the organism and its relation to body fluid. *Physiol. Bohemoslov.* **21**:295–304.

Schaefer, H., E. Bleicher, and F. Eckervogt. 1949. Weitere Beitrage zur elektrischen Reizung und zur Registrierung von elektrischen Vorgangen und der Atmung. *Arch. Ges. Physiol.* **251**:491–503.

Schwan, H. P. 1955. Electrical properties of body tissues and impedance plethysmography. *IRE Trans. Bio-Med. Electron.* **PGME-3**:32–46.

Schwan, H. P. 1963. Determination of biological impedances. In *Physical Techniques in Biological Research.* Vol. 6, Part B. Academic Press, New York and London, 425 pp.

Schwan, H. P., and C. F. Kay. 1957. Capacitative properties of body tissues. *Circ. Res.* **5**:439–443.

Schwan, H. P., and K. Li. 1953. Capacitance and conductivity of body tissues at ultra high frequencies. *Proc. IRE* **41**:1735–1740.

Severinghaus, J. W. 1971. Electrical measurement of pulmonary edema with a focusing conductivity bridge. *J. Physiol. (Proc. Physiol. Soc.)* **215**:53–55.

Severinghaus, J. W., C. Catron, and W. Noble. 1972. A focusing bridge for unilateral lung resistance. *J. Appl. Physiol.* **32**:526–530.

Sigel, H. 1953–1954. Prick threshold stimulation with square-wave current. *Yale J. Biol. Med.* **26**:145–154.

Sigman, E., A. Kolin, L. N, Katz, and K. Jochim. 1937. Effect of motion on the electrical conductivity of the blood. *Am. J. Physiol.* **118**:708–719.

Simonson, E. and K. Nakagawa. 1960. Effect of age on pulse wave velocity and ejection time in healthy men and in men with coronary heart disease. *Circulation* **22**:126–129.

Smith, J. J., J. E. Bush, V. T. Wiedmeier, and F. E. Tristani. 1970. Application of impedance cardiography to study of postural stress. *J. Appl. Physiol.* **29**:133–137.

Smith, McK., L. A. Geddes, and H. E. Hoff. 1967. Cardiac output determined by the saline conductivity method using an extra-arterial conductivity cell. *Cardiovasc. Res. Center Bull.* **5**:123–134.

Spitzka, E. A., and H. E. Radash. 1912. The brain lesions produced by electricity as observed after legal electrocution. *Am. J. Med. Sci.* **144**:341–347.

Steer, M. L. 1973. Limitations of impedance phlebography for diagnosis of venous thrombosis. *Arch. Surg.* **106**:44–48.

Sternbach, R. A. and B. Tursky. 1965. Ethnic differences among housewives in psychophysiological and skin potential responses to electric shock. *Psychophysiology* **1**:241–246.

Stewart, G. N. 1897–1898. Researches on the circulation time and on the influences which affect it. *J. Physiol.* **22**:158–183.

Stewart, G. N. 1921. The output of the heart in dogs. *Am. J. Physiol.* **57**:27–50.

Sugano, H., and M. Oda. 1960. A new method for blood flow measurement. *Japan. J. Pharmacol.* **10**:30–37.

Sullivan, G., and G. Weltman. 1963. The impedance oculogram—A new technique. *J. Appl. Physiol.* **18**:215–216.

Talibi, M. A., R. Drolet, H. Kunov, and C. J. Robson. 1970. A model for studying the electrical stimulation of the urinary bladder of dogs. *Brit. J. Urol.* **42**:56–65.

Tarjan, P. P. and R. McFee. 1968. Electrodless measurements of the effective resistivity of the human torso and head by magnetic induction. *IEEE Trans. Bio-Med. Eng.* **15**:275–278.

Tarjan, P. P. and R. McFee. 1970. Electrodless measurements of resistivity fluctuations in the human torso and head. *Ann. N.Y. Acad. Sci.* **170**:462–475.

Tasaki, I. 1952–1953. Properties of myelinated fibers in frog sciatic nerve in spinal cord as examined with microelectrodes. *Japan. J. Physiol.* **3**:73–94.

Taylor, D. H. 1962. The measurement of galvanic skin response. *Electron. Eng.* **34**:312–315.

Teorell, T. 1947. Applications of square wave analysis to bioelectric studies. *Acta Physiol. Scand.* **12**:235–254.

Tolles, W. E., and W. J. Carberry. 1959. The measurement of tissue resistance in psychophysiological problems *Proc. Int. Conf. Electron. Biol. Eng.* 43–49. Heffe & Sons, Ltd., London.

Tomberg, V. T. 1963. The high frequency spirometer. *Proc. Int. Cong. Med. Electron* Liege, Belgium.

Tomberg, V. T. 1964. Device and a new method of measuring pulmonary respiration. *17th Annual Conference on Biology and Medicine.* McGregor and Werner, Washington, D.C., 129 pp.

Tursky, B., P. D. Watson, D. N. O'Connor. 1965. A concentric shock electrode for pain stimulation. *Psychophysiology* **1**:296–298.

Tursky, B., and P. D. Watson. 1964. Controlled physical and subjective intensities of electric shock. *Psychophysiology* **1**:151–162.

Underwood, R. J., and D. Gowing. 1965. An electronic method of detecting blood volume changes. *Anesthesiology* **26**:199–203.

Ur, A. 1970. Determination of blood coagulation using impedance measurements. *Bio-Med. Eng.* **5**:342–345.

Valentinuzzi, M. E., L. A. Geddes, and L. E. Baker. 1971. The law of impedance pneumography. *Med. Biol. Eng.* **9**:157–163.

Van De Water, J. M., K. S. Kagey, and G. B. Dove. 1970. Clinical monitoring of thoracic fluid with electrical impedance. *Proc. 23rd Ann. Conf. Eng. Med. Biol.*, paper 25-4, p. 331.

Van De Water, J. M., I. T. Miller, E. N. C. Milne, G. F. Sheldon, and K. S. Kagey. 1970. Impedance plethysmography. *J. Thorac. Cardiovasc. Surg.* **60**:641–647.

Van De Water, J. M., P. A. Philips, L. G. Thouin, L. S. Watanabe, and R. S. Lappen. 1971. Bioelectric impedance. *Arch. Surg.* **102**:541–547.

Van De Water, J. M., W. C. Watring, L. A. Linton, M. Murphy, and R. L. Byron. 1972. Prevention of postoperative pulmonary complications. *Surgery* **138**:229–233.

Van der Berg, J., and A. J. Alberts. 1954. Limitation of electrical impedance plethysmography. *Circ. Res.* **2**:333–339.

Van Harreveld, A., and P. A. Biersteker. 1963. Acute asphyxiation of the spinal cord and other sections of the nervous system. *Am. J. Physiol.* **206**:8–14.

Velick, S., and M. Gorin. 1940. The electrical conductance of suspensions of ellipsoids and its relation to the study of avian erythrocytes. *J. Gen. Physiol.* **23**:753–771.

Waltz, F. M., G. W. Timm, and W. E. Bradley. 1971. Bladder volume sensing by resistance measurement. *IEEE Trans. Bio-Med. Eng.* **BME-18**:42–46.

Weltman, G., and D. C. Ukkestad. 1969. Impedance pneumograph recording across the arms. *J. Appl. Physiol.* **27**:907–909.

Whalen, R. E., C. F. Starner, and H. D. McIntosh. 1964. Electrical hazards associated with cardiac pacemaking. *Ann. N.Y. Acad. Sci.* **111**:922.

Wheeler, H. B., D. Pearson, S. C. Mullick. 1972. Impedance phlebography: Technique, interpretation and results. *Arch. Surg.* **104**:164–169.

White, H. L. 1947. Measurement of cardiac output by a continuously recording conductivity method. *Am. J. Physiol.* **151**:45–57.

Whitehorn, W. V., and E. R. Pearl. 1949. The use of change in capacity to record cardiac volume in human subjects. *Science* **109**:262–263.

Wiederhelm, C. A., and R. F. Rushmer. 1964. Pre and post-ateriolar resistance changes in the blood vessels of the frog's mesentery. *Bibl. Anat.* **4**:234–243.

Wiggers, H. C. 1944. Cardiac output and total peripheral resistance measurements in experimental dogs. *Am. J. Physiol.* **140**:519–534.

Wise, C. S. 1944. Fluid-displacement and pressure plethysmography. In *Methods in Medical Research,* , Vol. I. V. R. Potter (ed.). Year Book Publishers, Chicago.

Wolstenholme, G. E. W., and J. S. Freeman. 1954. *Peripheral Circulation in Man.* Little, Brown, Boston.

Yokota, T., and B. Fujimori. 1962. Impedance change of the skin during the galvanic skin reflex. *Japan. J. Physiol.* **12**:210–224.

Young, D. G., R. H. Cox, E. K. Stones, and W. J. Edman. 1967. Evaluation of quantitative impedance plethysmography for continuous flow measurement. III. Blood flow determinations *in vivo. Am. J. Phys. Med.* **46**:1450–1457.

Zajic, F., Z. Fejfar, L. Franc, and J. Brod. 1954. Impedance plethysmography. *Physiol. Bohemoslov.* **3**:355–361.

11

The Bioelectric Events

11-1. ORIGIN OF BIOELECTRIC EVENTS

Electrical potentials exist across the enveloping membranes of living cells, and many cells have the ability to propagate a change in these potentials. Nerve, muscle, and gland cells, as well as many plant cells, exhibit this phenomenon, which is related to the functioning of the cell. When such a cell responds to a stimulus, the membrane potential exhibits a series of reversible changes, called the action potential. Action potentials, unlike many other physiological events, call for no specialized transducers for their detection. Suitable electrodes, amplification, and appropriate display are the only requirements for their presentation.

Because each type of cell exhibits a characteristic electrical activity, measurement of this activity yields important information relating to cellular function. From this fact has developed the clinical study of bioelectric signals, which deals with the measurement of the electrical activity of large numbers of cells. Because dysfunction frequently reveals itself in the bioelectric signal, much diagnostic information can be obtained from such recordings. In this chapter are presented simplified explanations of the manner in which living cells develop action potentials and present them to electrodes.

Because many of the bioelectric signals can be detected at a distance from their source, the electrographic devices, by virtue of their ability to "peer" inside the body, can be likened to the x-ray, which reveals information hidden from view. In addition, the measurement of a bioelectric signal usually does not interfere with the event being measured, resulting in a true electrical representation of function. Moreover, because of the great practicality and ease of making electrographic recordings on human subjects, the techniques are ideally applicable to clinical medicine. There is little doubt that these features will lead to a considerable expansion of electrographic techniques.

Although the bioelectric signals recorded from different cells vary considerably in amplitude and form, they all have a common origin in the membrane potential, which is the potential difference that exists between the interior and exterior surfaces of the cell. The enveloping membrane serves as a semipermeable barrier to the passage of certain substances and ions. The resulting ionic gradient is maintained by virtue of metabolic energy expended by the cell. In mammalian nerve cells, for example, the concentration of potassium ion is approximately 30 times higher inside the cell than in the extracellular fluid. On the other hand, sodium ion is approximately 10 times more concentrated in the fluid bathing the outside of the cell than in the intracellular fluid; similar conditions obtain for other ions. The net result is a potential difference across the membrane with the inside negative with respect to the outside. Membrane potentials vary within wide limits, ranging from a few tens of millivolts to about 100 mV. Table 11-1 presents the resting membrane potentials of a variety of cells measured under the circumstances indicated.

In response to a stimulus of adequate intensity to cause local depolarization, many types of cells propagate this disturbance over their membranes. The process of depolarization, reverse polarization, and repolarization constitutes the action potential. In nerve, the propagated disturbance travels at a rate governed by the nerve fiber diameter and the temperature. The speed of propagation in the fastest nerves is approximately 150 m/sec, which represents the highest rate of propagation in any tissue. In muscle, propagation is much slower and contraction follows development of the action potential.

The genesis of the action potential can be understood by considering a single strip of irritable tissue (as in Fig. 11-1) forming the whole or part of a cell in which the membrane is intact and an ionic gradient exists to produce a membrane potential of 70 mV. This potential is measured by placing an electrode A on the intact surface of the cell and inserting a microelectrode[1] B into the cell. In Fig. 11-1(2), at the arrow, the microelectrode has penetrated the cell membrane, revealing the resting membrane potential at electrode A.

Assume now that a stimulus intense enough to depolarize the membrane is applied elsewhere to the same cell. An ionic current will flow from the surrounding polarized region to the depolarized area. This current is adequate to depolarize the adjacent regions, and a wave of depolarization will travel in all directions over the membrane. In most cells the process does not consist merely of depolarization; a slight reverse polarization also is found to occur, causing the outside of the portion of the cell, which is active, to be negative with respect to the inside. When this wave of depo-

---

[1] A microelectrode must be small with respect to the size of the cell so that its insertion will not produce cellular damage.

Table 11-1   Resting Membrane Potentials

Type of Tissue	Type of Environment	Membrane* Potential (mV)	Reference
Frog: myelinated axon	Excised—Ringer's	67.6 ± 1.4	Huxley and Stampfli (1951)
Rabbit: superior cervical ganglion cell	Excised—physiological solutions	65–80	Eccles (1955)
Cat: spinal motoneuron soma	*In vivo*	70	Coombs, Eccles, and Fatt (1955)
Cat: cortical pyramidal cell	*In vivo*	55	Phillips (1955)
Rat: skeletal muscle fiber	*In vivo*	99.8 ± 0.19	Bennett, Ware, Dunn, and McIntyre (1953)
Dog: papillary muscle	Excised	85	Hoffmann and Suckling (1953)
Dog: auricle	Excised	85	Hoffmann and Suckling (1953)
Dog: Purkinje fiber	Excised—Tyrode's	90	Draper and Weidmann (1951)
Guinea pig: intestinal smooth muscle fiber	Excised—physiological solutions	51.5–70	Holman (1958)
Kid: Purkinje fiber	Excised	94	Draper and Weidmann (1951)
Frog: ventricle	*In vivo*—Ringer's	62	Woodbury et al. (1950)
Squid: giant axon	Excised—sea water	45	Hodgkin and Huxley (1939)
Frog: skeletal muscle	Excised—Ringer's	92.2	Adrian (1956)
Frog: myoneural junction	Excised—Ringer's	90	Natsuk (1953)

* Interior of the cell is negative with respect to the exterior.

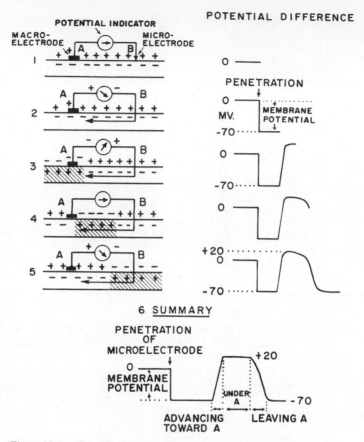

Figure 11-1. Genesis of the monophasic action potential.

larization-reverse polarization advances under electrode A [Fig. 11-1(3)], the potential indicator, which was previously indicating the membrane potential, shows a potential that drops to zero (depolarization of the membrane), then a potential that is in the opposite direction to the membrane potential, indicating that the region of reverse polarization is under A. This sequence of events appears on the right of Fig. 11-1(3).

As the wave of depolarization-reverse polarization advances, in its wake the metabolic activity of the cell causes recovery (reestablishment of the membrane potential) to occur. Thus as the wave passes electrode A [Fig. 11-1(4)], the membrane potential is becoming restored, and when full repolarization has occurred, the potential indicator reads the membrane potential again [Fig. 11-1(5)]. When the wave passes point B, the potential indicator shows no change because the electrode is inside the cell.

This sequence of events is summarized in Fig. 11-1(6), in which it is seen that the fundamental bioelectric event consists of a traveling wave of changing membrane polarity; first depolarization, then reverse polarization, followed by reestablishment of the membrane potential. Most cells exhibit a rapid depolarization and slower repolarization. Action potentials of short duration are called spikes. In many cells during recovery the rate of repolarization slows, and there appears another component called the negative afterpotential. Some cells overshoot their repolarization to produce what is called a positive afterpotential. Some even produce a second negative afterpotential before stabilization of the membrane potential occurs. In pacemaker cells, before the propagated action potential there occurs a spontaneous decay in membrane potential called the prepotential. The prepotential is representative of an unstable membrane potential, which upon reaching a critical value causes the cell to depolarize and a propagated action potential results. In summary, a bioelectric event derives its form from the manner in which a cell membrane depolarizes and repolarizes to produce a simple or complex action potential. Compilations of the various forms of action potentials have been presented by Grundfest (1947, 1966a and b), Hodgkin (1951), and Durnstock et al. (1963).

Figure 11-2 diagrams the sequence of events that a hypothetical cell may display. Depolarization is rapid; repolarization is slower and follows a time course characteristic of the type of cell, resulting not in a flat-topped action potential, as sketched in Fig. 11-1, but in a smooth curve, as in Fig. 11-2, where there are four of the types of potential change that may be exhibited by an irritable cell: (1) the prepotential, (2) the spike, (3) the negative afterpotential, and (4) the positive afterpotential.

During passage of the wave of depolarization, a small quantity of heat is liberated, the membrane impedance drops, and there is movement of ions across the cell membrane. Many of the extracellular ions enter the cell, and

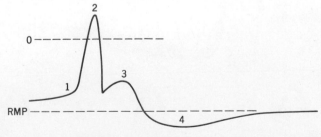

Figure 11-2.   Changes in membrane potential for a hypothetical cell, showing prepotential (1), spike (2), negative (3), and positive (4) after potentials; RMP is the resting membrane potential.

many of those in the cell move outward; the inward and outward movements do not occur simultaneously. During recovery there is a decrease in membrane permeability and the membrane potential is reestablished. Recovery is also characterized by a later reverse translocation of the ions that moved during excitation (depolarization). The rate of translocation of the various ions, and consequently, the form of the action potential, is characteristic for each type of cell.

The part of the cell that is occupied by the propagated wave of depolarization is unable to respond to a stimulus, and for this reason it is said to be refractory. However, during repolarization there is a cyclic variation in excitability, for a strong stimulus delivered early in the recovery phase will produce another response. Later, during the phase of the negative afterpotential (if it occurs), when the membrane is almost fully repolarized, a weaker stimulus will often produce a response. During a positive afterpotential (if it occurs), the effective stimulus would need to be stronger. Thus the action potential, in addition to indicating the time course of cellular activity, reveals the approximate time when it can be reactivated.

Figures 11-3 to 11-6 illustrate typical monophasic action potentials of

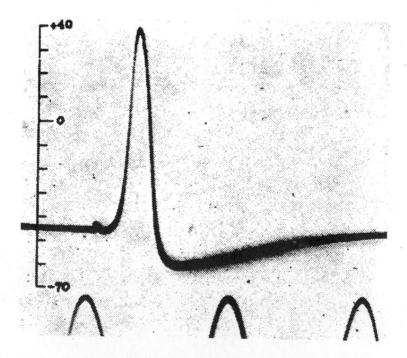

Figure 11-3. Membrane and action potential of giant axon of squid. Time pulses = 2 msec. [From Hodgkin and Huxley, *Nature* **144**:711 (1939). By permission.]

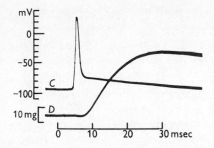

Figure 11-4. Action potential of a single skeletal muscle fibre in the frog (*C*) and the tension developed (*D*). [From Hodgkin and Horowicz, *J. Physiol.* **136**:18P (1957). By permission.]

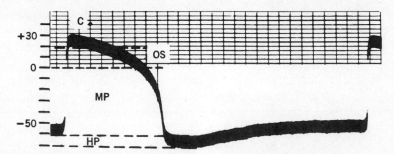

Figure 11-5. Membrane and action potential in a single cardiac muscle fiber in the frog. [From Woodbury et al., *Circulation* **1**:264–266 (1950). By permission of the American Heart Association.]

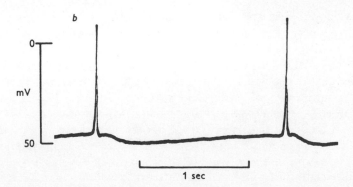

Figure 11-6. Membrane and action potential of single smooth muscle fiber of guinea pig gut. [From Holman, *J. Physiol.* **141**:466 (1958). By permission.]

various cells measured with microelectrodes. The monophasic action potential of a single nerve fiber of the squid is shown in Fig. 11-3. This fiber is so large (>100 μ) that it is relatively easy to make a microelectrode to study the membrane and action potentials. In addition, the large size permits cannulation and replacement of the axoplasm with solutions of known ionic content. As illustrated, the membrane potential measured in sea water at 20°C was 45 mV, and during the spike the membrane potential became nearly +40 mV. Thus the total amplitude of the action potential was 85 mV. During the recovery phase a positive afterpotential was recorded.

The action potential of a single frog skeletal muscle fiber and its relationship to the twitch appears in Fig. 11-4. In this experiment the resting membrane potential was −92 mV, and at the peak of the spike the potential difference was +30 mV. During recovery a negative afterpotential is clearly visible.

The membrane potential changes in frog cardiac muscle are plotted in Fig. 11-5. Starting from a resting value of about −55 mV, during peak activity the membrane potential became about +25 mV. Because recovery is prolonged in cardiac muscle, a relatively flat-topped monophasic action potential is produced. Clearly evident in this illustration is a positive afterpotential.

The electrical activity of smooth muscle of the guinea pig gut is presented in Fig. 11-6. During activity the membrane potential is seen to change from −46 to +10 mV. During recovery the afterpotentials previously mentioned can be seen.

11-2. RECORDING BIOELECTRIC EVENTS WITH EXTRACELLULAR ELECTRODES

Since body tissues and fluids are electrically conducting, there will be current flow in the environment of an active (depolarizing) and recovering (repolarizing) cell or cells. Therefore, suitably placed electrodes can be used to detect a voltage that reflects such a bioelectric event. The type of waveform detected depends on the size and location of the electrodes and the temporal nature of the depolarization-repolarization process exhibited by the cell or cells, often designated the "bioelectric generator."

There is no doubt that the potential appearing between the terminals of electrodes, which are strategically placed to record a bioelectric event, represents a difference in the potentials existing under each electrode. However, relating this extracellularly recorded action potential to the excursion in transmembrane potential is by no means simple or straightforward. Nonetheless, two useful theories have been created which provide reasonable explanations for the potentials detected by extracellular electrodes. The older "interference" theory postulates that the extracellular electrodes detect a voltage that is the difference in potential occurring under each electrode and that the potential under each resembles an attenuated version of the excursion in transmembrane potential. Thus these two potentials, which are separated temporally by the propagation time, "interfere" with each other.

The newer "dipole" theory postulates that excitation and recovery can be equated to the movement of sets of dipoles which exist in the boundary between active (depolarized) and recovered (polarized) tissue. The propagation of excitation is signaled by an array of dipoles traveling with their positive poles facing the direction of propagation; recovery is signaled by the movement of dipoles with their negative poles facing the direction of propagation. As will be seen, each theory is more applicable in some recording situations than in others. Several examples will be presented to illustrate the application of each theory.

11-3.   THE INTERFERENCE THEORY

11-3-1.   Electrode Axis Parallel to Excitation

The interference theory can be illustrated by considering a situation in which both electrodes are "active"; that is, they are both located on the surface of a strip of irritable tissue, as in Fig. 11-7. In this idealized situation it is assumed that the electrodes are small and widely separated. The dimensions were chosen so that the traveling wave of excitation and recovery in the tissue occupies a small fraction of the electrode spacing. In addition, the bioelectric event is considered as a simple monophasic action potential without prepotentials and afterpotentials.

In Fig. 11-7(1), when the tissue is inactive, both electrodes are in regions of equal positivity, and the potential difference seen by the indicator is zero. When the region under electrode A is excited, this electrode becomes negative with respect to electrode B and the indicator rises [Fig. 11-7(2)]. As the wave of excitation passes onward toward electrode B and occupies the region between the two electrodes, the region under A is recovered and that under B is not excited. Under these conditions no voltage is registered by the potential indicator [Fig. 11-7(3)], and the first (upward) phase of the monophasic action potential has been completed. As the wave of excitation occupies the region under electrode B, this electrode becomes negative with respect to A; hence the potential indicator falls [Fig. 11-7(4)]. As the wave of excitation passes B, recovery occurs; the membrane potential is reestablished, the potential indicator reads zero, and the downward phase of

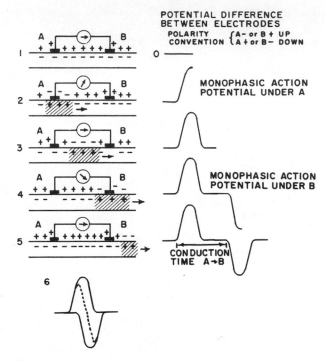

Figure 11-7.   Genesis of the biphasic action potential.

the action potential is completed [Fig. 11-7(5)]. Under these circumstances the time between the two phases of the action potential is determined by the speed of propagation in the tissue and the spacing of the electrodes. If the electrodes are closely spaced, the two monophasic action potentials will fuse to form a continuous and symmetrical biphasic action potential. If the temporal relations are such that the monophasic action potentials overlap, a smaller action potential will result. [see Fig. 11-7(6)].

Genesis of the biphasic action potential as just described is easy to demonstrate. For example, if two electrodes are placed on a strip of irritable tissue, as in Fig. 11-8, and the tissue is stimulated at one end, the traveling wave of depolarization and repolarization (action potential) will pass under electrode 1, then under electrode 2, describing a biphasic action potential. If now the distal electrode is moved further away, to positions 4 and 5, the two "interfering" phases of the biphasic action potential will be revealed. Moreover, by knowing the polarity indication of the recorder, it is possible to identify the direction of propagation of excitation because propagated excitation is, in reality, a traveling region of negativity.

11-3-2.   The Injury Potential

Between two points on the surface of intact, inactive, irritable tissue, there is no measurable potential difference. If the tissue under one electrode is depolarized, as by crushing or the application of potassium chloride (ca. 2%) solution, this region becomes negative with respect to the intact surface, and the potential difference measured between these areas is called the injury potential. Since this region is largely depolarized, it cannot be excited or recover. If the tissue becomes active elsewhere, there will be detected an excursion in potential that occurs under the electrode over uninjured tissue. Interestingly enough, the type of waveform obtained in this situation strongly resembles the excursion in transmembrane potential and arises from and returns to a baseline representing the magnitude of the injury potential.

The injury potential is particularly easy to demonstrate and is frequently encountered when a needle electrode is advanced into irritable tissue to record a bioelectric event. To demonstrate the development of an injury potential, it is expedient to use irritable tissue that is spontaneously active—for example, cardiac muscle. In Fig. 11-9 the electrical activity of a turtle ventricle was recorded with two 0.6% saline-filled wick electrodes connected to a direct-coupled amplifier. The polarity was arranged so that negativity of the basal electrode (1), and consequently, positivity of the

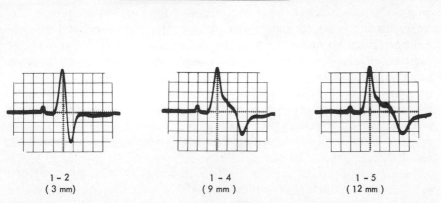

Figure 11-8. The effect of electrode spacing on the action potential of isolated frog sartorius muscle at room temperature: S = stimulus 0.5 msec; propagation velocity (calculated from record 1-5) = $12 \times 10^{-3}/6 \times 10^{-3}$ = 2 m/sec; time scale 2 msec. [From Geddes, *Electrodes and the Measurement of Bioelectric Events.* Wiley, New York, 1972.]

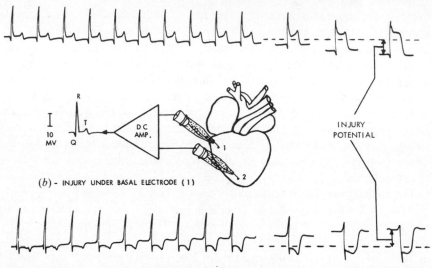

(a) - INJURY UNDER APICAL ELECTRODE (2)

(b) - INJURY UNDER BASAL ELECTRODE (1)

Figure 11-9. The injury potential. (a) Injury produced by placing a few drops of KCl under electrode 2, thereby depolarizing the tissue at this site; depression of the baseline indicates the development of injury under electrode 2. (b) Injury created under electrode 1 in a similar manner after injury was removed from under electrode 2.

apical electrode (2), caused the recording pen to rise. In the upper record, for the first few beats, both electrodes were over uninjured tissue. Then a drop of 2% potassium chloride solution was placed on the apical wick electrode, causing injury (depolarization) to develop. Note that there occurred a diastolic depression of the baseline as the region under electrode 2 became progressively negative, and the electrogram altered characteristically. Because the myocardium under electrode 2 had been rendered inactive by chemical injury, the activity recorded came mainly from the tissue under electrode 1, which shows that when this tissue became active (negative), the indicator rose, revealing the characteristic action potential of cardiac muscle, rising from and returning to a baseline that represents the injury potential.

For the first few beats in Fig. 11-9b, both electrodes were over uninjured tissue and the familiar R-T complex was seen. Then a drop of 2% potassium chloride solution was placed on the wick of electrode 1, causing injury (depolarization) to develop. Note that the diastolic baseline started to rise and the electrogram developed its characteristic change as the tissue under electrode 1 became depolarized. When depolarization began, electrical activity was recorded from the uninjured tissue under electrode 2, which, when it detects activity, causes the indicator to be deflected downward to exhibit the characteristic electrical waveform of cardiac activity falling from and returning to a baseline that has been elevated by an amount representing the injury potential.

It is interesting to note the similarity between the form of the cardiac monophasic action potential, produced by injury under a single electrode, and the excursion in transmembrane potential obtained (Fig. 11-5) when transmembrane electrodes are employed. Indeed, long before the action potential of cardiac muscle had been recorded with transmembrane electrodes, Burdon-Sanderson (1880) hypothesized that the ECG was created by the algebraic sum of two such oppositely directed monophasic action potentials displaced in time, as diagrammed in Fig. 11-13.

11-3-3.   Electrode Axis Perpendicular to Excitation

In the situations analyzed thus far, the electrodes were placed along the direction of depolarization and repolarization. If they are placed opposite each other on either side of the uniform strip of irritable tissue, as in Fig. 11-10(1), the indicator will show no potential difference. When the wave of excitation arrives at the electrodes [Fig. 11-10(2)], depolarization and reverse polarization will occur simultaneously under both electrodes, and the indicator will show no potential difference. As the wave of excitation passes onward and repolarization occurs [Fig. 11-10(3, 4)], the indicator will continue to show no potential difference.

The foregoing examples considered a uniform strip of irritable tissue in which the wave of excitation occupied a small portion of the tissue and was followed by recovery in a relatively short time. Although this situation is valid for nerve and skeletal muscle, it does not apply to cardiac muscle, in which the refractory period is long and the wave of excitation advances and occupies the whole of the tissue before recovery occurs. Moreover, in many circumstances recovery does not necessarily travel in the same direction as excitation. Therefore, the action potentials developed under these conditions are expected to be different from those previously discussed.

11-3-4.   Tissue with a Long Refractory Period

Figure 11-11(1) diagrams a strip of irritable tissue in which the refractory period is long. Assume that the tissue has been stimulated and that a wave of excitation advances and occupies the region under electrode A [Fig. 11-11(2)]. Thus A is negative with respect to electrode B, and the potential indicator rises. The wave of excitation continues to advance and ultimately occupies the region under electrode B. Because the refractory pe-

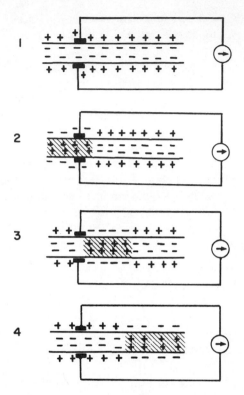

Figure 11-10.   Electrodes at right angles to direction of propagation.

riod is so long, recovery will not have occurred under electrode A; hence both electrodes are over active tissue, and the indicator shows no potential difference. Thus the first upward phase of the action potential will be described as in Fig. 11-11(3).

The sequence of events that follows depends on the manner in which recovery takes place. If the strip of irritable tissue is uniform, recovery follows in the same direction as excitation. If this situation obtains [Fig. 11-11(4)], recovery will occur first under electrode A. Under this condition electrode B is negative, A is positive, and the potential indicator falls. When recovery occurs under electrode B, the potential indicator reads zero and the second (downward) phase of the action potential is completed, as in Fig. 11-11(5).

In the sequence of events just described, the two phases of the action potential have a special meaning. The peak of the first upward monophasic action potential indicates excitation under electrode A. The end of this action potential shows that the whole tissue is active. The beginning of the downward wave indicates that recovery is starting under electrode A, and recovery under this electrode becomes complete when the peak of the downward action potential is reached. Completion of the downward action potential indicates full recovery of the tissue.

If the strip of irritable tissue is not uniform or if a metabolic gradient exists, the foregoing sequence of events will not occur. If, when all the tissue is active [Fig. 11-11(3)], recovery proceeds in the direction opposite to that of excitation, the second phase of the action potential will be different. In Fig. 11-11(6) recovery is shown to proceed from right to left, resulting in electrode B becoming positive with respect to A. Thus the potential indicator will rise, and the second phase of the monophasic action potential will be upward, that is, in the same direction as the first. As the tissue fully recovers, the second (upward) phase of the action potential is completed [Fig. 11-11(7)].

In the case just analyzed, the peak of the first upward phase described excitation under electrode A. At the end of the first monophasic action potential, when the indicator read zero, all the tissue was active. The beginning of the second upward phase indicated the start of recovery under elec-

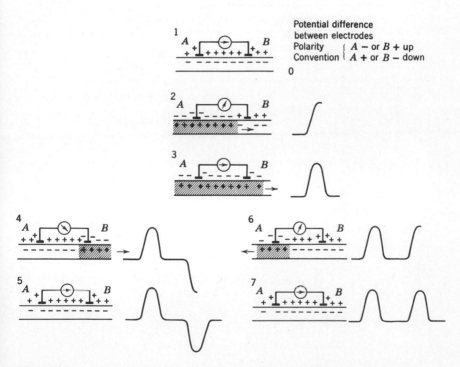

Figure 11-11.   Genesis of an action potential in a tissue with a long refractory period.

trode *B*, which was complete when the second upward monophasic action potential was completed.

Thus in irritable tissue, in which the refractory period is long, if the two phases of the action potential are in opposite directions, excitation and recovery travel in the same direction. If the two phases are in the same direction, excitation and recovery travel in opposite directions.

Figure 11-12 reveals how these fundamental circumstances underlie the genesis of the ECG when recorded with two electrodes on the heart. In Fig. 11-12*a* the ECG was obtained with a macroelectrode and a microelectrode which, in the first part of the record (Fig. 11-12*a*) rested on the outside of a cardiac muscle cell. On the left of the illustration can be seen the familiar QRS-T complex of the ECG. In the middle of the record the microelectrode was pushed into a single cardiac muscle cell and the ECG was replaced by a monophasic action potential. Figure 11-12*b* shows the relationship between the ECG and the simultaneously recorded monophasic action potential.

In Fig. 11-13 are monophasic action potentials recorded from a frog ventricle. Applying the interference theory, the recorder sees the algebraic temporal sum of the monophasic action potentials; the voltage recorded is the familiar R-T complex of the ECG. This situation is diagrammed in Fig. 11-13*c*. The solid line represents the summated ECG developed when excitation and recovery travel in the same direction; that is, the monophasic action potentials are alike but displaced in time. The dotted line in Fig. 11-13*b* illustrates the situation when recovery occurs earlier at the last electrode to become active. The effect is to make the T wave upward (dotted curve in Fig. 11-13*c*).

The ECG, as conventionally recorded, reflects the potential difference between a pair of electrodes on the surface of the body. The origin of this time-dependent potential difference resides in the muscle fibers that make up the two masses of the heart—the atria and the ventricles—each fiber producing its own action potential. Thus the ECG is the result of the temporal and spatial summation of the activities of all the myocardial fibers. Notwithstanding the obvious complexity of the resultant potential difference, it is interesting to see how the nature of the fundamental bioelectric generator, the monophasic action potential, reveals itself in recordings made with appropriately placed surface electrodes.

The manner in which initial polarity indicates direction of propagation of the wave of excitation can be demonstrated easily. For example, in the normal mammalian heart, because excitation of the ventricles advances generally from base to apex and the polarity for recording the ECG is chosen so that in lead II negativity of the right arm electrode (hence, positivity of the left leg) causes the indicator to deflect upward, the mono-

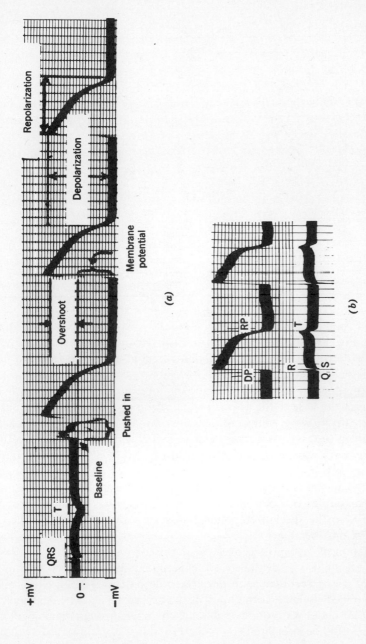

Figure 11-12. (*a*) Relationship of the electrocardiogram to the monophasic action potential. (*b*) Simultaneously recorded monophasic action potentials and the ECG. [From Hecht, *Ann. N.Y. Acad. Sci.* **65**:7 (1956–1957). By permission.]

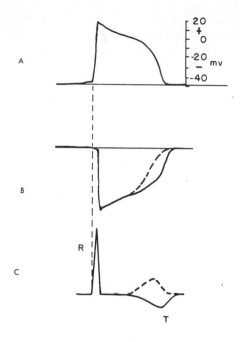

Figure 11-13. Summation of the monophasic action potentials to produce the ECG. (From Hoff and Geddes, *Experimental Physiology*, Baylor Medical College, Houston. By permission.)

phasic action potentials summate to cause the R wave of the ECG to be upward, as in Fig. 11-13c. If excitation travels in the opposite direction (apex to base), the downward monophasic action potential will occur first and the R wave will be inverted.

In the experimental animal, if excitation is forced to travel in the normal direction from the base to the apex, by application of a stimulus to the base of the heart, the R wave is upward, as shown by R' in Fig. 11-14. If excitation is forced to travel from apex to base by delivery of a stimulus to the apex, the primary wave of excitation, QS in Fig. 11-14, will be downward. Note that in both instances the wave of excitation (R' and QS) are longer in duration than the normally propagated waves of excitation because the evoked extrasystoles traveled in myocardium, which has a slower propagation rate than the specialized conduction system of the heart (bundle of His and Purkinje fibers).

The situation of hastened recovery of the tissue under the electrode last to be excited can also be demonstrated experimentally. Figure 11-15 shows the ECG of a dog recorded with one electrode on the right forelimb and the other applied directly to the apex of the left ventricle. The ventricular electrode (thermode) was a hollow metallic chamber through which cold or warm water could be circulated.

When warm water was circulated through the thermode (Fig. 11-15, left), local metabolism was increased and recovery was hastened. Under these conditions the T wave became large and upright. By circulating cold water through the electrode, recovery was prolonged; hence the T wave became inverted. This sequence of events appears on the right in Fig. 11-15. In the center of the record it can be seen that at an intermediate temperature the T wave disappeared, indicating that the recovery occurred simultaneously in the regions of the ventricles seen by both electrodes.

Thus it is apparent that the form of an action potential, as detected by the pair of electrodes on the surface of a strip of homogeneous irritable tissue, is dependent on the time course of depolarization, reverse polarization, and repolarization; the speed with which the depolarization travels in the tissue; the amount of tissue occupied by the wave of excitation; and the orientation of the electrodes with respect to the direction of propagation of the wave of excitation, and recovery.

11-4. DIPOLE THEORY

Since active tissue is electronegative with respect to an inactive or recovered area, a boundary exists which is characterized by an array of positive and negative charges (see Fig. 11-16a). The boundary between active and inactive tissue can be represented by a dipole, and because environmental tissues and fluids can conduct current, potential fields will be established, as in Fig. 11-16b.

The potential field surrounding a current dipole in an infinite volume conductor is represented in Fig. 11-17. If the dipole moves along its axis, its field will accompany it, and the potential (V_p) at a nearby point (with respect to an indifferent electrode located in a region of zero potential) will start to rise, then fall to zero (when the dipole center is nearest the point), increase in the negative direction, then decrease as the dipole moves farther away. Thus a positive-negative diphasic wave will be described as in Fig. 11-17 ($d = 1$) as the dipole passes the measuring point. If the point is

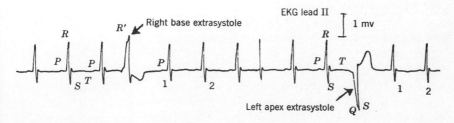

Figure 11-14.   Normal canine ECG, showing induced venticular basal (R') and apical (QS) systoles.

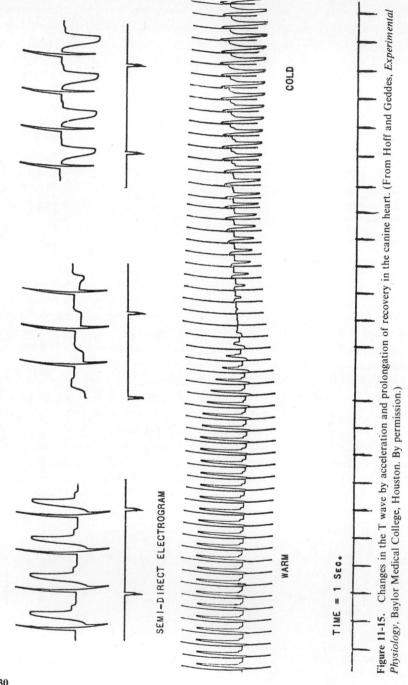

SEMI-DIRECT ELECTROGRAM

WARM

COLD

TIME = 1 SEC.

Figure 11-15. Changes in the T wave by acceleration and prolongation of recovery in the canine heart. (From Hoff and Geddes, *Experimental Physiology*, Baylor Medical College, Houston. By permission.)

430

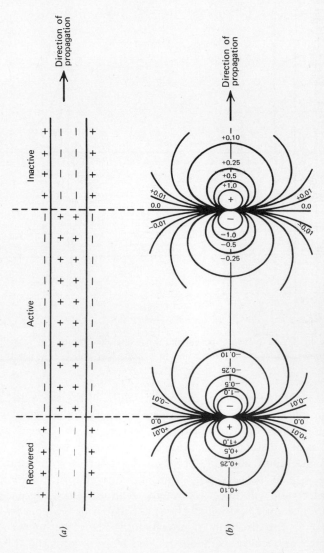

Figure 11-16. Application of the dipole concept to represent excitation and recovery. Because active tissue is electronegative to inactive and recovered tissue, the boundaries of active tissue can be equated to dipoles. The dipole of excitation travels with its positive pole facing the direction of propagation of excitation. The dipole of recovery travels with its negative pole facing the direction of propagation of recovery.

431

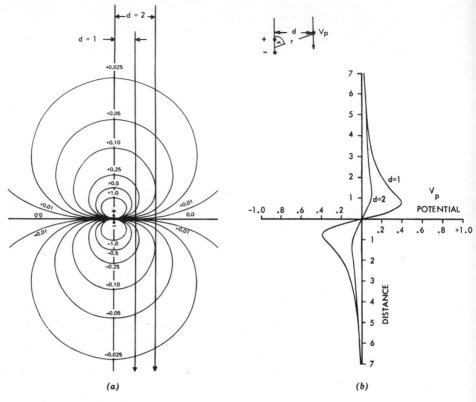

Figure 11-17. The dipole and its field of potential: (*a*) potential distribution; (*b*) potential encountered by exploring electrode moving along lines (*d* = 1, *d* = 2) parallel to the dipole axis.

more distant, (*d* = 2), the potential excursion will be in the same direction but decreased in amplitude. This sequence of events describes what is obtained with "monopolar" recording; that is, one electrode is near active tissue, the other is at a distance in a region of no potential change.

According to the dipole concept, propagated excitation is equated to a dipole traveling with its positive pole facing the direction of propagation. Thus a nearby electrode will detect a positive-negative biphasic potential as excitation passes. Recovery (repolarization) is equated to a dipole with its negative pole facing the direction of propagation. Therefore, at a nearby point, the passage of recovery will be signaled by a negative-positive biphasic potential. If excitation and recovery are widely separated, a complex tetraphasic waveform (Fig. 11-18*a*) would be expected for the passage of excitation recovery. If, on the other hand, excitation occupied only a small amount of tissue, the potential fields of the two dipoles will overlap and a triphasic waveform (Fig. 11-18c) will be obtained.

It is interesting to note that in many situations of "monopolar" recording the waveform seen is quite similar to that in Fig. 11-18c. However, certain important limitations must be borne in mind regarding the physiological application of the dipole concept. For example, although the boundary between active and inactive tissue is sharp enough to allow use of the dipole concept, the boundary between active and recovering tissue is much more diffuse and irregular; hence, the dipoles of excitation and recovery do not have the same strength or spatial distribution. Moreover, the dipoles of excitation and recovery increase and decrease in strength temporally, and the amount of tissue occupied by excitation is a property of the type of tissue; hence, the "separation" of the dipoles of excitation and recovery will reflect this fact along with the speed of propagation of recovery and excitation. When applying the dipole concept to explain the genesis of a waveform, it is wise to remember these important physiological factors.

The dipole concept was first applied to nerve by Bernstein's pupil, Hermann (1879); it was later applied by Craib (1927), Wilson et al. (1934), and Macleod (1938a and b) to cardiac muscle. Verification of its applicability to human electrocardiography has been presented by Woodbury et al. (1950). Lorente de Nó (1947), in an elegant series of experiments, mapped out the dipole potential field surrounding active and recovered regions in frog sciatic nerve.

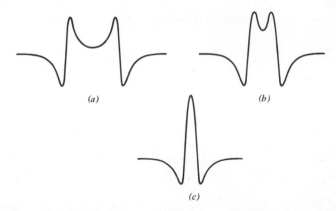

(a)   (b)

(c)

Figure 11-18. Theoretical waveforms obtainable by a dipole of excitation and recovery passing a local electrode with the reference electrode in a region of zero potential. From (a) to (c) the dipoles of excitation and recovery are progressively closer. The waveform in (c) is frequently encountered with monopolar recording.

11-5. POTENTIAL DISTRIBUTION AROUND BIOELECTRIC GENERATORS

After measuring the potential differences between leads placed on various points on the surface of the body, Waller (1889) postulated that the potential distribution at the peak of the R wave due to ventricular activity could be attributed to an equivalent dipole, as in Fig. 11-19. Since Waller's time many investigators have plotted the isopotential lines at various instants in the cycle of activity of bioelectric generators. Electrocardiographic isopotential lines appearing on the thorax at different instants during atrial and ventricular excitation and recovery were mapped in

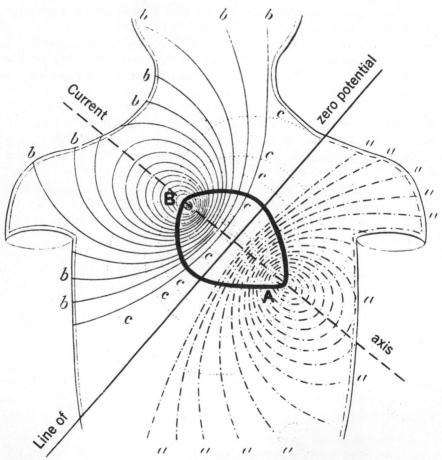

Figure 11-19. Waller's concept of the distribution of potential on the human thorax resulting from ventricular activity. [From Waller, *Phil. Trans. Roy. Soc.* **180B**:169–194 (1889). By permission of the Royal Society.]

human subjects by Nahum et al. (1951), Mauro et al. (1952), Nahum et al. (1952–1953), Simonson (1952), Frank (1955, 1956–1957), Nelson (1956), Tasaki (1959), Flaherty et al. (1967), Spach et al. (1966); in the dog by Maruo et al. (1952), Taccardi (1962), Horan et al. (1963), and Nelson et al. (1965); and in the monkey and lamb by Nelson et al. (1965).

Such isopotential maps represent the potential distribution during one instant in the cardiac cycle. A complete display of the electrical activity for the whole cardiac cycle would require the plotting of instantaneous potential distributions at each instant in atrial and ventricular activity and recovery, that is, during the P, Tp, QRS, and T waves. Thus, it is apparent that the isopotential lines are time varying. Figure 11-20 illustrates the time variance of the surface potential distribution during the ventricular depolarization process as described by the QRS wave of the ECG.

It should be obvious that the availability of a temporal series of isopotential maps derived for excitation and recovery of any bioelectric source identifies the source of potential and allows derivation of the voltage-time curve obtained with electrodes located anywhere in the mapped potential field. The voltage appearing between a pair of electrodes in the potential field is, of course, the difference in the potentials under each electrode.

Electroencephalographic isopotential lines have been plotted for various cerebral states. Two of the earliest to investigate this method of localizing active regions of the brain were Adrian and Matthews (1934). The study was continued by Brazier (1949), who presented a series of diagrams constructed from the EEG records of normal and abnormal subjects. Two of her diagrams from normal subjects appear in Fig. 11-21. Figure 11-21*a* shows the scalp potential distribution during an instant in the development of the alpha rhythm, the normal background activity that characterizes the awake, relaxed subject. Clearly evident is the focal location of this rhythm in the occipital region. Figure 11-21*b* shows the location of the origin of a low-frequency source in the sleeping subject.

Many penetrating theoretical studies have been carried out on the surface distributions of potentials for dipoles in irregularly shaped volume conductors. Those interested in this aspect of this field should consult the papers by Wilson and Bayley (1950), Frank (1953a), Okada (1956, 1957), Geselowitz (1960), Brody et al. (1961), Hlavin and Plonsey (1963), and Plonsey (1963).

11-6.   THE TRANSMEMBRANE AND EXTRACELLULAR POTENTIAL

When a strip of irritable tissue in a living organism becomes active, this region is electronegative with respect to the tissue that is inactive (or has

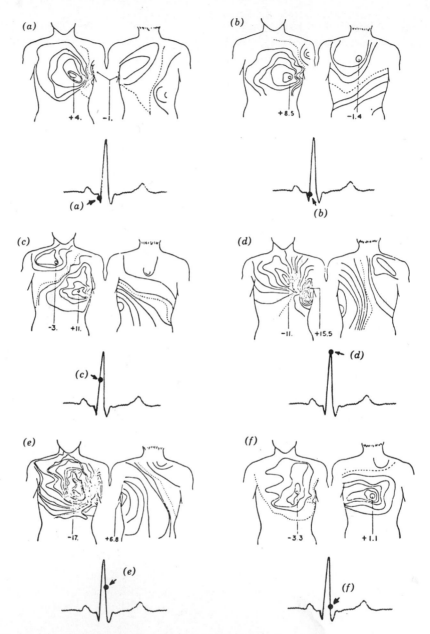

Figure 11-20. Thoracic potential distribution at various instants in the ventricular depolarization process. Lead I is shown for identification purposes. (From Nahum, in Fulton (ed); *Textbook of Physiology*, 17th ed. W. B. Saunders Co. Philadelphia, (1955). By permission of the author and publisher.)

436

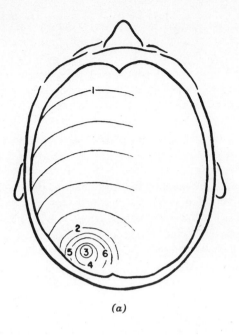

(a)

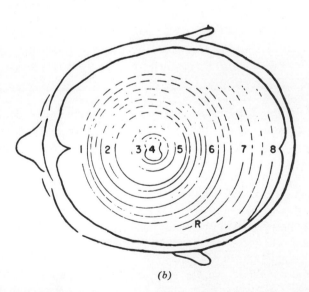

(b)

Figure 11-21. Potential distribution on the head due to electrical activity of the brain: (*a*) surface potential distribution of an alpha rhythm; (*b*) surface potential distribution at one instant during sleep. [From Brazier, *EEG Clin. Neurophysiol. Suppl.* **2**:38–52 (1949). By permission of Masson & Cie, Publisher.]

recovered). Therefore, current will flow in the anisotropic environmental volume conductor constituted by tissues and fluids, each of which has its own conductance. Consequently, the spatial distribution of current will not resemble that surrounding a dipole in a volume conductor. Nonetheless, a potential field will be established by the current flow, and a voltage can be measured between an exploring (active) electrode placed in the field and another (reference) electrode in a region of zero potential. However, the waveform of the voltage detected by the extracellular active electrode is quite different from the form of the excursion in transmembrane potential when the tissue becomes active and recovers. It would be convenient if there were a simple method to relate the extracellular action potential to the excursion in transmembrane potential. Unfortunately, this relationship can only be established for very simple cases in which the geometry of the active tissue and the environment are simple and the environmental volume conductor is isotropic. Nonetheless, the first steps have been taken to establish the nature of this relationship. In his book on bioelectric phenomena, Plonsey (1969) discusses the difficulties in using the core-conductor (cable) model and in applying field theory to the solution of biological problems based on this model. Excellent papers on the cable analog, which is best applied to a long strip of irritable tissue, were presented by Huxley and Stampfli (1944), Tasaki (1959), Clark and Plonsey (1966), and Geselowitz (1966). The applications of field theory were presented by Lorente de Nó (1947), Clark and Plonsey (1968), and Plonsey (1969). In the application of field theory to determine the extracellular potential distribution, it is necessary to solve the Laplace equation, and the main difficulty centers around specification of the boundary conditions.

The solutions of the equations based on the cable analog and those applying field theory are obviously different. Nonetheless, both contain a term which is the second derivative of the transmembrane potential, although other factors are also present. If a simple monophasic waveform for the excursion in transmembrane potential V(t) is chosen, as in Fig. 11-22, it is possible to differentiate it twice to obtain a waveform that will demonstrate the principal differences between the transmembrane and extracellular potential, recorded with a monopolar electrode. Note that the second derivative is a triphasic action potential, having an upward wave much shorter than that of the excursion in transmembrane potential.

There is considerable debate regarding the exact relationship between the transmembrane potential and the form of the extracellular action potential, but the work thus far tends to confirm that the form resembles that of a second derivative of the transmembrane potential. Figure 11-23 presents a compilation of transmembrane potential recordings and extracellular action potentials. The extracellular action potentials have the general ap-

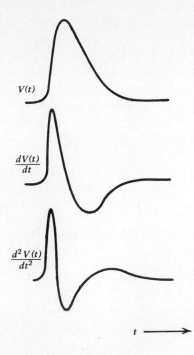

Figure 11-22. Idealized transmembrane potential excursion $V_{(t)}$, its first derivative $dV(t)/dt$, and its second derivative $d^2V(t)/dt^2$.

pearance of the second derivative of the excursion in transmembrane potential.

11-7. ELECTROMYOGRAPHY (EMG)

Electromyography is the study of the electrical activity of muscle; clinical electromyography (or EMG) is the name applied to the investigation of the electrical activity of normal and diseased skeletal muscle with extracellular electrodes. It is important to note that electrical studies are also made of the other two types of muscle, namely, cardiac and smooth. Electrocardiography (ECG) is concerned with the electrical manifestations of heart muscle; there is no special name assigned to electrographic study of smooth muscle, although such studies are made of the urinary bladder, ureters, stomach, intestine, sphincters, and other smooth-muscle organs.

Clinical electromyography provides important information on the physiological status of skeletal muscle and its nerve supply. In cases of muscle paralysis, it allows identification of the site of the lesion, that is, within the brain (upper motor neuron) or spinal cord (lower motor neuron), its axon, the end plate, and muscle fiber. Upper motor neuron dysfunction, due to stroke, hysteria, malingering, trauma, or other causes, although

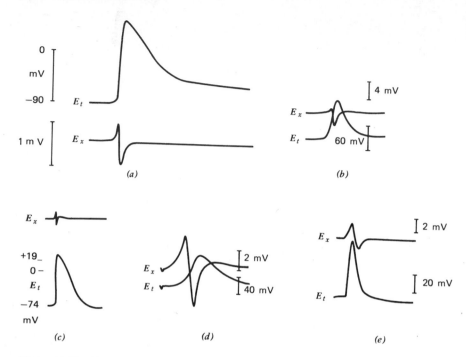

Figure 11-23. Transmembrane (E_t) and extracellular action potentials (E_x) obtained from different irritable tissues. (a) Frog semitendinous muscle. [Redrawn from Hakansson, *Acta Physiol Scand.* **39**:291–312 (1957).] (b) Toad sartorius muscle. [Redrawn from Murakami et al., *Jap. J. Physiol.* **11**:80–88 (1961).] (c) Rabbit atrium. [Redrawn from Williams, *Nature* **183**:1341–1342 (1959).] (d) Crayfish giant axon. [Redrawn from (e) Single spinal motoneurone. [Redrawn from Freygang, *Gen. Physiol.* **42**:749–760 (1959).]

resulting in paralysis, does not produce the same electromyographic signs seen with disease of the spinal motor nerve cell and its associated axon and muscle fibers. When a motor nerve cell or its axon degenerates, or when the nerve fiber to a muscle is severed, the previously innervated muscle fibers are paralyzed and cannot be contracted voluntarily or reflexly. A normally innervated muscle shows no electrical activity at rest; when voluntarily or reflexly contracted it produces action potentials. Following denervation, a muscle is paralyzed; but after a time, which is species-dependent (Table 11-2), the individual muscle fibers start to contract and relax independently (i.e., to fibrillate), producing a characteristic type of rhythmic action potential called fibrillation waves, which signal that the nerve supply has been interrupted. These random and asynchronous contractions produce no net muscle tension, and they continue as long as there is muscle tissue present and denervation persists. If reinnervation does not occur, the

Table 11-2 Appearance Time for Fibrillation Potentials in Denervated Skeletal Muscle*

Species	Muscle	Appearance Time (days)
Mouse	Peroneal	3.5
Rat	—	4
Rabbit	—	6
Monkey	Brachio-radialis	8
Man	Brachio-radialis	18

* From G. Weddell, *Lancet* 1: 236–239, 1943.

muscle fibers atrophy and the fibrillation potentials disappear. If reinnervation occurs, the muscle fibers cease to atrophy, and the fibrillation potentials gradually disappear, being replaced slowly by normal muscle action potentials, which appear when a voluntary effort is made or when the muscle is contracted reflexly. It is important to realize that during reinnervation a characteristic polyphasic (nascent) action potential can be detected with voluntary contraction, long before there are visible signs of muscular contraction. Figure 11-24a illustrates a typical normal muscle action potential; Figs. 11-24b and 11-24c show, respectively, fibrillation potentials and a typical electromyographic picture during reinnervation when primitive muscle action and fibrillation potentials are present.

The type of equipment used to record clinical electromyograms merits special consideration because of the small area of the active electrodes and the short duration and rapid rise of the electromyographic signals. Direct graphic recording instruments cannot be employed to obtain recordings of

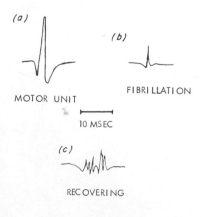

(a)

(b)

MOTOR UNIT

FIBRILLATION

10 MSEC

(c)

RECOVERING

Figure 11-24. Normal motor unit potential (a) and fibrillation waves (b); the latter are characteristically present in denervated muscle. During early reinnervation (c), recovering, low-amplitude, short-duration polyphasic action potentials appear during a voluntary contraction effort; at this time muscle contraction is seldom visible.

diagnostic significance; instead, a cathode ray oscilloscope is used with an amplifier having a high input impedance (several megohms) and an adequate bandwidth (ca. 2–5000 Hz). The repetition rate of the sweep of the oscilloscope is usually fixed at about 7 sweeps/sec and the sweep speed is controllable from 20 to 2 msec/cm. Minimum performance recommendations for electromyographs are presented at the end of this chapter.

It is convenient to use a loudspeaker to provide aural monitoring since the diagnostic information is contained in waveform and repetition rate. With very little experience, the ear can be trained to detect normal motor unit action potentials, which produce a thumping sound; fibrillation potentials give a characteristic ticking, clicking, or crackling sound. Although it is easy to recognize these and other characteristic waveforms, 'considerable skill and experience are needed to assess their significance in terms of the presence of neuromuscular disease or dysfunction.

In general, the clinical electromyographer applies the reference and ground electrodes to the subject, as shown in Fig. 11-25. Then while the investigator watches the oscilloscope and listens to the loudspeaker, the needle electrode is quickly advanced into the muscle to be examined. Insertion of the needle usually causes mechanical stimulation of subjacent muscle (or nerve) fibers, and a short burst of action potentials will be heard and also seen on the oscilloscope. The character of these insertion

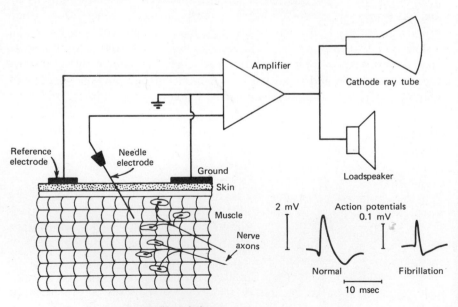

Figure 11-25.   Electromyographic technique.

potentials depends on the status of the muscle. If normally innervated, the action potentials will resemble normal motor units, which will disappear within a few seconds if the muscle is at rest. Prolonged or absent insertion potentials is a sign of muscle abnormality. When the needle electrode is positioned close to contracting motor units, the action potentials obtained are 1 to 10 msec in duration and 50 to 3000 μV in amplitude.

Proper location of the electrode tip is greatly facilitated by the sound in the loudspeaker. As active fibers are approached, the sound becomes characteristically sharper and much more distinct. If the muscle is denervated and enough time has passed (Table 11-2) for fibrillation potentials to develop, the insertion potentials are a train of short-duration fibrillation waves, which continue at a much slower rate (1 to 10 per second), thereby providing the diagnostic sign of denervation. Subsequent mechanical movement of the needle often sets off a train of positive-wave potentials, when the needle electrode is in injured muscle.

To comprehend the various waveforms obtained in electromyographic studies, it is necessary to have an understanding of neuromuscular physiology, which is concerned with the manner by which muscular contraction occurs. The following abbreviated account provides the essential details.

The contractile unit of skeletal muscle is the muscle fiber, which is a single multinucleated cylindrical cell about 50 μ in diameter; when stimulated, the fiber is capable of shortening (contracting) and developing force. A whole muscle consists of parallel bundles (fascicles) of muscle fibers. Each muscle fiber is in turn composed of fibrils, which are bundles of filaments of contractile protein; the filaments are about 150 Å in diameter. The structural arrangement of the contractile filaments causes skeletal muscle to exhibit cross striations visible with a low-power microscope. For this reason it is often called striated muscle.

Activation of each skeletal muscle fiber occurs in response to an action potential traveling along a motor nerve fiber (axon) which innervates the muscle fiber. Depending on the location and function of the muscle, each axon may innervate one muscle fiber (as in the extraocular muscles) or as many as 600 to 1200 muscle fibers (as in the case of the postural muscles): Fig. 11-25 illustrates an innervation ratio of 3:1. The combination of the motor nerve cell in the spinal cord, its axon, and the muscle fibers that it innervates is the basic functional unit of the muscular system and is called the motor unit. When the nerve action potential reaches the specialized tissue junction between the nerve and muscle (the myoneural junction or motor end plate), a quantum of chemical transmitter (acetylcholine) is released. This transmitter causes a local depolarization of the subjacent polarized membrane of the muscle fiber and initiates an action potential that is propagated over the entire muscle fiber; a single contraction (twitch) follows within about one millisecond. The transmitter is quickly neutralized by acetylcholine esterase and the end plate is ready to receive another quantum of transmitter. Meanwhile, during the contraction, the membrane of the muscle fiber starts to recover, and recovery is complete even before the full force of contraction is reached. Figure 11-4 illustrates the temporal relationship between the twitch and the excursion in transmembrane potential. Since recovery is so rapid in skeletal muscle, many closely spaced stimuli can be delivered, and the contractions will fuse into a sustained or tetanic contraction, as in Fig. 11-26.

The force developed by a muscle is graded in two ways. It is now apparent that a single action potential in an axon of the motor nerve will produce a twitch in all the muscle fibers that it innervates. If more axons are activated, at the same time, more muscle fibers will be stimulated, and the twitch will develop more force. On the other hand, if a single axon is stimulated more frequently, the twitches will fuse into a tetanic contraction, which develops several times more force than does the twitch. Therefore, the force of muscular contraction is graded by controlling the number of axons that are stimulated and the frequency of stimulation in each axon.

In clinical electromyography, muscle action potentials are recorded with a small-area (active) electrode located near a contracting muscle fiber and the reference electrode located at a distance. Therefore, the waveform obtained with such an extracellular recording method will not resemble the

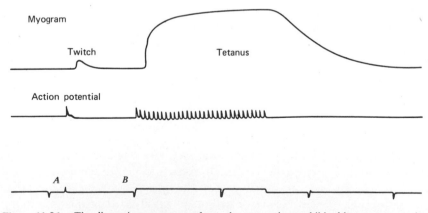

Figure 11-26. The discontinuous nature of muscle contractions exhibited by a myogram (upper) and an electromyogram (lower) obtained from a frog gastrocnemius muscle by delivering single and repetitive stimuli to the sciatic nerve. A single stimulus (*A*) provides a single action potential and a twitch; (*B*) repetitive stimulation at 20 per second evoked an action potential for each stimulus and a sustained (tetanic) contraction. (Time marks, 1 sec.)

excursion in transmembrane potential because the active electrode measures the potential change caused by extracellular current flow within the muscle, which acts as an inhomogeneous volume conductor. Depending on the medium surrounding the active tissue, the waveform detected approximates the second time derivative of the transmembrane potential. Katz and Miledi (1965) presented an interesting record (Fig. 11-27) which illustrates this point. Microelectrodes were inserted into a frog sartorius muscle immersed in saline at 20°C; one microelectrode was used for stimulation, the other recorded the transmembrane potential with respect to a reference electrode in the saline. The extracellular recording electrode was about 6 mm from the tendon. The excursion in transmembrane potential is a typical monophasic action potential rising quickly from the resting membrane potential, overshooting (reversing polarization), and slowly returning to the resting membrane potential. The extracellular action potential is triphasic and resembles the second derivative of the transmembrane potential.

The electrical activity of skeletal muscle can be recorded by placing two disk electrodes on the surface of the skin along the axis of a contracting skeletal muscle. The voltage appearing between the electrodes is the algebraic sum of all the action potentials of the contracting and recovering muscle fibers between the electrodes. The frequency and the peak voltage exhibit a nonlinear relationship with the force developed by the muscle. The frequency of the action potentials ranges from zero at rest to several hundred hertz during a maximal contraction. Although this noninvasive technique is of value in kinesiology studies, it is too imprecise for the diagnosis of neuromuscular diseases that require a needle electrode, paired with a surface (reference) electrode (Fig. 11-25) or a monopolar or bipolar coaxial hypodermic electrode (see Chapter 9). Using these subcutaneous electrodes, a muscle can be examined for the presence of normal motor units or fibrillation potentials. It is important to understand that the amplitude and duration of the action potentials are dependent on the type of electrode employed and the muscle under investigation.

At the beginning of this section, it was stated that clinical electromyography (in which a needle and a skin-surface electrode are used) provides useful information on the innervation status of skeletal muscle. A few examples are now presented to illustrate how diagnostic information is provided by the EMG. For example, in myasthenia gravis—a condition in which the muscle fibers are normally innervated but transmission of impulses across the myoneural junction is impaired—muscular contraction can be sustained only for short periods. In severe cases there is widespread paralysis involving the respiratory muscles. With this disease, because the muscle fibers are normally innervated, there are no fibrillation potentials at

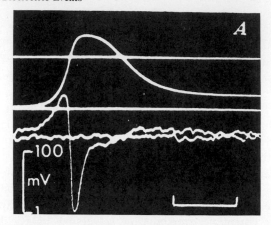

Figure 11-27. Simultaneous transmembrane potential (upper) and extracellular action potential (lower) recorded from a monopolar electrode near a frog gastrocnemius muscle. The length of the vertical calibration bar represents 100 mV for the transmembrane recording and 1 mV for the extracellular recording. The muscle was stimulated by an intracellular electrode. [From Katz and Miledi, *Proc. Roy. Soc.* (*London*) **161B**:453–495 (1964–1965). By permission.]

rest. Insertion of the needle electrode produces a train of insertion potentials as in the case of a normal muscle. With voluntary contraction, normal potentials arise, but do not persist because of impaired transmission at the myoneural junction. If the disease is severe, the frequency and voltage of the normal motor units are reduced. The diagnosis of myasthenia gravis is confirmed by the administration of a short-acting acetylcholine esterase inhibitor, which temporarily enhances myoneural transmission and provides an essentially normal EMG on voluntary contraction.

Muscular dystrophy is a degenerative disease of muscle in which there is atrophy of some fibers, swelling of others, an increase in sarcolemmal nuclei and connective tissue separations, with the deposition of fat between other fibers that become hypertrophied. On insertion of the needle electrode, there is a vigorous discharge of low-amplitude, short-duration, high-frequency (dystrophic) potentials. At rest, there are no fibrillation waves because there is usually no nerve damage (see below). With voluntary contraction, the action potentials are low in amplitude, short in duration (1–2 msec), and high in frequency (up to 40/sec); they produce a high-pitched whirring sound in the loudspeaker. As a result of the loss of contractile elements in the motor units, more motor units are brought into action to provide the necessary force; hence, the increased frequency of discharge with voluntary effort is not surprising. On relaxation there is electrical silence. With sustained contraction, the electrical activity alternately increases and decreases as the muscle begins to fatigue, at which time there is a marked reduction in electrical activity. Depending on the severity of the disease, normal motor unit potentials may also be recorded. Fibrillation potentials are rarely seen and, if present, result from nerve interruption due to fibrotic muscle encroaching on nerve fibers within the muscle.

Myotonia is a degenerative disease of muscle in which the individual muscle fibers are hyperexcitable and the whole muscle does not relax readily. Insertion of the needle electrode evokes an intense discharge of regular, high-frequency action potentials which may persist for a few seconds or as long as nearly one minute. This pattern of electrical discharge produces a characteristic initial thunderstorm-like sound in the loud-speaker. Similar discharges can be evoked by tapping the muscle or the needle electrode. When relaxation does occur, there is electrical silence and no fibrillation potentials are recorded. During voluntary contraction, normal motor unit activity is recorded along with short-duration discharges from the diseased muscle fibers.

From this brief introductory description of the type of electrical activity recorded in normal skeletal muscles and in several common neuromuscular diseases, it should be evident that if a muscle is denervated, either by disease or trauma affecting the spinal motor neuron or its axon, there will occur paralysis, atrophy of the muscle fibers previously innervated, and fibrillation potentials. In man, such potentials appear about three weeks following denervation; they persist as long as muscle fibers are present. The fibrillation potentials slowly disappear as reinnervation occurs, or when the muscle fibers disappear. On the other hand, with diseases that affect muscle fibers' (myopathies), fibrillation potentials are absent, and the electrical activity recorded depends on the type of muscle disease.

The reader who is interested in pursuing the study of electromyography in depth should consult the following original papers: Weddell et al. (1944), Kugelberg (1947), Jasper and Ballem (1949), Denny-Brown (1949), Petersen and Kugelberg (1949), Landau (1951), Lundervold and Li (1953), Buchtal et al. (1954), and Liberson (1962). Among the useful clinical textbooks on electromyography are those by Pearson (1961), Licht (1961), Norris (1963), and Marinacci (1965), and the review of electromyography by Simpson (1973).

11-8. ELECTROCARDIOGRAPHY

Regardless of how it is recorded, the electrocardiogram merely reflects the propagation of electrical depolarization and repolarization over the various contractile chambers of the heart. Propagation of excitation (depolarization) is the trigger for releasing the stored contractile energy in cardiac muscle. It must be recognized that situations are commonly encountered in which there is an uncoupling of the excitation-contraction mechanism, and excitation can occur without contraction. In addition, a premature ventricular electrical excitation may not be followed by a mechanical contraction strong enough to open the aortic or pulmonic valves. In this circumstance, the number of R waves of the ECG is greater than the number of arterial pulses.

The term "electrocardiogram" is specifically reserved for a record of the electrical activity of the heart obtained with body-surface electrodes. "Cardiac electrogram" is the term employed when electrodes are placed directly on the heart to detect its electrical activity. A semidirect cardiac electrogram describes a record of the electrical activity of the heart obtained with one direct-heart electrode and one body-surface electrode. These terms are not always used properly, but the correct definitions should be noted. Finally, the English-language abbreviation is ECG, rather than EKG (which derives from the German Elektrokardiogramm). To avoid confusion, electroencephalographers now use ECoG (rather than ECG) to designate the electrocorticogram, which is a recording of the electrical activity of the exposed outer surface (cortex) of the brain (see Section 11-10).

All hearts consist of a series of contractile chambers, suitably equipped with valves that allow blood to be propelled in one direction. Each contractile chamber produces electrical action and recovery potentials associated with mechanical contraction and relaxation (recovery). The general rule is that the bioelectric event precedes the mechanical event. Each contractile chamber, or a region within it, exhibits spontaneous rhythmicity. That special region of the heart with the highest degree of rhythmicity is the pacemaker that normally sets the cardiac frequency; in the mammalian heart this is a region of modified muscle tissue called the sinoatrial (SA) node. The pacemaker rate is affected by temperature and the net neural bias. With these generalizations, it is possible to understand the action of a wide variety of hearts.

Neither the interference nor the dipole theories totally explain all the waveforms encountered in clinical electrocardiography. The simplest hypothesis equates the propagation of excitation as the advance of an array of positive charges (dipoles) with negativity trailing. The conventions employed to record this electrical event are given in Figs. 11-28 and 11-29; for the polarities indicated, an upward deflection signals the advance of excitation toward the positive electrode. Recovery is indicated by the approach of an array of negative charges (dipoles). If recovery progresses in the same direction as excitation, a downward deflection is obtained in leads shown in Figs. 11-28 and 11-29.

A convenient method of studying the cardiac cycle employs the electrocardiogram as a timing reference. This technique will be applied to the cardiac cycle of the mammalian heart, which contains two distinct atria (which contract together) and two separate ventricles, which also contract together shortly after atrial contraction.

Excitation from the atria is propagated to the ventricles by way of a tissue bridge called the atrioventricular (A-V) node, which has a low propagation velocity and therefore delays the spread of excitation to the ventricles. Excitation of the ventricular musculature occurs by way of the A-V node, bundle of His, and Purkinje fibers. It is largely the spread of electrical activity over the surface of the heart that constitutes the electrocardiogram.

The mammalian ECG can be dissected into two major components, one associated with the propagation of excitation and recovery over the atria; the other, with events occurring in the ventricles, the main pumping chambers of the heart. Excitation of the atria gives rise to the P wave, after which atrial contraction propels blood from the atria into the ventricles; this event is sometimes accompanied by the fourth heart sound. An atrial recovery wave exists, but is rarely seen because it is obscured by ventricular excitation, which is signaled by the QRS wave. During the latter part of the QRS wave, ventricular contraction commences which closes the A-V valves (giving rise to the first heart sound). Slightly thereafter, blood is pumped into the lungs by the right ventricle and into the aorta by the left ventricle. Recovery of the ventricles is preceded by the T wave. When ventricular pressure falls below the outflow pressure, the outflow valves (pulmonic and aortic) close, suddenly giving rise to the second heart sound. When ventricular pressure falls below atrial pressure, ventricular filling occurs, which often gives rise to a third heart sound. The evolution of the ECG during movement of the atria and ventricles is depicted in Fig. 11-30; the relationship between the ECG and the events of the cardiac cycle just described appear in Fig. 11-31. Thus, examination of the various components of the ECG identifies the sequence of excitation and recovery of the heart. The configuration of the ECG and the durations of the various waves carry important physiologic and diagnostic information. The ECG should therefore be viewed as the timing signal for the events of the cardiac cycle.

Although Einthoven originally employed the familiar letters P, QRS, and T to designate the waves of the electrocardiogram, there soon occurred considerable confusion regarding their use in a variety of leads. Pardee (1940) proposed the system that has been adopted universally to describe the intervals and durations of the various waves.

To localize the direction (vectors) of excitation and recovery of the atria and ventricles, and to estimate the extent of injury (such as might result from insufficient coronary circulation), a variety of electrode arrays is em-

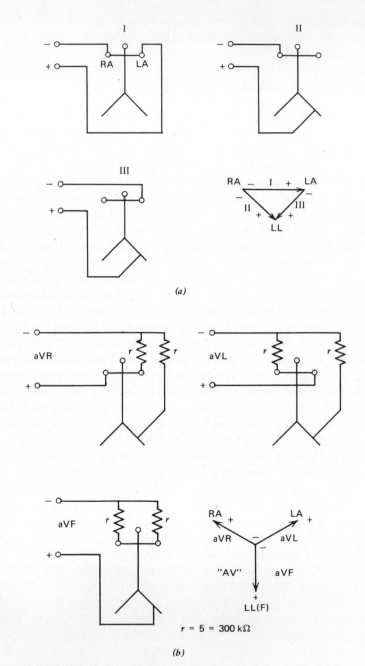

Figure 11-28. ECG frontal plane leads: (*a*) limb leads, (*b*) augmented limb leads, (*c*) frontal plane vectors.

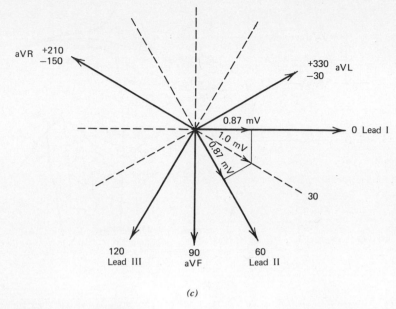

(c)

Figure 11-28   (Continued)

ployed. The electrode placements are based on easily located anatomical "landmarks," the most popular of these arrays illustrated in Figs. 11-28 and 11-29. The standard (I, II, III), augmented (aVR, aVL, aVF), and precordial (V) leads are routinely recorded by electrocardiographers. By visual inspection of the recordings and knowledge of the direction represented by each lead, it is possible to locate the mean vectors of excitation and recovery to within 15 degrees. The rule is that the isoelectric lead (or equal positive and negative deflection) is at right angles to the direction of the event (excitation or recovery). To identify the direction in which the cardiac vector points, it is merely necessary to look at the polarity in a lead that is orthogonal to the lead with zero net amplitude. If there is no lead array in which the net amplitude is zero, interpolation must be employed by inspection of the leads with the minimum net amplitude.

The concept that underlies the vector representation was proposed by Einthoven et al. (1913), who imagined the heart to be at the center of an equilateral triangle with the apices at the right and left shoulders and the pubis. The leads to these points were placed on the right and left arms and both feet; later only the left foot was used. With this electrode array, it is possible to represent excitation or recovery (of the atria and ventricles) as a vector whose components are amplitudes projected on lead I (RA-LA), lead II (RA-LL) and lead III (LA-LL), as in Fig. 11-32. Thus if the amplitudes

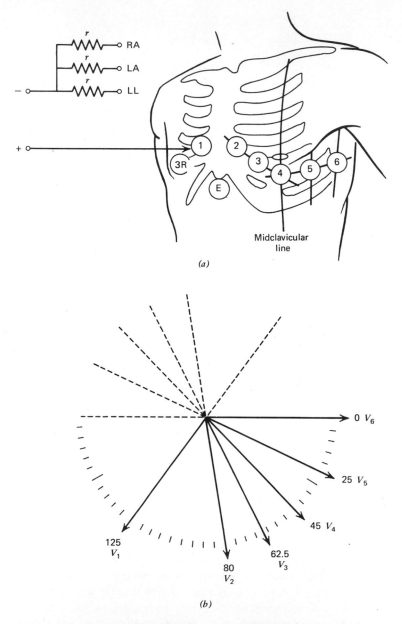

(a)

(b)

Figure 11-29. The precordial leads: (a) r = 5 to 300 kΩ. (b) Horizontal plane vectors.

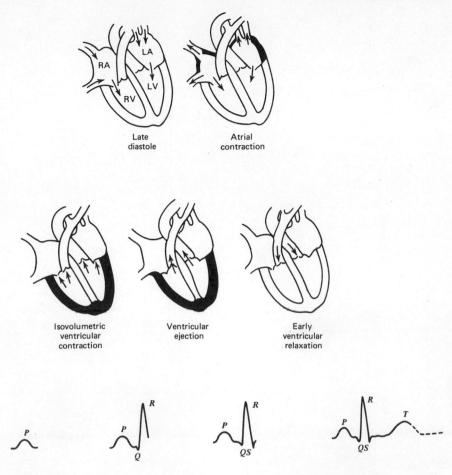

Figure 11-30. Evalution of the electrocardiogram during mechanical activity of the heart.

in two of the three leads are known, the magnitude and direction of the cardiac vector is known (see Fig. 11-32). From this concept of a 120-degree triaxial reference system came Einthoven's law, which states that the amplitude in lead II equals the algebraic sum of the amplitudes in leads I and III. This statement is true only for this triaxial system (Valentinuzzi et al., 1970).

The technique for locating cardiac vectors can be illustrated by referring to Fig. 11-28c, which shows a cardiac vector (which could represent excitation or recovery in either the atria or ventricles), with a magnitude of 1.0 mV and a direction of 30 degrees. Dropping perpendiculars from the tip of the vector to any of the other lead directions will give the amplitude in that

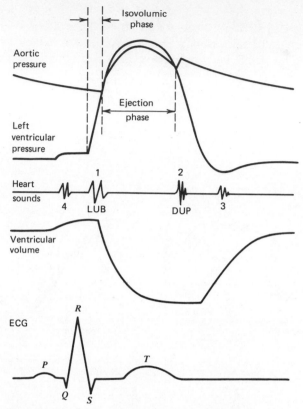

Figure 11-31.   Some of the events of the cardiac cycle.

lead. Since the vector direction is 30 degrees, its amplitude in lead III is zero, indicating that it is orthogonal to this lead. The amplitude is 0.87 mV in leads I and II, as in Fig. 11-28. Note that deflections are upward when the perpendicular from the tip of the cardiac vector intersects the solid lines, and downward when the intersection falls on the dashed lines.

This discussion has centered on mean cardiac vectors; it has not been mentioned that the maximum and minimum amplitudes do not occur simultaneously in all leads, as was correctly pointed out by Einthoven et al. (1913). Therefore, the technique of obtaining mean amplitudes for the vector components by simple subtraction is merely a practical convenience to allow easy estimation of a mean vector. In reality, at each instant in the cardiac cycle, vector components can be obtained and the instantaneous vectors can be determined. A line joining the extremities of the instantaneous vectors will describe a loop whose major vector usually approximates the mean cardiac vector obtained as described previously. A continuous record of the instantaneous vectors constitutes the study of vector-cardiography, which is described in the next section.

In electrocardiographic monitoring, a variety of standard and nonstandard leads (Fig. 11-33) are used to obtain a large-amplitude QRS wave, free from muscle or body-movement artifacts. Thus electrodes are frequently placed on the chest or back. One lead that enjoys considerable popularity is the MX (manubriumxiphoid) array (Lian and Golblin, 1936; Geddes et al., 1960) in which the electrodes are located at the ends of the sternum. With this lead, there are no contracting skeletal muscles between the electrodes; in addition, the electrodes are close to the heart, which provides a large-amplitude ECG. Although the MX lead is very convenient for estimating heart rate, by counting QRS waves, it is not the best lead for

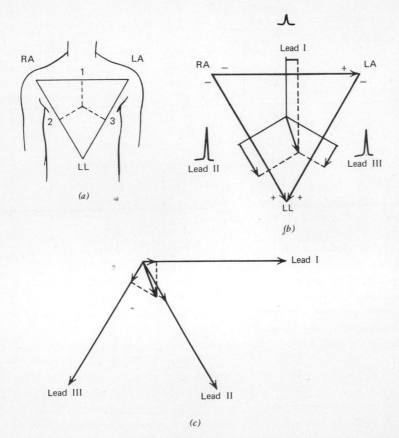

Figure 11-32. Einthoven's triangular representation of the three limb leads (*a*), their use to locate a cardiac vector (*b*), and the simplified method of representing the lead axes (*c*).

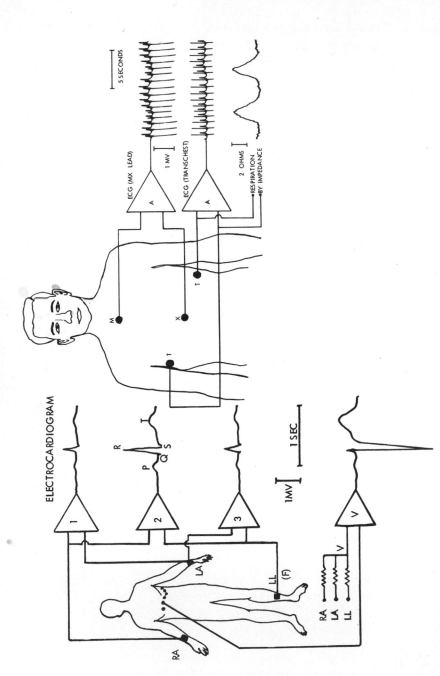

Figure 11-33. Commonly used ECG lead configurations: left, the standard limb and precordial (*V*) leads along with typical waveforms; above, two lead systems (MX or manubrium-xiphoid and TT or transthoracic). The MX lead is readily applicable to exercising subjects. With the transthoracic lead, the ECG and respiration can be recorded from the same pair of electrodes. [Redrawn from Geddes, *IEEE Spectrum* **9**:41–48 (1972).]

identification of metabolic changes in the ventricles, as revealed by the T wave.

Another ECG lead that enjoys some popularity employs one electrode on the thorax just below the right axilla; the other electrode is on the left side of the chest on the midaxillary line and at the level of the fifth or sixth rib. With this transthoracic (TT) array, which approximates lead II, a large amplitude ECG can be obtained and the same electrodes can be used for recording respiration by the impedance method (Geddes et al., 1962).

With a single-channel ECG recording, which shows clear P, R, and T waves, it is possible to obtain a considerable amount of valuable information regarding cardiac activity. For example, the presence of an orderly sequence of P, R, and T waves with a normal range of intervals and durations denotes normal cardiac excitation and recovery. The ECG during sudden cardiac slowing in an impaired heart is presented in Fig. 11-34, along with femoral artery blood pressure. Note that the ECG complex marked X is essentially normal in configuration, yet the force of ventricular contraction was insufficient to open the aortic valve and eject blood. Intermittent interruption of the propagation of excitation between the atria and ventricles is shown in Fig. 11-35, along with carotid artery blood pressure. At A there is 2:1 atrioventricular block (2 P waves for each normal QRS-T complex). Immediately thereafter, total A-V block occurred, as evidenced by the P waves continuing without causing ventricular excitation; however, the ventricles produced two extrasystoles (X_1 X_2)

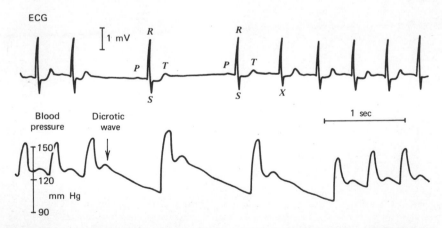

Figure 11-34. Lead II ECG and femoral artery pressure during sudden vagal slowing of a hypoxic canine heart. Note that during slowing the ECG for beat X exhibited a normal configuration, but the force of ventricular contraction was insufficient to open the aortic valve and eject blood.

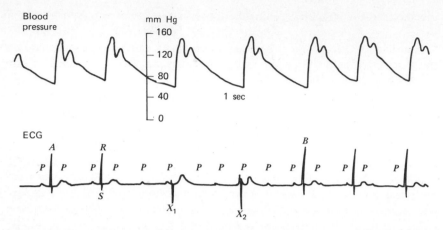

Figure 11-35. Lead II ECG and carotid artery blood pressure in an anesthetized dog. At *A*, 2:1 A-V block is present, followed by total A-V block, during which two apical extrasystoles (X_1, X_2) occurred. At *B*, 2:1 block was reestablished; during this sequence there was minimal change in the blood pressure record.

initiating from a focus in the apical region, illustrated by the downward QRS waves, which have no fixed relationship with the P waves. At *B*, 2:1 A-V block was reestablished. Note that only a minor disturbance in pulse rate and blood pressure accompanied these events. Total A-V block with apical ventricular pacemaker is represented in Fig. 11-36, which was derived from the same animal. Note that the QRS waves are all inverted

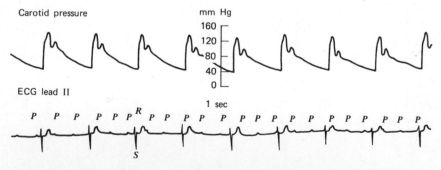

Figure 11-36. Lead II ECG and carotid artery blood pressure in an anesthetized dog illustrating that total A-V block is present, as shown by absence of fixed relationship between the P and QRS waves. Note that an apical ventricular pacemaker had developed, as evidenced by the downward QRS waves in the ECG. The blood pressure record, of course, gives no clue regarding this disturbed cardiac rhythm in which pacemaker activity is normal, as indicated by the regularly occurring P waves.

and there is no fixed relationship between the atrial P and the ventricular RS waves.

Ventricular extrasystoles occurring at the apex and base (just below the atria) are identified in Fig. 11-37, which displays lead II ECG and femoral artery blood pressure. Note that both the left apical and right basal extrasystole failed to develop enough contractile force to open the aortic valve and produce a blood pressure pulse, as evidenced by the pulse deficit. Also, there is a period of alternating strong and weak beats (pulsus alternans) with a normal ECG, following the right basal extrasystole.

As demonstrated earlier, the ventricles have the capability of originating beats with an appreciable degree of automaticity. Figure 11-38 illustrates one interesting type of arrythmia known as bigeminus rhythm. Note that a ventricular extrasystole (R–S–T) regularly follows each normal beat. The blood pressure shows that the ventricular extrasystoles did not result in ejection of blood, as shown by the carotid artery pressure recording. Thus the ECG shows twice the number of ventricular excitations as blood-pressure pulses.

Fibrillation is that condition in a cardiac chamber in which all fibers contract and relax randomly; consequently, there is no pumping action associated with a fibrillating chamber. Since atrial contraction contributes only a small amount to ventricular filling, loss of this component by atrial fibrillation is relatively unimportant in the nonexercising subject. However, the fibrillating atria bombard the A-V node with propagated excitations, resulting in a rapid and irregular ventricular rate. In fact, the rate is so high that filling is compromised and cardiac output is reduced because many ventricular contractions do not eject blood, as evidenced by a pulse deficit.

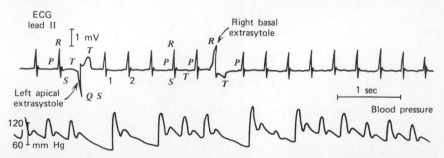

Figure 11-37. Lead II ECG and femoral artery blood pressure in an anesthetized dog. The induced left apical and right basal extrasystoles failed to result in a ventricular contraction forceful enough to open the aortic valve, as evidenced by the pulse deficits in the blood pressure record. Note the period of pulsus alternans with a normal ECG following the right basal extrasystole and the absence of a pulse following normal beat 2.

ECG lead II

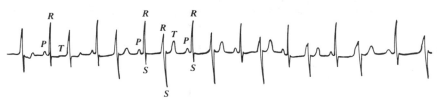

1 sec

Blood pressure

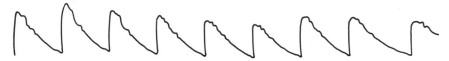

Figure 11-38.   Lead II ECG and carotid artery blood pressure in an anesthetized dog which is exhibiting bigeminus rhythm. Following every normal P, QRS-T complex is a ventricular extrasystole. Since there are twice as many ventricular excitations as blood pressure pulses, it is clear that the extrasystole did not result in an ejection of blood from the left ventricle. In addition, the focus of the extrasystole varied throughout the period of recording.

The ECG permits easy identification of the presence of atrial fibrillation. The atrial P waves are absent, being replaced by fibrillation (f) waves. Figure 11-39 is a record of atrial fibrillation that ceased spontaneously in a dog. The top channel displays a direct atrial electrogram, the second is lead II ECG, and the third is femoral artery blood pressure. While the atria are fibrillating, there are no P waves, and only very small amplitude f waves are visible in lead II. It is quite apparent that there are more ventricular excitations (R waves) than blood pressure pulses during atrial fibrillation. When atrial fibrillation ceased and sinus rhythm was restored, the P waves reappeared, as is shown clearly in lead II, and the tachycardia and pulse deficit both disappeared.

Ventricular fibrillation results in the loss of cardiac output, hence blood pressure. Asystole of the ventricles exhibits the same condition; however, the ECG allows instant differentiation, for in asystole there are no QRS–T waves, whereas with ventricular fibrillation, the QRS–T waves are replaced by random irregular electrical activity. Figure 11-40 illustrates the ECG and blood pressure prior to and during the precipitation of ventricular fibrillation.

Ventricular fibrillation is incompatible with life and if not reversed within a few minutes, irreversible damage occurs in the central nervous system. While preparations are made for defibrillation, cardiac compression (open- or closed-chest) and artificial respiration must be applied. Defibrillation is achieved by the passage of a single pulse of current through the ventricles (by transchest or directly applied electrodes) to depolarize the cardiac tissue totally and to allow the pacemaker (normally the SA node) to resume pacing.

The ECG shows striking changes when the heart muscle is deprived of an adequate supply of blood, as may occur from narrowing or occlusion of a branch of the coronary arteries. The cells in an area deprived of circulation cannot sustain their metabolic activities, and membrane integrity is lost; this results in the presence of a depolarized area that is electrically negative with respect to healthy tissue. The injured area, which manifests itself as an injury potential in the ECG, is inexcitable and develops no contractile

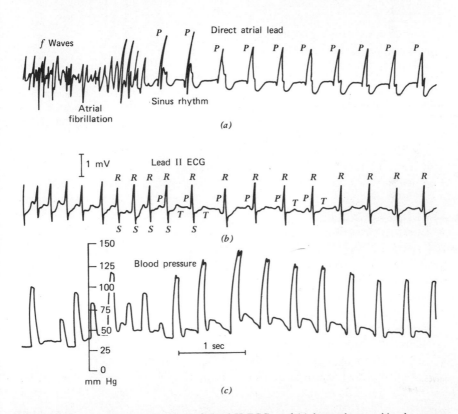

Figure 11-39. (*a*) Atrial electrogram, (*b*) lead II ECG, and (*c*) femoral artery blood pressure in the dog during atrial fibrillation (left) and normal sinus rhythm (right). Note that during atrial fibrillation there are no P waves in lead II, and there is a tachycardia and pulse deficit. When sinus rhythm returned, the P waves appeared in lead II, and the tachycardia and pulse deficit both disappeared.

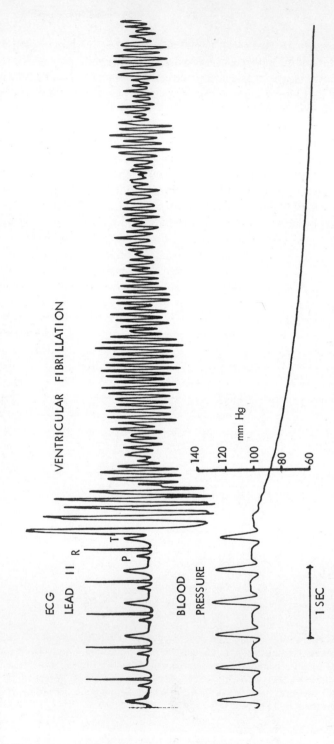

Figure 11-40. The precipitation of ventricular fibrillation in the dog by applying repetitive electrical stimuli to the right ventricle. Note the replacement of the QRS-T complex by fibrillation waves and the sudden fall in blood pressure.

force. With the passage of time the injured area is converted to scar tissue and the injury potential disappears from the ECG.

The type of waveform exhibited by the ECG when myocardial injury is present is often explained by the interference theory, which holds that the voltage appearing between the terminals of the ECG electrodes is due to the summation of the monophasic myocardial action potentials seen by each electrode, as idealized in Fig. 11-13. Injury eliminates some of the monophasic action potentials and produces a persistent diastolic depolarization; consequently, the region between the R and T waves is no longer isoelectric, being above or below the baseline, depending on the location of the injury and polarity for the particular lead.

A typical example of alteration in the ECG due to coronary artery occlusion appears in Fig. 11-41. On the left is the control electrocardiogram of a dog; one electrode was placed on the left forelimb and the other was on the chest over the apical region. Negativity of the left forelimb electrode is displayed as an upward deflection in the recording. Note that the segment between the end of the R wave (i.e., the S wave) and the beginning of the T wave is isoelectric. A myocardial infarction was created by ligating the left interventricular coronary artery, which resulted in considerable injury (hence persistent depolarization) to the apex of the left ventricle. The absence of excitation in this area reveals itself by an upward displacement in the S–T segment, on the right of Fig. 11-41. This is the classical electrographic sign of early myocardial infarction. However, the upward displacement of the S–T segment is in reality a persistent (diastolic) depression of the baseline due to depolarization of the injured area.

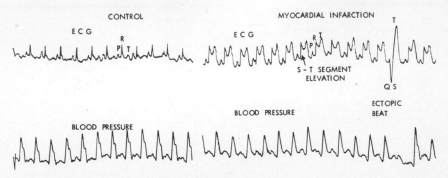

Figure 11-41. Electrocardiogram obtained from a dog with one electrode (−) on the left forelimb and the other (+) on the left chest wall in the region of the apex beat. On the left is the control record in which the segment between the end of the R wave (i.e., S wave) and the beginning of the T wave is isoelectric. On the right is the ECG after ligation of the left interventricular coronary artery. Presence of apical injury is indicated by the elevation in the S–T segment, which is the classical sign of myocardial infarction.

Parenthetically, it is interesting to note that the first evidence of an electrocardiac signal was demonstrated by Koelliker and Mueller in 1856 using the rheoscopic frog; it was first recorded in 1876 by Marey and Lippmann using the capillary electrometer. Human electrocardiograms were recorded by Waller in 1887, also using the capillary electrometer. Dissatisfaction with the capillary electrometer led Einthoven to develop his string galvanometer in 1903. During this time, when cardiology was being born, cardiac action was recorded using pneumatic pulse pickups and the smoked-drum kymograph. Although useful diagnostic information was obtained in this manner, the ability of the electrocardiogram, recorded with the string galvanometer, to demonstrate the sequence of excitation and recovery was soon recognized and pulse recording was abandoned. By the 1920s string electrocardiographs were in use clinically. Direct-writing recorders started to supplant string galvanometers in the early 1940s. Although the ECG proved very useful in the diagnosis of arrythmias, its greater value in identifying the presence of injury (myocardial infarction) was not established until the late 1930s.

11-9. VECTORCARDIOGRAPHY

The idea of locating the electrical axis of the ventricles by measuring potential differences appearing between limb electrodes was clearly demonstrated by Waller (1887). Almost a quarter-century later, Einthoven (1913) postulated that in the human thorax the heart was almost in the center of an equilateral triangle in which the apices were the right and left arms (shoulders) and both feet (pubic area). He soon found that only the left foot was necessary and abandoned use of the right foot.

Einthoven knew very well that he was recording only a component of ventricular depolarization in a (frontal) plane parallel to the anterior surface of the body. In addition, on the triangle he plotted only a single line to represent the ventricular (manifest) vector of excitation, reflecting the R wave, although he knew that the R wave reached its peak at different times in the different leads. The notion that a series of instantaneous vectors could be drawn to describe the ventricular depolarization process was due to Williams (1914), who used the Einthoven triangle to plot the synchronous values of the amplitudes during the QRS wave derived from the limb leads.

It remained for Mann (1920) to introduce the concept of the vector loop by plotting the locus of the tips of the instantaneous values of the QRS and T vectors, as recorded by the three limb leads, to obtain loops which he called monocardiograms. Figure 11-42a illustrates the loop formed by joining the tips of the instantaneous vectors obtained for every 10-msec in-

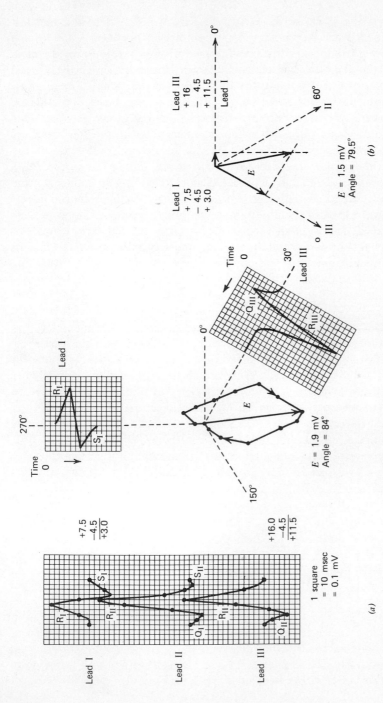

Figure 11-42. (a) The vector loop for the R wave of the ECG obtained by joining the tips of the instantaneous vectors obtained at each 10 msec throughout the QRS wave. (b) The mean QRS vector obtained by using the net amplitude in leads I and III. (Redrawn from Geddes, *Electrodes and the Measurement of Bioelectric Events*, Wiley, New York, 1972.)

465

terval during the QRS wave. Figure 11-42*b* gives the derivation of the mean cardiac R wave vector using the net amplitudes for leads I and III.

In 1925 Mann built an instrument to record monocardiograms directly; later (1931) he demonstrated their value in the diagnosis of bundle-branch block, which was difficult to identify in the ECG at that time. A description of his instrument did not appear until 1938. Probably because no cathode ray tubes were available, Mann constructed an ingenious galvanometer consisting of a single mirror, which was deflected by three coils mounted with their axes 60 degrees apart, each axis corresponding to one of the leads as represented by the Einthoven triangle. A photographic record of the deflection of a light beam reflected from the mirror produced these early vectorcardiograms, although this name was not to be used until later.

The Braun cathode ray tube was introduced to vectorcardiography by Schellong et al. (1937), who used a two-axis tube to obtain vector loops (vectordiagrams) in the frontal, horizontal, and sagittal planes (Fig. 11-43). Hollmann and Hollmann (1938) employed a cathode ray tube with three pairs of deflection plates with 60-degree orientation and called the records that they obtained triograms (Fig. 11-44). Sulzer and Duchosal (1938) used the Braun tube to display what they called planograms derived from electrodes placed to record frontal, sagittal, and horizontal components of the ECG. Studies were carried out by Arrighi (1939) to locate the best electrode placement for the sagittal projection lead. His selection is shown in Fig. 11-45. At the same time Wilson and Johnston (1938) employed a cathode ray tube with their "central terminal" (Fig. 11-46) to make the Einthoven triangle method practical for clinical vectorcardiography. In this paper Wilson initiated the use of the word vectorcardiogram.

Because the electrocardiograph was in fairly widespread use and provided extremely valuable information on the condition of the heart, the vectorcardiograph was expected to provide more and different data about the

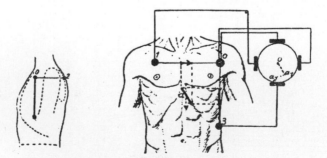

Figure 11-43. Schellong's method of producing vectordiagrams. [From Schellong et al., *Z. Kreislaufforsch.* **29**:497 (1937). By permission.]

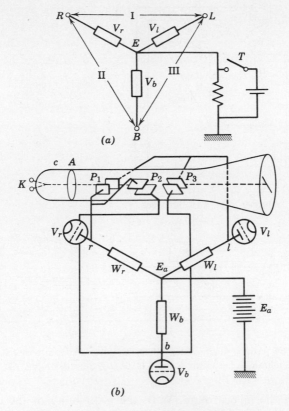

(a)

(b)

Figure 11-44. The Hollmann method of presenting triograms. [From W. and H. E. Hollmann, *Z. Krieslaufforsch.* **29**:546 (1937). By permission.]

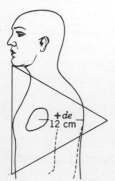

Figure 11-45. Arrighi's sagittal electrode placement. [From F. Arrighi, *Prensa Med. Arg.* **26**:253 (1939). By permission.]

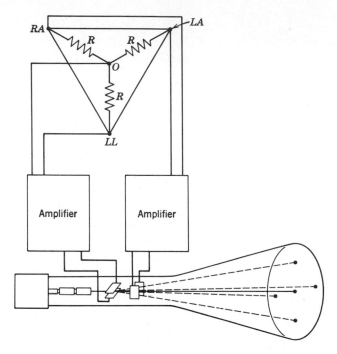

Figure 11-46. The vectorcardiogram derived from Wilson's central terminal. [From F. N. Wilson and F. D. Johnston, *Am. Heart J.* **16**:14 (1938). By permission.]

functioning of the myocardium. With the availability of the cathode ray tube and high-fidelity voltage amplifiers after 1945, there arose a new interest in multiplane (spatial) vectorcardiography. To record such VCGs, many patterns of electrode location were proposed, most of which could be traced back to the reasoning behind the Einthoven triangle. However, before long it was realized that the basic assumptions in Einthoven's simple equilateral triangle were not entirely valid; for example, the heart is not at the center of an equilateral triangle with apices where the limbs join the trunk, nor is the resistivity of the tissues and fluids surrounding the heart uniform in all directions. Among the first to question the validity of Einthoven's concept were Burger and van Milaan (1947), who constructed a torso model, filled it with copper sulfate, and implanted a dipole generator in it in the position occupied by the heart as determined by x-ray studies on human subjects. Even in this homogeneously conducting model, the potentials of the three limb leads were not those predicted on the basis of Einthoven's triangle. These investigators then altered their model by inserting masses of material to simulate the lungs (a bag of moist sand) and spinal column (cork), and showed that the potentials recorded by the limb leads were those represented by a scalene triangle having angles of 96 degrees at the right arm, 56 degrees at the left arm, and 28 degrees at the left leg.

Despite knowledge that the torso is irregular in shape and anisotropic, many body-surface electrode arrangements were developed to obtain voltages from which the ventricular vector loop could be located spatially with reference to the electrode array. The electrode locations were usually chosen on the basis of equal distance from the "center" of the ventricles. The lines joining the electrodes formed the boundaries of a solid figure, which was often used to identify the electrode array. Controversy over the ability of a particular electrode reference frame to locate the "cardiac vectors" has continued to the present time.

On the basis of considerable clinical experience with vectorcardiography, Sulzer and Duchosal (1945) advocated the two electrode schemes appearing in Figure 11-47. Although both gave similar loops, they preferred the system of Fig. 11-47b, which became known as the double-cube system.

Wilson et al. (1947), after studying the potential distribution of an electrically driven dipole placed in a cadaver heart, introduced the equilateral tetrahedral reference frame (Fig. 11-48). With this system, limb electrodes and the central terminal were used to obtain the frontal plane projection. From a back electrode and the central terminal was derived the sagittal projection. The relative voltages appearing between the various electrode pairs were in nearly all instances those predicted from the geometry of the torso. With such evidence the tetrahedral system gained considerable support.

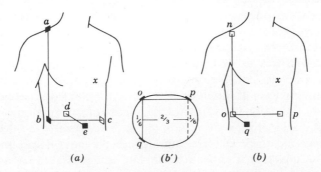

Figure 11-47. Sulzer and Duchosal's reference frames. [From R. Sulzer and P. W. Duchosal, *Cardiologia* 9:10–120 (1945). By permission.]

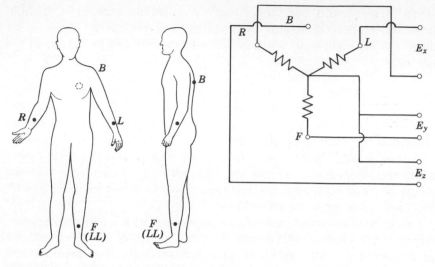

Figure 11-48. Wilson's tetrahedral reference frame. (Redrawn from G. Burch et al., *Spatial Vectorcardiography*, Lea and Febiger, Philadelphia.)

Grishman et al. (1951), after obtaining clinical records with the Wilson tetrahedral, the Arrighi triangle, and the Duchosal reference frames, were led to develop the cubic electrode arrangement shown in Fig. 11-49. The no. 1 electrode was placed "near the right posterior axillary line at the level of the first and second lumbar vertebrae"; no. 2, in the left posterior axillary line; no. 3, over the right anterior axillary line; and no. 4, over the left scapula. With this arrangment the authors claimed that the heart was as equidistant from the electrodes as the thorax allowed and that the electrodes were easily located anatomically.

Although all reference frames provided reasonable VCGs, the QRS and T loops derived from normal subjects exhibited a remarkably wide range of magnitudes and orientations, even when the same vectorcardiographic reference frame was used. In addition, the data obtained with different reference frames were not easily comparable. It is not difficult to find possible reasons for this situation. At least two concerted attempts have been made to identify the variables by means of investigations in which electrically driven dipoles were implanted into electroyte-filled human torso models and the resulting body-surface potential distributions were studied. The investigations by Schmitt and Simonson (1955) and Frank (1956) are fine examples of this technique. From their studies both investigators developed orthogonal lead systems for spatial vectorcardiography.

Schmitt's SVEC III system and Frank's VCG lead system are presented in Figs. 11-50 and 11-51, respectively. Both systems are used clinically.

In Schmitt's system 14 active electrodes are employed. The voltage that represents the X component of the cardiac vector is derived from the right- and left-arm electrodes, along with components derived from chest and back electrodes placed at the level of the fifth intercostal space. The Y component is obtained from the head and left-leg electrodes, and the Z component from eight electrodes located on the chest and back at the third and sixth interspace.

Seven active electrodes are used with Frank's system (Fig. 11-51). The X component is derived from an array of electrodes that surround the heart approximately at the level of the fifth interspace. The Y component is obtained from the neck and left-leg electrodes, and the Z component from the voltage appearing between an array of three electrodes on the anterior of the chest and one electrode in the back and one on the midaxillary line. To provide more accurate location of the level for the chest and back electrodes, Frank developed a three-electrode exploring tool and presented instructions for its use.

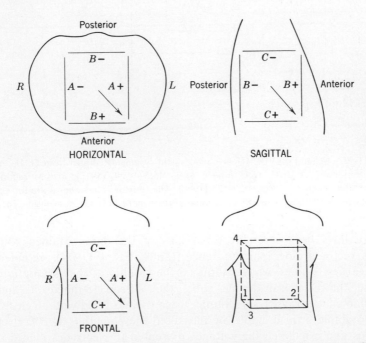

Figure 11-49.   The cubic reference system employed by Grishman. [Adapted from Grishman et al., *Am. Heart J.* **41**:483–493 (1951). By permission.]

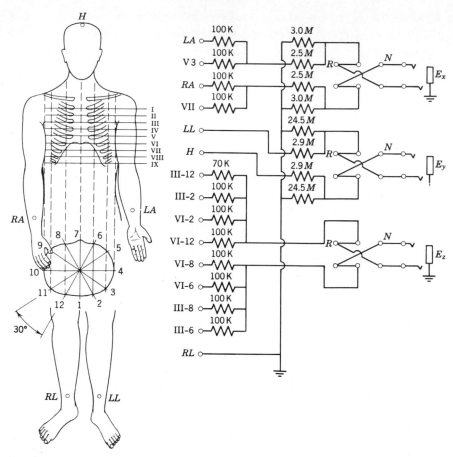

Figure 11-50. Schmitt's SVEC III orthogonal lead system. [Redrawn from O. H. Schmitt and E. Simonson, *A.M.A. Arch. Intern. Med.* **96:**574–590 (1955), and as reported by Pipberger and Wood, *Cir. Res.* **6:**239–24 (1958). The resistor values shown are for an input impedance of 10 MΩ to ground. (By permission of the American Heart Association, Inc.)]

There have been several comparisons of the data obtained with the various vectorcardiographic reference frames. Frank (1954) presented one of the earliest studies, which examined the validity of the assumptions underlying the Duchosal double cube, the Wilson tetrahedron, and the Grishman cube arrays. Using human torso models filled with an electrolyte and containing a fixed dipole, he measured the potentials at 200 electrode positions and calculated the voltages presented to electrodes placed in the locations specified by the three reference frames. He found that "the scalar lead shapes of the Wilson tetrahedron deviate, on the average, by approximately 15% from the torso dipole variations, but the scalar lead shapes of the systems of Duchosal and Grishman show significantly larger discrepancies." He also found that the standardization factors employed in the Wilson system were too large, particularly with respect to the head-to-foot dipole component (by a factor of 2.3), and added, "Certain fortuitous features of the Wilson system enable a modification of the standardization factors which leads to results that are fairly satisfactory for a dipole located in the center of the heart. This system which possesses certain other advantages would appear to deserve further study."

The practical value of Wilson's system was also investigated by Abildskov and Pence (1956), who compared data obtained by means of Wilson's tetrahedron with those obtained with the corrected tetrahedron as advocated by McFee and Johnston (1954). In 75 subjects they found that although the data were similar with both methods, the scatter was less with the corrected tetrahedron. Brody (1957) carried out another study on a series of human subjects using the scalene tetrahedron and Wilson's equilateral tetrahedron, discovering that although the scalene tetrahedron was based on sound experimentally determined data, "the mean spatial QRS-

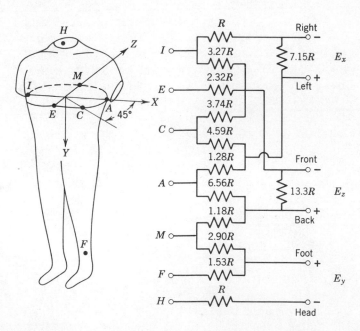

Figure 11-51. Frank's vectorcardiographic lead system. [From E. Frank, *Circulation* **13**:737–749 (1956). By permission of the American Heart Association.]

and T-vector loci exhibited slightly less scatter and better coefficients of correlation within the uncorrected frame of reference," and that "the corrected frame of reference does not appear to possess sufficient merit to warrant its routine application to the analysis of mean QRS- and T-vector orientation." In another investigation of Wilson's tetrahedral system, Burger et al. (1956) applied their scalene triangle correction and compared data collected on a series of 96 patients with their own reference frame. They found good agreement between the two methods, using the electrode locations advocated by Wilson only when their correction was applied. It is probably because of such studies in which deviations from the "ideal" value turn out to be clinically unimportant that the Wilson method still enjoys considerable support.

The Schmitt, Frank, Helm, and McFee (corrected Einthoven triangle) systems have also been exposed to close scrutiny by Langner et al. (1958). The importance of the differences depends on how critical the reader may be. Langner found that for the Z lead the systems were interchangeable in more than 90% of the cases for the QRS and T loops in regard to shape and orientation. For the X lead the systems were interchangeable in all cases for the QRS loop and in 90% for the T loop. In another study involving 4 normal and 182 elderly subjects, Simonson et al. (1959) compared the QRS and T loops obtained with eight popular orthogonal-lead systems to find large differences between these systems. However, they stated, "most types of pathology can be recognized in any of the lead systems." Although their extensive study was carefully executed, they were reluctant to advocate the superiority of one system over another.

Nonogawa (1966) called attention to the important fact that many of the popular electrode reference frames were derived from torso models of Caucasian adults. He wondered whether these frames were applicable to the Oriental torso. Therefore, he constructed Caucasian and Oriental torso models into which he placed electrically excited dipoles and obtained VCG data with the Frank, Schmitt SVEC III, McFee, Polygraph III, and Grishman lead systems. He concluded that in each of the $X, Y,$ and Z axis leads the Schmitt and Frank systems were similar. The other lead systems showed larger differences. However, he also concluded that "these VCG systems, in their original networks, can be applied to the Japanese without appreciable error."

With such variety of reference frames and the lack of clear-cut clinical evidence to indicate the superiority of one reference system over another to identify specific myocardial diseases, it is difficult to set forth criteria that would lead to the adoption of a single method. Information on this interesting field can be found in the monographs by Grant and Estes (1951), Grishman (1952), Goldberger (1953), Burch et al. (1953), Grant

(1957), Kowarzykowic and Kowarzykowic (1961), Pozzi (1961), Uhley (1962), Guntheroth (1965), and Lamb (1965). Pozzi's (1961) monograph contains an excellent bibliography of the original papers, which describe the various vectorcardiographic lead systems and potential distributions around the heart of the human subject and in models of the human torso. The bibliography also lists studies in which field mapping was carried out with various dipole models.

In considering the merits of one reference frame over another, it is useful to remember that most of the carefully examined reference frames were derived from human torso models in which electrically driven dipoles were implanted. Although this is a good starting point, the situation in the actual human subject is quite different. Not only do human torsos come in a wide range of shapes and sizes, but the tissues between the heart and body-surface electrodes have quite different electrical properties. Even within a single tissue the resistivity is not the same in all directions. Therefore, there still remains the need to conduct more cadaver experiments such as those carried out by Wilson et al. (1947) to evaluate the magnitude of the distortions produced by the intrathoracic contents.

Traditionally, the VCG is displayed in Cartesian coordinates on a two-axis cathode ray tube. Usually a single photograph is taken of each cardiac cycle. From such pictures the magnitude and orientation of the P-, QRS-, and T-vector loops are determined. Timing of the vector loops is accomplished by blanking the beam with a triangular pulse to indicate the direction of development of the loop. Continuous moving picture records of the same presentation produce figures that are grossly distorted.

With the conventional cathode ray tube presentation, an adequate display for the large, rapidly developing QRS loop requires the use of a high-intensity beam. When this situation obtains, there is a bright halo around the P and T loops. Between heart beats the bright stationary spot soon damages the cathode ray tube screen. To overcome this defect, Briller et al. (1950) described a method of obtaining a triggering signal from the P wave of the ECG to turn on the cathode ray tube beam only for the duration of the QRS or the T wave. Becking et al. (1950) reported a most practical method of brightening the cathode ray tube trace in proportion to the velocity of the excursion of the beam. This technique not only protects the screen between heart beats, but also provides a means of obtaining photographs with high contrast. Isaacs (1964) described a method similar to Briller's in which the R wave was used to trigger delay generators that could be manually set to turn on the cathode ray tube beam for all or part of the next heart beat. A combination of the techniques described by these investigators would undoubtedly improve display of the loops.

An interesting three-dimensional display system was described by Ishitoya et al. (1965). With this method the X, Y, and Z signals derived by using the Frank system were applied to three galvanometers with their deflection axes mutually perpendicular. A light beam was reflected from the first galvanometer to the second and to a screen on the third beside which was a half-silvered mirror used to view the screen. Three illuminated mutually perpendicular axes were placed behind the half-silvered mirror, and the whole assembly was mounted in a lightproof box. The spatial orientation of the vector loops with respect to the three axes could be clearly seen by an observer looking into a viewing hole.

The use of polar coordinates for presentation of the VCG was described by Dower et al. (1965). Instead of a conventional cathode ray tube display, they employed an analog computer which continuously calculated the spherical coordinates (r, θ, ϕ) and presented them on a graphic record. Although such a presentation is not easy to comprehend, it does retain the important PR, QRS, and QT time intervals, which are lost in the conventional Cartesian coordinate vector-loop presentations.

There is no doubt that the cathode-ray tube presentation of the spatial VCG provides an intellectually pleasing display and clearly illustrates the phase differences between the voltages in the leads from which it is derived. The major piece of information that it presents is the direction of depolarization and repolarization of the atria and the ventricles. The most prominent feature, the QRS loop, is usually so large that it is difficult to see the P and T loops. Beam brightness-controlling techniques offer some solution to this problem.

There is not unanimity of opinion regarding the best location for body-surface electrodes and choice of weighting networks. A reference frame designed to give orthogonal components for ventricular depolarization (QRS) may not indicate repolarization (T) with the same accuracy. Moreover, the same reference frame may be quite inappropriate for atrial depolarization and repolarization. From these loops, as they are displayed on the conventional two-axis cathode ray tube, it is impossible to determine the important time durations and intervals (PR, QRS, and QT), which contain a considerable amount of diagnostic information. Although conduction disturbances and ectopic beats identify themselves clearly in the VCG, they are equally well indicated by the ECG. Injury to the myocardium, as shown by S-T segment deviations, is better displayed in the ECG by precordial leads.

The preceding discussion appears to indicate that the VCG has limited clinical value and will not replace the ECG in routine electrocardiography, particularly since mean cardiac axes can be visually estimated using the 6 limb and 6 precordial leads as described in the preceding section. As a teaching device the VCG has much to offer. Its ability to display the rate of depolarization and repolarization is far superior to that of the ECG. Especially well displayed by the VCG are the small, beat-by-beat changes in these quantities. Expanded clinical use of the VCG will depend on the clinical value of the information it produces. So many reference frames are employed, however, that the time when the full usefulness of the VCG is established will probably be delayed.

11-10. ELECTROENCEPHALOGRAPHY (EEG)

The electrical activity of the brain is recorded with three types of electrodes—scalp, cortical, and depth. With scalp electrodes the recording is called an electroencephalogram (EEG). When electrodes are placed on the exposed surface (cortex) of the brain, the recording is called an electrocorticogram (ECoG). Electrodes also may be advanced into the brain, in which case the term "depth recording" designates the technique. It is interesting to note that there is surprisingly little damage to the brain with depth recording. Whether obtained from the scalp, cortex, or depths of the brain, the potentials recorded represent the activity of numerous neurons in which fluctuating membrane and action potentials are occurring. These three different techniques are therefore examples of extracellular recording.

The fact that the brain exhibits spontaneous electrical activity was reported by Caton (1875, 1887), who used Thomson's reflecting galvanometer (see Fig. 11-79a) connected to electrodes applied to a variety of different animals. His choice of this instrument was fortunate since it had a frequency response (to about 5 Hz) which was adequate for the reproduction of the dominant rhythm of the animals he studied. Caton was not able to make graphic recordings from the animals, although he did provide convincing verbal descriptions of the electrical activity displayed as variations in the position of a luminous spot on a screen. It was about a half-century later when the electrical activity of the human brain was recorded by Berger (1929), who employed a string galvanometer (see Fig. 11-87) connected to scalp electrodes. Berger's first and succeeding papers were largely unnoticed until Adrian and Matthews (1934) in Great Britain and Jasper and Carmichael (1935) in the United States reviewed them and confirmed Berger's findings, thereby introducing electroencephalography to the English-speaking world. In both investigations, full credit was given to Berger for the discovery. A complete account of the development of electroencephalography was reported under the editorship of Rémond (1971), and an excellent account of Berger's work, including a translation of his papers, was presented by Gloor (1969).

11-10-1.   Electrode Locations

Scalp electrodes are employed in conjunction with both "monopolar" and bipolar recording techniques. Figure 11-52 illustrates both techniques for connecting a four-channel EEG to a subject. With "monopolar" recording, one side of each amplifier is connected to a reference electrode, often located on the ear lobe. With bipolar recording, the amplifiers are connected between pairs of scalp electrodes in a regular order. With both types of recording, one-half the number of channels is connected to electrodes on one side of the head; the remaining channels are connected to electrodes on the opposite side of the head. In this way, the electrical activity from homologous areas of the brain can be compared at a glance. Additional data are obtained with bipolar scalp-to-scalp recordings.

In clinical electroencephalography, 21 electrodes are applied to the head in what is known as the 10-20 system, illustrated in Fig. 11-53. This array was described by Jasper (1958), who chaired the meeting of the International Federation of EEG Societies, which developed this standard placement.

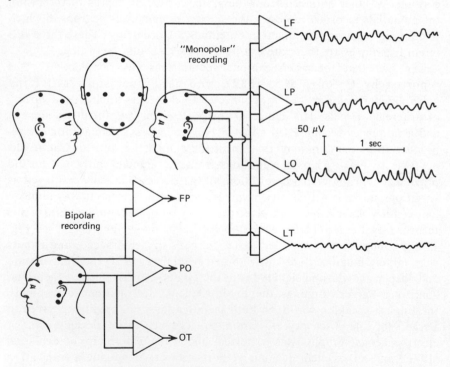

Figure 11-52.   Method of connecting the recording channels for "monopolar" and bipolar recording. With "monopolar" recording, the reference electrode is on the earlobe, chin, or neck.

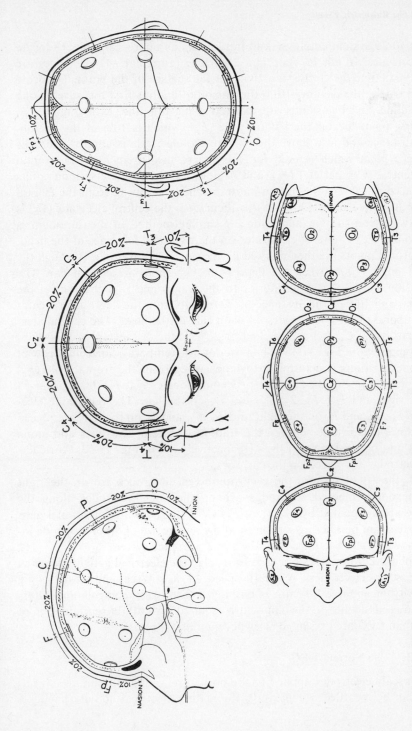

Figure 11-53. The 10-20 electrode system recommended by the International Federation of EEG Societies. [From H. Jasper, *EEG Clin. Neurophysiol.* **10**:371–375 (1958). By permission.]

The 10-20 system employs skull landmarks as reference points to locate the electrodes. In all, 19 scalp and 2 earlobe (auricular, A) electrodes are used to examine the electrical activity of the surface of the brain. To locate the electrodes, the distance from the nasion to inion is first measured along the midline, and five points are marked along this line, as in Fig. 11-53. The first point locates the frontal pole (F_p), which is 10% of the nasion-inion distance and just above the nasion. No electrode is applied over this reference point which is used for subsequent measurements. The frontal (F_z), central (C_z), parietal (P_z), and occipital (O_z) midline electrode points are spaced by 20% of the nasion-inion distance measuring from the frontal pole (F_p), as in Fig. 11-53. With this technique, the central electrode (C_z) is midway between nasion and inion. A similar method of measurement is used to place two rows of electrodes on the right and left sides of the head. The coronal points are then marked by measuring the distance (through the central point C_z) between the depression just in front of each ear. The depression is easily located anterior to the tragus and is at the root of the zygoma, and 10% of this distance measured up from the depression locates the temporal (T_4, T_3) electrodes on each side of the head. The central electrode positions (C_4, C_3) are marked at 20% of the distance above the temporal points, as in Fig. 11-53. Then the lowest (temporal) horizontal row of electrode positions is determined by measuring from the frontal pole (F_p) to the inion (see Fig. 11-53); this procedure locates F_{p2}, F_8, T_4, T_6, and O_2 on the right and F_{p1}, F_7, T_3, T_5, and O_1 on the left. The remaining electrodes (F_4, C_4, and P_4 on the right and F_3, C_3, and P_3 on the left) are placed along lines equidistant between the midline and temporal lines and along frontal and parietal coronal lines, respectively, as in Fig. 11-53. Auricular (A) electrodes are placed on the earlobes.

With the 10-20 system, the even-numbered electrodes are on the right and the odd-numbered electrodes are on the left. Electrodes along the midline are designated by a Z (i.e., F_z, C_z, P_z). There are intentional gaps in the subscript numbering system to allow for the use of other electrode locations, which can be added with the same reference system.

Graphic recording pens are used to display the electrical activity detected by the scalp electrodes. A chart speed of 3 cm/sec and a recording sensitivity of about 7 μV/mm is employed. Step gain controls and filters are also used; details on the bandwidth required for faithful reproduction of the human EEG are presented elsewhere in this chapter.

11-10-2.   The Normal EEG

With scalp electrodes applied to the normal relaxed adult human subject, there can be recorded a constantly fluctuating electrical activity having a dominant frequency of about 10 Hz and an amplitude in the range of 20 to 200 μV. This activity, which is called the alpha rhythm, ranges in frequency from about 8 to 12 Hz and is most prominent in the occipital and parietal areas; it may occupy as much as one-half the record. The alpha rhythm increases in frequency with age from birth and attains its adult form by about 15 to 20 years of age. The alpha rhythm is most prominent when the eyes are closed and in the absence of concentration. The frequency of the alpha rhythm is also species-dependent; Fig. 11-54 illustrates typical alpha rhythm patterns of guinea pig, cat, monkey, and man. Opening the eyes, to engage in patterned vision, or performing such cerebral activity as mental arithmetic, diminishes or abolishes the alpha rhythm. Figure 11-55 presents an outstanding example of this phenomenon in the cat and man.

   Although the alpha rhythm is the most prominent electrical activity, other frequencies are present in the normal human subject. For example, there is a considerable amount of low-voltage, higher-frequency (beta) activity present ranging in frequency from 18 to 30 Hz. It is most frequently found in the frontal part of the brain. However, the normal electroencephalogram contains waves of various frequencies (in the range of 1 to 60 Hz) and amplitudes, depending on the cerebral state. To improve communication between electroencephalographers, a terminology has been developed to describe waveforms and their frequencies; Table 11-3 presents a glossary of these terms.

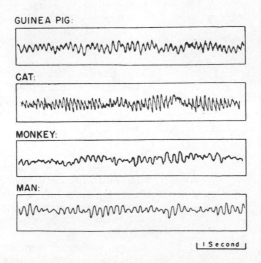

GUINEA PIG:

CAT:

MONKEY:

MAN:

⌊ I Second ⌋

Figure 11-54.   Typical alpha rhythm patterns of different subjects. (From M. A. B. Brazier, *Electrical Activity of the Nervous System.* Pitman, London, 1951. By permission.)

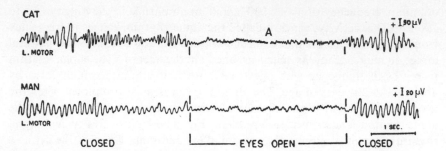

Figure 11-55. Blocking of the alpha rhythm in the cat and man by opening the eyes. (From M. A. B. Brazier, *Electrical Activity of the Nervous System.* Pitman, London, 1951. By permission.)

Table 11-3   EEG Waveform Terminology

Waveform	Frequency (Hz)	Remarks
Alpha rhythm	8–12	Parietal-occipital; associated with the awake and relaxed subject; prominent with eyes closed
Beta rhythm	18–30	More evident in frontal-parietal leads; seen best when alpha is blocked
Delta	1–3.5	Associated with normal sleep and present in children less than 1 year old; also seen in organic brain disease
Theta	4–7	Parietal-temporal; prominent in children 2 to 5 years old
Sleep spindle (sigma)	12–14	Waxing and waning of a sinusoidal like wave having the envelope that resembles a spindle; seen during sleep.
Lambda	Transient	Visually evoked, low-amplitude, occipital wave, resulting from recognition of a new retinal image
Spike and wave	ca. 3	Sharp wave (spike) followed by rounded wave associated with petit-mal epilepsy.
V or vertex wave	Transient	Spike about 150–250 msec in duration recorded over the vertex
K-complex	Transient	Vertex wave sometimes followed by a spindle; often seen in sleep and in response to auditory stimulus
Mu (arcade)	8–12	Central dominant, resembling a half-sinusoid (i.e., an arch with the apex downward when recorded with scalp to reference electrode)

The cerebral state profoundly affects the electroencephalogram in the normal subject. Figure 11-56 illustrates the typical changes that occur with sleep, which is perhaps the best example. As the subject goes to sleep, the higher-frequency activity that is associated with alertness or excitement, and the alpha rhythm that dominates the waking record in the relaxed state, are replaced by a characteristic cyclic sequence of changes that now constitute the focus of a new specialty devoted to sleep physiology, in which the EEG is used to identify different stages of sleep.

An interesting spectrum of cyclic physiological changes occurs during a prolonged period of sleep. In fact, deviation from these normal changes often indicates the presence of brain pathology. Sleep laboratories are being created wherein the EEG and several other physiological events are recorded continuously throughout the sleep period. Excellent accounts of the physiological changes that accompany sleep and the criteria for identifying the depth of sleep have been presented by Rechtschaffen and Kales (1968) and Williams et al. (1974).

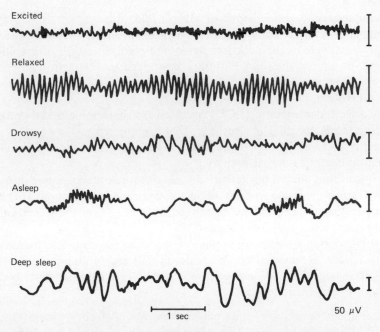

Figure 11-56. The electroencephalographic changes that occur as a human subject goes to sleep. The calibration marks on the right represent 50 μV. (From H. H. Jasper, in *Epilepsy and Cerebral Localization,* W. G. Penfield, and T. C. Erickson (eds.). Charles C. Thomas, Springfield, Ill., 1941. By permission.)

The physiological variables recorded to describe the depth sleep are the EEG, eye movements (EOG), ECG, and the EMG; respiration is sometimes recorded also. Three "monopolar" channels of EEG contribute important information regarding the cerebral state. Electrodes are connected to O_2–A_1 to monitor the alpha activity, C_4 (or P_4)–A_1 to detect sleep spindles, V waves, and K-complexes; F_4–A_1 is used to monitor slow-wave activity. Note that the three scalp electrodes (even-numbered subscripts) on the right-hand side of the head are paired with one on the contralateral earlobe (A_1). During light sleep, there are slow, disconjugate eye movements; to obtain these, the electrooculogram (EOG) is recorded using two monopolar channels connected to a reference electrode on an earlobe or mastoid process. One of the active electrodes is located 1 cm above and medial to the outer canthis of one eye; the second is 1 cm below and medial to the outer canthus of the other eye. Eye movements that are conjugate appear out of phase; therefore, use of this technique permits easy identification of artifacts in the recording. It is important to note that other electrode arrays are used in sleep EEG studies, and complete standardization has not been achieved.

The assessment of the degree of muscle relaxation is determined by recording the electrical activity (EMG) of neck muscles. Electrodes are applied to each side of the neck just below the chin. This type of graphic recording, of course, does not faithfully reproduce muscle action potentials. However, the only information desired is assessment of the degree of muscular relaxation.

The electrocardiogram (ECG) is used to determine heart rate by counting the R waves. The electrodes that are applied to the arms serve to detect the ECG and EMG if the arm muscles contract, thereby providing another indicator of muscle activity.

Respiration is sometimes recorded with a thoracic strain gauge or by the use of transthoracic electrodes and an impedance pneumograph. If the latter apparatus is used, the ECG can be obtained from the same pair of transthoracic electrodes (see Chapter 10).

Several scoring systems are applied to the sleep recordings to identify the depth of sleep. Rechtschaffen and Kales (1968) and Williams et al. (1974) have presented detailed accounts of them. The method described by Williams et al. is as follows.

Stage 0. The awake (W) state before the onset of sleep. At least 30 sec of 8 to 12 Hz occipital activity with a minimum amplitude of 40 μV peak-to-peak.

Stage 1. Less than 30 sec of 8 to 12 Hz, 40 μV peak-to-peak occipital activity, and no more than one well-defined spindle or K-complex; if an individual does not display clear 8 to 12 Hz activity, muscle-artifact and eye-movement tracings are used.

Stage 2. At least two well-defined spindles, or at least two K-complexes, or one of each; no more than 12 sec of 1 to 3 Hz, 40 μV peak-to-peak, or greater, slow waves.

Stage 3. At least 13 sec of 1 to 3 Hz, 40 μV peak-to-peak activity, but less than 30 sec of this activity.

Stage 4. At least 30 dominant sec of 1 to 3 Hz, 40 μV peak-to-peak activity.

As the subject goes from the wakeful (stage 0 or *W*) relaxed state, in which alpha rhythm dominates the EEG recording, gradual changes occur. With drowsiness (stage 1), alpha activity diminishes and theta (4 to 8 Hz) activity appears, along with some faster activity. Usually slow eye movements can be recorded. With light sleep (stage 2), the theta activity increases and sleep spindles, V waves, and K-complexes appear. Sleep spindles are bursts of waxing and waning 12 to 14 Hz activity; the V (or vertex) wave is an electronegative sharp wave occurring generally at the vertex and lasting about 150 msec; the K-complex is a vertex wave, sometimes followed by a spindle in response to an auditory stimulus. In moderately deep sleep (stage 3), V waves and delta waves (less than 4 Hz) dominate the record. In deep sleep (stage 4) the record is dominated by low-frequency delta waves with a frequency of less than 4 Hz. Throughout the night, periods of rapid-eye-movement (REM) sleep occur, accompanied by body movements. Dreaming has been shown to be associated with REM sleep.

Based on the scoring method just described, the depth of sleep for typical normal adults has been plotted throughout the night. Fig. 11-57 presents an

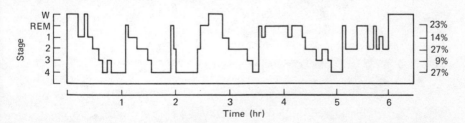

Figure 11-57. Depth of sleep, expressed in stages, versus duration of sleep, expressed in hours. Depth of sleep varies cyclically throughout the night, becoming very light (REM, or rapid-eye-movement stage) at times. Note that the time spent in the deepest stage of sleep (4) decreases after the first few hours. (Redrawn from L. G. Kiloh, A. J. McComas, and J. W. Osselton, *Clinical Electroencephalography*. Butterworths, London, 1972. By permission.)

example of how the depth of sleep varies cyclically during a night's sleep. Note that the time spent in deep sleep diminishes after about 2.5 hr, and just before awakening there are many oscillations in the depth of sleep.

Rapid, deep breathing, at a rate of about 30/min for about 3 min (hyperventilation), dramatically alters the EEG in normal subjects (Fig. 11-58). This act reduces the venous plasma carbon dioxide from a normal value of 60 to about 54 vol % (Morrice, 1956). The EEGs of children are especially responsive to hyperventilation. A typical response consists of large-amplitude, bilaterally synchronous, frontally prominent, slow theta activity; the frequency usually decreases with increasing hyperventilation. The lack of bilateral symmetry is an indication of abnormality. Controlled hyperventilation is used as a diagnostic technique to activate irritable and destructive foci, as well as generalized convulsive disorders, including petitmal epilepsy.

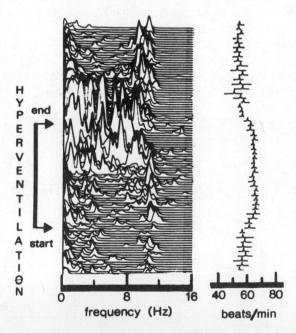

Figure 11-58. Combined compressed spectral array (CSA) of the electroencephalogram and the heart rate (ECG rate) of a subject hyperventilating for 173 sec. The vertical bars on the ECG rate record indicate the highest and lowest rates during the 4-sec periods of analysis. The heart rate increased just after hyperventilation and the EEG spectrum did not alter until halfway through the period of hyperventilation. Note that the interbeat variation in heart rate is reduced during the accelerated EEG phase and is markedly increased after the period of hyperventilation. (Record kindly provided by Dr. R. G. Bickford, University of California, San Diego, 1974.)

Anesthesia profoundly alters the electroencephalogram in a manner that is dependent on the type and amount of anesthetic employed and the species. The characteristic responses to a variety of anesthetic agents have been reported by Faulconer and Bickford (1960), Brechner et al. (1962), and Sadove et al. (1967). However, despite the differences among the various anesthetic agents, some important similarities accompany anesthesia. The first change that occurs is replacement of the alpha rhythm with low-voltage, high-frequency activity, which accompanies the analgesia and delirium stages. Thus the EEG resembles that of an alert or excited subject, although the subject is not appropriately responsive to stimuli; usually the responsiveness is excessive and/or inappropriate. From this point on, the type of EEG obtained with deepening anesthesia depends on the type of anesthetic and the species. However, when a deeper level of anesthesia is reached, the EEG waveform becomes less dependent on the species and the type of anesthetic. Large-amplitude slow waves begin to dominate the record, and with deepening anesthesia their frequency is reduced and they begin to occur intermittently. With very (dangerously) deep anesthesia, the record is flat (i.e., isoelectric). Complicating interpretation of the EEG in anesthesia are the effects of hypoxia, hypercapnia, and hypoglycemia, all of which mimic deep anesthesia.

Even though in the surgical stages of anesthesia the EEG spectrum is closely dependent on the type of anesthetic and species, it is relatively easy to learn to use the EEG as an indicator of depth of anesthesia by correlating the waveforms with the clinical signs that indicate depth. As an example of the correlation of EEG pattern with anesthesia depth, Bickford (1950) described a servosystem in which the EEG controlled the depth of anesthesia. The technique employed an integrator that summated the EEG activity from one channel; when a critical level of volt-seconds was reached, a thyratron fired, discharging the integrating capacitor and injecting an incremental dose of anesthesia to the vein of an animal that had been anesthetized previously.

11-10-3. The Compressed Spectral Array

Since the physiological state of a subject is reflected in the EEG, attempts have been made to provide band-pass filters and frequency analyzers to display those frequencies in the EEG that correlate best with the status of the subject. A useful display method was described by Bickford et al. (1972), who developed an on-line method of performing an analysis of the EEG frequency components in the 1- to 16-Hz band. One complete analysis was performed every 4 sec. A small digital computer was used to process the data and generate the display, which is called a "compressed spectral array" (CSA).

The CSA display technique employs an $X-Y$ plotter, whose X- axis represents the frequency range; the Y- axis, for one spectral analysis, represents energy. Immediately after the first 4-sec analysis period, the second begins and the $X-Y$ plotter is advanced by about 1 mm along the Y axis; then it writes out the second 4-sec scan. The process is repeated as long as it is desired to analyze an EEG channel. Thus the X axis of a compressed spectral array represents the frequency range extending from 1 to 16 Hz, and the Y axis indicates the energy of the various components present during one 4-sec scan. Each scan line on the Y axis also represents data analyzed 4 sec later. Hidden-line suppression is used to provide more clarity in the display. A typical compressed spectral array of a subject being monitored during hyperventilation appears in Fig. 11-58.

11-10-4.   Clinical Value of the EEG

The electroencephalogram sees its most valuable service in clinical medicine as a screening test for intracranial pathology. Parenthetically, the clinical correlation of EEG waveforms is much ahead of the rigorous physiological explanation of these phenomena. Thus the utility of electroencephalography rests principally on recognition of patterns of frequency, voltage, and waveform.

The EEG has its greatest value as an aid in the diagnosis and differentiation of the many types of epilepsy, a condition in which groups of neurons in the brain become hyperirritable and, depending on their location, produce both sensory, motor and autonomic manifestations. The epilepsies associated with cortical lesions are often detected by the scalp EEG. The EEG in epileptics is usually abnormal between and during attacks. The EEG often provides information on the localization of the area (or areas) of abnormal neuronal activity. In epilepsy, in general, the characteristic finding is of spikes (i.e., short-duration waves), alone or in association with other waves. For example, in petit-mal epilepsy, in which there is a transient alteration of consciousness (often not easily detected), the EEG shows a characteristic 3-per-second spike-and-wave activity.

Space-occupying lesions, such as tumors, subdural hematomas, and abscesses, give evidence of their presence by slow (delta) waves and depression of normal rhythms in the EEG, which allows localization and an estimate of the extent of the lesion. Such lesions are ideally localized with the bipolar recording technique (Fig. 11-52). If one of the electrodes common to two channels is over the slow-wave focus, there is a phase reversal in the recordings of these two channels.

Injury to the brain accompanies the application of high accelerative and decelerative forces; loss of consciousness and amnesia usually results. The type of posttrauma EEG relates to the extent of neuronal and/or vascular damage. In general, however, a depression in cortical activity and low-frequency activity accompanies such injury. Serial EEGs, taken over a prolonged period of time, provide useful prognostic information.

It is not the purpose of this section to discuss all the physiologic, pharmacologic, and clinical aspects of electroencephalography. Rather, an attempt has been made to show how recordings of the electrical activity of the brain, obtained from scalp electrodes, can provide useful clinical information. However, it is important to be aware that results of the EEG examination are always considered in the context of other clinical findings.

Electroencephalography enjoys a small, but secure, place in clinical medicine, and the interpretation of the EEG for its content of diagnostic information is the province of the well-trained and experienced electroencephalographer, who is aware that an abnormal EEG can be obtained from a normal subject; therefore, he exercises careful clinical judgment when interpreting the EEG.

11-11. THE ELECTRODERMAL PHENOMENA

Skin containing sweat glands (Fig. 11-59) exhibits two phenomena that arise in response to an attention-getting or alerting stimulus. The two

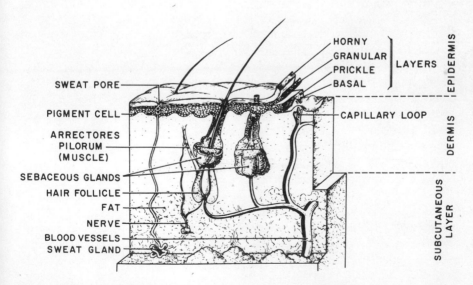

Figure 11-59.   Cross section of facial skin. (From G. L. Sauer, Charles C. Thomas, Springfield, Ill., 1965. By permission.)

phenomena (Fig. 11-60) are a decrease in resistance and a change in potential; the accurate measurement of each requires special attention to the type and location of the electrodes, the electrolytes used with them, and the characteristics of the measuring instrument. The change in resistance is still referred to as the exosomatic response, and the change in potential is frequently designated the endosomatic response. It is particularly distressing that many different names and symbols are used to describe these two phenomena. Standardization of symbols and terminology is still the subject of considerable debate, even though the phenomena have been investigated for almost a century.

The resistance change (or its reciprocal, conductance), or exosomatic response, was discovered by Féré (1888), who reported a transient decrease in resistance between electrodes applied to the anterior surface of an arm and leg of a hysterical subject who was presented with a variety of visual and acoustic stimuli. Féré suggested that the phenomenon could be of value in psychophysiological studies. Since Féré's time, the skin has been mapped to identify those regions which provide the maximum change in resistance in response to an alerting stimulus. Table 11-4 summarizes such data obtained by Edelberg (1967).

The potential change, or endosomatic response, was described by Tarchanoff (1890). This bioelectric event is almost universally called the skin-potential response. Significantly, its measurement requires placement of

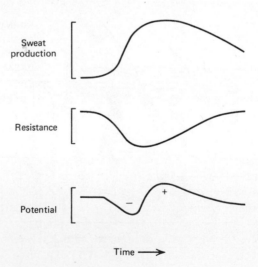

Figure 11-60. Relationship between simultaneously recorded sweat production, skin resistance, and skin potential in response to a strong emotion-provoking stimulus. [Redrawn from C. W. Darrow, *Psychophysiology* 1:31–38 (1964).]

Table 11-4   Relative Skin Conductance Level and Relative Skin Resistance Response (SRR) for Electrodes Placed at Various Sites on the Body: Values Expressed with Respect to Palmar Surface of the Finger*

Site	Number of Subjects	Relative Skin Conductance	Number of Subjects	Relative SRR
Finger				
Palmar	All	1.00	All	1.00
Dorsal	14	0.64	20	0.90
Hand				
Palmar (thenar, hypothenar, and center)	12	1.21	6	1.38
Dorsal	5	0.32		
Wrist				
Volar	11	0.38	5	0.13
Dorsal	5	0.36		
Foot				
Dorsal	14	0.53	9	0.20
Medial, over abductor hallucis muscle	8	1.26	15	1.70
Lateral			5	0.68
Plantar				
Heel	8	1.32	14	0.88
Arch	9	0.91	10	0.60
Ball	8	0.89	14	0.61
Toe	8	1.27	3	0.38

* From R. Edelberg, Electrical properties of the skin. In C. Brown, *Methods of Psychophysiology*. Williams and Wilkins Co., Baltimore, 1967. (By permission.)

one electrode over an area supplied with sweat glands (active site) and the other over an area devoid of them (or one that is rendered inactive by skin penetration or abrasion to obtain a reference site). If both electrodes are placed on sites that are equally active (i.e., they produce the same potential change), the potential difference between the electrode terminals will be zero. The relative activity of various body sites has been mapped out by Edelberg (1967), whose data are presented in Table 11-5. Note that the inner aspect of the earlobe appears to be the least active intact site. Abrasion of the skin, as by a cut, use of a needle electrode, or the application of Shackel's (1959) skin-drilling technique provides a relatively inactive site.

Table 11-5 Skin Potential and Relative Skin Potential Response for Electrodes Applied to Various Areas of the Body: The "Indifferent" or "Inactive" Electrode Was Located over a Skin-Drilled Site

Site	Number of Subjects	Skin Potential	Number of Subjects	Relative Skin Potential Response
Finger				
Palmar	25	−39.0	00	1.00
Dorsal	13	−24.8	12	0.57
Forearm				
Over ulnar bone, 2 in. from elbow	13	−15.2	12	0.07
Ear				
Inner aspect of earlobe	25	−14.1	24	0.05
Leg				
Over tibial bone, 2 in. above junction with foot	13	− 9.2	39	0.18
Foot				
Dorsal			7	0.23
Lateral, near sole			6	1.52
Medial, over abductor hallucis muscle	13	−36.2	12	1.94
Plantar				
Heel			12	3.87
Ball			12	1.89

From R. Edelberg, Electrical properties of the skin. In C. Brown, *Methods in Psychophysiology*. Williams and Wilkins Co., Baltimore, 1967. (by permission.)

To render a skin site inactive, it is only necessary to penetrate the epidermis down to the stratum malpighi, which is the germinal layer consisting of the basal and prickle cells. No blood is drawn with Shackel's skin-drilling technique. When so drilled, the site appears shiny at first and soon becomes wetted with tissue fluid.

As stated previously, the electrodermal phenomena have been studied for about a century, yet there is no standardization for the terms used to describe the conductive and voltaic properties of the skin. Terms employing "reflex" and "response" such as galvanic skin reflex or response (GSR), psychogalvanic reflex or response (PGR), skin potential reflex or response (SPR), skin resistance (SR), skin resistance level (SRL), skin resistance response (SRR), skin conductance (SC), skin conductance level (SCL), skin conductance response (SCR), and many others are used, often imprecisely. However, attempts are now being made to encourage psychophysiologists and others to adopt a consistent terminology. Venables and Martin (1967) and Edelberg (1972) (who reported on the terminology recommended by a committee of the Society for Psychophysiological Research) have presented terms that are very reasonable and descriptive. To this list, the authors have added two terms permitting description of the alternating current properties of the skin; Table 11-6 presents this terminology. Wang (1957) suggested that the term "response" has been used rather than "reflex," which has a special meaning physiologically. The authors wish to add that to be consistent with engineering practice, the symbol Z should be used for impedance and Y for its reciprocal, admittance.

11-11-1.   Skin Resistance Response (SRR)

The transient reduction in skin resistance (or increase in conductance) that accompanies an alerting stimulus can be recorded with one or both electrodes on active sites. Whether linear resistance or conductance changes are recorded depends on the type of circuit employed. Skin resistance level (SRL) and the changes it undergoes (skin resistance response, SRR) are measured with the constant-current circuit. The constant-voltage circuit measures skin conductance level (SCL) and its changes (SCR). Each type of circuit has properties that make it suitable for a particular application. The advantages and disadvantages of each are discussed subsequently.

Before describing the two types of circuit, it is necessary to recognize the importance of the type of electrode metal and electrolyte employed; as Edelberg et al. (1960, 1962) have pointed out, both can alter the magnitude of the change in skin resistance. Although lead and zinc, and even aluminum electrodes, have been used in the past with various electrolytes, their suitability is seriously questioned. Edelberg et al. (1960, 1962) have shown conclusively that calcium chloride, ammonium chloride, potassium sulfate, aluminum chloride, and zinc chloride enhanced the resistance change produced by alerting stimuli. The magnitude of the enhancement at a site was influenced by the direction of the current. Very dilute detergents, acetic acid, and alkali decreased the skin-resistance response. In addition, Edelberg (1967) pointed out that standard electrode preparations used for other purposes (e.g., ECG, EEG) are not suitable for recording skin resistance responses. Likewise, attention must be given to the choice of

Table 11-6 Terminology for the Electrodermal Phenomena

Basal or "Tonic" Level	Abbreviation	Dynamic or "Phasic" Response	Abbreviation	Units
Skin Potential (level)	SP or SPL	Skin potential response	SPR	mV
Skin Resistance (level)	SR or SRL	Skin resistance response	SRR	Ω
Skin Conductance (level)	SC or SCL	Skin conductance response	SCR	mhos
Skin Impedance (level)	SZ or SZL	Skin impedance response	SZR	Ω
Skin Admittance (level)	SY or SYL	Skin admittance response	SYR	mhos

metal, since it can react with the electrolyte to produce a salt that could enhance or depress the resistance response. At present, bare or chlorided silver appears to be the electrode surface preferred by many psychophysiologists. The electrolyte of choice is a weak sodium chloride solution that approximates perspiration (0.1–0.3% NaCl). With this solution current direction is unimportant. Edelberg (1967) advocated the use of 0.3% NaCl (i.e., 0.05 M) in a starch paste to which was added a preservative. Complete details for preparing two such pastes are presented in his report. For short-term recording, a dilute NaCl solution is satisfactory.

Although mentioned infrequently, the magnitude of the skin-resistance response is greatly affected by temperature. Maulsby and Edelberg (1960) and Edelberg (1972) reported that the resistance change decreased by about 5% per degree centigrade reduction in temperature. These authors found considerable individual differences in response; nonetheless, this fact emphasizes the need for controlling or reporting the environmental temperature.

In addition to the types of electrode and electrolyte and the temperature of the site, current density is important in determining the magnitude of the skin resistance response. If there were no physiological considerations, increasing the current would produce a larger recordable signal for the same percentage change in resistance or conductance; however, a limit is imposed by important physiological considerations. Edelberg et al. (1960) conducted a series of studies in which a test site was compared with a control site. They found that the skin resistance response increased linearly up to a current density of about 11 μA/cm², but with a current density of 100 μA/cm² the skin resistance response was reduced by about one-quarter. Therefore, as a design figure, a current density of about 10 μA/cm² represents an optimum value.

With a very low current density, the voltage change that represents the endosomatic signal (skin potential response) may be recorded along with that due to the resistance change, if one electrode is on an active and the other on an inactive site. This point is elaborated in the section dealing with the endosomatic response. Before approaching this subject, it is important to be aware that the current used to obtain the skin resistance response flows through one electrode-subject interface in one direction and through the other in the opposite direction. Therefore, depending on the direction of the current, the potential recorded as the skin potential response could include either series-aiding or series-opposing voltages produced by the potential rise or drop associated with the current flow used to measure the resistance.

Because current flows through the two electrode-electrolyte junctions in opposite directions, two different electrolytic processes may take place if the current density is high enough. In the case of silver-silver chloride electrodes, this situation admits the possibility of adding chloride to the anode and removing it from the cathode. With other metals, consideration should be given to the type of electrolytic products that may be formed, since potentiation or depression of the skin resistance response may occur at either electrode, depending on current direction and the activity of the site over which each electrode is placed. Studies, such as those described by Edelberg et al. (1960) and Edelberg and Burch (1962) using control and test sites with forward and reverse current and with one electrode on an active and the other on an inactive site, will provide decisive information in a particular recording situation.

11-11-2. Equivalent Circuit

Before the operation of the constant-current and constant-voltage circuits can be discussed, explanations are required regarding the circuit appearing between the terminals of a pair of electrodes used to measure the exosomatic or endosomatic response. Although the equivalent circuit is complex, it consists of three portions, which represent (1) the electrode-electrolyte interface, (2) the skin, and (3) the body tissues and fluids. Figure 11-61 presents an oversimplified model of these three equivalent circuits as they appear between the terminals (1, 2) of a pair of electrodes placed on the skin.

The electrode-electrolyte interface contains resistive $(R_w R_f)$ and capacitive (C_w) components and a half-cell potential $(E_{1/2})$. The magnitude of the resistive component R_w decreases with increasing area and current density; it also decreases as the frequency of the measuring current is increased. The capacitive component (C_w) increases with area, hence its reactance decreases with area; the reactance of C_w also decreases with current density and as the frequency used to measure it is increased. The resistance R_f depends inversely on area; it is usually high, it represents the direct-current resistance of the electrode-electrolyte interface, and it accounts for the electrolytic process. The half-cell potential $(E_{1/2})$ depends on the species of metal, the type and concentration of the electrolyte, and the temperature. A discussion of these factors is presented in Chapter 9. In a practical situation the impedance of the electrode-electrolyte interface is usually low compared with the magnitude of the other impedances encountered in electrodermal studies.

The equivalent circuit for the skin has been simplified to show a resistance R_{sc} (for the stratum corneum, or dry, horny layer) and a capacitor C_{sc} in which the stratum corneum and subjacent membranes represent the leaky dielectric, and the two "plates" are the electrode above

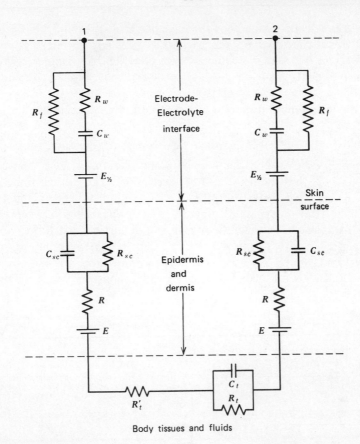

Figure 11-61. Approximate equivalent circuit for electrodes placed on the skin to record the electrodermal phenomena.

and the conducting body tissues and fluids below. The magnitude of R_{sc} is of course dependent on the type of electrolyte used and the secretion of sweat. The resistance R represents the resistance of membranes that change their permeability, thus contributing to the skin resistance response. A potential (E) has been included to represent the voltage that changes to produce the skin potential response. Similar models consisting of variable voltages and variable resistances were proposed by Edelberg (1967) and Lykken et al. (1968). In the case of the skin resistance response, both R and R_{sc} decrease in response to an alerting stimulus; the change in R_{sc} is probably brought about by the secretion of sweat.

Subcutaneous body tissues and fluids can be represented by resistive and capacitive components; the latter is due to cell membranes and the former is due to intra- and extracellular electrolytes. The origin of this circuit (R'_t R_t C_t) was discussed extensively by Cole (1933), and it is attractive because it exhibits an impedance-frequency characteristic quite similar to that of a specimen of living tissue.

11-11-3. Constant-Current Circuit for Resistance Measurement

With the constant-current circuit (Fig. 11-62a), the voltage (e) appearing between the electrode terminals (1, 2) is linearly proportional to the skin-resistance level (R_o) and the skin resistance response (ΔR). The essential requirement is that the resistor (R_i) in series with the voltage source (E) be much higher (e.g., 100 to 1000 times) than the equivalent resistive component (R_o) of the total impedance (Z_{12}) appearing between the electrode terminals (1, 2); thus, the magnitude of current that flows will be determined by R_i rather than R_o, even though R_o may vary among subjects. Figure 11-62a shows a passive constant-current source obtained by placing a high value of resistance (R_i) in series with a constant voltage supply (E).

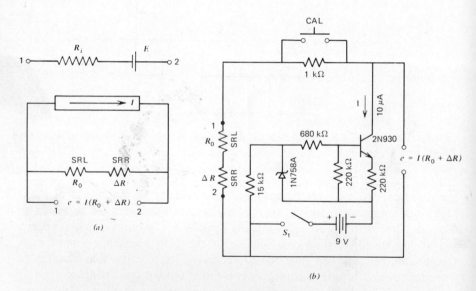

Figure 11-62. Constant-current circuits for measurement of skin resistance level (SRL) and skin resistance response (SRR). (*a*) Simple, constant-current generator, created by using a voltage source (E) with a resistance (R_i), which is high with respect to the skin resistance level (R_0), and the changes it exhibits (ΔR) which constitute the skin resistance response (SRR). (*b*) Constant-current circuit created by placing the subject ($R_0 + \Delta R$) in series with the collector of a transistor (2N930). The current (I) flowing through the subject is 10 μA and is controlled by the base bias on the transistor derived from the 680 and 220 kΩ resistors arranged in series.

Although this technique is convenient and inexpensive, the voltage required to obtain the desired current through the subject is often quite high. There are, however, active constant-current circuits available in which much less supply voltage is needed. For example, the collector circuit of a transistor or the appropriate configuration of an operational amplifier constitutes excellent constant-current circuits. Figure 11-62b illustrates a simple, low-cost, constant-current circuit used by Geddes et al. (1974). The equivalent impedance of this circuit is 500 MΩ, and it maintains a constant current for a resistance range extending from 0 to 1.5 MΩ. The current value is set by adjustment of the resistors that apply bias to the base of the transistor.

With the constant-current circuit, the desired signal is obtained directly from the electrode terminals (1, 2) using a recording instrument with an input impedance that is high with respect to R_o. The voltage (e) across the electrode terminals is given by

$$e = I(R_0 + \Delta R),$$

but
$$I = \frac{E}{R_i} \quad \text{when} \quad R_i \gg R_0 \quad \text{and} \quad \Delta R \ll R.$$

$$e = \frac{E}{R_i} R_0 + \frac{E}{R_i} \Delta R.$$

With the constant-current circuit, the voltage across the electrode terminals (1, 2) consists of a large constant voltage ER_o/R_i representing the basal skin resistance, and a smaller one $E\Delta R/R_i$ that represents the skin resistance response (ΔR) due to the altering stimulus. If both electrodes are over active sites, ΔR is doubled. As long as R_i is much greater than the total resistance (R_o) between the electrode terminals, the change in voltage, which reflects the skin resistance response, is independent of the skin resistance level.

In a typical application, the skin resistance response amounts to from 100 to perhaps 5000 Ω and stands on a constant resistance baseline of 10 to 50 kΩ. Figures 11-60, 11-65, and 11-66 illustrate typical skin resistance responses. Note that the resistance change is monophasic, consisting of a rapid decrease and a slower increase to the original baseline. A decrease in skin resistance is very frequently displayed as an upward deflection on the record.

11-11-4.   Constant-Voltage Circuit for Conductance Measurement

With the constant-voltage circuit (Fig. 11-63), a low-impedance voltage source (E) is used. The current (I) that flows is linearly proportional to the applied voltage and the conductance (G_0), which is the skin conductance

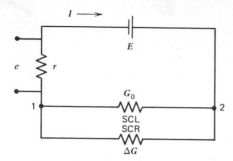

Figure 11-63. Constant-voltage circuit used for skin conductance measurement. The current due to the skin conductance level (G_0) and its changes (ΔG), which constitute the skin conductance response, are measured by recording the voltage (e) which appears across the resistor (r), which is many times smaller than I/G_0.

level in the absence of a skin conductance response (SCR). The skin conductance G_0 is the reciprocal of the direct-current resistance component (R_0) of the impedance appearing between the electrode terminals (1, 2). Thus $I = E\, G_0$.

An alerting stimulus will cause a small increase in conductance (ΔG); therefore, the general expression for the current is

$$I = E(G_0 + \Delta G).$$

Measurement of current is usually accomplished by recording the voltage (e) appearing across a resistance (r) which is added to the circuit and is very much smaller than $1/G_0$; in practice, the resistance (r) is in the range of 10 to 100 Ω. The voltage across r is therefore

$$e = Ir = rE(G_0 + \Delta G),$$
$$= rEG_0 + rE\,\Delta G.$$

The small conductance-change signal ($rE\Delta G$), which is the skin conductance response, stands on a larger skin conductance level signal that amounts to rEG_0. In a practical situation, the actual current that flows through the subject is dependent on G_0, which depends on electrode area and the subject's resistance level; hence, care must be exercised in the choice of a voltage (E) that will not send excessive current through low-resistance subjects.

In practice, a basal skin conductance of 0.1×10^{-3} mho/cm² represents the low resistance range for typical subjects (Edelberg, 1967), with perhaps a value of 0.01 to 0.002×10^{-3} mho/cm² being representative for high-resistance skin. A survey of the published literature on skin conductance was presented by Pfeiffer (1968). Hence for a 1-cm² electrode, the voltages that will provide 10 μA of current are 0.1 and 1.0 to 5 V, respectively. Therefore, careful consideration must be given to the choice of voltage with respect to the area of the electrodes if it is desired to maintain the current density at 10 μA/cm², the value recommended by Edelberg et al. (1960).

11-11-5. Amplifier Input Impedance

The input impedance of the amplifier connected to record skin resistance or conductance merits special consideration because the requirements are quite different for the two phenomena. In the case of measurement of skin resistance (see Fig. 11-62a), the amplifier used to record the resistance-dependent voltage (e) must have an input impedance that is high with respect to the skin resistance level R_0. Note that the output impedance (R_i) of the constant-current generator is high with respect to R_0. When measuring skin conductance, as in Fig. 11-63, the conductance-dependent signal (e), which appears across r, must be measured with an amplifier whose input impedance is high with respect to r, which is in turn much smaller than the basal resistance (R_0) of the subject, which is $1/G_0$. If a high-sensitivity current-measuring device with a resistive input resistance equal to or less than r is available, it can be substituted for r.

With both the constant-current (resistance measurement) and constant-voltage (conductance-measurement) circuits, the signal due to a resistance or conductance change is very small in comparison to the standing voltage representing the basal skin resistance or conductance level. In practice, the standing voltage is smaller with the constant-voltage method. With each circuit, the standing voltage must be canceled at some point in the system, permitting the much smaller signal produced by the physiological event to be amplified and suitably recorded. Since the insertion of a series-opposing voltage sometimes presents practical problems, the use of an adequately large coupling capacitor is common. The price paid in using a capacitor is the loss of dc or "baseline" information, providing only changes in resistance (SRR) or conductance (SCR). A practical circuit for eliminating the large standing potential at its source is the Wheatstone bridge (Fig. 11-64). One side of the bridge is constituted by the subject and the series resistor R_i or r, the magnitude of which depends on whether resistance or conductance is to be measured. The other side of the bridge consists of a potentiometer (P); its value is usually chosen so that approximately the same current flows through it as through the subject and the series resistor (R_i or r). When the bridge is balanced for basal values of R_0 or G_0, the voltage $E_{13} = 0$. Changes in E_{13} from the zero value are produced by an appropriate physiological stimulus. This output signal (E_{13}) is connected directly to a differential amplifier, which in turn drives a display device. Adjustment of the potentiometer rotor (3) allows presentation of zero voltage to the amplifier for any resistance or conductance level. The potentiometer is therefore the balance control for the Wheatstone bridge. Whether the bridge circuit provides a signal that represents resistance or conductance depends on the magnitude of the resistance (R_i or r) in series with the subject. With respect to the subject resistance (R_0), a high value of

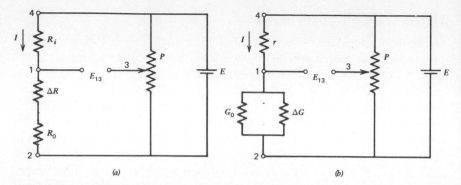

Figure 11-64. Wheatstone bridge circuits arranged for linear indication of skin resistance. (a) constant-current skin resistance ($R_i \gg R_0 + \Delta R$); (b) constant-voltage skin conductance ($r \ll 1/(G_0 + \Delta G)$).

series resistance (R_i) provides linear resistance recording (Fig. 11-62); a low value (r) provides linear conductance recording (Fig. 11-63). This important component must be chosen properly. In the past, sufficient attention has not always been given to this point, and in reading some reports it is not possible to tell whether the recordings represent linear resistance or conductance changes.

When using the Wheatstone bridge, and a differential amplifier to record skin resistance or conductance, consideration should be given to the need to use an isolated source (E) to supply current to the subject and to the ability of the differential amplifier to tolerate an appreciable common-mode (offset) signal. It is highly desirable to employ a separate source to apply current to the subject and to energize the differential amplifier to avoid the risk of providing multiple current paths through the subject and input circuit of the amplifier. For example, referring to Fig. 11-64, the input of the amplifier is connected to points 1 and 3, and in a practical situation it is often necessary to ground point 2 or 4 to reject common-mode signals, such as 60-Hz interference. When this is done, even with the bridge balanced (i.e., $E_{13} = 0$), there is an appreciable standing potential (E_{12} or E_{14}, depending on whether point 2 or 4 is grounded). In operation, the differential amplifier must be able to tolerate this common-mode offset voltage if its common terminal is connected to either 1 or 4.

11-11-6. Bandwidth Requirements

If basal skin resistance or conductance levels are to be recorded, direct-coupled systems are required (i.e., the sinusoidal frequency response must extend to 0 Hz); however, if only changes in skin resistance or conductances are of interest, capacitive coupling with a time constant of 5 sec or longer, as advocated by Edelberg (1967), provides adequate fidelity. This value for the time constant corresponds to a lower sinusoidal frequency limit (for 70% amplitude) of 0.03 Hz.

The high-frequency response required for faithful reproduction of the electrodermal phenomena has not been investigated extensively, possibly because there are so many graphic recording systems that obviously respond much faster than skin resistance and conductance changes. Measurement of the most rapidly changing components of skin resistance and conductance recordings reveals that a rise time (10–90%) of about 0.1 sec is typical. The equivalent sinusoidal high-frequency response is therefore 5 Hz. Thus a bandwidth extending from 0 to above 5 Hz will allow faithful reproduction of skin resistance or conductance levels and their changes. If only changes are of interest, a bandwidth extending from 0.03 to 5 Hz is satisfactory.

11-11-7. Characteristics of the Constant-Current and Constant-Voltage Circuits

The type of circuit selected by an investigator depends primarily on the projected use for the data, the size of signal desired, and the electrophysiological model chosen. Extensive discussions on the characteristics and advantages of one method over the other have been presented by Darrow (1964), Wilcott and Hammond (1965), Edelberg (1967), and Lykken and Venables (1971); selection of the best is by no means a settled issue. If indication of the presence or absence of a response is sufficient, both the constant-current (resistance) and constant-voltage (conductance) circuits are suitable, with the practical exception that the former provides a signal about tenfold larger than the latter. When skin resistance or conductance levels are to be recorded, the size of the bucking voltage required is higher with the skin resistance method. With the constant-current (resistance) circuit, the input impedance of the amplifier must be on the order of many megohms in order to be much higher than the skin resistance level. The input impedance of the amplifier used with the constant-voltage (conductance) system need only be high with respect to the low value of resistance in series with the subject (r in Fig. 11-63).

If it is assumed that the secretion of sweat is the major contributor to the decrease in resistance, and that the sweat glands are arranged in parallel under the active electrode, the conductance method is the one of choice because the increase in conductance is linearly related to the number of actively secreting sweat glands (Darrow, 1934; Thomas and Korr, (1957)). Thus with an increase in number of active sweat glands, current flow through an active site is not changed by other sites becoming active. According to Lykken (1971), the conductance change is relatively independent of the basal or tonic skin conductance level. With the constant-current circuit, Darrow (1964) has shown that the change in resistance decreases with decreasing skin resistance level. This situation follows from peripheral considerations; however, since a decreased skin resistance is associated with an increase in central response to the stimulus, this effect counteracts the peripheral manifestation.

With the constant-voltage (conductance) method, current is limited only by the skin resistance level of the subject and the internal resistance of the current source, and precautions must be taken to avoid using excessively high current densities ($>10 \, \mu A/cm^2$) when low skin resistance levels are encountered. With the constant-current (resistance) method, the current is always the same, regardless of the skin resistance level of the subject. However, with a very high skin resistance, the constant-current system may generate a high voltage drop across the skin, which will cause the resistance to fall (Wilcott and Hammond, 1965).

In some instances it is desirable to use the skin resistance electrodes to detect a bioelectric event, such as the ECG. Use of the conductance method places a short circuit across the electrodes, rendering the pair useless for any other purpose. However, the impedance of a constant-current source is high; therefore, one or both electrodes can be used to record a bioelectric event, providing its amplitude and/or frequency spectrum will allow separation of the skin resistance signal. Use of the same fingertip "dry" silver electrodes for the simultaneous measurement of changes in skin resistance and the ECG was described by Geddes et al. (1975); Fig. 11-65 presents a typical recording made using this technique in which the subject was asked to take deep breaths to produce large-amplitude skin resistance responses. Figure 11-66 is a typical recording of skin resistance responses and instantaneous heart rate, obtained in the same way during a simple lying test. Here the subject was asked to think of a number between 6 and 10 and say "no" to every interrogation. The subject lied about number 8, which was the number he had selected.

Although the skin resistance response is usually recorded using direct current, sinusoidal alternating current has also been employed. Such applications are described in Chapter 10. The studies carried out thus far make it clear that the magnitude of the resistance change decreases with increasing frequency. However, insufficient data exist to indicate the optimum frequency range. There is evidence that use of a frequency of 100 Hz provides a reasonably good skin resistance response and eliminates bothersome galvanic electrode potentials (Edelberg, 1974).

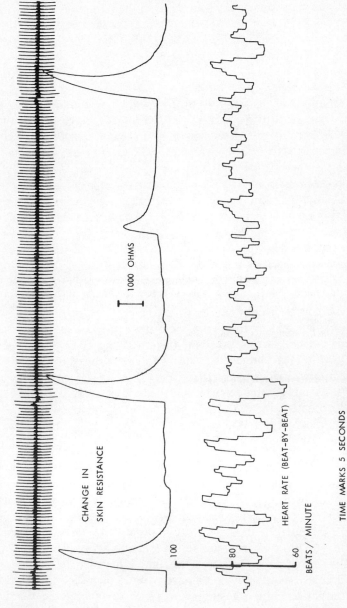

Figure 11-65. The electrocardiogram (ECG) and skin resistance response obtained from the same pair of dry silver electrodes applied to the volar surfaces of the tips of the second fingers. The instantaneous heart rate was derived from the ECG. [From Geddes et al., *Med. Biol. Eng.* 1975 (January). By permission].

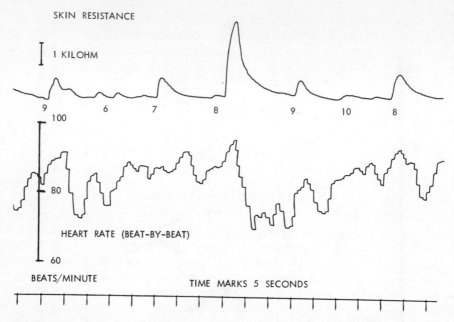

Figure 11-66. Typical record of changes in skin resistance and beat-by-beat heart rate during a simple lying test in which the subject was asked to concentrate on any number between 6 and 10 and say "no" to each number guessed by the interrogator. Note that the amplitude of the skin resistance change was greatest for number 8. Note also the considerable reduction in heart rate following the first response to number 8.

11-11-8. Skin Potential Response (SPR)

As stated previously, with the endosomatic method one electrode is placed on an active site, the other on an inactive site. The active sites most frequently employed are the sole of the foot, palm of the hand, and the volar surface of a finger tip (often the second finger is employed). Table 11-5 presents data on the relative activities of the various body sites. Chlorided-silver electrodes, with a weak electrolyte of known composition approximating that of sweat (ca. 0.3% NaCl), are frequently employed. With an electrode over an area rich in sweat glands (active site) and one on an inactive site, the potential of the active site is negative by an amount that varies from a few to 50 or 60 mV; the actual magnitude depends on many factors. An alerting stimulus produces an initial increase in negativity followed by a decrease (positive wave) and sometimes by a second negative wave. The first negative and the positive waves were designated the *a* and *b* waves by Forbes (1936); however, this terminology is not widely used.

The skin potential level drifts slowly for about 15 min following application of the electrodes, and the change is believed to be due to hydration of the tissues by the electrolytic preparation. This phenomenon is under active investigation (Edelberg, 1968; Fowles and Venables, 1970) and becomes important when the skin potential level is to be used as a measure of the level of alertness.

Edelberg (1972) pointed out that the several phases of the skin potential response are affected differently by various electrolytes. However, at this time there are insufficient data to permit making strong recommendations. Presumably, weak electrolytes, such as those used for skin resistance responses (i.e., 0.3% NaCl), do not enhance or depress the skin potential response.

The temperature of the active site affects the skin potential response; a reduction in temperature decreases the amplitude and affects the negative and positive phases differently. Yokota et al. (1959) showed that the positive phase was absent (with electrodes placed on the palm and dorsum of the hand) when the temperature was decreased to 20°C and reappeared at 30°C. At 40°C the amplitude was increased. The negative phase was most prominent at 20°C (Yokota et al., 1959). These facts suggest that attention should be given to maintaining and reporting the temperature of the site or the environment.

With one electrode on an active site and the other over an inactive site, there are at least two electrode-electrolyte potentials, the skin potential and perhaps an injury potential, if the inactive site has been created by marked abrasion of the skin; thus the algebraic sum of these voltages appears between the electrode terminals and is presented to the input of the recording apparatus. If it is desired to record this skin potential level (SPL) and the changes it experiences in response to an alerting stimulus (SPR), it is necessary to employ a bucking or canceling voltage in the input circuit of the recording apparatus because the typical change in skin potential is quite small (on the order of millivolts) and the skin potential level (plus electrode and injury potential) may be many tens of millivolts, hence may block the amplifier. If only changes in skin potential (SPR) are desired, capacitive coupling with an adequately long time constant (ca. 5 sec) eliminates the need for using a bucking voltage. In both cases the amplifying apparatus must have an adequately high input impedance for the size of the electrodes employed. In a typical situation, an input impedance greater than 2 MΩ can be used with electrodes having an area of about 1 cm^2.

A typical skin potential response is shown in Fig. 11-60, along with the change in resistance and secretion of sweat. Note that the waveform of the response is biphasic, the active area becoming initially more negative with respect to the inactive site. The type of waveform is not always symmetrical nor biphasic; polyphasic patterns have been reported (Edelberg, 1972).

At this point, a few remarks are in order regarding the endosomatic method. Of paramount importance is the need to locate one electrode in an active site and the other in an inactive site. Since voltage is measured, the technique is easily standardized, calibration being achieved by the application of a step-function of voltage on the order of 1 mV. Apart from specifying the electrode type, size, and site, there are no other important variables (presuming that the amplifying system has an adequately high input impedance and adequate bandwidth). If these criteria are met, precise control of electrode area is relatively unimportant unless it becomes so small that R_0 begins to approach the input resistance of the amplifier. If the calibrating signal is maintained for about 20 sec, the time constant of the recording apparatus will be recorded if capacitive coupling is used. Of course, if direct coupling is used, the recorder will remain deflected as long as the calibrating signal is present. If direct coupling is used to obtain the skin potential level, very stable electrodes are required along with provision for an adjustable canceling or bucking voltage. Depending on the electrode locations and suitable separation of component frequencies with appropriate circuitry, one or both of the electrodes can be used to detect another bioelectric event.

11-11-9. Origin of the Electrodermal Phenomena

Although the skin resistance and skin potential responses (SRR and SPR) have been investigated for almost a century, there are insufficient data to formulate an acceptable explanation for them. The many theories and models advanced thus far have been described very fairly by Edelberg (1972), whose review is recommended reading for those wishing to delve further into this subject. Although no single explanation is tenable, certain facts are well accepted. For example, the SRR and SPR both require the presence of active sweat glands (Richter, 1927), which in man are brought into action by the sympathetic nervous system via the neural transmitter acetylcholine. Thus the sweat glands are sympathetic-cholinergic, and their activity is blocked by atropine, which raises the skin resistance level and abolishes both the SRR and SPR. Likewise, interruption of the sympathetic nerve supply to the sweat glands abolishes the SRR and the SPR. From this point on, it becomes increasingly difficult to make definite statements. For example, there is no doubt that these two responses reside in the superficial layers of the skin, but the precise level has not been established. Abrasion of the skin down to the granular layer abolishes both responses. Although it is obvious that sweat secretion will lower skin resistance, visible (surface) sweating is not necessary for the production of a skin resistance response. One group of investigators believes that sweat rises in the ducts, spreads laterally, hydrating the stratum corneum and reducing its resistance. However, there appears to be evidence that epidermal membranes become permeable in response to neural stimuli, resulting in a decrease in resistance and change in membrane potential, and both contribute to the skin resistance and skin potential response. In addition, some investigators believe that there is a presecretory and a secretory potential associated with the activity of a sweat gland and its duct, which, along with sweat expulsion, enhance the detection of a skin potential (and resistance) response. Which of these phenomena dominates or is subordinate in the genesis of the electrodermal phenomena awaits further investigation. However, it is not necessary to have the results of such studies to use the electrodermal phenomena as indicators of activity of the sympathetic division of the autonomic nervous system.

11-12.   ELECTROOCULOGRAPHY

It is well known that placing two orthogonal pairs of electrodes around an eye will permit measurement of potentials that can be used to identify the direction of gaze with respect to the head. The bioelectric event underlying these signals is a standing potential, measurable between the cornea and the posterior pole (fundus) of the eyeball. Thus the eyeball resembles a dipole that can move in an inhomogeneous volume conductor (the head), as illustrated in Fig. 11-67. The polarity of the potential depends on the type of eye, and the magnitude of the potential increases above a basal value with increasing illumination; this increase forms the basis for electroretinography, which is described in a subsequent section of this chapter.

Apparently the first to report an electrical potential associated with the eye was duBois-Reymond, who in 1849 made measurements on the tench, a European freshwater fish of the carp family. Marg's (1951) translation of the report is as follows: "With the eye on its side, the cornea and optic nerve could be brought into contact with the electrodes. From this it was shown that an arbitrary point in the surface of the eyeball was positive with respect to the cross-section of the nerve." From this description it is not possible to discover how much the optic nerve injury potential contributed to what is now known to be the standing potential between the cornea and the back of the eyeball. DuBois-Reymond's experiment was repeated by Dewar and M'Kendrick (1876) and Dewar (1877), using rabbit, cat, dog, pigeon, owl, goldfish, rock fish, stickleback, frog, toad, snake, crab, and lobster eyes connected via duBois-Reymond's nonpolarizable electrodes to a Thomson reflecting galvanometer. In addition, they observed a change in the standing potential with illumination of the retina. In a postscript to their

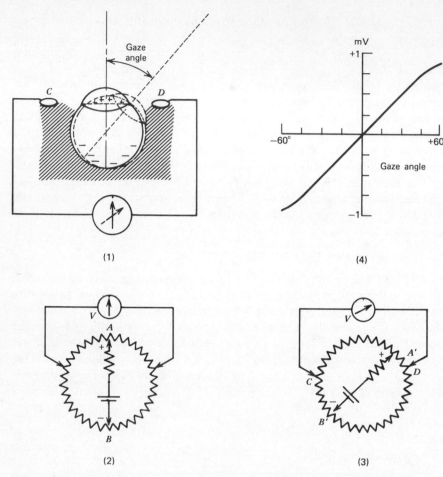

Figure 11-67. The corneoretinal potential (1) and its representation as an equivalent circuit (2, 3) for forward and right gaze; (4) represents a typical voltage versus gaze angle relationship. (Redrawn from "Electrodes for Recording Primary Bioelectric Signals," ASD Tech. Rept. 61-437, USAF, Wright-Patterson, AFB, Ohio.)

paper they reported having located Holmgren's (1865–1866, 1870–1871) reports (in Swedish) describing similar studies. These early investigators reported galvanometer deflections rather than voltages, probably because the volt had not been universally adopted as the unit for potential.

Most of the early investigators who had used galvanometers and "nonpolarizable" electrodes to measure the response of the eye to light noted the presence of a steady potential when the retina was not illuminated; this potential was measurable between an electrode on the cornea and one behind the eye, or at an indifferent site on the body. Evidence of the corneo-retinal potential in the human subject came from studies reported by Dewar and M'Kendrick, who were interested in the response of the eye to light. Yet they demonstrated that eye movements could be recorded and stated:

"Having succeeded in detecting the action of light on the retina of the living warm-blooded animal without any operative procedures, it appeared possible to apply a similar method to the eye of man. For this purpose, a small trough of clay or paraffin was constructed round the margin of the orbit, so as to contain a quantity of dilute salt solution when the body was placed horizontally and the head properly secured. Into this solution the terminal of a non-polarisable electrode was introduced, and in order to complete the circuit the other electrode was connected with a large gutta-percha trough containing salt solution, into which one of the hands was inserted. By a laborious process of education it is possible to diminish largely the electrical variation due to the involuntary movements of the eye-ball, and by fixing the eye on one point with concentrated attention, another observer, watching the galvanometer, and altering the intensity of the light, can detect an electrical variation similar to what is seen in other animals. This method, however, is too exhausting and uncertain to permit of quantitative observations being made."

Notwithstanding, Dewar and M'Kendrick were the first to demonstrate an eye-position-dependent signal.

Actual measurement of the standing corneofundal potential has been made infrequently. Several authors have reported a magnitude of 6 to 12 mV, without indicating how the measurement was made. Perhaps the best review of the literature that is concerned with the standing potential was presented by Kohlrausch (1931); a translation and summary of his conclusions were given by Marg (1951), who reported:

"1. In vertebrates the cornea is positive relative to the retina. In in-vertebrates, however, the anterior of the eye is negative. This corresponds to the difference in orientation of the retinas of subphylum Vertebrata and the retinas of the invertebrates, the visual cells pointing outward in the former and inward in the latter.

"2. The polarity of the standing potential is increased by light (the illumination potential) whether the animal has a positive cornea (vertebrate) or not (invertebrate).

"3. There is a sudden discontinuity in potential at the ora serrata, which is found as one measures the topographic distribution of voltage.

"4. Under certain influences, such as ionic changes or mechanical insults, there are independent changes of the standing and the illumination potential.

"5. One finds a similar alteration in both the standing and the illumination potential under other influences, such as changes in carbon dioxide and oxygen tensions, temperature and electrical stimuli."

Even before the magnitude and true origin of the corneofundal potential were established, it was put to practical use to detect eye position using periorbital electrodes. Schott (1922) and Meyers (1929) appear to have been the first to achieve success using the string galvanometer; Schott employed a wire and a button electrode (both of copper) placed nasally (on the caruncle) and temporally on the conjunctiva in the outer canthus of the cocainized eye. A spectacle frame was used to stabilize the electrodes, and the cocaine diminished electrode irritation. Schott's interest lay in recording nystagmus, rather than eye position. Meyers applied a pair of horseshoe-shaped electrodes located bitemporally with the open part facing the eye. He noted that not only lateral deviations of the eye were recorded, but vertical movements could be detected with electrodes above and below one eye. Although he obtained recordings of opposite polarity when the direction of the gaze was reversed, he did not study the relationship between recorded amplitude and deviation of the eyes from the central fixation point, probably because his interest was the study of nystagmus. Incidentally, he named the technique "electro-nystagmography," but erroneously attributed the source of the potential to a summation of action potentials of the ocular muscles. Likewise, Jacobson (1930) attributed the electrooculographic signals to the contraction of ocular muscles. Wrong as this was later shown to be, Jacobson appears to have been the first to mention that eye position signals could be obtained with closed eyes.

Up to this time there appear to have been three theories regarding the origin of the signal that reflects eye position. Some thought that contraction of the muscles causing deviation of the eyeball produced action potentials that were summated and detected by the electrodes. Others thought that because string galvanometers were used and there was current flow, a change in interelectrode resistance caused the galvanometer to be deflected as the eyes were deviated. Another group thought that a standing potential existed between the cornea and back of the eyeball, and movement of the eye varied the voltage presented to periorbital electrodes. It was not long before these three theories were subjected to experimental test. In a single paper Mowrer et al. (1935–1936) clearly showed that the source of the electrooculographic signal was the standing potential that exists between the cornea and fundus of an eye with a functioning retina. The manner by which they dispelled all doubts is interesting for the clear logic of the presentation. For example, the investigators reasoned that if resistance change produced the signal, transtemporal electrodes should detect the same resistance change for deviation of the eyes to the right and left; therefore, the galvanometer should be deviated in the same direction for right and left deviations. Experiment showed that the galvanometer was deflected in opposite directions, with left and right deviations of the eyes. To add further proof to the fallacy of resistance change being an important contributor, they recorded the electrooculogram with a high input impedance amplifier connected ahead of a string galvanometer; with this arrangement virtually no current was drawn from the subject, and a left and right gaze produced oppositely directed deflections on the recording.

To prove that summated muscle action potentials were not the basis of the electrooculographic signal, Mowrer et al. (1935–1936) pointed out that contracting muscle is electronegative to resting tissue, and with transtemporal electrodes, a gaze to the right produced a positive polarity at the right-temporal electrode; if the signal were due to summated muscle action potentials, the polarity should be negative. In addition, summation of action potentials would produce a jagged deflection in the recording; this was never seen. To add even more proof, they placed transtemporal electrodes on a deeply anesthetized cat and deviated the eyes passively by attaching a probe to the anesthetized cornea. The galvanometer showed deflections related to the direction of deviation of the eyeballs; under this condition, deviation was produced without muscular contraction. To prove that the electrooculogram so produced was not due to reflex contraction of the ocular muscles, they showed that destruction of the retina, by intraocular injection of a 5% solution of chromic acid, completely abolished the voltage produced by passive movement of the eyes. Finally, they showed that the electrooculogram was produced by a standing potential measurable between the cornea and fundus of the eye by removing the eye and measuring a potential between electrodes in these locations; the cornea was found to be positive with respect to the back of the eyeball; however, they did not report the magnitude of the potential differences.

Now that the existence of a corneofundal potential has been established, it is of value to examine the appropriateness of the model in Fig. 11-67. If the corneofundal potential is equated to a dipole in a volume conductor, the potential detected by a pair of electrodes placed on the skin, above and below or lateral to an eye, ought to be zero with the gaze directed forward, varying as the sine of the gaze angle measured when the gaze is deflected along the axis of an electrode pair—provided the head does not seriously distort the dipole field. This model can be simplified by considering the electrooculographic generator (the corneofundal potential A, B) to be a battery that moves within a circular resistor. The potential-measuring electrodes are represented by taps (*C, D*) on the circular resistor [Fig. 11-67 (2)].

Many studies have been carried out to determine the voltate-versus-gaze angle relationship. In the early days of electrooculography, Fenn and Hursh (1937) reported that the voltage detected by bitemporal electrodes is related to the sine of the angle of deviation from the central fixation point. Since that time, others have sought to confirm or refute this relationship; many have shown that, within limits, the voltage is linearly related to the horizontal angle of gaze. That the electrooculogram did reflect eye position was verified by Hoffman et al. (1939), using a binocular corneal reflection technique and photographic recording; they concluded that "the electrical method is reliable enough to be used in psychological research." In support of this belief, Halstead (1938) reported being able to detect vertical and horizontal eye movements as small as one degree. Even though the potential measured between bitemporal electrodes was found to be related to eye position, Byford (1963) reported that comparisons with an optical eye-tracking device showed that the electrooculographic method was undependable in a few of the subjects being tested.

Among those who have reported a linearity of voltage with angle of gaze are Leksell (1939) for ±40°, Mackensen and Harder (1954) for ±30°, Kris (1957, 1958) for ±5 to ±60°, and Kris (1960) for ±30°; Mackensen and Harder's data showed a good correspondence with the sinusoidal relationship up to 40°. Law and Devalois (1958) wrote that a linear relationship existed between 0.5 and 15°, and North (1965) stated that the electrooculographic voltage did not follow a sinusoidal relationship with gaze angle; Leksell (1939) and Shackel (1960, 1967) reported that both a linear and a sinusoidal relationship are good approximations.

In a recent study by Geddes et al. (1973), a comparison was made between the linear and sinusoidal relationship for horizontal gaze deflection by measuring the potential appearing between a pair of dry silver electrodes located at the outer canthus of each eye. Precise control of gaze direction was obtained by using a semicircular frame (perimeter) equipped with 13 miniature neon lamps, located at every 10 degrees of gaze direction and placed in front of the subject's head (see Fig. 11-68). The head position was stabilized by a chin support. The subject first directed his gaze at the illuminated neon lamp at the central fixation point (CFP) directly in front of him. Then the operator extinguished the CFP lamp and illuminated any other lamp; the subject directed his gaze to the newly lit lamp, and afterward the CFP lamp was illuminated. The test was repeated five times for each gaze angle to the left and right from 0 to 60 degrees. The voltage (*e*) readings obtained for each gaze angle (θ) were plotted versus gaze angle

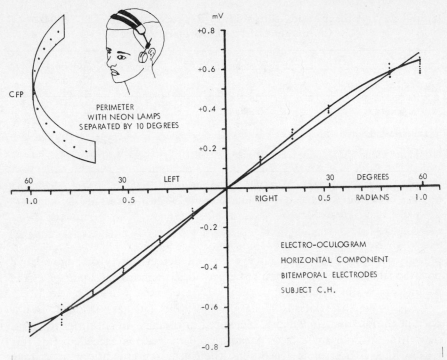

Figure 11-68. Voltage versus horizontal-gaze direction in man, using bitemporal electrodes. [From Geddes et al., *Med. Biol. Eng.* **11**:73–77 (1973). By permission.]

and, for each subject, least-squares fits were obtained for linear ($e = E\theta$) and for sinusoidal ($e = E_m \sin \theta$) representations. A set of data for a typical subject appears in Fig. 11-68, along with the linear and sinusoidal representations. The data for 22 subjects were analyzed and are summarized in Table 11-7. This study revealed that for gaze angles up to ±60 degrees, the sinusoidal representation was superior to the linear representation; the former exhibited a standard error of estimate (SEE) of 0.029 and the latter a value of 0.037. However, for a gaze angle of ±45 degrees, the linear representation is sufficiently accurate for practical purposes.

Although the dipole concept is very useful for modeling the standing corneofundal potential, it should be mentioned that Kris (1960) has shown that whereas electrodes placed lateral to the canthus of the eyes detect only the horizontal component of lateral gaze, an electrode pair placed on the supraorbital margin and the infraorbital ridge do not detect purely a vertical component of gaze direction. In other words, two electrodes pairs

Table 11-7 Linear and Sinusoidal Representations for Horizontal Component of the EOG of Each Eye*

	Linear Representation† $e = E\theta$	Sinusoidal Representation† $e = E_m \sin\theta$
Average value	$e = 0.600\theta$	$e = 0.684 \sin\theta$
Maximum value	$e = 1.05\theta$	$e = 1.21 \sin\theta$
Minimum value	$e = 0.364\theta$	$e = 0.413 \sin\theta$

* From Geddes et al., *Med. Biol. Eng.* 11:73–77, 1973.

† The values for E and E_m are in millivolts, the angle θ is measured in radians (1 radian = 57.3 degrees).

placed orthogonally around an eye do not detect purely orthogonal eye position signals. Of the two pairs of electrodes, the horizontal pair gives the purest component signal.

In assessing the relationship between voltage and gaze angle, it is important to note that $\sin\theta$ and θ, measured in radians, do not differ by more than 10% until an angle of 0.75 radian (43 degrees) is exceeded. For this reason, if a 10% error is acceptable, the linear representation for voltage versus gaze angle is adequate up to this limit. For gaze angles larger than this figure, for theoretical and practical reasons the sinusoidal representation offers a better correlation between voltage and horizontal eye position.

Despite the considerable use made of the electrooculogram, there is no universally agreed-on terminology to describe location of the electrodes about one or both eyes. Two of the pioneer investigators in this field, Miles and Lindsley, proposed the use of lead systems; however, Miles (1939) applied periorbital nasal and temporal electrodes around each eye to record horizontal movements only. Leads 1 and 2 detected the horizontal component of the EOG for the left and right eye, respectively; lead 3 identified the bitemporal (eyes-in-series) electrode pair, lead 4 was recorded between the two nasal electrodes, and lead 5 designated the connection for both eyes in parallel. Lindsley and Hunter (1939) employed lead 1 to designate nasal and temporal electrodes about the right eye, lead 2 to identify the supra- and infra-orbital electrodes of the right eye, lead 3 to specify the bitemporal electrode array, and lead 4 to identify a right eye oblique lead employing supraorbital and nasal-electrode sites.

Since electrodes are almost always placed lateral to and above and below the eyes to detect horizontal and vertical displacements, it would seem appropriate to create a simple, easily remembered terminology to simplify communication among investigators in this rapidly expanding field. For example, using V and H to designate vertical and horizontal electrodes (hence, eye-movement direction), and L and R as subscripts referring to left and right eyes, the following simple notation may be of assistance; it can be extended readily to designate other less-used electrode arrangements. For example, H_{R+L} would signify addition of the horizontal components of the EOG for both eyes; likewise, H_{R-L} would indicate subtraction of these two signals. Similarly, H_{RLP} could mean the parallel connection of the horizontal electrodes about each eye. Likewise, V_{R+L}, V_{R-L}, and V_{RLP} are designations for the series-aiding, opposing, and parallel connections of the vertical electrodes about the eyes.

11-13.   ELECTRORETINOGRAPHY (ERG)

In the dark, a standing measurable potential exists across the various layers of the retina. When the retina is illuminated, cyclic changes occur in this potential, a recording of which constitutes the electroretinogram (ERG). Although the bioelectric generators responsible for the phenomenon lie within the various layers of the retina, the ERG can be recorded by placing one electrode on the cornea and the other at the back (fundus) of the eye, or at a distance on the surface of the body. Sometimes the reference (body-surface) electrode is placed over the mastoid process, occasionally on the forehead or cheek. The various types of corneal electrodes were described by Sundmark (1959). Fig. 11-69 shows several types that have been used; one of these, the "contact glass" electrode described by Riggs (1941) and Karpe (1945), saw extensive clinical service. Sundmark presented quantitative data for the optimum design for such electrodes. At present, a contact lens is used to carry the corneal electrode, which often incorporates a chlorided silver wire, a substance which can exhibit its own photoelectric effect. Usually a short-acting anesthetic is applied to the cornea to eliminate irritation in response to application of the electrode.

The ERG of the human and animal eye is by no means a simple bioelectric event. Although it arises in the retina, this structure is complex, consisting of photosensitive receptors (rods and cones), nerve cells, and pigment cells, all of which can exhibit bioelectric phenomena. Each human retina has about 120 million rods and 7 million cones, four types of nerve cells (bipolar, ganglion, horizontal, and amacrine), along with pigment and glial cells. Animals with excellent night (scotopic) vision have retinas dominated by rods (previously designated E retinas); others that see poorly in the dark but well in daylight (photopic vision) have retinas dominated

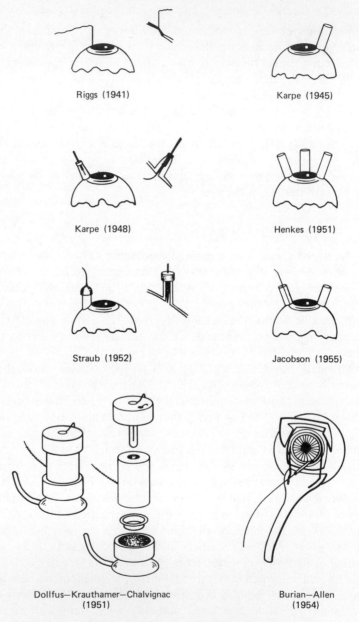

Riggs (1941)

Karpe (1945)

Karpe (1948)

Henkes (1951)

Straub (1952)

Jacobson (1955)

Dollfus—Krauthamer—Chalvignac
(1951)

Burian—Allen
(1954)

Figure 11-69. Various types of corneal electrodes used to detect the electroretinogram. [From E. Sundmark, *Acta Ophthalmol.* **37**:8–40 (1959). By permission.]

by cones (previously designated I retinas). Most animals, including man, have mixed retinas.

As stated in the section on electrooculography, the ERG was apparently discovered by duBois-Reymond (1849) in the carp. This photobioelectric phenomenon was confirmed by Holmgren (1865–1866, 1870–1871) in the eye of the frog, viper, rabbit, dog, and cat. About the same time, and independently, Dewar and M'Kendrick (1876) and Dewar (1877) recorded the ERG from the eye of the rabbit, cat, dog, pigeon, owl, goldfish, rock fish, stickleback, frog, toad, snake, crab, and lobster. They also showed that the response to illumination depends on the color of the light stimulus. Finally they succeeded in recording the ERG of man; their description of this feat appears in the section on electrooculography. That the photobioelectric signal was due only to the retina was demonstrated by Holmgren (1870–1871) and Kühne and Steiner (1880), the latter investigators concerning themselves with isolated retinas.

The type of the ERG recorded with an electrode on the cornea and one on the surface of the body depends on many factors; perhaps the most important relates to the environmental conditions (i.e., whether the eye has been light or dark adapted). A typical ERG obtained in response to a 2-sec burst of high-level illumination of the retina with white light is shown in Figure 11-70. The letter designations (a, b, c) for three of the four waves were provided by Einthoven[2] and Jolly (1908). In the vertebrate eye, retinal illumination causes the corneofundal potential to first decrease slightly (a wave); then it exhibits a marked increase, which describes the prominent b wave. The combination is often designated the "on effect." With sustained illumination of the retina, the potential falls, then rises slowly to describe the c wave. When the illumination is removed, a d wave or "off effect" is frequently recorded. The relative magnitudes of these waves depend on the illumination intensity, the degree of light or dark adaptation, and the type of retina. In response to a brief flash (ca. 50 msec) of light, only the a and b waves are recordable.

Granit (1962) presented a most comprehensive description of the ERG for dark- and light-adapted cone and rod-dominated retinas; Fig. 11-71 is his illustration. From numerous experimental techniques that used light and dark adaptation, variation of light intensity, color and duration, anesthesia, hypoxia, and drugs, it has been possible to show that the complex cornea-body surface photobioelectric potential is made up of at least

---

[2] It is interesting to note that Einthoven first used these letters for the principal waves of the ECG. Very soon thereafter he labeled the ECG waves P, Q, R, S, and T. The a, b, c designation has been retained for the electroretinogram.

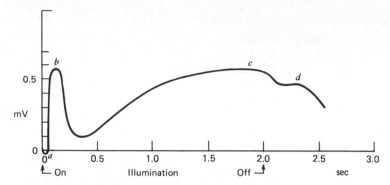

Figure 11-70. Typical human electroretinogram in response to a long-duration (2-sec) light stimulus of high intensity. (Redrawn from M. Sosonow and E. Ross, "Electrodes for Recording Primary Bioelectric Signals," ASD Tech, Rept. 61-437, Aeromedical Laboratory. Wright-Patterson AFB, Ohio.)

three components designated PI, PII, and PIII, which reflect different slow and fast retinal processes. The reader who is interested in pursuing study of the meanings of these components is directed to Granit's review (1962).

As stated earlier, the ERG is often recorded in response to a short-duration (ca. 50 msec or less) stimulus, and in this situation only the a and b waves are obtained. It was also stated that most retinas contain two types of photoreceptors, rods and cones; the former are receptors for night (scotopic) vision and the latter for day (photopic) vision. Each receptor type has a different spectral sensitivity, the rods being primarily blue-green sensitive and the cones being primarily orange-red sensitive. Adrian (1945) presented an excellent study demonstrating the separate ERGs of the rods and cones. Using himself as the subject, he recorded the ERG using a corneal-cheek electrode array. Single flashes (25 msec) of light of different colors were used to illuminate the retina which was first light adapted, then dark adapted. Adrian's results (Fig. 11-72) indicate that in the light-adapted eye, which yields a cone-dominated response, the ERG was maximum for orange-red light and no response was obtained for blue light. In the dark-adapted eye, which yields a rod-dominated response, the ERG was maximum for blue-green light and the smallest amplitude was obtained for deep-red light. Note that the amplitudes and time courses of the ERGs for light- and dark-adapted eyes are different.

The degree of contribution of each of the retinal cell types in the genesis of the ERG is by no means settled. There is agreement that the photoreceptors (rods and cones) and the bipolar cells play an important role. It is therefore apparent that since the presence of an ERG is indicative of a functioning retina, the ERG ought to be of value as a diagnostic tool.

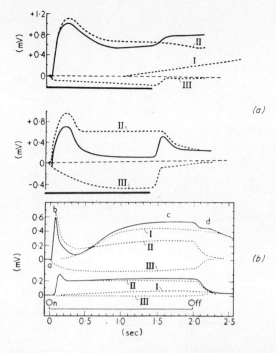

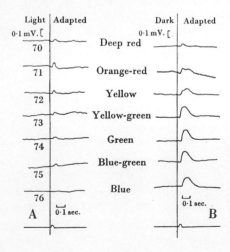

Figure 11-71. (*a*) The I (cone) electroretinogram of dark-adapted (upper) and light-adapted (lower) eyes. (*b*) The E (rod) electroretinogram in response to two intensities (upper, 14; lower, 0.14 mL). The PI, PII, and III, components appear as dashed curves. (From R. Granit, in *The Eye*, H. Dawson, ed. Academic Press, New York, 1962. By permission.)

Figure 11-72. The electroretinograms of man in response to single flashes of light of various colors presented to the light-adapted (A) and dark-adapted (B) eye. Bottom tracings show the duration of the flash of light. [From E. D. Adrian, *J. Physiol.* **104**:84–104 (1945). By permission.]

However, before discussing this topic, a few comments are in order regarding the manner in which visual information reaches the cortex where light and form are discriminated.

As stated previously, the retina of a human eye contains about 120 million rods and 7 million cones; thus there are 127 million photoreceptors. These receptors are complexly interconnected in the retina and synapse, first with bipolar, then ganglion cells. Axons of the ganglion cells exit the globe and constitute the optic nerve, which contains only about a million fibers. Most of the fibers of the optic nerve synapse again with neurons in the lateral geniculate nucleus of the thalamus. Fibers arising from this structure project to the visual (occipital) cortex, the primary processing area for visual information. How, in the presence of more receptors than centrally communicating pathways, visual acuity is so good, remains a mystery.

Despite the close linkage of the ERG with the visual process and despite the ease of recording the ERG in the human, clinical use of the ERG for diagnosis is just beginning to emerge, and several studies have been carried out to demonstrate its clinical usefulness. For example, Sachs (1929) found that the ERG amplitude was smaller in response to red-light stimulation in subjects who are color blind to red light (protanopes). Karpe (1945) conducted a carefully controlled study of the ERG in patients with known visual defects. The technique employed a bright flash of light, about 40 msec in duration, and recorded the ERGs from dark-adapted eyes using a saline-filled cup (contact glass) electrode paired with one on the forehead. With this technique he found a reduced ERG amplitude in subjects with diseases that affected the rods. He also reported that a difference in ERG amplitude greater than 25% between the eyes is indicative of retinal pathology; a difference of 10% is within normal limits. According to Ito (1973), the ERG amplitude is remarkably decreased in subjects with retinal pigment degeneration and with retinal detachment. He stated that the ERG is often recorded before and after the surgical removal of congenital cataracts to confirm retinal function.

Perhaps the clinical use of the ERG is limited because applying the technique to the human subject is time-consuming and not without some risk to the subject since it is necessary to desensitize the cornea by the topical application of an anesthetic and the protective reflex is temporarily depressed. Because the retina can be examined visually with an ophthalmoscope, the changes produced by disease are often quite obvious to the trained observer. Moreover, the subject can be interrogated, and the history often provides the necessary diagnostic information.

A method of recording a potential that reflects the ERG and does not impose discomfort or hazard on the subject was described by Arden et al.

(1962) and Arden and Kelsey (1962). This technique makes use of the dependence of the amplitude of the EOG signal, detected by horizontally located periorbital electrodes, on the magnitude of the corneofundal (retinal) potential and the angle of gaze. By having the subject shift his gaze repeatedly between two fixed, lighted reference points, separated by an angle of 34.5 degrees, the peak-to-peak amplitude of the EOG becomes a function of the corneoretinal potential and can be recorded with an ordinary capacity-coupled amplifier with an adequately long time constant (greater than 2 sec).

Arden and his co-workers devised tests in which the peak-to-peak amplitude of the EOG was plotted for periods up to 2 hr following sustained changes in ambient illumination. During the test, the subject executed horizontal eye movements between the fixation points. The eye movements were made with a frequency of 2 per second for 10 sec each minute. A typical plot, obtained by illuminating a dark-adapted eye, is given in Fig. 11-73a. The type of potential variation obtained following a sudden decrease in ambient illumination of a light-adapted eye is shown in Fig. 11-73b. The initial maxima and minima are called the light rise and trough. Arden and his co-workers reported that the ratio of peak-to-trough voltage is independent of electrode location and provides an index of the functional capacity of the pigment epithelium. In normal eyes, the ratio is greater than 1.85.

Arden and his associates have shown that their tests are well suited to detect pathologic processes in the eye. For example, quite different plots are obtained with retinitis pigmentosa, absence of rod vision, retinal detachment, and choroid lesions. Since clinicians are only beginning to collect data using this technique, it is too soon to make evaluative statements.

11-14. MAGNETOGRAPHY

The movement of electric charge is accompanied by a magnetic field. During excitation and recovery in irritable tissue, there is a translocation of charge (ions) across cell membranes. Therefore, this charge movement will give rise to a magnetic field that can be detected and recorded with suitable apparatus. The authors have applied the name "magnetography" to studies concerned with recording the magnetic component of the action potential produced by irritable tissue. Because electrograms (bioelectric voltages recorded with electrodes) and magnetograms have a common origin, they reflect the same event. However, each provides a different type of information. Whether magnetograms, with their directional characteristics, will provide useful physiological and diagnostic information is yet to be established. The highly desirable and outstanding characteristic of magneto-

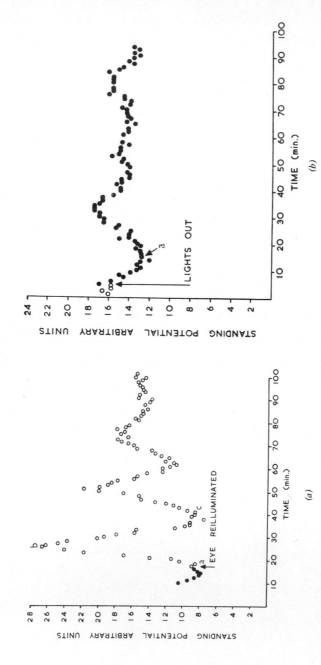

Figure 11-73. Variations in the peak-to-peak amplitude of the EOG for a horizontal gaze angle of 34.5 degrees on illumination of the normal dark-adapted eye (*a*) and in response to decreasing illumination of the normal light-adapted eye (*b*). The magnitudes of these waveforms track changes in the corneoretinal potential. The amplitudes and periods of the waves are characteristically altered by disease. [From G. B. Arden and J. H. Kelsey, *Brit. J. Ophthalmol.* **46:**449–467 (1962). By permission.]

grams is that no electrodes are required for their detection. However, magnetic field detecting systems of extremely high sensitivity are needed. Moreover, successful recording of magnetograms requires that adequate means must be secured to attenuate environmental magnetic fields. Typically, magnetograms from active tissue provide a field strength that is less than one-millionth of that of the earth's magnetic field.

Magnetograms from isolated frog nerve were recorded by Seipel and Morrow (1960). Stratbucker et al. (1963) measured the changing magnetic field associated with the beating of an isolated guinea pig heart by recording the voltage induced in a coil of 17,640 turns wrapped on a toroid that was concentric with the heart located in a volume conductor. The voltage induced in the coil resembled the first time derivative of the ECG which was detected by apex-base electrodes in the volume conductor. The human magnetocardiogram (MCG) was recorded by Baule and his associates (1963, 1965, 1970), who introduced the parallel-coil technique (Fig. 11-74a), which was employed by many later workers. With such coil-detecting systems, the magnetocardiogram is expected to resemble the first time derivative of the ECG, as shown in Fig. 11-74b. Safonov et al. (1967) and Cohen and his colleagues (1967a and b, 1969, 1972) also used the parallel-coil method to record the human MCG. With considerable initial difficulty (1968), and relative ease later, the human magnetoencephalogram was reported by Cohen (1972).

The most successful and potentially useful magnetograms recorded to date are those from the human heart, the first of which were recorded by Baule and associates (1963, 1965, 1970) using two coils 30 cm long and 9 cm in diameter placed normal to the thorax. Each coil contained one million turns wound on a ferrite core. The coils were connected in series and provided a peak voltage (ca. 30 μV) proportional to the rate of change of the magnetic field. Safonov et al. (1967) employed a similar technique except that the detector and subject were placed in a magnetically shielded iron enclosure with walls 1.5 in. thick. Cohen (1967a) described an improved magnetically shielded enclosure for magnetography which employed moly-permalloy. To the inner shell was applied a layer of aluminum 0.19 in. thick. The cubical housing measured 86 × 88 × 88 in. Subjects from whom magnetograms were to be recorded were placed in this enclosure. The magnetic detector consisted of several coils (each 200,000 turns, 5 cm long, and 8 cm in diameter) placed on a ferrite core and covered with a brass cylinder to provide electrostatic shielding. The detector was mounted securely in front of the thorax of the subject. With an overall bandwidth extending from 0 to 30 Hz, quite acceptable MCGs were recorded. In a subsequent paper, Cohen et al. (1971) employed a more sophisticated shielded enclosure and a superconducting magnetometer (SQUID) of the Josephson type (see review by

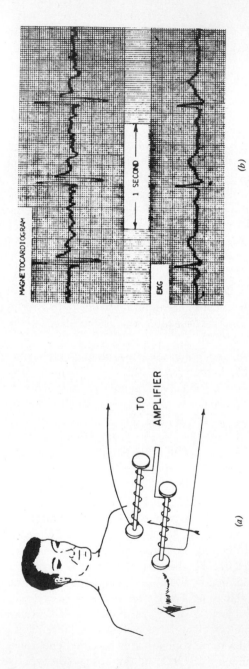

Figure 11-74. (*a*) Method first employed to detect the magnetic component of the cardiac action potential; (*b*) magnetocardiogram and electrocardiogram. Each of the two pickup coils consisted of 2 million turns of wire wound on a dumbbell-shaped ferrite core about one foot long. [From G. Baule and R. McFee, *Am. Heart J.* **66**:95–96 (1963). By permission.]

Doyle, 1971) to detect MCGs in dogs during experimental myocardial infarction created by inflating a cuff around a coronary artery branch. With an effective bandwidth of 0 to 40 Hz, control and infarction MCGs were obtained. Figure 11-75 is a typical example of the canine MCG before and after producing the infarct by occlusion of the left anterior descending coronary artery. Note the change that resembles the S–T segment shift characteristically seen in the electrocardiogram with myocardial infarction (see p. 463).

Truly remarkable magnetoencephalograms on the order of 1×10^{-9} G were reported by Cohen (1972), who employed an improved triply shielded room and a superconducting SQUID magnetometer. Figure 11-76 presents a typical example of the MEG and EEG obtained from a human subject with the magnetic detector about 2 cm from the back of the head. The low noise level and calibration (2×10^{-8} G) indicate that a remarkable degree of sensitivity has been obtained for magnetography.

Magnetograms give evidence of events occurring below the surface of the body, and such events may not always be detectable with surface electrodes. Magnetography now offers the opportunity to measure direct-current fields, a measurement that is difficult with electrodes because of their half-cell potentials. Since magnetography does not call for the use of electrodes, no contact with the subject is required; this feature may be valuable in some situations. For example, in the case of severely burned subjects in whom it is desired to measure cardiac and brain activity, magnetography is ideally suited.

Another area of application of magnetography may be the determination of pathways for externally injected current. At present, it is extremely difficult to assess the path traversed by current flowing through anisotropic body tissues. The magnitude and direction of the fields such currents produce can be investigated by magnetography.

Before   During

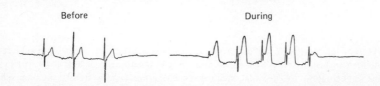

Figure 11-75.   Magnetocardiograms obtained from the dog by use of a superconducting magnetometer placed in front of the chest. The control (before) and during occlusion of the left anterior descending coronary artery are shown. Note that injury is indicated by the equivalent of an S-T segment elevation. This illustration can be compared with the ECG in myocardial infarction shown in Fig. 11-41. Courtesy of D. Cohen, Frances Bitter National Magnet Laboratory, Massachusetts Institute of Technology.

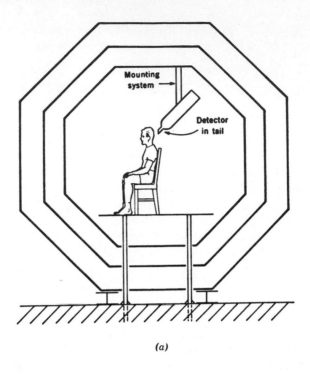

(a)

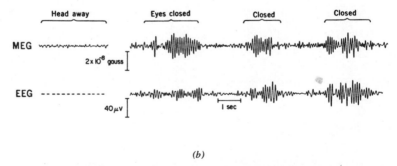

(b)

Figure 11-76. (a) Method of obtaining magnetoencephalograms by enclosing a subject in a triply shielded enclosure and using a superconducting magnetometer as a detector. (b) Typical magnetoencephalogram (MEG) and electroencephalogram (EEG) from a human subject. [From D. Cohen, *Science* **175**:664–665 (1972). By permission.]

11-15. BIOELECTRIC EVENTS: HISTORICAL POSTSCRIPT

The electrical activity of nerve and that accompanying the contraction of skeletal and cardiac muscle were known long before there were instruments adequate for their accurate reproduction. Galvani's three important experiments (ca. 1800) have been recounted frequently (Fulton and Cushing, 1936; Hoff, 1936; Walker, 1937) because they led directly and immediately to the development of current electricity and to an intense interest in bioelectricity, even though Galvani's explanation for them was incorrect, as demonstrated by Volta (Geddes and Hoff, 1971). In fact it was the Galvani-Volta controversy that led directly to the discovery of current electricity, giving birth to electrical engineering. Of Galvani's three experiments, only the third, which described contraction of the gastrocnemius muscle without the use of metals, need concern us here, for it was the only one that demonstrated the existence of a true bioelectric potential. This experiment, sketched in Fig. 11-77 (a), consisted of observing a twitch in a rheoscopic[3] frog preparation when the sciatic nerve was laid over a cut muscle so that contact was made between the intact and cut surfaces. Between the cut (injured) and the intact surfaces appeared the injury potential, which was of sufficient magnitude to stimulate (on contact) the sciatic nerve of the rheoscope and produce a twitch in the muscle. In a primitive way this experiment demonstrated the existence of the membrane potential.

Carlo Matteucci (1842a and b) used the rheoscopic frog to first demonstrate the existence of an action potential accompanying muscular contraction. His experiment, sketched in Fig. 11-77b, consisted of laying the sciatic nerve N_2 of a rheoscopic frog over the surface of a muscle M_1 in which the nerve N_1 was intact. Repetitive stimulation of nerve N_1 caused muscle M_1 to develop action potentials and twitches. The muscle action potentials stimulated nerve N_2 of the rheoscopic frog, causing twitches in its muscle M_2. Thus was demonstrated the first electromyographic signal.

The electrical activity accompanying the heart beat was also discovered with the rheoscopic frog by Koelliker and Mueller (1856) in the manner shown in Fig. 11-77c. When these investigators laid the nerve N over the beating ventricle of a frog heart, the muscle M twitched once and sometimes twice. Stimulation of the nerve obviously occurred with depolarization and repolarization of the ventricles. Because at that time there were no rapidly responding galvanometers, Donders (1872) recorded the twitches of

---

[3] "Current-seeing" preparation, consisting of an isolated sciatic nerve-gastrocnemius muscle used before invention of the galvanometer to demonstrate the existence of an electric potential.

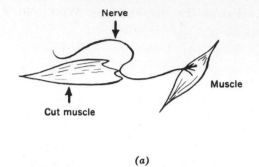

(a)

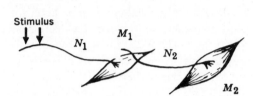

(b)

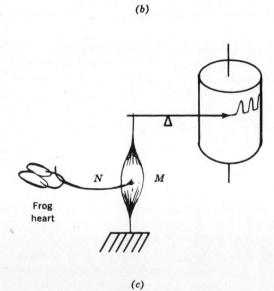

(c)

Figure 11-77. The beginnings of bioelectricity: (a) Galvani; (b) Matteucci; (c) Koelliker, Mueller, and Donders.

the rheoscope to provide a graphic demonstration of the existence of an electrocardiographic signal (Fig. 11-77c).

The first measurements of bioelectric potentials by means of a physical instrument were those of Nobili (1828), who measured the injury current by connecting his astatic galvanometer (Fig. 11-78) to electrodes on the cut and intact surfaces of a pile of frog muscles. The next to measure myoelectric potentials was du Bois-Reymond (1843), who postulated that a difference of potential existed between the interior and the exterior of muscle, another prediction of the existence of a membrane potential. Connecting a galvanometer to electrodes on the fingers of the two hands, he noted a deflection when the muscles of one arm were contracted; this was probably the first demonstration of the human electromyogram.

True voltage-time graphs of the bioelectric signals were made long before rapidly responding indicators were available. The actual waveform of the nerve action potential was determined by Bernstein (1868), using the rheotome;[4] this was perhaps one of the earliest applications of the sampling method. In this technique, developed by the Russian physicist Lenz (1849, 1854), a commutator briefly connected a slowly responding galvanometer (such as those shown in Fig. 11-79a, b); the device averaged the voltage at different instants after a tissue had been stimulated by completion of a circuit, using a second pair of contacts on the commutator. A graph of the average values of voltage and time after the stimulus permitted Bernstein to plot the true voltage-time curve of the nerve action potential, lasting 0.6759 msec. Figure 11-80 illustrates Bernstein's rheotome and the nerve action potential he obtained with it.

Using the rheotome, Marchand (1877), Englemann (1878), and Burdon-Sanderson and Page (1879) plotted accurate representations of the waveform of the ventricular component of the electrocardiogram. The record obtained by Burdon-Sanderson and Page, which clearly reveals what are now called the R and T waves, is shown in Fig. 11-81. From this study came the proposal that the ventricular electrogram is the sum of two interfering monophasic action potentials. This theory provided an understanding of the respective relationships of the R wave to excitation and the T wave to recovery of the ventricles (Fig. 11-13).

The first instrument to provide a continuous record of a rapidly changing bioelectric event was the capillary electrometer[5] developed by Marey (1876). This device (Fig. 11-82a) consisted of a mercury-sulfuric acid interface enclosed in a capillary tube. Current, obtained from electrodes on an irritable tissue, changed the charge distribution at the interface and altered

[4] See Hoff and Geddes (1957).
[5] Geddes and Hoff (1961).

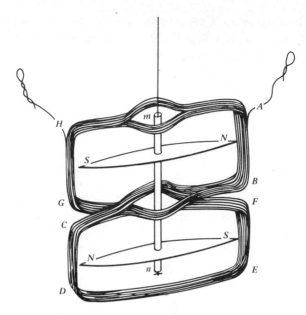

Figure 11-78. Nobili's astatic galvanometer, consisting of two magnets mounted rigidly to a suspension with their poles in opposite directions. Thus the suspension would not align itself with the earth's magnetic field. The magnets were surrounded by coils wound in opposite directions. The frog (injury) current flowing through the coils caused the suspension to be deflected from its zero position by an amount proportioned to the current. [From C. L. Nobili, *J. Chem. Phys.* **45**:249–256 (1825) (supplement added by Schweigger). By permission.]

the contour of the mercury meniscus. By the use of a high-intensity light and an optical system, the variations in the contour of the meniscus were photographed to display the first spontaneously occurring bioelectric signals, the tortoise and frog cardiac electrograms appearing in Figs. 11-82b and 11-82c.

The capillary electrometer was the first instrument to display the ECGs of animals and man as they arose spontaneously. Using this electrometer, Burdon-Sanderson and Page (1878, 1879) stated again that the R and T waves of the ventricles could be explained by the "interference" between two monophasic action potentials, representing the bioelectric event under each electrode. This they did by first injuring the tissue under one of the electrodes (Fig. 11-83a) on a frog ventricle, thus obtaining a monophasic action potential. Then with electrodes on the intact surface of the ventricle, they cooled the region under the distal electrode, thereby delaying recovery and prolonging the duration of this monophasic action potential and making the T wave more prominent and downward, as in Fig. 11-83b. From such experiments they proved their interference theory enunciated several years earlier.

Fig. 11-83c shows that the R wave of the cardiac electrogram represents the temporal difference in excitation of the two regions under the recording electrodes and the T wave represents the temporal difference in recovery under the two electrodes. Delaying repolarization of the tissue under the last region to be excited caused the T wave to be increased in downward amplitude (see Fig. 11-83c). As mentioned earlier, this theory has limited applicability to electrocardiography when body-surface leads are used, but it provided dramatic information regarding the waveform of the cardiac electrogram and showed that the R and T waves are related to excitation and recovery, respectively, and that the duration of the refractory period is long in cardiac muscle.

Waller (1887, 1889) discovered that the capillary electrometer could be used to record the electrocardiogram of animals and man without opening the thorax. A copy of one of his human records (Fig. 11-84) illustrates the motion of the ventricles as represented by the apex cardiogram (h–h), along with the electrocardiogram (e–e) recorded from chest-to-back leads. Al-

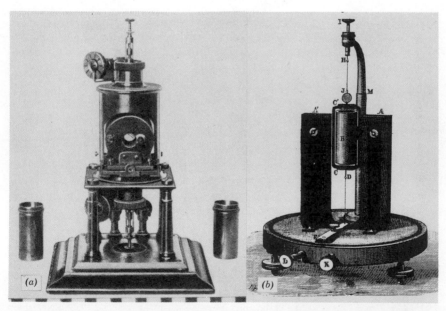

Figure 11-79. Two of the galvanometers used by the early electrophysiologists. (a) Thomson's (moving magnet) reflecting galvanometer (1858) used by Caton to record the electroencephalogram of a rabbit (1875). (b) The d'Arsonval (moving coil) galvanometer, used frequently with the rheotome to plot the waveform of action potentials. Thomson's galvanometer carries UK patent number 329, dated 1858. d'Arsonval's galvanometer was described in *C.R. Acad. Sci. (Paris)* **94**:1347–1350 (1882).

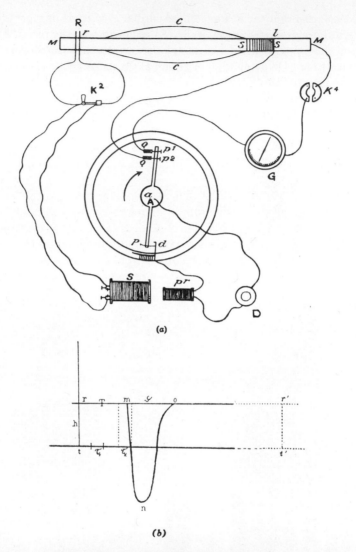

Figure 11-80. (*a*) Bernstein's rheotome, 1876; (*b*) the nerve action potential. [From H. E. Hoff and L. A. Geddes, *Bull. Hist. Med.* **31**(3):212–347 (1957). By permission.]

though the electrocardiogram only partially resembles those obtained today, it nonetheless contains the essential details of ventricular activity— an R wave (small downward spike) followed by a T wave (smooth, rounded, downward wave). It is also clear that the R wave precedes ventricular contraction and the T wave precedes ventricular relaxation. To better illustrate this point, Waller recorded the ventricular myogram and electrogram of an exposed kitten heart and obtained a similar record.

In Waller's investigation of the animal and human electrocardiograms, he was led to investigate the effect of electrode location on the amplitude of the electrocardiogram. Waller wrote:

"An investigation made last year upon my own person gave the following results:

"Leading off from the surface of the body by the several limbs and from the mouth, I found that some combinations were favourable, while others were unfavourable* to the demonstration of the cardiac variation [the electrical signal]. The favourable combinations were the

"Front of chest and back of chest,
Left hand and right hand,
Right hand and right foot,
Right hand and left foot,
Mouth and left hand,
Mouth and right foot,
Mouth and left foot."

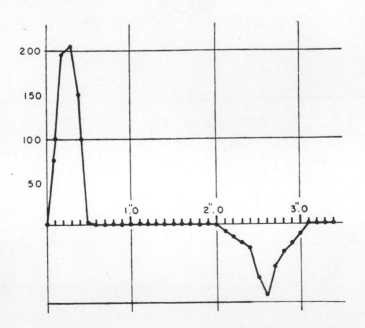

Figure 11-81. Burdon-Sanderson's record of the ECG, made by using the rheotome. [From J. Burdon-Sanderson and F. J. M. Page, *J. Physiol.* **2**:384–435 (1880). By permission.]

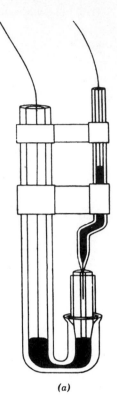

(a)

T

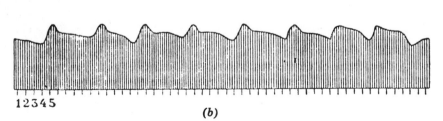

1 2 3 4 5

(b)

G

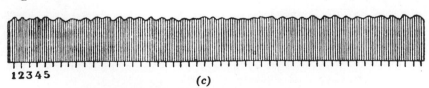

1 2 3 4 5

(c)

536

"The unfavourable combinations were:

Left hand and left foot,
Left hand and right foot,
Right foot and left foot,
Mouth and right hand."

* "I use the terms "favourable" and "unfavourable" for the following reason: With a moderately sensitive electrometer no variation is seen with an unfavourable combination and a small variation is seen with a favourable combination; with a very sensitive electrometer a small variation is seen with an unfavourable, and a comparatively large variation with a favourable combination."

From the amplitudes obtained with these "favourable" and "unfavourable" leads, Waller proposed that as a result of the electrical activity of the ventricles, isopotential lines could be mapped out on the surface of the body (Fig. 11-19). He also showed that measurement of this potential distribution would permit determining the electrical axis of the ventricles. These properties were used later by Einthoven (1913) in his work on vectorcardiography.

The first nerve action potentials were recorded by Gotch and Horsley using the capillary electrometer. Figure 11-85 illustrates the records they obtained. Because they wanted to be sure that the signals recorded by the capillary electrometer were not artifacts from the induction coil stimulator, they made a separate record of the stimulus to show that the make (m) and break (b) shocks moved the mercury meniscus in opposite directions. The nerve action potentials evoked by both make and break shocks always moved the mercury meniscus in the same direction, thereby proving the physiological origin of the waves recorded in Fig. 11-85 (top).

Although the capillary electrometer was used to record skeletal muscle action potentials, great difficulty was encountered because of the long response time and the need to apply the correction technique described by Burch (1892). Moreover, it was difficult practically to excite skeletal muscle electrically and eliminate stimulus artifact. In addition, the waveforms of muscle action potentials had been determined previously with the

---

Figure 11-82. (a) The capillary electrometer. (b) and (c) The first electrocardiograms. Tracing (b) is Marey and Lippmann's tortoise electrocardiogram. It is difficult to be certain of the identity of the waves because the authors did not provide enough information on the location of the electrodes. Quite probably the waves shown here are the R and T waves. Tracing (c) is Marey and Lippmann's frog auricular electrogram. If, as the authors say, the time divisions are $1/25$ sec, the auricular rate was 5/sec or 300/min, which is excessively fast for a frog heart. Very possibly the auricles were in a state of fibrillation, and if so, this is one of the earliest records of auricular fibrillation. [From L. A. Geddes and H. E. Hoff, *Arch. Intern. Hist. Sci.* **56–57**:275–290 (1961).]

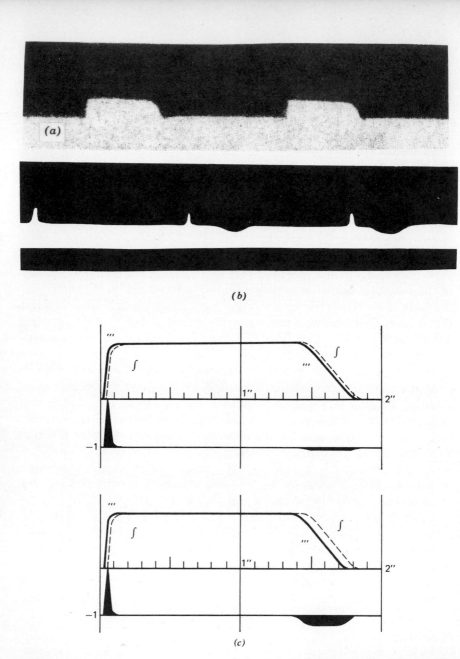

Figure 11-83. Capillary electrometer recordings of the frog heart. (*a*) Monophasic action potential obtained by injuring the tissue under one electrode; (*b*) the effect of prolonging recovery by cooling under one electrode, thereby lengthening the duration of the monophasic action potential and increasing the amplitude of the downward T wave; (*c*) the interference theory (i.e., the R and T waves are created by the temporal interference of two monophasic action potentials, one occurring under each electrode). [(*a*), (*b*), and (*c*) from J. S. Burdon-Sanderson and F. J. M. Page, *J. Physiol.* **4**:327–338 (1883).] (By permission)

538

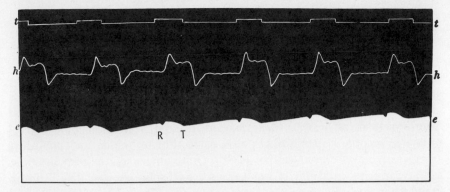

Figure 11-84. The first human electrocardiogram (*e–e*) recorded by Waller, employing the capillary electrometer. The recording above (*h–h*) is the apex cardiogram, which illustrates that the R wave precedes ventricular systole and the T wave precedes ventricular diastole. The R and T designations have been added by the authors for identification purposes. [From A. D. Waller, *J. Physiol.* **8**:229–234 (1887). By permission.]

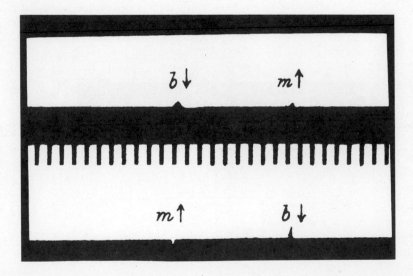

Figure 11-85. Nerve action potentials (upper) and stimulus (lower) recorded with the capillary electrometer. [From Gotch and Horsley, *Proc. Roy. Soc.* (*London*) **108B**:169–194 (1889). By permission.]

rheotome. For these reasons, and because better bioelectric recorders were soon to appear, there are few good records of muscle action potentials taken with the capillary electrometer. Although the records obtained by the capillary electrometer could be corrected to provide true voltage-time graphs, this unnecessary inconvenience, along with the erratic behavior of the electrometer, so infuriated Einthoven that he set himself to the task of developing a rapidly responding recording instrument. To show how the true waveform of the electrocardiogram differed from the capillary electrometer record, he applied his own correction technique and published comparative recordings (see Fig. 11-86). Quite obviously, the response time of the capillary electrometer was too long to display the fine details in the human electrocardiogram.

Einthoven used the telegraphic recorder of Ader (1897) as the starting point for his new recorder. The improvements he made consisted of using a strong electromagnet, rather than a permanent magnet as in the Ader instrument, and a silvered quartz filament, rather than a fine wire as used by Ader. Finally, Einthoven employed an optical system to allow

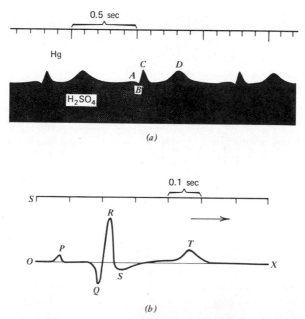

Figure 11-86. A capillary electrometer record (*a*) and its corrected version (*b*) presented by Einthoven to show the inadequacy of the electrometer in displaying rapidly changing waveforms. [From F. A. Willius and T. E. Keys, *Cardiac Classics*, C. V. Mosby Co., St. Louis, Mo., 1941.]

photographic recording of the sidewise motion of the quartz filament as the bioelectric currents traversed it. Figure 11-87a is Einthoven's (1903) sketch of his string galvanometer; Fig. 11-87b illustrates an electrocardiogram and the immersion electrodes used to obtain it. Contact with the subject was made by means of saline-filled buckets containing a metallic electrode. Figure 11-87b shows the connection for lead I (right arm–left arm). It was soon recognized that use of these bucket immersion electrodes meant that the patient had to get out of bed, a stressful procedure. To remove this requirement, plate electrodes and strong electrolytic pastes, containing abrasives, were soon developed. Parenthetically, it is interesting to note that Einthoven used the same chart speed as Marey (2.5 cm/sec) and many of the leads reported by Waller.

Although amplifier-type electrocardiographs with mirror galvanometers were demonstrated in the early 1930s[6], they did not gain popularity because of their excessively short time constants. Their records, when compared with those of the string galvanometer, consequently exhibited distortions having clinical implications. Introduction of the hot-stylus recorder by Haynes (1936) and its use with an amplifier having a long time constant resulted in the apppearance of practical direct-writing electrocardiographs; since 1945, these devices have displaced the Einthoven string galvanometer.

The electrical activity of the brain was first recorded by Caton (1875), who used a Thomson reflecting galvanometer (Fig. 11-79a, UK patent 329, dated 1858) connected to electrodes placed on the head of a rabbit. Caton's choice of this animal was fortuitous because the frequencies of the brain waves are low (less than 5 Hz) and they could be recorded adequately by Thomson's galvanometer, which was developed with a short response time to allow rapid recording of telegraphic signals. The galvanometer consisted of a tiny magnet (a piece of magnetized watch spring) that carried a mirror and was suspended in the center of a fixed coil to which the current was applied. Unfortunately, Caton's papers contain no electroencephalographic recordings.

It was not until 1929 that the first human electroencephalogram was recorded by Berger, who employed an Einthoven string galvanometer (Fig. 11-87a) connected to scalp electrodes. By the early 1940s electroencephalography had become a clinical tool, and from the beginning, multichannel ink-writing instruments were employed.

The need for a rapidly responding recorder for transient bioelectric events led Gasser and Erlanger (1922) to introduce physiologists to the

---

[6] See Pardee (1929-30), Ernstence and Levine (1928–1929), Caldwell et al. (1932), Mann (1931–1932), and D'Zuma (1931).

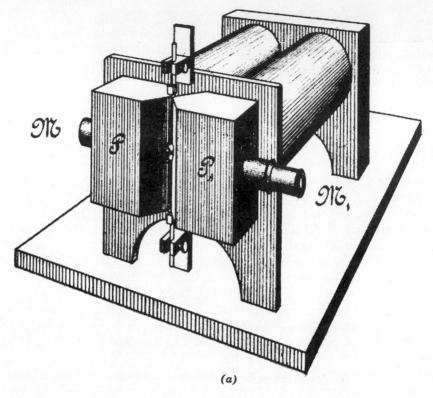

(a)

Figure 11-87. (*a*) Einthoven's string galvanometer. (*b*) Method of using the device with immersion electrodes to record lead I (right-left arm) electrocardiogram. [From W. Einthoven, *Arch. Int. Physiol.* **4**:132–164 (1906). By permission.]

Braun tube, one of the first cathode ray tubes. Their use of the cathode ray tube predated its use in electrical engineering. In their pioneering study Gasser and Erlanger built their own amplifiers and circuitry to operate the Braun tube, with which they obtained high-fidelity recordings of nerve action potentials.

Figure 11-88*a* illustrates the Gasser-Erlanger method for stimulating a nerve trunk and starting the sweep capacitor *C* charging, thereby causing the luminous spot (produced by the electron beam) to traverse the screen. The compound action potential (under electrode 1) was amplified by a vacuum tube amplifier and displayed as a vertical deflection on the screen. All electrical activity under electrode 2 was abolished by injury.

The type of record obtained by Gasser and Erlanger (see Fig. 11-88*b*) illustrates the various action potentials developed by the *A*, *B*, and *C* fibers

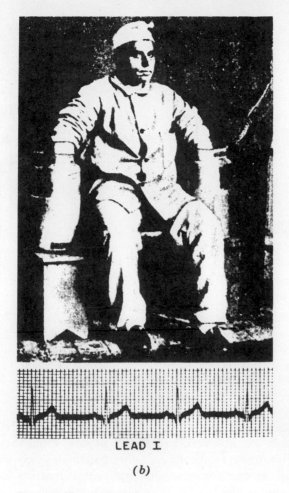

LEAD I

(b)

Figure 11-87   (Continued)

as their excitations arrived under electrode 1. From this Nobel Prize winning study, they showed that excitation is propagated with a velocity that is dependent on the diameter of the nerve fiber.

The other great study on the peripheral nervous system was carried out by Adrian without the benefit of the oscilloscope. In this definitive work, which established the "law of the nervous system," Adrian and his colleagues showed that intensity is signaled by the frequency of nerve impulses in a given nerve fiber and also by the number of nerve fibers active in communicating information. He also showed that in a single nerve fiber, all

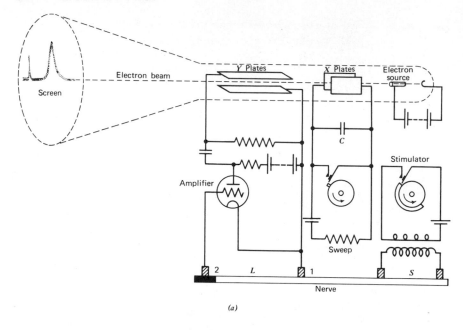

Electron beam

Screen

Y Plates

X Plates

Electron source

C

Amplifier

Stimulator

Sweep

2   L   1   S

Nerve

(a)

Figure 11-88. (*a*) Erlanger and Gasser's equipment; (*b*) recordings of the compound action potential of a nerve trunk, which showed that propagation velocity depends on nerve fiber diameter. (From J. Erlanger and H. S. Gasser, *Electrical Signs of Nervous Activity*, University of Pennsylvania Press, Philadelphia, 1973. By permission.)

action potentials are identical, irrespective of how often they occur. He made these discoveries by recording action potentials from single sensory nerve fibers as the receptor was stimulated with increasing intensity. The frequency of the action potentials was monitored with a capillary electrometer driven by a vacuum tube amplifier as in Fig. 11-89; the potentials were also monitored as clicks in headphones (P_1) or a loudspeaker (*LS*) connected to an amplifier (*B*). Adrian (1932) offered the following as the reason for his success: "The revolution in technique has come about, not from any increase in the sensitivity of galvanometers and electrometers, but from the use of amplifiers (like those employed in radio) to amplify potential changes."

The pioneering studies of Gasser and Erlanger and Adrian and his colleagues paved the way for the later investigations of Weddell et al. (1943, 1944), who developed the basic information on which clinical electromyography is based.

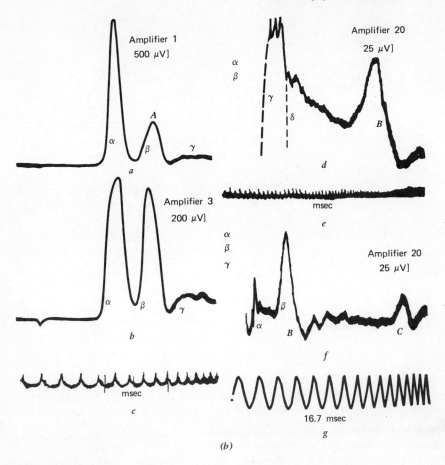

Figure 11-88   (Continued)

11-16.   EQUIPMENT STANDARDS

Despite successes in obtaining faithful records of many bioelectric events, only three have attained a prominent position in clinical medicine: the electrocardiogram, the electroencephalogram, and the electromyogram. Although these three events can be recorded with many different kinds of instruments, clinical use has imposed standards on techniques of recording and display. Such standards are necessary to guarantee not only that recordings made on a subject in one laboratory will be identical with those made on the same subject in another, but that all will be obtained with instruments known to be capable of faithful reproduction. In the United States minimum performance recommendations for many devices have

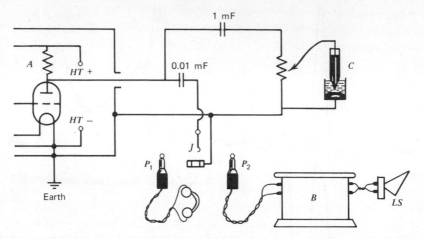

Figure 11-89. Amplifier (*A*) and capillary electrometer (*C*) used by Adrian to record the frequency of nerve action potentials. Aural monitoring was achieved by connecting headphones or a loudspeaker (*LS*) to the amplifier output via jack (*J*) and plugs P_1 and P_2, respectively. With this simple apparatus, Adrian discovered the fundamental law of the nervous system—namely, intensity is signaled by the frequency of nerve impulses. [From E. D. Adrian and D. W. Bronk, *J. Physiol.* **66**:81–101 (1928). By permission.]

been set by various professional societies in consultation with scientists who are considered to be leaders in their fields. These recommendations are usually published in reports of the Council on Physical Medicine of the American Medical Association in its journal and in the journals of the specialty societies. Those who want ECG, EEG, and EMG recordings to have clinical value and desire to make such records with instruments other than those which have been approved should check the specifications in these reports.

11-16-1.   Electrocardiography

For faithful reproduction of the ECG, minimum requirements have been set to guarantee the adequate low- and high-frequency responses and to standardize the speed of the recording chart and the sensitivity of the recording device. Such requirements have been reported by the Council on Physical Medicine of the AMA (1950) and the American Heart Association (1938, 1943); see also Wilson (1954) and the most recent report (1967) of the American Heart Association. Interestingly enough in all of these reports, the recommended chart speed is that which Einthoven used (25 mm/sec); it was derived from Marey's studies. The sensitivity (1 mV/cm) was adopted by Einthoven.

The most recent recommendations for the ECG, promulgated by the American Heart Association (1967), provide a tremendous amount of useful information and should be consulted for details. The following excerpts from this report are designed to provide the essential information for those who want to record the ECG faithfully using other than standard, commercially available electrocardiographs, virtually all of which now exceed these minimum performance recommendations.

"A. *Direct-Writing Electrocardiographs*

"1. System performance, linearity, and distortion. The deviation of the recorded output from an exact linear representation of the input signal shall not exceed 5% of the peak-to-peak output for amplitudes between 5 and 50 mm. For peak-to-peak amplitudes below 5 mm, this deviation shall not exceed 0.25 mm. The input signal may be comprised of frequency components between 0.05 and 100 Hz in any combination. For signals containing frequency components above 50 Hz, the peak-to-peak output amplitudes contributed by these components need be no greater than 5 mm to meet this performance requirement.

"2. Input range. The instrument shall meet specifications with input amplitudes up to 10 millivolts peak-to-peak and shall function accurately for any input signal and electrical or mechanical offset so long as the ideal response will require the writing point to remain on the ruled portion of the recording chart.

"3. Input impedance and current. In each position of the lead switch the magnitude of the input impedance over the working frequency range shall be no less than 500,000 ohms between any single patient electrode and ground. This measurement is to be made with all patient electrodes grounded except the one under consideration. The instrument shall not cause currents greater than 1.0 microampere to flow in the circuits to the patient. Because of offset potentials which may exist at the electrodes, the instrument shall be capable of meeting all specifications when differential offset voltages up to 100 millivolts and common mode offset voltages up to 200 millivolts are present.

"4. Central terminal. The magnitude of the deflections in all leads, including the augmented leads, referred to the central terminal, must not deviate from their correct values by more than an additional 2% from the allowable deviations specified in paragraph A1. [Original text includes a footnote referring to the use of 300,000-Ω resistors in the averaging network.]

"5. Gain. The gain is to be adjustable from the panel of the instrument in three clearly labeled fixed steps, having the following values:
10 mm per millivolt

5 mm per millivolt

20 mm per millivolt

Any continuous or vernier gain adjustment should be available as a restricted access control to be operated, for example, by screwdriver. Since the need to use this adjustment may often be caused by deterioration of the calibrating (standardizing) signal (par. A13), a note to this effect should be placed near this control.

"6.   Stability of gain and base line. To verify stability of gain and base line, the following test may be performed: Connect the right leg (RL) terminal, in each instance through a resistor of 20,000 ohms, to the terminals of the right arm (RA), the left arm (LA), the left leg (LL), and the chest.

"(a)   With the lead selector switch on Lead I and the sensitivity switch on 20 mm per millivolt, turn the machine on after it has not been used for at least 1 hour. After 3 minutes, center the trace. During the next 12 minutes the baseline should not drift more than 10 mm. During the following 45 minutes, the base line should not drift more than an additional 2 mm. After 1 hour, turn the lead selector switch through all positions. In each case the baseline level after the reset button has been pressed should not shift by more than 1 mm from its value in Lead I.

"(b)   With the lead selector switch on Lead I and the sensitivity switch on 20 mm per millivolt, turn the machine on after it has not been used at least 1 hour. After 3 minutes, center the baseline. Press the 1 millivolt calibration button. The deflection of approximately 20 mm should differ by less than 1 mm from the deflection measured after 1 hour.

"(c)   Turn the instrument off. Turn it on again 1 hour later. The deflection measured in the Lead I position after 1 hour's warm-up should differ by less than 0.5 mm from that measured in step b.

"7.   Overload. There shall be no damage to the instrument when it is subjected to 1.0 volt at any frequency from 47 to 63 Hz applied for 2 seconds to the input terminals with the controls set at any sensitivity or lead position.

"8.   Frequency response [Fig. 11-90]. In addition to the linearity and distortion requirements specified in paragraph A1, the following design characteristics are acceptable with constant amplitude sinusoidal input signals:

"(a)   From 0.14 to 50 Hz, the response shall be flat to within $\pm 6\%$ (+0.5 dB). The response down to 0.05 Hz shall not be reduced by more than 30% (-3 dB) from the response at 0.14 Hz. This requirement corresponds to a "time constant" of at least 3.2 seconds, where ""time constant" refers to the time required for a direct current step input (such as the calibration voltage) to decay to 36.8% of its original magnitude.

"(b)   With an amplitude response of 5 mm peak to peak at 50 Hz, the

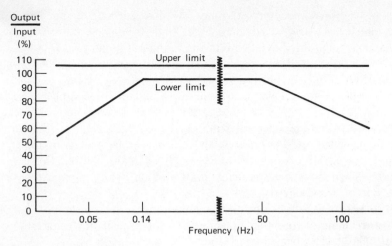

Figure 11-90. Recommended minimum frequency response of direct-writing electrocardiographs; response of recorder is between upper and lower limits, as indicated. [From Recommendations for Standardizations of Leads as Specifications for Instruments in Electrocardiography and Vectorcardiographics, *Circulation* **35**:583–602 (1967). By permission.]

response to constant amplitude sinusoidal input signals up to 100 Hz shall not be reduced by more than 30% (-3 dB), leaving an amplitude of at least 3.5 mm at 100 Hz.

"(c)   The response shall at no frequency exceed the restraints specified for the range of 0.14 to 50 Hz.

"9.   Common mode rejection. For each position of the lead switch with the recorder gain set at 10 mm per millivolt, and with all active electrode leads connected together, a potential difference of 100 millivolts peak-to-peak applied between them and the right leg lead shall cause no more than 1.0 mm peak-to-peak deflection for frequencies from 45 to 65 Hz. In a like manner the application of 10 millivolts shall cause no more than 1.0 mm peak-to-peak deflection at any frequency. This specification must be met when a resistance of 5,000 ohms is placed in series with any one electrode lead.

These requirements correspond to a common mode rejection of 1,000:1 at frequencies between 45 and 65 Hz, and 100:1 at any other frequency.

"10.   Noise level. Upon simulating a subject by means of completely shielded resistors of 25,000 ohms placed between each patient lead and ground, the output noise, with the recorder calibrated to 10 mm per millivolt shall not exceed the equivalent of 0.1 mm root mean square in any position of the lead switch (10 microvolts root mean square referred to the input).

"11.   Radio frequency interference. Manufacturers are urged to minimize interference from radio and other high frequencies through proper design of circuits, shielding, and filtering in the power supply.

"12.   Grounding. Line-operated electrocardiographs shall be supplied with a three-terminal, powerline plug. The existence of multiple connections between a subject and a line-operated electrocardiograph creates the potential hazard of uncomfortable or even lethal electric shock. Protection of the patient and the operator from currents greater than 5 milliamperes must be provided by fuses or circuitry to furnish equal protection under any of the following circumstances present singly or in any combination:

"(a)   When the subject is inadvertently or purposely grounded by connection to a second device.

"(b)   When defective or frayed insulation of the power cord of any transformer, motor, or other line-operated component may make the case containing the electrocardiograph "hot."

"(c)   When an incorrectly wired, three-wire receptacle is used to energize the electrocardiograph.

"(d)   When an internal short circuit or component failure may occur in the amplifier connected to the patient.

"(e)   When the subject may be wired directly to the instrument case.

Since satisfactory recording in electrically noisy locations may be possible only by connecting the instrument directly to a ground more suitable than can be obtained through the power-line plug, provision for this alternate mode of operation must be made. With or without such a connection, leakage of current back to the power-line ground or to the auxiliary ground for either polarity of the power line, must be less than 50 microamperes.

Currents considerably less than 5 milliamperes in magnitude may cause ventricular fibrillation in a patient when a saline-filled catheter or other externally accessible, artificial conducting connection to the heart is present. The user must be warned of the potential hazard of a line-operated or battery-operated electrocardiograph under these special circumstances since the protection against electrical shock ordinarily afforded by the instrument may be inadequate.

"13.   Calibration ("standardization"). The standardizing voltage shall be a signal of 1.0 millivolt $\pm 2\%$ with a time constant no less than 100 seconds and an output impedance of 1,000 ohms or less, which can be applied continuously to the inputs by a switch on the panel of the instrument. When a multichannel recorder is used, means shall be provided for the simultaneous application of the calibration signal to all channels. The instrument shall be capable of recording this standardizing voltage as follows:

"(a)   Superimposed in series while recording the electrocardiogram from any lead position, and

"(b)   With the patient disconnected from the instrument.

In addition, the standardizing signal shall be available through a suitable connector to provide for checking of its accuracy.

If a battery is used for obtaining the standardizing voltage, the instrument shall be provided with an indicator (a push-to-test control is suggested) to alert the user when the battery needs replacement; for example, battery is no longer capable of supplying the standardizing voltage to the required accuracy.

"14.   Speed and speed accuracy. A minimum of 2 speeds, 25 mm per second and 50 mm per second, shall be available. Accuracy of speed shall be $\pm 2\%$ when operating from a 60-cycle source.* Time markings at intervals of 1 second $\pm 2\%$ shall be recorded at all speeds at an edge of the time rulings of the recording paper by a device operating independently of the transport mechanism of the recorder.

"15.   Recording paper. The recording paper shall be ruled with 1.0 mm divisions along both the time and voltage axes. Every fifth division shall be ruled darker than the others. The 1.0 mm divisions shall not deviate by more than $\pm 1\%$ from 1.0 mm in either axis. The ruled divisions shall cover a total of 5 cm in width, and recordings shall be rectilinear. These dimensional accuracies shall be met throughout a temperature range from 10°C to 50°C and for relative humidities from 10 to 80%.

"16.   Skew

"(a)   Skew of recording, due to all causes, shall not exceed 0.1 mm of horizontal displacement per 1.0 cm of vertical deflection.

"(b)   In multichannel recording, it is especially important to ensure temporal alignment of traces. Therefore, with the amplifiers for each channel set to the same frequency response limits, all traces shall fall dynamically within a 0.5 mm band of the ideal (zero skew) response at all transport speeds for the entire frequency range of the instrument.

"17.   Recorded output. The vertical width of the undeflected trace shall not exceed 1.0 mm at any paper transport speed. Both the upstroke and downstroke of the writing device at rates of deflection less than 1,000 mm per second shall leave a visible, continuous trace with sharp edges.

"18.   Auxiliary output. A jack shall be available for gaining access to the output. The signal at this jack shall have a driving capability of at least

---

* Accuracy requirements of $\pm 2\%$ have been specified to permit use of synchronous timing devices and synchronously operated paper transports. If such devices are used, they will be unable to meet the accuracy requirement when the line frequency deviates appreciably from 60 cycles; therefore, a note to this effect should be placed on the instrument.

1.0 milliampere for loads of 1,000 ohms or more at ±1.0 volt, full scale. The output impedance shall be less than 100 ohms. The output characteristics shall be the same as specified herein except that the frequency response shall extend to at least 1,000 Hz (1 dB down). This output shall have a dc offset voltage no greater than ±1 volt, which can be centered at zero volts. No damage shall occur to the instrument when the output is short circuited. Upon removal of the short circuit, the instrument shall be capable of meeting specifications.

"19.   Trace reset. A capability for trace reset must be provided by a switch or button on the instrument. After a pulse of 10 millivolts has been applied to the input for 10 seconds at a gain of 20 mm per millivolt, depressing this button shall cause the trace to return to within 1 mm of its initial position within 0.5 second. Releasing the button after it has been depressed for not more than 0.5 second shall result in no more than 1 mm of additional displacement.

"20.   Powerline variations. For instruments operating at 60 Hz and 120 volts, all specifications shall be met when used in the range of powerline voltages from 95 to 135 volts and frequencies from 57 to 63 Hz. A disturbance of ±5 volts in the power line should not cause a deflection greater than that which would be obtained with an input signal of ±50 microvolts. For battery-powered instruments, an indicator shall be provided to alert the operator when the batteries need replacement or recharging.

"21.   Temperature and altitude. The instrument shall meet all specifications over the temperature range of 10°C to 50°C, at altitudes from 0 to 3,000 meters above sea level, and at relative humidities of 5% to 95%.

"22.   Electrode impedance. It is desirable that any paste or jelly and electrode combination which is used results in a skin-to-electrode impedance of 5,000 ohms or less, measured at 60 Hz with currents not exceeding 100 microamperes.*

"23.   Standardization of controls, cables, legends, and recording format. Electrocardiographs meeting this specification shall be equipped with the following controls labeled as shown in quotation marks.

| "Paper Speed" | Two-position switch | "25 mm/s" |
| | | "50 mm/s" |

* Electrodes of small size such as used in pediatric practice, inadequate preparation of the skin, or poor quality electrode paste may lead to considerably higher skin-to-electrode impedances, particularly at lower frequencies. Resulting signal distortions may be reduced to acceptable levels by use of other than conventional input circuitry, e.g. buffer amplifiers for each active electrode.

"On-Off"	Two-position switch	(Light or flag indicating equipment is on.)
"1 mV"	Push button	
"Lead"	Multiposition switch	"0," "I," "II," "III," "aV$_R$," "aV$_L$," "aV$_F$," "V"
"Center"	Potentiometer	
"Reset"	Push button or switch	
"Gain vernier"	This potentiometer shall be a recessed control behind a hinged plate.	
"Sensitivity"	Three-position switch	"5 mm/mV," "10 mm/mV." "20 mm/mV"

The following cable legends and colors shall be used:

"RA"	Right arm	white
"LA"	Left arm	black
"LL"	Left leg	red
"RL"	Right leg	green
"C"	Chest	brown

11-16-2.   Electroencephalography

In 1948 the Council on Physical Medicine of the AMA reported on the minimum requirements for acceptable direct-reading electroencephalographs. The report was based on earlier recommendations of the American EEG Society. More recently, international agreement on minimum performance standards has been reached, and in 1956, the International Federation of EEG Societies drew up a set of recommendations for EEG equipment. It was not their intent to create rigid standards; rather, in their own words, "Users as well as manufacturers of electroencephalographs may take these recommendations as being a collection of opinions of what is desired in such apparatus." Under the chairmanship of Knott, the committee report (1958) described many features of EEG machines in detail. From this report the following high-priority requirements have been selected to inform those who wish to obtain EEG recordings of clinical significance with other than EEG equipment.

"1. Linearity, Deflection of Pens. The maximal deflection of the pen should be at least 2 cm., peak to peak, with a linearity of 10 per cent of applied signal, or 0.25 mm., whichever is larger, at all frequencies from 1 to 60 cycles per second.

"2. Amplification

"(a) At maximum gain, 1.0 μV input should give not less than 1 mm deflection, over the full range of working frequencies.

"(b) The ratio between maximum deflection proportional to the input voltage, and the minimum visible deflection, should not be less than 40 to 1, at all frequencies from 1 to 60 cycles per second.

"(c) The total maximum attenuation should be not less than 1,000 to 1. A step attenuator, with steps of not more than one-half, should be provided; and there should be a variable equalizing control capable of equalizing within 5 percent.

"(d) It is desirable that a "Master" gain control be provided.

"3. Frequency Response

"(a) Between the limits of 1 and 65 cycles per second, the amplitude response should be plus or minus 10 percent, or 0.25 mm, whichever is larger. If the response extends beyond 60 cycles per second, then the amplitude should not increase by more than 20 percent of the response at 60 cycles per second.

"(b) The longest time constant (time taken for a step function of input to fall to 37 percent of initial deflection) should be at least 0.3 second.

"(c) Appropriate means for separately adjusting the high and low frequency response within the working range should be provided.

"(d) There may be need for extending the upper and lower frequency limits of equipment: such extension by manufacturers should be encouraged.

"(e) The manufacturer should make clear to the user that the overall phase shift will vary with the choice of time constant. Figures for the total phase change in the complete system (amplifiers and pens) should be supplied. With identical time constants there should be no visible differences in the phase shifts between channels.

"4. Coupling of Controls. The operation of any one control should not alter the effective setting of any other control by more than 5 per cent.

"5. Noise Level. With the inputs connected through 5000 ohms, and the controls set to give a full-scale deflection with 10 μV, and frequency response set as at 2 (a), no intermittent or transient deflections greater than 4 μV should appear more often than, on the average, once per minute and none greater than 2 μV once per second.

"6. Discrimination. With the input terminals connected together, a sine wave input, over the frequency range of 1 to 60 cycles per second applied between them and ground, should not produce a deflection greater than that produced by a signal of one-thousandth of the former potential, applied between the input terminals. This should be preserved with a 10,000 ohm resistance inserted in one input lead, to allow for asymmetry of electrode resistance.

"7. Relationships between Channels

"(a) Interchannel coupling. With controls on all channels set for equal amplitude outputs, an input to any one channel should not produce a deflection in any other channel greater than 1 percent of that produced in the first, with the input terminals of the other channels connected through 10,000 ohms to ground.

"(b) Similarity between channels. When all step controls are equally set and amplification in each channel is the same, an EEG signal applied to the inputs of all channels should give outputs which appear identical.

"8. Recorder

"(a) The paper should travel from right to left and should be visible for 60 cm to the left of the recording pen.

"(b) The speed of the paper mechanism should include 30 mm per second (plus or minus 2 percent), with 15 mm and 60 mm per second selectable during operation.

"(c) Where means are provided for registering the vertical alignment of the pens, this should be possible without the use of special tools or without the need for bending the writer arms.

"(d) A time marker might be desirable, and if provided should be independent of the paper drive mechanism itself.

"(e) At zero deflection, the writing points of the recorders should line up perpendicularly within plus or minus 0.5 mm.

"(f) The arc distortion of the recording pens should be not more than that produced by a pen 10 cm long.

"(g) The distance between adjacent recording pens should be such that the deflection of paragraph A-1 can be obtained without mechanical interference between them.

11-16-3. Electromyography

There appear to be no universally adopted minimum requirements for acceptable electromyographs, although there is considerable agreement on the need for such standards.[7] At the 1954 meeting of the Committee on

[7] See Lambert (1954), in Committee on Instrumentation and Techniques. For practical reasons the overall frequency response in clinical instruments may be less than that required to guarantee faithful reproduction of the EMG. Buchtal et al. (1954) reported that an overall frequency response extending from 2 to 10,000 Hz was necessary.

Instrumentation and Technique of the American Association for Electromyography and Electrodiagnosis, there was composed a document entitled "Information Concerning the Formulation of Minimal Requirements for Electromyographs for Clinical Use." This document listed several specifications that probably reflected the characteristics of good-quality electromyographs of that time.

The committee recognized the difficulty in setting up standards in a new field in which techniques were varied. Nonetheless it recommended that when needle electrodes were employed, the following criteria were to be satisfied. The maximum overall recording sensitivity should be 5 microvolts per millimeter of deflection of the indicating device. Recognizing that, although a frequency response uniform over the range of 2 to 10,000 Hz would be ideal, difficulties encountered during the taking of routine EMGs dictated that a somewhat narrower frequency response would be adequate. The Committee stated:

"3(a)   The overall frequency response of the system shall be such that between 40 and 3000 cps the deflections at all frequencies shall be within 10 percent of the average of the maximal and minimal deflections within this range.

"3(b)   Overall time constant (RC) should be not less than 5 milliseconds. This implies a square wave response which declines to 0.37 of its peak value in 0.005 second."

The Committee recognized the importance of a high input impedance in view of the small-area needle electrodes ordinarily used. It therefore recommended as follows:

"8.   The impedance between each input lead and the ground connection of the preamplifier, without the input cable, shall be at least 500,000 ohms in parallel with not more than 25 $\mu\mu$F[pF]. The input cable shall not add more than 250 $\mu\mu$F. These values are minimal requirements for use with needle electrodes having an exposed tip of not less than 0.1 millimeter in diameter; for needles having a smaller tip area and a relatively high impedance, the input impedance of the preamplifier should be greater. Microelectrodes require a cathode follower input for undistorted recording."

Because the EMG signals are low in amplitude a differential input stage is required to provide the necessary amplification. In recognition of this fact, the committee recommended that a high discrimination ratio (common mode rejection ratio) be provided:

"7.   Discrimination ratio refers to the ratio of the deflection produced by a signal applied between the two input terminals to that produced by the

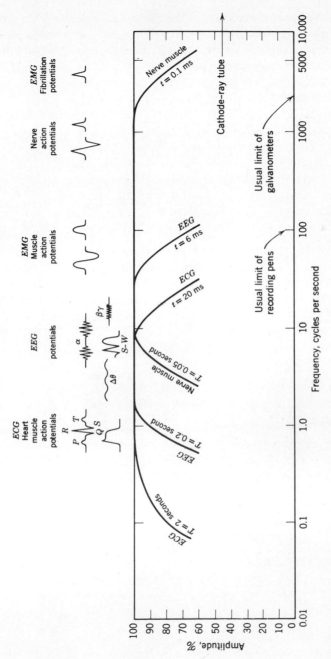

Figure 11-91. Frequency spectrum and waveforms of clinically recorded bioelectric events.

557

same signal applied between ground and the two input terminals connected together. The discrimination ratio of the instrument shall be at least 2000 to 1. A greater ratio is desirable, particularly when the instrument is recommended for use in unshielded rooms."

11-16-4. Conclusion

To provide the reader with a perspective of the three bioelectric phenomena now recorded clinically, Fig. 11-91 has been composed as a means of presenting frequency-response data and techniques for recording and display.

There is no doubt that in the near future, governmental regulations will be promulgated which relate to the safety and minimum performance standards for the bioelectric recording instruments that have proven clinical usefulness. It may even be possible to achieve international agreement in minimum performance requirements for instruments for specifically designated tasks. Although the highest fidelity is always requested, the reader should recognize that fidelity and cost are closely interrelated. The real difficulty in specifying the degree of fidelity centers around quantitating the amount of clinically useful information that is lost by a progressive reduction in fidelity.

REFERENCES

Abildskov, J. A., and E. D. Pence. 1956. Comparative study of spatial vectorcardiograms with the equilateral tetrahedron and a corrected system of electrode placement. *Circulation* **13**:263–269.

Ader, M. 1897. Sur un nouvel appareil enregistreur pour cables sous-marins. *Comptes Rendus* **124**:1440–1442.

Adrian, E. D. 1967. See *Nobel Prize Winners in Medicine and Physiology (1901–1965)* T. L. Sourkes (ed.) Abelard-Schuman, London.

Adrian, E. D. 1945. The electric response of the human eye. *J. Physiol.* **104**:84–104.

Adrian, E. D., and D. W. Bronk. 1928. The discharge of impulses in motor nerve fibers. Part 1. *J. Physiol.* **66**:81–101.

Adrian, E. D., and B. H. C. Matthews. 1934. The Berger rhythm: Potential changes from the occipital lobes in man. *Brain* **57**:355–385.

American Heart Association. 1938. Joint Recommendations of the American Heart Association and the Cardiac Society of Great Britain and Ireland. Standardization of the precordial leads. *Am. Heart J.* **15**:107–108.

American Heart Association. 1943. Committee for the Standardization of precordial leads. *JAMA* **121**:1349.

American Heart Association. 1967. Report of Committee on Electrocardiography. Recommendations for standardization of leads and specifications for instruments in electrocardiography and vectorcardiography. *Circulation* **35**:583–602.

Arden, G. B., A. Barrada, and J. H. Kelsey. 1962. New clinical test of retinal function based upon standing potential of the eye. *Brit. J. Ophthalmol.* **46**:449–467.

Arden, G. B., and J. H. Kelsey. 1962. Some observations on the relationship between the standing potential of the human eye and the bleaching and regeneration of visual purple. *J. Physiol.* **161**:205–226.

Arrighi, F. P. 1939. El eje electrico del corazon en el espacio. *Prensa Med. Arg.* **26**:253–283.

Baule, G. M. 1965. Instrumentation for measuring the heart's magnetic field. *Trans. N.Y. Acad. Sci.* **27**:689–700.

Baule, G., and R. McPhee. 1963. Detection of the magnetic field of the heart. *Am. Heart J.* **66**:95–96.

Baule, G., and R. McPhee. 1970. The magnetic heart vector. *Am. Heart J.* **79**:223–236.

Becking, A. G. T., H. C. Burger, and J. B. van Milaan. 1950. A universal vector cardiograph. *Brit. Heart J.* **12**:339–342.

Bennett, A. L., F. Ware, A. L. Dunn, and A. R. McIntyre. 1953. The normal membrane resting potential of mammalian skeletal muscle measured *in vivo. J. Cell. Comp. Physiol.* **42**:343–357.

Berger, H. 1929. Über das Elektronkephalogramn des Menschen. *Arch. Psychiat. Nervenkr.* **87**:527–570.

Berger, H. 1967. On the electroencephalogram of man. (trans. by P. Gloor). *EEG Clin. Neurophysiol.* **Suppl. 28**:1–350.

Bernstein, J. 1868. Über den zeitlichen Verlauf der negativen Schwankung des Nervenstroms. *Arch. Ges. Physiol.* **1**:173–207.

Bickford, R. G. 1950. Automatic electroencephalographic control of general anesthesia. *EEG Clin. Neurophysiol.* **2**:93–96.

Bickford, R. G., T. W., Billinger, N. I. Fleming, and L. Stewart. 1972. The compressed spectral array (CSA)—A pictorial EEG. *Proc. 1972 San Diego Biomed. Symp.*

Brazier, M. A. B. 1949. A study of the electric fields at the surface of the head. *EEG Clin. Neurophysiol. Suppl.* **2**:38–52.

Brechner, V. L., R. D. Walter, and J. B. Dillon. 1962. *Practical Electroencephalography for the Anesthesiologist.* Charles C. Thomas, Springfield, Ill., 107 pp.

Briller, S. A., N. Marchand, and C. E. Kossman. 1950. A differential vectorcardiograph. *Rev. Sci. Instr.* **21**:805–811.

Brody, D. A. 1957. An analysis of the plane and spatial electrocardiographic indices of normal subjects as referred to an orthogonalized lead system. *Am. Heart J.* **53**:125–131.

Brody, D. A., J. C. Bradshaw, and J. W. Evans. 1961. A basis for determining heart lead relations of the equivalent cardiac multipole. *IRE Trans. Bio-Med. Electron.* **BME-8**:139–143.

Buchtal, F., C. Guld, and P. Rosenflack. 1954. Action potential parameters in normal human muscle and their dependence on physical variables. *Acta Physiol. Scand.* **32**:200–229.

Burch, G. J. 1892. On the time-relations of the excursions of the capillary electrometer, with a description of the method of using it for the investigations of electrical changes. *Phil. Trans. Roy. Soc. London,* **183**:81–106.

Burch, G., J. A. Abildskov, and J. A. Cronvitch. 1953. *Spatial Vectorcardiography.* Lea and Febiger, Philadelphia, 173 pp.

Burdon-Sanderson, J., and F. J. M. Page. 1878. Experimental results relating to the rhythmical and excitatory motions of the ventricle of the heart of the frog and the electrical phenomena which accompany them. *Proc. Roy. Soc. (London)* **27**:410.

Burdon-Sanderson, J., and F. J. M. Page. 1879. On the time relations of the excitatory process in the ventricle of the heart of the frog. *J. Physiol.* **2**:384–435.

Burger, H. C., and J. B. van Milaan. 1946. Heart vector and leads. *Brit. Heart J.* **8**:157–161.

Burger, H. C., and J. B. van Milaan. 1947. Heart vector and leads. Part II. *Brit. Heart J.* **9**:154–160.

Burger, H. C., J. B. van Milaan, and W. Klip. 1956. Comparison of two systems of vectorcardiography with an electrode to the frontal and dorsal sides of the trunk respectively. *Am. Heart J.* **51**:26–33.

Byford, G. H. 1963. Non-linear relations between the corneo-retinal potential and horizontal eye movements. *J. Physiol.* **168**:14P–15P.

Caldwell, S. H., C. B. Oler, and J. C. Peters. 1932. An improved form of electrocardiograph. *Rev. Sci. Instr.* **3**:277–286.

Caton, R. 1875. The electric currents of the brain. *Brit. Med. J.* **2**:278.

Caton, R. 1887. Researches on the electrical phenomena of cerebral gray matter. *Trans. IX Internat. Med. Congr.* **3**:247–249.

Clark, J., and R. Plonsey. 1966. A mathematical evaluation of the core conductor model. *Biophys. J.* **6**:95–112.

Clark, J., and R. Plonsey. 1968. The extracellular potential field of the single active nerve fiber in a volume conductor. *Biophys. J.* **8**:842–864.

Cohen, D. 1967a. A shielded facility for low-level magnetic measurements. *J. Appl. Phys.* **38**:1295–1296.

Cohen, D. 1967b. Magnetic fields around the torso: production by electrical activity of the human heart. *Science* **156**:652–654.

Cohen, D. 1968. Magnetoencephalography: Evidence of magnetic fields produced by alpha-rhythm currents. *Science* **161**:764–786.

Cohen, D. 1972. Magnetoencephalography. *Science* **175**:664–666.

Cohen, D., and L. Chandler. 1969. Measurements and a simplified interpretation of magnetocardiograms from humans. *Circulation* **39**:395–402.

Cohen, D., and D. McCaughan. 1972. Magnetocardiograms and their variation over the chest in normal subjects. *Am. J. Cardiol.* **29**:678–685.

Cohen, D., J. C. Normann, F. Molokhia, and W. Hood. 1971. Magnetocardiography of direct currents: S-T segment and baseline shifts during experimental myocardial infarction. *Science* **172**:1329–1332.

Cohn, R. 1949. *Clinical Electroencephalography.* McGraw-Hill, New York, 639 pp.

Cole, K. S. 1933. Electrical conductance of biological systems. *Cold Spring Harbor Symp. Quant. Biol.* **1**:107–116.

Committee on Electrocardiography. 1954. American Heart Association. Recommendations for standardization of electrocardiographic and vectorcardiographic leads. *Circulation* **10**:564–573.

Committee on Instrumentation and Technique of the American Association for Electromyography and Electrodiagnosis. 1954. Chairman E. H. Lambert. 11 pp. (Personal communication.)

Coombs, J. S., J. C. Eccles, and P. Fatt. 1955. The electrical properties of the motoneurone membrane. *J. Physiol.* **130**:291–325.

Council on Physical Medicine. 1948. Tentative minimum requirements for acceptable direct reading electroencephalographs. *JAMA* **138**:958–959.

Council on Physical Medicine and Rehabilitation. 1950. Minimum requirements for acceptable electrocardiographs. *JAMA* **143**:654–655.

Craib, W. H. 1927. A study of the electrical field surrounding active heart muscle. *Heart* **14**:71–109.

Darrow, C. W. 1934. Quantitative records of cutaneous secretory reactions. The significance of skin resistances in the light of its relation to the amount of perspiration. *J. Gen. Psychol.* **11**:435.

Darrow, C. W. 1964. The rationale for treating the change in galvanic skin resistance response as a change in conductance. *Psychophysiol.* **1**:31–38.

Denny-Brown, D. 1949. Interpretation of the electromyogram. *Arch. Neurol. Psychiat.* **61**:99–128.

Dewar, J. 1877. The physiological action of light. *Nature* **15**:433–435.

Dewar, J., and J. G. M'Kendrick. 1876. On the physiological action of light. *Trans. Roy. Soc. Edin.* **27**:141–166.

Donders, F. C. 1872. De secondaire contracties onder den involed der systolen van het hart, met en zonder vagus-prikkfung. *Utrecht Rijksuniv. Phys. Lab. Onder Zoekinjen,* **1**, Suppl. 3:246–255.

Dower, G. E., H. E. Horn, and W. G. Ziegler. 1965. The polarcardiograph. *Am. Heart J.* **69**:355–381.

Doyle, O. 1971. Josephson junctions leave the lab—But only a few at a time. *Electronics* **44**:38–45.

Draper, M. H., and S. Wiedmann. 1951. Cardiac resting and action potentials recorded with an intracellular electrode. *J. Physiol.* **115**:74–94.

du Bois-Reymond, E. 1843. Vorläufiger Abriss einer Untersuchung über dem sogenannten Froschstrom und über die electromotorische Fische. *Ann. Phys. Chem.* **58**:1–30.

du Bois-Reymond, E. R. 1849. Untersuchungen über Thierische Electrizität. G. Reimer, Berlin.

du Bois-Reymond, E. 1849. Intelligence and misc. articles (translation of duBois-Reymond's article). Deflection of the magnetic needle by volition. *Phil. Mag.* **34**:543–545.

Duchosal, P., and J. R. Grosgurin. 1952. The spatial vectorcardiogram obtained by use of a trihedron and its scalar comparisons. *Circulation* **5**:237–248.

Duchosal, P. W., and R. Sulzer. 1949. *La Vectorcardiographie.* Karger, Basle, Switzerland, and New York, 172 pp.

Durnstock, G., M. E. Holman, and C. L. Prosser. 1963. Electrophysiology of smooth muscle. *Physiol. Rev.* **43**:482–528.

D'Zuma, A. P. 1931. A new electrocardiograph. *JAMA* **96**:439–440.

Eccles, R. M. 1955. Intracellular potentials recorded from a mammalian sympathetic ganglion. *J. Physiol.* **130**:572–584.

Edelberg, R. 1967. In *Methods in Psychophysiology.* C. Brown (ed.). Williams & Wilkins Co., Baltimore.

Edelberg, R. 1968. Biopotentials from the skin surface: The hydration effect. *Ann. N.Y. Acad. Sci.* **148**:252–262.

Edelberg, R. 1972. Electrical activity of the skin. In *Handbook of Psychophysiology*. N. S. Greenfield, and R. D. Sternback (eds.). Holt, Rinehart & Winston, New York.

Edelberg, R. 1974. Personal communication.

Edelberg, R., and N. R. Burch. 1962. Skin resistance and galvanic skin response. *Arch. Gen. Psychiat.* 7:163–169.

Edelberg, R., T. Greiner, and N. R. Burch. 1960. Some membrane properties of the effector in the galvanic skin response. *J. Appl. Physiol.* 15:691–696.

Einthoven, W. 1903. Ein neues Galvanometer. *Ann. Phys.* 12, Suppl. 4:1059–1071.

Einthoven, W., G. Fahr, and A. deWaart. 1913. Über die Richtung und die manifeste Grosse der Potentialschwankungen in menschlichen Herzen und über den Einfluss der Herzlage auf die Form des Elektrokardiogramms. *Pfluger's Arch.* 150:275–315.

Einthoven, W. G. Fahr, and A. de Waart. 1950. On the direction and manifest size of the variations of potential in the human heart and on the influence of the position of the heart on the form of the electrocardiogram. Translated by H. E. Hoff, and P. Sekelj, *Am. Heart J.* 40:163–211.

Einthoven, W., and W. A. Jolly. 1908. The form and magnitude of the electrical response of the eye to stimulation by light at various intensities. *Quart. J. Exp. Physiol.* 1:373–416.

Englemann, T. W. 1878. Über das electrische Verhalten des thätigen Herzens. *Arch. Ges. Physiol.* 17:68.

Ernstence, A. E., and S. A. Levine. 1928–1929. A comparison of records taken with the Einthoven string galvanometer and the amplifier type electrocardiograph. *Am. Heart J.* 4:725–731.

Faulconer, A., and R. G. Bickford. 1960. *Electroencephalography in Anesthesiology*. Charles C. Thomas, Springfield, Ill., 90 pp.

Fenn, W. O. and J. B. Hursh. 1937. Movements of the eyes when the lids are closed. *Am. J. Physiol.* 118:8–14.

Féré, C. 1888. Note sur des modifications de la résistance électrique sous l'influence des excitations sensorielles et des émotions. *C. R. Soc. Biol.* 40:217–218.

Flaherty, J. T., M. S. Spach, J. P. Bonneau, R. V. Canent, R. C. Barr, and D. C. Sabiston. 1967. Cardiac potentials on body surface of infants with anomalous left coronary artery (myocardial infarction). *Circulation* 36:345–358.

Forbes, T. W. 1936. Skin potential and impedance responses with recurring shock stimulation. *Am. J. Physiol.* 117:189–199.

Fowles, D. C., and P. H. Venables. 1970. The reduction of palmar skin potential by epidermal hydration. *Psychophysiology* 7:254–261.

Frank, E. 1953a. Theoretical analysis of the influence of heart dipole eccentricity on limb leads, Wilson central-terminal voltage and the frontal plane vectorcardiogram. *Circ. Res.* 1:380–388.

Frank, E. 1953b. A comparative analysis of the eccentric double-layer presentaton of the human heart. *Am. Heart J.* 46:364–378.

Frank, E. 1954. A direct experimental study of three systems of spatial vectorcardiography *Circulation* 10:101–113.

Frank, E. 1955. Absolute quantitative comparison of instantaneous QRS equipotentials on a normal subject with dipole potentials on a homogeneous torso model. *Circ. Res.* 3:243–251.

Frank, E. 1956. An accurate, clinically practical system for spatial vectorcardiography. *Circulation* **13**:737–749.

Frank, E. 1956–1957. Spread of current in volume conductors of finite extent. *Ann. N.Y. Acad. Sci.* **65**:980–1002.

Freygang, W. H., and K. Frank. 1959. Extracellular potentials from single spinal motoneurones. *J. Gen. Physiol.* **42**:749–759.

Fulton, J. F., and H. Cushing. 1936. A bibliographical study of the Galvani and the Aldini writings on animal electricity. *Ann. Sci.* **1**:239–268.

Gasser, H. S., and J. Erlanger. 1922. A study of action currents of nerve with the cathode ray oscillograph. *Am. J. Physiol.* **62**:496–524.

Geddes, L. A., J. D. Bourland, R. W. Smalling, and R. B. Steinberg. 1974. Recording skin resistance and beat-by-beat heart rate from the same pair of dry electrodes. *Psychophysiology.* **11**:394–397.

Geddes, L. A., J. D. Bourland, G. Wise, and R. Steinberg. 1973. Linearity of the horizontal component of the electro-oculogram. *Med. Biol. Eng.* **11**(1):73–77.

Geddes, L. A., and H. E. Hoff. 1961. The capillary electrometer. *Arch. Internat. Hist. Sci.* **56–57**:275–290.

Geddes, L. A., and H. E. Hoff. 1971. The discovery of bioelectricity and current electricity (the Galvani-Volta controversy). *IEEE Spectrum* **8**(12):38–46.

Geddes, L. A., M. Partridge, and H. E. Hoff. 1960. An EKG lead for exercising subjects. *J. Appl. Physiol.* **15**:311–312.

Geselowitz, D. B. 1960. Multipole representation for an equivalent cardiac generator. *Proc. IRE* **48**:75–79.

Geselowitz, D. B. 1966. Comment on the core conductor model. *Biophys. J.* **6**:691–692.

Gibbs, F. A., and E. L. Gibbs. 1950, and 1964. *Atlas of Electroencephalography.* Wesley Press, Cambridge, Mass., 3 vols.

Gloor, P. 1967. Trans. of Berger's papers. *EEG. Clin. Neurophysiol.* **Suppl. 28**:1–350.

Gloor, P. 1969. Hans Berger; on the electroencephalogram of man. *EEG Clin. Neurophysiol. Suppl. 28.*

Goldberger, E. 1953. *Unipolar Lead Electrocardiography and Vectorcardiography.* Lea and Febiger, Philadelphia, 601 pp.

Granit, R. 1962. Neurophysiology of the retina. In *The Eye*, vol. 2. H. Davson (ed.). Academic Press, New York.

Grant, R. P. 1957. *Clinical Electrocardiography—The Spatial Vector Approach.* McGraw-Hill, New York, 225 pp.

Grant, R. P., and E. H. Estes. 1951. *Spatial Vector Electrocardiography.* Blakiston Co., Philadelphia, 145 pp.

Grishman, A. 1952. *Spatial Vectorcardiography.* W. B. Saunders, Philadelphia, 217 pp.

Grishman, A., E. R. Borun, and H. L. Jaffe. 1951. Spatial vectorcardiography. *Am. Heart J.* **41**:483–493.

Grundfest, H. 1947. Bioelectric potentials in the nervous system and in muscle. *Ann. Rev. Physiol.* **9**:477–506.

Grundfest, H. 1966a. Comparative electrobiology of excitable membranes. *Adv. Comp. Physiol. Biochem.* **2**:1–116.

Grundfest, H. 1966b. Heterogeneity of excitable membranes; electrophysiological and pharmacological evidence and some consequences. *Ann. N.Y. Acad. Sci.* **137**:901–949.

Guntheroth, W. G. 1965. *Pediatric Electrocardiography.* W. B. Saunders, Philadelphia, 150 pp.

Hakansson, C. H. 1957. Action potentials recorded intra and extracellularly from the isolated frog muscle fiber in Ringer's solution and in air. *Acta Physiol. Scand.* **39**:291–312.

Halstead, W. C. 1938. A method for the quantitative recording of eye movements. *J. Psychol.* **6**:177–180.

Haynes, J. R. 1936. A heated stylus for use with waxed recording paper. *Rev. Sci. Instr.* **7**:108.

Hecht, H. H. 1956–1957. Normal and abnormal transmembrane potentials of the spontaneously beating heart. *Ann. N.Y. Acad. Sci.* **65**:700–740.

Helm, R. A. 1957. An accurate lead system for spatial vectorcardiography. *Am. Heart J.* **53**:415–424.

Hermann, L. 1879. Allgemeine Muskelphysik. *Handbuch der Physiologie der Bewegunsapparate* **1**:1–260.

Hill, D., and G. Parr. 1950. *Electroencephalography: A Symposium on Its Various Aspects.* Macdonald & Co., London, 438 pp.

Hill, D., and G. Parr, 1963. *Electroencephalography: A Symposium on Its Various Aspects,* Macmillan, New York, 509 pp.

Hlavin, J. M., and R. Plonsey. 1963. An experimental determination of a multipole representation of a turtle heart. *IEEE Trans. Bio-Med. Electron.* **BME-10**:98–105.

Hodgkin, A. L. 1951. The ionic basis of electrical activity in nerve and muscle. *Biol. Rev. Cambridge Phil. Soc.* **26**:339–409.

Hodgkin, A. L., and P. Horowicz. 1957. The differential action of hypertonic solutions on the twitch and action potential of a muscle fiber. *J. Physiol.* **136**:17P-18P.

Hodgkin, A. L., and A. F. Huxley. 1939. Action potentials recorded from inside a nerve fiber. *Nature* **144**:710–711.

Hoff, H. E. 1936. Galvani and the pre-Galvani electrophysiologists. *Ann. Sci.* **1**:157–172.

Hoff, H. E., and L. A. Geddes. 1957. The rheotome and its prehistory: A study in the historical interrelation of electrophysiology and electromechanics, *Bull. Hist. Med.* **31**:212–347.

Hoff, H. E., and L. A. Geddes. *Experimental Physiology* (2nd ed.). Baylor University College of Medicine, Houston.

Hoffman, A. C., B. Wellman, and L. Carmichael. 1939. A quantitative comparison of the electrical and photographic techniques of eye-movement recording. *J. Exp. Psychol.* **24**:40–53.

Hoffmann, B. F., and E. E. Suckling. 1953. Cardiac cellular potentials: Effect of vagal stimulation and acetylcholine. *Am. J. Physiol.* **173**:312–320.

Hollmann, H. E., and W. Hollmann. 1938. Das Einthovensche Druckschema als Grudlage neuer elektrokardiograpischen Registriermethoden. *Z. Klinik. Med.* **134**:732–753.

Holman, M. E. 1958. Membrane potentials recorded with high resistance micro-electrodes. *J. Physiol.* **141**:464–488.

Holmgren, F. 1865–1866. Method at objektivera effekten of liusintryck po retina. Upsala Lakareforenings Forhanklingar, 1865–1866. *Acta Soc. Med. Upaslein.* **1**:177–184 (in Swedish).

Holmgren, F. 1870–1871. On the retinal current *Acta Soc. Med. Upsalein.* **6**:419 (in Swedish).

Horan, L. G., N. C. Flowers, and D. A. Brody. 1963. Body surface potential distribution. *Circ. Res.* **13**:373–387.

Hughes, R. R. 1961. *An Introduction to Electroencephalography.* J. Wright, Bristol, 118 pp.

Huxley, A. F., and R. Stampfli. 1944. Evidence for saltatory conduction in peripheral myelinated nerve fibers. *J. Physiol.* **108**:315–339.

Huxley, A. F., and R. Stampfli. 1951. Direct determination of membrane resting potential and action potential in single myelinated nerve fibers. *J. Physiol.* **112**:476–495.

Isaacs, J. H. 1964. A study of electrical fields. The differential vectorscope. *Am. J. Med. Electron.* **2**:34–40.

Ishitoya, J. T. Sakurai, I. Aita, and K. Sasaki. 1965. A new type of spatial vectorcardiograph *Tohoku J. Exp. Med.* **85**:1–8.

Ito, H. 1973. Personal communication.

Jacobson, E. 1930. Electrical measurement of neuromuscular states during mental activity. *Am. J. Physiol.* **95**:694–702.

Jasper, H. H. 1958. International Federation of Societies for Electroencephalography and Clinical Neurophysiology. Appendix IX. The ten-twenty electrode system of the International Federation. *EEG Clin. Neurophysiol.* **10**:371–375.

Jasper, H. H., and G. Ballem. 1949. Unipolar electromyograms of normal and denervated human muscle. *J. Neurophysiol.* **12**:231–244.

Jasper, H. H. and L. Carmichael. 1935. Electric potentials from the intact human brain. *Science* **81**:51–53.

Karpe, G. 1945. The basis of clinical electroretinography. *Acta Ophthalmol.* **23** (suppl. **23–24**):1–116.

Katz, B., and R. Miledi. 1965. Propagation of electric activity in motor nerve terminals. *Proc. Roy. Soc. (London)* **161B**:453–482.

Kerwin, A. J. 1953. The effect of frequency response of electrocardiographs on the form of electrocardiograms and vectorcardiograms. *Circulation* **8**:98–110.

Kiegler, J. 1964. *Electroencephalography in Hospital and General Consulting Practice.* Elsevier, Amsterdam, 180 pp.

Kiloh, L. G., A. J. McComas, and J. W. Osselton. 1972. *Clinical Electroencephalography,* 3rd ed. Butterworths, London, 239 pp.

Knott, J. 1958. Report of the Committee on Apparatus. International Federation of EEG Societies. *EEG Clin. Neurophysiol.* **10**:378–380.

Koelliker, R. A., and J. Mueller. 1856. Nachweis der negativen Schwankung des Muskelstroms am natürlich sich contrahirenden Muskel. *Verhandl. Phys. Med. Ges. Wurzburg* **6**:528–533.

Kohlrausch, A. 1931. Elektrische Erscheinungen am Auge. *Handb. Norm. Pathol. Physiol.* **12**(2):1394–1496.

Kowarzykowic, H., and Z. Kowarzykowic. 1961. *Spatial Vectorcardiography.* Pergamon Press, Oxford, 254 pp.

Kris, C. 1957. Electrical measurement of eye movement during perception. *Proc. Int. Congr. Psychol. Amsterdam, 1957,* New Holland, Amsterdam, pp. 247–249.

Kris, C. 1958. A technique for electrically recording eye position. WADC Technical Report 58–60, 33 pp. (ASTIA Document AD 209385, USAF Wright-Patterson, AFB, Ohio).

Kris, C. 1960. Vision: Electro-oculography. In O. Glasser, *Medical Physics,* vol. 3. Year Book Publishing, Chicago, pp. 692–700.

Kügelberg, E. 1947. Electromyograms in muscular disorders. *J. Neurol. Neurosurg. Psychiat.* **10**:122–136.

Kühne, W., and J. Steiner, 1880. Über das elektromotorische Verhaltender Netzhaut. Untersuchungen. auf der physiologischer Institut der Univ. Heidelberg 1880, 3:327.

Lamb, L. E. 1965. *Electrocardiography and Vectorcardiography.* W. B. Saunders, Philadelphia, 609 pp.

Landau, W. M. 1951. Comparison of different needle leads in EMG recording from a single site. *EEG Clin. Neurophysiol.* 3:163–168.

Langner, P. H. 1952. The value of high fidelity electrocardiography using the cathode, ray oscillograph and an expanded time scale. *Circulation* 5:249–256.

Langner, P. H., R. Okada, S. R. Moore, and H. C. Fies. 1958. Comparison of four orthogonal systems of vectorcardiography. *Circulation* 17:46–54.

Law, T., and R. L. Devalois. 1958. Periorbital potentials recorded during small eye movements. Papers of the Michigan Academy of Science, Arts, and Letters, vol. 43, pp. 171–180.

Leksell, L. 1939. Clinical recording of eye movements. *Acta Chir. Scand.* **82**:262–270.

Lenz, E. 1849, 1854. Über den Einfluss der Geschwindigkeit des Drehens auf den durch magneto-electrische Machinen erzeugten Inductronsstrom. *Ann. Physik. Chem.* 1849, **152**:494–523; 1854, **92**:128–152.

Lian, C. and V. Golblin. 1936. Intérèt nosographique et pratique de la derivation precordiale auriculaire s 5. *Archives des Maladies du Coeur des Vaisseaux et du Sang* 29:721–734.

Liberson, W. T. 1962. Report on the standardization of reporting and terminology in electromyography. *EEG Clin. Neurophysiol.* **22**:107–172.

Licht, S. H. 1961. *Electrodiagnosis and Electromyography.* E. Licht, New Haven, Conn., 470 pp.

Lindsley, D. B., and W. S. Hunter. 1939. A note on polarity potentials from the human eye. *Proc. Natl. Acad. Sci. (U.S.)* **25**:180–183.

Lorente de Nó, R. 1947. *A Study of Nerve Physiology.* Rockefeller Institute, New York, Part 2, Chap. 16.

Lundervold, A., and C-L. Li. 1953. Motor units and fibrillation potentials as recorded with different kinds of needle electrodes. *Acta Psychiat. Neurol. Scand.* **28**:201–212.

Lykken, D. T., R. D. Miller, and R. F. Strahan. 1968. Some properties of skin conductance and potential. *Psychophysiology.* **8**:253–268.

Lykken, D. T., and P. H. Venables. 1971. Direct measurement of skin conductance: A proposal for standardizations. *Psychophysiology* 8:656–672.

Mackensen, C., and S. Harder. 1954. Untersuchunger zur elektrischen Aufzeichnung von Augenbeiwegungen. *von Graefe's Arch. Ophthalmol.* **155**:397–412.

Macleod, A. G. 1938a. The electrogram of cardiac muscle: an analysis which explains the regression or T deflection. *Am. Heart J.* **15**:165–186.

Macleod, A. G. 1938b. The electrocardiogram of cardiac muscle. *Am. Heart J.* **15**:402–413.

Mann, H. 1920. A method of analyzing the electrocardiogram. *Arch. Intern. Med.* **25**:283–294.

Mann, H. 1931. Interpretation of bundle-branch block by means of the monocardiogram. *Am. Heart. J.* **6**:447–457.

Mann, H. 1931–1932. A light weight portable EKG. *Am. Heart J.* **7**:796–797.

Mann, H. 1938. The monocardiograph. *Am. Heart J.* **15**:681-689.

Marchand, R. 1877. Beiträge zur Kentniss der Reizwelle und Contractionswelle des Herzmuskels. *Arch. Ges. Physiol.* **15**:511.

Marey, E. J. 1876. Des variations électriques des muscles du coeur en particulier étudiées au moyen de l'électromètre de M. Lippmann. *Comptes Rendus* **82**:975-977.

Marg, E. 1951. Development of electro-oculography. *Arch. Ophthalmol.* **45**:169-185.

Marg, E., and G. G. Heath. 1955. Localized electroretinograms from isolated poikilothermic retinas. *Science* **122**:1234-1235.

Marinacci, A. A. 1965. *Clinical Electromyography.* San Lucas Press, Los Angeles, 199 pp.

Matteucci, C. 1824a. Correspondence. *Comptes Rendus* **159**, Suppl. **2**:797-798.

Matteucci, C. 1842b. Sur un phénomène physiologique produit par les muscles en contraction. *Ann. Chim. Phys.* **6**: Suppl. **3**:339-343.

Maulsby, R., and R. Edelberg. 1960. The interrelationship between the galvanic skin response, basal resistance and temperature. *J. Comp. Physiol. Psychol.* **53**:475-479.

Mauro, A., L. H. Nahum, and R. Sikand. 1952-1953. Instantaneous equipotential distribution on the thoracic surface of human subjects with cardiac pathology. *J. Appl. Physiol.* **5**:698-704.

Mauro, A., L. H. Nahum, R. S. Sikand, and H. Chernoff. 1952. Equipotential distribution for the various instants of the cardiac cycle of the body surface of the dog. *Am. J. Physiol.* **168**:584-591.

McFee, R., and F. D. Johnston. 1954. Electrocardiographic leads. III. Synthesis. *Circulation* **9**:868-880.

Meyers, I. L. 1929. Electronystagmography. *Arch. Neurol. Psychiat.* **21**:900-918.

Miles, W. R. 1939. The steady polarity potential of the human eye. *Proc. Natl. Acad. Sci. (U.S.)* **25**:25-36.

Morrice, J. K. W. 1956. Slow wave production in the EEG with reference to hyperpnoea, carbon dioxide and autonomic balance. *EEG Clin. Neurophysiol.* **8**:49-72.

Mowrer, G. H., T. C. Ruch, and N. E. Miller. 1935-1936. *Am. J. Physiol.* **114**:423-428.

Murakami, M., K. Watanabe, and T. Tomita. 1961. Effect of impalement with a micropipette on the local cell membrane. *Japan J. Physiol.* **11**:80-88.

Nahum, L. H., A. Mauro, H. M. Chernoff, and R. J. Sikand. 1951. Instantaneous equipotential distribution on surface of the human body for various instants in the cardiac cycle. *J. Appl. Physiol.* **3**:454-464.

Nahum, L. H., A. Mauro, H. Levine, and D. G. Abrahams. 1952-1953. Potential field during the S T segment. *J. Appl. Physiol.* **5**:693-697.

Nelson, C. V. 1956. Human thorax potentials. *Ann. N.Y. Acad. Sci.* **65**:1014-1050.

Nelson, C. V., E. T. Angelakos, and P. R. Gastonguay. 1965. Dipole moments of dog, monkey and lamb hearts. *Circ. Res.* **17**:168-177.

Nobili, C. L. 1828. Comparison entre deux galvanomètres les plus sensibles, la grenouille et le multiplicateur à deux aiguilles suivi de quelques resultats nouveaux. *Ann. Chim. Phys.* **38**, Suppl. **2**:225-245.

Nonogawa, A. 1966. Comparison of five different vectorcardiographic systems. *Japan. Circ. J.* **30**:1009-1016.

Norris, F. H. 1963. *The EMG.* Grune and Stratton, New York, 134 pp.

North, A. W. 1965. Accuracy and precision of electro-oculographic recording. *Invest. Ophthalmol.* **4**:343–348.

Okada, R. H. 1956. Potentials produced by an eccentric current dipole in a finite-length circular conducting cylinder. *IRE Trans. Bio-Med. Electron.* **7**:14–19.

Okada, R. H. 1957. An experimental study of multiple dipole potentials and the effects of inhomogeneities in volume conductors. *Am. Heart J.* **54**:567–571.

Pardee, H. E. B. 1929–1930. The distortion of the EKG by capacitance. *Am. Heart J.* **5**:191–196.

Pardee, H. E. B. 1940. Nomenclature and description of the electrocardiogram. *Am. Heart J.* **29**:1–12.

Pearson, R. B. 1961. *Handbook of Clinical Electromyography.* Meditron Co., El Monte, Calif., 72 pp.

Petersen, I., and E. Kugelberg. 1949. Duration and form of action potential in the normal human muscle. *J. Neurol. Neurosurg. Psychiat.* **12**:124–128.

Phillips, C. G. 1955. The dimensions of a cortical motor point. *J. Physiol.* **129**:20P-21P.

Plonsey, R. 1963a. Current dipole images and reference potentials. *IEEE Trans. Bio-Med. Electron.* **BME-10**:1–8.

Plonsey, R. 1963b. Reciprocity applied to volume conductors and the ECG. *IEEE Trans. Bio-Med. Electron.* **BME-10**:9–12.

Plonsey, R. 1969. *Bioelectric Phenomena.* McGraw-Hill, New York.

Pozzi, L. 1961. *Basic Principles in Vector Electrocardiography.* Charles C. Thomas, Springfield, Ill., 292 pp.

Rappaport, M. B., C. Williams, and P. D. White. 1949. An analysis of the relative accuracies of the Wilson and Goldberger methods for registering unipolar and augmented unipolar and augmented unipolar electrocardiographic leads. *Am. Heart J.* **37**:892–917.

Rechtschaffen, A., and Kales, (eds.). 1968. *A Manual of Standardized Terminology, Techniques and Scoring System for Sleep Stages of Human Subjects.* Government Printing Office, Washington, D.C. National Institutes of Health Publication No. 204.

Rémond, A. 1967. Handbook of Electroencephalography. *EEG Clin. Neurophysiol.* **Suppl. 28**:1–350.

Rémond, A. (ed.) 1971. *Handbook of Electroencephalography and Clinical Neurophysiology.* Elsevier, Amsterdam, vol. 1.

Report of the Committee on Electrocardiography, American Heart Association. 1954. *Circulation* **10**:564–573.

Richter, C. P. 1927. A study of the electrical skin resistance and the psychogalvanic reflex in a case of unilateral sweating. *Brain* **50**:216–235.

Riggs, L. A. 1941. Continuous and reproducible records of the electrical activity of the human retina. *Proc. Soc. Exp. Biol. Med.* **48**:204–207.

Sachs, E. 1929. Die Aktionsstrome des menschlichen Auges, ihre Bezichung zu Reiz und Empfundung. *Klin. Wochenschr.* **8**:136–137.

Sadove, M. S., D. Becka, and F. A. Gibbs. 1967. *Electroencephalography for Anesthesiologists and Surgeons.* Lippincott, Philadelphia, 95 pp.

Safonov, V. M., V. M. Provotorov, V. M. Lube, and L. I. Yakimenkov. 1967. Method of recording the magnetic field of the heart (magnetocardiography). *Bull. Exp. Med.* **64**:1022–1024.

Schellong, F., S. Heller, and E. Schwingel. 1937. Das Vektordiagramm. 1. Z. *Kreislaufforsch.* **29**:497–509.

Schellong, F., and E. Schwingel. 1937. Das Vektordiagramm. II. Z. *Kreislaufforsch.* **29**:596–607.

Schellong, F., E. Schwingel, and C. Hermann. 1937. Die praktisch-klinische Methode der Vektordiagraphie und des normale Vektordiagramm. *Arch. Kreislaufforsch.* **1**:1.

Schmitt, O. H., and E. Simonson. 1955. The present status of vectorcardiography. *AMA Arch. Intern. Med.* **96**:574–590.

Schott, E. 1922. Über die Registrierung des Nystagmus und anderer Augenbewegungen vermittels des Saitengalvanometers. *Deut. Arch. Klin. Med.* **140**:79–90.

Seipel, J. H., and R. D. Morrow. 1960. The magnetic field accompanying neuronal activity. *J. Wash. Acad. Sci.* **50**:1–4.

Shackel, B. 1959. Skin-drilling: A method of diminishing galvanic skin potentials. *Am. J. Psychol.* **72**:114–121.

Shackel, B. 1960. Pilot study in electro-oculography. *Brit. J. Ophthalmol.* **44**:89–113.

Shackel, B. 1967. In P. H. Venables and I. Martin (eds.). *A Manual of Psychophysiological Methods.* North Holland, Amsterdam, pp. 300–334.

Simonson, E. 1952. The distribution of cardiac potentials around the chest in one hundred and three normal men. *Circulation* **6**:201–211.

Simonson, E. 1961. *Differentiation Between Normal and Abnormal in Electrocardiography.* C. V. Mosby Co., St. Louis, 328 pp.

Simonson, E., O. Schmitt, and H. Nakagawa. 1959. Quantitative comparison of eight vectorcardiographic lead systems. *Circ. Res.* **7**:296–302.

Simpson, J. A. 1973. Electromyography: Neuromuscular diseases. *Handb. EEG Clin. Neurophysiol.* **16B**:5–162.

Spach, M., W. P. Silberg, J. P. Borneau, R. C. Barr, E. C. Long, T. M. Gallie, J. B. Gabor, and A. G. Wallace. 1966. Body surface isopotential maps in normal children. *Am. Heart Jn.* **72**:640–652.

Stewart, L. 1961. *Introduction to the Principles of Electroencephalography.* Charles C. Thomas, Springfield, Ill., 55 pp.

Stratbucker, R. A., C. M. Hyde, and S. E. Wixson. 1963. The magnetocardiogram—A new approach to the fields surrounding the heart. *IEEE Trans. Bio-Med. Electron.* **BME-10**:145–149.

Straus, H. 1952. *Diagnostic Electroencephalography.* Grune and Stratton. New York, 282 pp.

Subcommittee on Instrumentation. 1967. Recommendations for standardization in electrocardiography and vectorcardiography. *IEEE Trans. Bio-Med. Eng.* **BME-14**:60–68.

Sulzer, R., and P. W. Duchosal. 1938. Applications de la planographie. *Arch. Mal. Coeur Vaisseaux.* **31**:682–685, 686–696.

Sulzer, R., and P. W. Duchosal. 1945. Principes de cardiovectorgraphie. *Cardiologia* **9**:106–120.

Sundmark, E. 1959. The contact glass in human electroretinography. *Acta Ophthalmol.* **37** (suppl. 52–58):8–40.

Taccardi, B. 1962. Distribution of heart potentials on dog's thoracic surface. *Circ. Res.* **11**:862–869.

Taccardi, B. 1963. Distribution of heart potentials on the thoracic surface of normal human subjects. *Circ. Res.* **12:**341–352.

Tarchanoff, J. 1890. Über die galvanischen Erscheinungen in der Haut der Menschen bei Reizungen der Sinnesorgan und bei verschiedenen Formen der psychischen Thatigkeit. *Arch. Deut. Ges. Physiol.* **46:**46–55.

Tasaki, I. 1959. Conduction of the nerve impulse. In *Handbook of Neurophysiology*, vol. 1. J. Field, H. W. Magvien, and V. E. Hill (eds.). American Physiological Society, Washington, D.C. pp. 75–121.

Thomas, P. E. and I. M. Korr. 1957. Relationship between sweat gland activity and electrical resistance of the skin. *J. Appl. Physiol.* **10:**505–510.

Uhley, H. N. 1962. *Vector Electrocardiography*. Lippincott, Philadelphia, Pa., 339 pp.

Valentinuzzi, M. E., L. A. Geddes, H. E. Hoff, and J. Bourland. 1970. Properties of the 30° hexaxial (Einthoven-Goldberger) system of vectocardiography. *Cardiovasc. Res. Center Bull.* **9:**64–72.

Venables, P. H. and I. Martin. 1967. Skin resistance and skin potential. In P. H. Venables and I. Martin (eds.). *A Manual of Psychophysiological Methods*. North Holland, Amsterdam.

Vigoroux, R. 1879. Sur le rôle de la résistance électrique des tissus dans l'électrodiagnostic. *C. R. Soc. Biol.* **31:**336–339.

Walker, W. C. 1937. Animal electricity before Galvani. *Ann. Sci.* **2:**83–113.

Waller, A. D. 1887. A demonstration on man of electromotive changes accompanying the heart's beat. *J. Physiol.* **8:**229–234.

Waller, A. D. 1889. On the electromotive changes connected with the beat of the mammalian heart and of the human heart in particular. *Phil. Trans. Roy. Soc. London* **180B:**169–194.

Weddell, G., B. Feinstein, and R. E. Prattle. 1943. The clinical application of electromyography. *Lancet* **1:**236–239.

Weddell, G., B. Feinstein, and R. E. Prattle. 1944. The electrical activity of voluntary muscle in man under normal and pathological conditions. *Brain* **67:**178–257.

Wilcott, R. C., and L. J. Hammond. 1965–1966. On the constant-current error in skin resistance measurement. *Psychophysiol.* **2:**39–41.

Williams, E. M. V. 1959. Relation of extracellular to intracellular potential records from single cardiac muscle fibers. *Nature* **183:**1341–1342.

Williams, H. B. 1914. On the cause of the phase difference frequently observed between homonymous peaks of the electrocardiogram. *Am. J. Physiol.* **35:**292–300.

Williams, R. L., I. Karacan, and C. J. Hursh. 1974. *The EEG of Human Sleep*. Wiley, New York, 169 pp.

Wilson, F. N. 1954. Recommendations for standardization of electrocardiographic and vectorcardiographic leads. *Circulation* **10:**564.

Wilson, F. N., and R. H. Bayley. 1950. The electric field of an eccentric dipole in a homogeneous spherical conducting medium. *Circulation* **1:**84–92.

Wilson, F. N., and F. D. Johnston. 1938. The vectorcardiogram. *Am. Heart J.* **16:**14–28.

Wilson, F. N., F. D. Johnston, and C. E. Kossman. 1947. The substitution of a tetrahedron for the Einthoven triangle. *Am. Heart J.* **33:**594–603.

Wilson, F. N., F. D. Johnston, A. G. Macleod, and P. S. Barker. 1934. Electrocardiograms that represent the potential variations of a single electrode. *Am. Heart J.* 9:447–458.

Woodbury, L. A., J. W. Woodbury, and H. H. Hecht. 1950. Membrane resting and action potentials of single cardiac muscle fibers. *Circulation* 1:264–266.

Yokota, T., T. Takahashi, M. Kondo, and B. Fujimori. 1959. Studies in the diphasic waveform of the galvanic skin reflex. *EEG Clin. Neurophysiol.* 11:687–696.

12

Semiconductor Transducers

In general, a semiconductor device is one in which the electrical characteristics are dependent on the properties of a P-N junction. However, devices that contain the primary semiconductor materials (silicon and germanium) are sometimes designated semiconductor devices. Thus, some strain gauges and photodetectors often have the term semiconductor as a prefix. But many interesting and important semiconductor (P–N) devices can be put to work to detect physiological events. Mention has already been made of two of these, the junction photocell and the phototransistor (see Chapter 5). This chapter describes three other important devices—the light-emitting diode, the optical isolator, and the Pitran, a pressure-sensitive transducer.

12-1. THE LIGHT–EMITTING DIODE (LED)

It is frequently necessary to have a cool light source with a long life. In many physiological applications, the color of the light is important, and filtering to obtain the desired color causes a reduction in the light output for a given power input to the light source. The light-emitting diode (LED) is an ideal candidate for such applications and promises to see increasing use in a large number of colorimetric and noncolorimetric transduction applications.

Certain semiconductor diodes emit light when they are forward biased because the electrons in the material are raised to the conduction energy level and then fall back to recombine with holes. When the electrons fall back, energy is released as radiation. The color (wavelength) of the radiation is dependent on the difference between the valence and conduction-band energies, which in turn is a property of the material. In the design of LEDs, the materials are carefully chosen to obtain the desired radiation. Light-emitting diodes are available which emit infrared, red, orange, yellow, and green light; a large number emit infrared radiation. The cur-

rent-voltage characteristic for several light-emitting diodes and their radiation spectra, along with the spectral sensitivity of the average human eye,
are illustrated in Fig. 12-1. Some manufacturers employ wave-changing
techniques to obtain a color other than that emitted by the semiconductor
material. With this technique, the emitted radiation is used to excite a
phosphor which produces light of the desired color; this technique is employed in conventional fluorescent lighting.

Light-emitting diodes are available in a variety of configurations and are

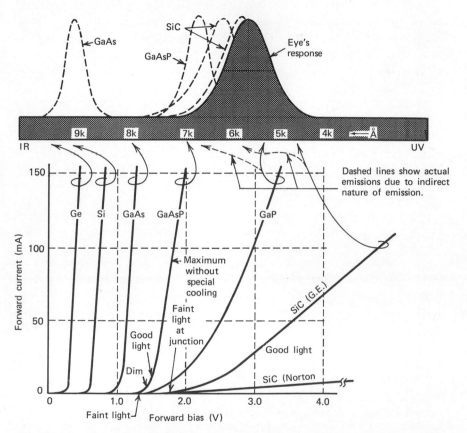

Figure 12-1. Current-voltage characteristics of various light-emitting diodes and their
spectral emission characteristics. Such devices are commercially available from Monsanto,
Electronic Special Products, 800 N. Lindberg Blvd., St. Louis, Mo. 63166; Hewlett-Packard,
620 Page Mill Rd., Palo Alto, Calif. 94304; General Electric, Miniature Lamp Dept., Nela
Park, Cleveland, Ohio 44112; Norton Research Corp., 70 Memorial Dr., Cambridge, Mass.
02142; RCA Electronic Components, Harrison, N.J. 07029; Texas Instruments Incorporated,
Semiconductor Components Div., Box 5012, Dallas, Tex. From *Electronic Design News* 1968
(October) page 54. (By permission.)

best seen head-on. In some models a hemispherical lens is applied to focus the beam; in others the light is emitted from a bright, pointlike source. Some LEDs emit light in the form of a bright line. LEDs must be classed as low-power devices (typically 100 mW); higher power units are available, but a heat sink is usually required for cooling. Over a limited range, the light output varies linearly with current.

The current-voltage curve of a typical LED reveals that it is a low impedance device (Fig. 12-2a). In addition, the range of voltage over which the device can be operated safely is quite narrow. Figure 12-2b indicates the range over which light output is linear with current, and Fig. 12-2c shows the light output (ϕ) (relative to the output at 20mA) with increasing current. Because the typical LED has a steep current-voltage curve, it must (Fig. 12-2a) be driven by a current source so that the correct operating point can be maintained easily.

The LED is a rapidly responding (microseconds to nanoseconds) light emitter in which the light output is linear with applied current over a limited range. Therefore, precautions must be taken when using it as an analog device; it sees its best service in digital circuits (i.e., when the information is carried by an off–on sequence of light flashes).

The relationship between the spectral output of light-emitting diodes to that produced by other light sources is plotted in Fig. 12-3. Also shown are the transmission characteristics of a variety of materials through which radiant energy must often pass. In viewing this chart, it should be recalled that the visible spectrum ranges from 350 to 700 mμ or 3500 to 7000 Å. Red light has a wavelength of about 600 mμ, the infrared spectrum is beyond 700 mμ, and the wavelength of the ultraviolet spectrum is shorter than blue light, or about 350 mμ.

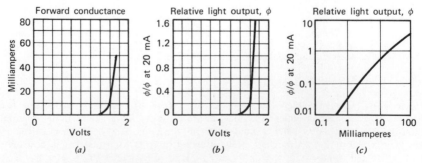

Figure 12-2. (a) Forward conductance and (b) and (c) relative light output characteristics of a typical gallium arsenide-phosphide light-emitting diode (LED).

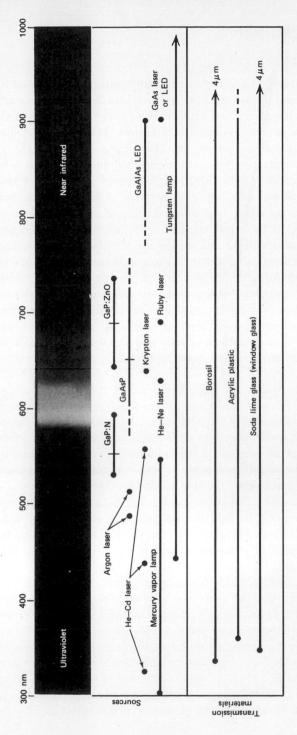

Figure 12-3. Spectral emission characteristics of light emitters and absorption characteristics of various materials. [Redrawn from H. E. Hardeman, *Electronics* **46**:109–114 (1973).]

12-2. OPTOELECTRONICS

Many circuit design problems are readily solved by the use of light-emitting devices and light sensors, and a completely new specialty has developed which is concerned with the use of light detectors and electrically driven emitters of electromagnetic radiation. The term "optoelectronics" designates the activities in this field. The combination of a light source and miniature photodetectors for reading punched cards and tape is a familiar example of optoelectronics. More sophisticated is the use of laser beams for communication, distance measurement, and producing holographic images. In fact, the whole field of television and motion pictures might well become a part of this new area of specialization. Another area in optoelectronics deals with the design and use of solid-state letter and number displays. The numerical displays in most electronic calculators are constituted by light-emitting diodes. A simple optoelectronic device consisting of a light emitter and detector, called an optical isolator, allows coupling information from one circuit to another without electrical connection, the information being carried by a beam of visible or invisible light. There is no doubt that the field of optoelectronics will expand, and from it we can expect the creation of many new devices.

12-3. OPTICAL ISOLATORS

The combination of a photodetector and a source of light constitutes an optical isolator; sometimes it is called a photon coupler. At first glance it might seem that an excessively inefficient route has been taken by using a signal to produce light, then using a photodetector to detect the light and recover the signal. However, this technique provides complete electrical isolation between the two circuits, allowing both to be at quite large differences in potential. In fact, the insulation in some optical isolators will withstand a difference in potential in the kilovolt range. Optical isolation is also used to eliminate ground-loop and common-mode signals that arise in many circuits.

Desirable as the benefits from optical isolation may be, it must be recognized that optical couplers are nonlinear devices; that is, the presentation of a signal to the light emitter will not provide the same signal from the photodetector unless special precautions are taken. This operating characteristic is due to the components of most optical isolators—namely, a light-emitting diode to produce the photons (electromagnetic radiation) and a photojunction photocell as the detector. Although the response time of both devices is short (microseconds to nanoseconds), and the response of the detector is linear with light intensity, the emitter (LED) provides a linear light output only over a limited range of current applied to it (see Section 12-1). Thus, optical isolators see their most value in digital circuits (e.g., those in which information is carried by a sequence of on–off pulses). The wavelength of the radiant energy is not an important consideration beyond the need to provide the appropriate detector, and many optical isolators employ infrared radiation as the coupling agent.

Although optical isolators are designed primarily for digital systems, it is possible to use them as analog devices because there is a region in which the output of the light emitter is linear with applied current. Figure 12-4 illustrates a method that employs two optical isolators ($LED1, 2; PJ1, 2$) to obtain linear operation. The input signal (E_{in}) is amplified by a unity-gain amplifier, which provides a signal for the LED-driving amplifier. The output of amplifier A_1 is fed into a similar amplifier (A_2) connected for unity-gain operation and provides an inverted signal to drive a second LED-driving amplifier. Therefore, the light emitted by the two LEDs is always 180 degrees out of phase. The operating points of the LEDs are chosen for linear operation (i.e., light output is linear with current). The light output, detected by the junction photocells ($PJ1, 2$), is applied to a differential amplifier (A_3), which enlarges the photon-coupled signal. It should be apparent that the

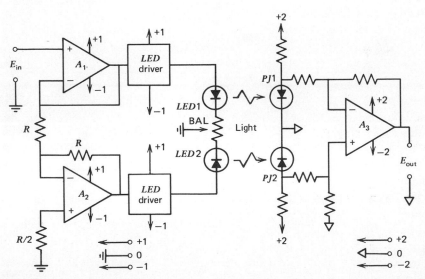

Figure 12-4. The use of an optical isolator (LED 1, 2, and PJ 1, 2) to provide coupling without direct electrical connection. The signal is coupled by modulating the light output of the light emitting diodes (LED 1, 2) and detecting the light by two junction photocells (PJ 1, 2).

system just described uses the two LEDs in push-pull, class-A operation. The system will exhibit a bandwidth, extending from zero to a high frequency, which need be limited only by the response time of the optical isolator (*LED*1, 2 and *PJ*1, 2).

One very practical use for the combination of a light emitter and detector is in resistance-capacity coupled amplifiers with long time constants, as are frequently used in the life sciences. Large-amplitude signals block such amplifiers, and it is necessary to wait many seconds until the voltages on the coupling capacitors return to their operating values. Quick return to the operating point can be accomplished by the use of shorting switches to reestablish the voltage levels. Switch contacts bounce, often causing undesired transients. The wiring associated with switches would add considerable capacitance, and thereby reduce the high-frequency response of the amplifier. Rapid reestablishment of the operating point can be attained without penalty by using a photoconductive cell mounted in front of a controllable light source. It will be recalled (see Chapter 5) that the dark resistance of a typical photoconductive cell is extremely high (hundreds of megohms), and when illuminated, the resistance drops to a few hundred ohms. Thus, by mounting a photoconductor in front of a small pilot light or LED (and with the whole assembly placed in a lightproof case), a high-quality, remotely controlled switch can be obtained. When the photoconductive cells in several such devices are connected across the input terminals of differential resistance-capacitance coupled amplifiers, as in Fig. 12-5, the voltages on the coupling capacitors can be quickly restored to the operating values by depressing a pushbutton (*TR*) which illuminates all the light bulbs (*L*) in front of the photoconductive cells (*PC*).

This brief discussion of optoelectronic techniques is designed to make the reader aware of a few methods for solving some unusual problems. The widespread availability of miniature, low-cost photoemitters and photodetectors now provides the researcher with an array of components that can be applied to solve a wide variety of problems.

12-4. THE PITRAN

The Pitran[1] is a silicon N–P–N planar transistor in which the emitter-base junction is mechanically coupled to a diaphragm that forms part of the TO-46 case; Fig. 12-6 illustrates the transistor, and a cutaway view gives the essential operational details. When pressure (P_1) is applied to the diaphragm, the electrical properties of the emitter-base junction are al-

---

[1] Stow Laboratories, Inc., Hudson, Mass.

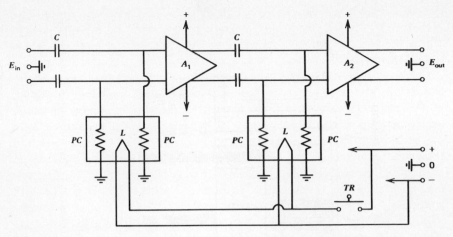

Figure 12-5. The use of photoconductive cells (*PC*) adjacent to light sources (*L*) to provide quick trace restoration (*TR*) in capacitively (*C*) coupled amplifiers. Depression of the trace restore switch (*TR*) illuminates the photoconductors and reduces their resistance to a few hundred ohms, thereby shortening the coupling time constants.

tered; when connected as in Fig. 12-7*a*, a larger, linear collector-emitter voltage (V_{CE}) is obtained, as in Fig. 12-7*b*.

The phenomenon underlying operation of the Pitran was described by Rindner (1962) and Rindner and Braun (1963), who found that localized stress applied to a P-N junction caused a large reversible change in both forward and reverse current. This phenomenon, now called the "anisotropic stress effect," occurs at P-N junctions of silicon and germanium. Although the underlying mechanism is not fully understood, the effect is explained on the basis of a change in the gap between energy levels or by a change in generation-recombination of charges.

In the Pitran, the anisotropic stress effect is used in a transistor in which the application of stress to the emitter-base junction reduces the forward current gain by as much as 4 orders of magnitude. The output capacitance is also varied by the application of stress, allowing use of this parameter to control an oscillator to provide a signal in which a pressure change is converted to a frequency change. Other transistor parameters are also altered by the application of stress and may be used appropriately.

The manufacturer provides nine different Pitrans covering a pressure range extending from 0.1 to 20 psi. In addition, there is access to both sides of the diaphragm; therefore, the pressure range listed is applicable to differential pressure measurement. The maximum deflection of the diaphragm is 2 μin. and the equivalent volume displacement is 4×10^{-8}in.^{3}. The

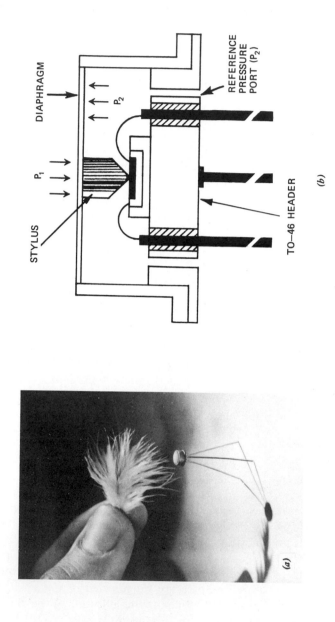

Figure 12-6. (a) The Pitran. (b) Cutaway view showing how pressure is applied to the base-emitter junction to alter its electrical characteristics. (Courtesy of Stow Laboratories, Hudson, Mass.)

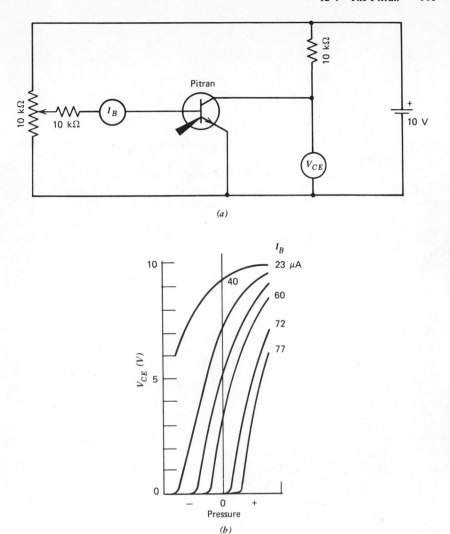

(a)

(b)

Figure 12-7. (a) Method of connecting the Pitran to obtain a change in collector to emitter voltage (V_{CE}) with the application of pressure. (b) Relationship between collector-emitter voltage (V_{CE}) versus pressure for various base currents applied to a typical Pitran. (Courtesy of Stow Laboratories, Hudson, Mass.)

mechanical resonant frequency is 150 kHz. The sensitivity, expressed as the change in output voltage (V_{CE}) for the application of a given pressure (ΔP), depends on the base current (I_B) and the model number; Fig. 12-7a presents a typical circuit configuration. In general, with a supply of voltage of about 10, an output of several volts can be obtained for the maximum pressure range for each model (Fig. 12-7*b*). Like all semiconductor devices, the Pitran is quite sensitive to temperature changes, a factor which assumes major importance when small pressure changes are being measured. However, the use of two matched Pitrans in a differential type of circuit (see Fig. 12-8) provides considerable immunity from changes in temperature and variations in power supply voltage.

Probably because the device is so new, there have been few biological applications of the Pitran, although many suggest themselves immediately. The differential pressure capabilities of the Pitran were employed by Darling et al. (1972) to record the oscillation amplitude in a pressurized blood-pressure cuff wrapped around a member. One side of the Pitran diaphragm was exposed to mean cuff pressure plus oscillations; the other side was presented with mean cuff pressure. Therefore, the output of the Pitran represented the amplitude of the volume pulsations in the segment under the cuff. This technique is the oscillometric method of measuring segmental volume, and Darling et al. (1972) applied it to study patients with vascular disease.

Although the Pitran is a pressure transducer, its pressure-sensitive diaphragm can be coupled to a lever system to detect force. This technique was employed by Jacobs et al. (1973), who desired a high-sensitivity, linear, low-noise, rapidly responding, stable transducer for the measurement of the contractile force of strips of ventricular muscle from the hamster. The

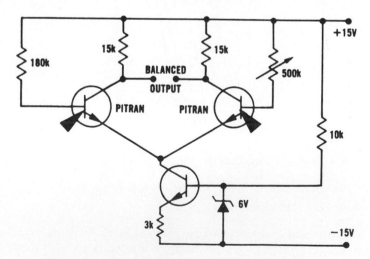

Figure 12-8. Differential circuit for obtaining temperature stabilization using two Pitrans. The constant-current source in the emitter circuit provides immunity from changes in power supply variation.

muscle strips were placed in a temperature-controlled physiological solution and coupled to a lever, one end of which was in the solution. The other end of the lever was above the solution, and the pressure-sensitive diaphragm of a PTM 2 Pitran could be brought in contact with it by way of a micrometer drive assembly. With the Pitran connected to an operational amplifier (741C), an overall sensitivity of 16.78 mV output was obtained for a force of 1 mg. The output was linear within 5%, and the overall frequency response extended from 0 to 5 kHz. Drift, due to temperature changes, was minimized because the Pitran was mounted just above the level of the physiological solution, therefore in a relatively constant temperature environment.

Pinto and Fung (1973) also employed a Pitran as a rapidly responding, sensitive force transducer to investigate the viscoelastic properties of rabbit papillary muscle. The Pitran was mounted in series with the device, which applied force to the specimen; a second transducer measured displacement. The light weight and short response time of the Pitran allowed detection of rapidly changing forces. There was some drift due to the Pitran at the high sensitivity required; however, this was overcome by combining the Pitran signal with a slowly responding force transducer coupled to the specimen.

From the few examples cited, it can be seen that the Pitran is a useful rapidly responding transducer for pressure and force. Although now rather expensive, there is no doubt that, like other semiconductor devices, its price will come down with volume production.

REFERENCES

Darling, R. C., J. K. Raines, B. J. Brener, and W. G. Austen. 1972. Quantitative segmental pulse volume recorder. *Surgery* 22:873–887.

Jacobs, H. K., D. P. McConnell, A. R. Rowley, and F. E. South. 1973. A force transducer for cardiac muscle strips. *J. Appl. Physiol.* 35:436–438.

Pinto, J. G., and Y. C. Fung. 1973. Mechanical properties of the heart muscle in the passive state. *J. Biomechan.* 6:597–616.

Rindner, W. 1962. Resistance of elastically deformed shallow P-N junctions. *J. Appl. Phys.* 33:2479–2480.

Rindner, W., and I. Braun. 1963. Resistance of elastically deformed shallow P–N junctions. II. *J. Appl. Phys.* 34:1958–1970.

13

Criteria for the Faithful Reproduction of an Event

For the familiar three-part system (transducer, processor, and reproducer) used to measure the time course of a physiological event, it is possible to set forth general conditions which, if satisfied, will guarantee faithful reproduction of the event. It is necessary either to appropriately impose the same conditions on the three parts of the channel or to incorporate any necessary compensation so that the overall system will meet the criteria if the individual parts do not. In such a system three criteria must be fulfilled. Because of the extreme importance of these criteria, their meaning must be clearly understood. Even though many of the underlying factors are of necessity technical and complex, simple examples can be chosen to illustrate their importance.

Any system designed for faithful reproduction of an event must possess these characteristics:

1. Amplitude linearity.
2. Adequate bandwidth.
3. Phase linearity.

The first requisite, amplitude linearity, calls for the input-output characteristic to be linear in the working range. If, for example, the input is doubled in the positive direction, the output indication also must be doubled. If the operating range extends into the reverse direction, negative inputs must be reproduced by a linear output indication in the negative direction.

13-1. FOURIER SERIES

Before the second and third criteria can be discussed, it is necessary to establish the relationship between sine waves and waves of nonsinusoidal form. All periodic waves of nonsinusoidal form are designated complex

584

waves. By the use of the Fourier series it is possible to show that any periodic complex wave can be dissected into a series of sine and cosine waves that when added will reproduce the original complex wave. The sine and cosine waves that have the same frequency as the complex wave constitute the components of the fundamental or first harmonic. Those having twice and thrice the frequency constitute the second and third harmonics, and so on. The foregoing can be restated by saying that a periodic complex wave can be represented by an infinite series consisting of a constant, plus harmonically related sine and cosine waves. Expressed mathematically, the series for the function $F(t)$ may be written as follows:

$$F(t) = \frac{a_0}{2} + a_1 \cos wt + a_2 \cos 2wt + a_3 \cos 3wt + \ldots + a_n \cos nwt$$

$$+ b_1 \sin wt + b_2 \sin 2wt + b_3 \sin 3wt + \ldots + b_n \sin nwt,$$

where

$$a_n = (1/\pi) \int_0^{2\pi} F(t) \cos nwt \, dt,$$

$$b_n = (1/\pi) \int_0^{2\pi} F(t) \sin nwt \, dt,$$

$$w = 2\pi f$$

(where f is the fundamental frequency of the complex wave in hertz).

To use the series to describe a waveform, it is necessary to calculate the coefficients $a_0 \ldots a_n$ and $b_0 \ldots b_n$, some of which may be zero. However, for purposes of this study it is neither necessary nor profitable to perform the calculations to demonstrate the validity of the series. Many waves have been analyzed and the coefficients published. Selection of two examples, the square wave and the blood pressure curve, will suffice to show the value of the concept.

One of the most difficult waveforms to reproduce is the square wave (Fig. 13-1a), which instantaneously changes its value from zero to a fixed value, maintains this value for a time before reversing itself below zero by the same amount and for the same time, and returns abruptly to zero again. When this wave is analyzed for its harmonic content, some of the coefficients are zero, and the series reduces to the fundamental and an infinite series of odd harmonics in which the amplitudes of the higher-frequency components decrease; that is, these components contribute less to the resynthesis of the original wave. Table 13-1 lists a few of the harmonic amplitudes for the square wave.

In Fig. 13-1b the first and the third harmonic components have been

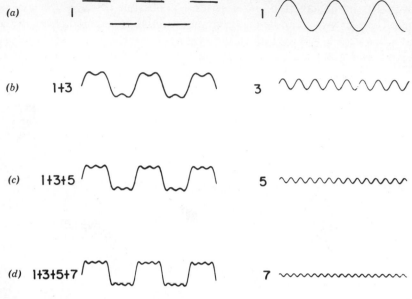

Figure 13-1.   Synthesis of a square wave.

summated to yield the curve labeled 1 + 3. In this case, even with only two components, the beginnings of the square wave are apparent. When the first, third, and fifth components are summated (Fig. 13-1c), a better representation of the original wave is obtained (1 + 3 + 5). By adding the first, third, fifth, and seventh components, an even better likeness of the original wave (Fig. 13-1d) is obtained (1 + 3 + 5 + 7). The addition of more and more harmonics would further improve the reproduction; the addition of an infinite number of the ever-diminishing-amplitude high-frequency components would reconstitute the original wave.

Table 13-1   Harmonic Amplitudes of Square Wave

Harmonic	Amplitude	Amplitude (%)
Fundamental	1	100
3rd	⅓	33
5th	⅕	20
7th	⅐	14

The arterial pressure pulse is a good example of the utilitarian value of harmonic analysis. Hansen (1949), using a high-fidelity system, recorded the arterial pulse wave and applied harmonic analysis to it. His data (redrawn), plotted in Fig. 13-2a, show the degree of fidelity obtainable by summating the first six harmonics. The arterial pressure waveform is designated (a), and the waveform resulting from summing the first six harmonics is labeled (b). The amplitudes of the higher-frequency components

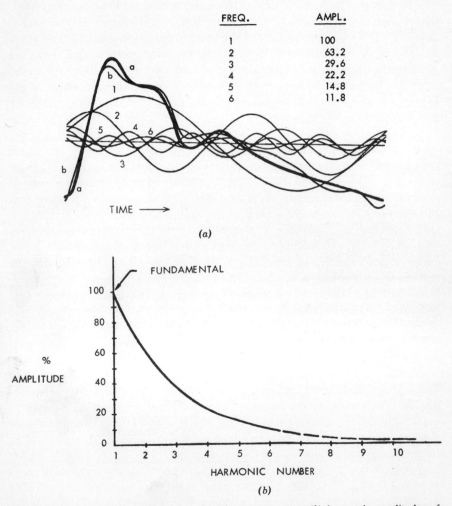

FREQ.	AMPL.
1	100
2	63.2
3	29.6
4	22.2
5	14.8
6	11.8

(a)

(b)

Figure 13-2. (a) Fourier analysis of a blood pressure curve; (b) harmonic amplitudes of components of a blood pressure pulse. (From data obtained by A. T. Hansen, *Pressure Measurement in the Human Organism,* Technisk Forlag, Copenhagen, 1949. By permission.)

are progressively smaller with increasing harmonic numbers, the sixth being present with an amplitude of slightly more than 10%. Figure 13-2*b* illustrates this point.

To obtain a more faithful reproduction, addition of many more of the smaller-and-smaller-amplitude high-frequency components would be necessary. Thus the amount of frequency response required is closely related to the degree of fidelity desired.

From these relatively simple examples two very important conclusions can be drawn. The first is that the frequency of the periodic complex wave determines the frequency of the fundamental component. The second is that the fidelity of reproduction of the quickly changing parts of the wave is determined by the number of high-frequency components added. Thus the bandwidth required for reproduction of the two waves analyzed would extend from below the fundamental frequency of the complex wave to the highest harmonic deemed important for adequate reproduction of the sharp portions of the complex wave.

In the two examples cited, the waves chosen were symmetrical about the time axis. If they were not, the analysis would have shown the same components with one notable exception: the constant a_0 would have a value other than zero, for a_0 is the average amplitude over a complete period. It is easily proved mathematically, and indeed is obvious, that a train of unidirectional pulses must have an average value other than zero. In the case of the arterial pressure wave, a_0 would be the mean pressure. Therefore, to reproduce a train of unidirectional pulses, it is necessary to provide a uniform frequency response extending from 0 Hz to a value high enough for full reproduction of the highest harmonic deemed important. In practice, the high-frequency response is made to include the tenth harmonic and sometimes higher harmonics.

13-2. AMPLITUDE AND PHASE DISTORTION

Perhaps of more importance than the cases in which the criteria are satisfied are those in which some criteria are not met. The following examples illustrate some of the possible types of distortion. Because the square wave is one of the most difficult to reproduce, it is useful to examine the effects of alteration of the amplitudes of the harmonics on the reproduction of this waveform. Terman (1943) showed that if only the low-frequency components are attenuated, the square wave will have a concave top, as sketched in Fig. 13-3*a*. On the other hand, if the low-frequency components are enhanced, the top of the square wave will be convex, as in Fig. 13-3*b*.

If the harmonics are present in their proper amplitudes, but are merely displaced in time, a characteristic type of distortion occurs. Time dis-

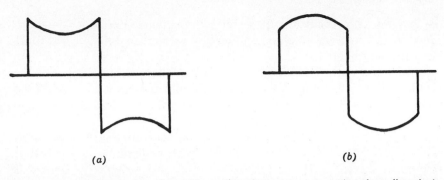

Figure 13-3. Amplitude distortion: (*a*) loss of low-frequency response (no phase distortion); (*b*) increased amplification of low frequencies (no phase distortion). (From F. E. Terman, *Radio Engineers Handbook,* 1st ed., McGraw-Hill, New York, 1943. By permission.)

placement is not customarily expressed in seconds; it is usually stated in angular measure (radians or degrees) as a phase lag or lead. For example, if the time displacement for a given frequency f is t, and since the period T corresponds to 360 degrees, the phase lag or lead ϕ in degrees is $t/T \times 360$ degrees. Since $T = 1/f$, one can express the phase lag or lead in terms of frequency; that is, $\phi = tf \times 360$ degrees. Thus with equal time displacements for all frequency components ($t = k$), $\phi = kf$; that is, the phase shift must be linear with frequency. It is also possible to state this requirement by specifying that in relation to some reference (e.g., the fundamental), the components must be transmitted through the system such that they bear exactly the same phase relationship one to another at the output as existed at the input.

Figure 13-4 illustrates the effect of phase distortion on the reproduction of the square wave. The harmonic components are present in their correct amplitudes, but time displacements have been caused to occur. In Fig. 13-4*a* the fundamental leads the higher harmonics, and in Fig. 13-4*b* the reverse condition exists. In each case the resulting reproduction is indicated by dashed lines.

Phase distortion can be present when only minimal loss of amplitude response occurs. Terman (1943) called attention to the fact that in many networks, such as those used to couple amplifier stages, when the low-frequency sine wave response is 99.94%, a 2-degree phase-shift error is encountered which results in a 10% tilt to the top of the square wave of the same frequency.

Because phase shift and loss of amplitude response are usually inseparable, it is often difficult to appreciate the effect of each of these types of distortion. To demonstrate the practical importance of this fact, Geddes (1951) constructed a variable-frequency oscillator that produced a sine

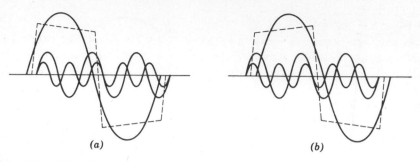

(a)   (b)

Figure 13-4. Phase distortion: (*a*) phase leads at low frequency (no amplitude distortion); (*b*) phase lags at low frequency (no amplitude distortion).

wave having a notch at its peak positive amplitude. The location of the notch (square pulse) was fixed, but the frequency of the complex wave was variable. This wave was used to test electroencephalographs to estimate their ability to reproduce faithfully the familiar spike-and-wave complex found in recordings from patients with petit-mal epilepsy.

The wave was applied to one of several EEG machines meeting existing standards; the frequency was varied and the output recorded. Figure 13-5*a* is a sketch of the input waveform. The other sections of the figure represent the reproduction achieved at various frequencies. In Fig. 13-5*b*, recorded at 1 Hz, it is obvious that there is a 45-degree phase shift. Increasing the frequency to 2 and 3 Hz (Figs. 13-5*c* and 13-5*d*) places the spike more nearly in its correct position, where it appears when the frequency is 6 Hz. However, although the phase distortion is minimal (Fig. 13-5*e*), at 6 Hz the amplitude of the spike has decreased because the system had inadequate high-frequency response to pass the high-frequency components contained in the spike.

The practical significance of phase distortion was demonstrated by Saunders and Jell (1959), who recorded the effect in a unique way by using two identical channels of an EEG machine. The output of the first channel was attenuated and fed into the second; the output of both channels appeared on the same record. They first tested the system for phase distortion, using a 3-Hz sine wave. On a typical EEG machine in which a 3-Hz sine wave was attenuated insignificantly, they recorded a time delay between channels amounting to 51.3 msec or 55.4 degrees. This testing technique demonstrated the phase shift in the second channel only. Next, in a practical study, stimulus-response waves, eye-blink artifacts, and spike-and-wave patterns were observed to exhibit time distortions when the recordings from the two channels were compared. A time separation of 75 msec between the spike and wave recorded on the first channel was reduced to 63 msec after passing through the second channel.

From the examples given, it is apparent that the three criteria—amplitude linearity, frequency response, and phase linearity—must be satisfied to guarantee the faithful reproduction of an event. Amplitude linearity occurs when output and input are proportional. Frequency response is usually described in terms of bandwidth, which is designated as the frequency range between the lowest and highest sine wave frequencies at which a satisfactory amplitude response is obtained. It is also frequently designated as the spectrum between the two frequencies at which the output amplitude has fallen to 70% of the midfrequency response. In some instances the 50, 90, or 95% points are specified.

13-3. THE STEP FUNCTION

For practical testing of a system, the step function is of considerable value. It is a waveform that changes abruptly from one level to another and is frequently employed as a calibration signal in many bioelectric recording instruments. Since the sine wave frequency response curves of most devices are given by equipment manufacturers, it is illuminating to apply the step function to systems with known frequency response curves to determine the relationship between sinusoidal and step-function responses.

If the step function shown in Fig. 13-6a is applied to a simple system that

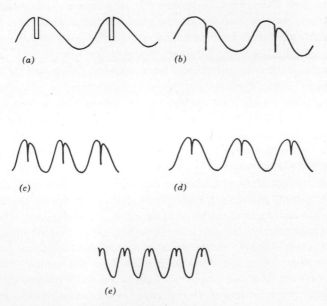

(a)   (b)

(c)   (d)

(e)

Figure 13-5. Amplitude and phase distortion.

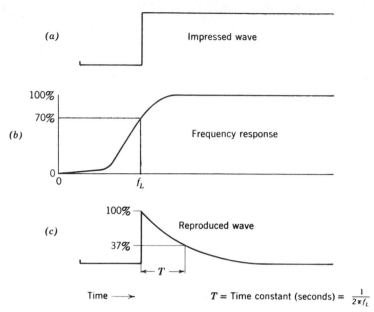

Figure 13-6.   Relationship between time constant and low-frequency response.

does not possess a sine wave frequency response extending to 0 Hz (Fig. 13-6*b*) but has an infinite high-frequency response, the reproduced wave is of exponential form (see Fig. 13-6*c*). The decay time is described as the time taken for the amplitude to fall from 100% to 37% amplitude. This time, measured in seconds, is called the time constant. The time constant is related to the sine wave frequency response by the following relationship:

$$T = \frac{1}{2\pi f_L},$$

where T is time constant in seconds, and f_L is frequency on the sine wave curve at which the response is 70%.

Often in the recording of physiological and bioelectric events, as a result of the intermittent activity of a variety of cells and organs, short-duration asymmetrical (with respect to the time axis) or completely monophasic pulses are presented to the reproducing apparatus. A harmonic analysis of such waveforms reveals the presence of a first term (a_0) in the Fourier series. Therefore, faithful reproduction of such events requires the use of a system with a frequency response extending to 0 Hz, that is, a dc response. Frequently it is not practical to meet this requirement. Under many circumstances a reasonable reproduction of the event can be obtained with a processing system having a time constant that is very long with respect to the duration of the event. This technique is employed in the instruments which record many of the bioelectric events, such as the ECG, EEG, and EMG.

The effect of time constant on the reproduction of a single monophasic flat-topped pulse is illustrated in Fig. 13-7. The percentage drop (tilt) on the top of the reproduced wave is compared with the ratio of the duration of the pulse to the time constant of the circuit passing it. For simplicity of illustration, the calculations were based on a single-section R-C circuit.

It is readily apparent that a 10% tilt is encountered if the duration of the pulse is approximately one-tenth of the time constant of the circuit. Increasing the time constant of the circuit or decreasing the pulse duration would reduce the percentage tilt.

There is also an undershoot following the pulse. The magnitude is equal to the amount of the tilt. If the pulse duration is many times longer than the time constant, the familiar biphasic condenser charge and discharge current wave is seen.

To further improve the reproduction of short-duration square pulses when using amplifiers without dc response, investigators often add phase- and amplitude-compensating networks, designed to flatten the top of the pulse. This technique is employed in most ECG amplifiers. A good treatment of this subject is given by Valley and Wallman (1948) in the chapter dealing with pulse amplifiers.

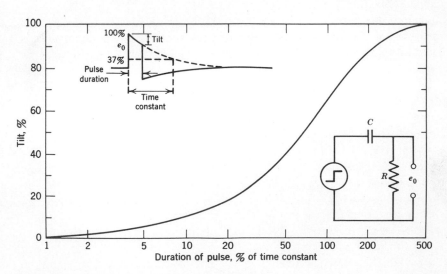

Figure 13-7.   Square pulse response of an R-C circuit.

If the step function (Fig. 13-8a) is impressed on a simple system having a low-frequency response extending to 0 Hz and a high-frequency response not extending to an infinitely high frequency (Fig. 13-8b), the type of response shown in Fig. 13-8c is encountered. It can be seen that the reproduced wave does not attain its final value instantly, but takes a finite time to reach it. This rise or response time is frequently described as the time in seconds for the amplitude to rise from 10 to 90% of its final value. The rise time is related to the high-frequency sine wave response by the following expression:

$$t = \frac{1}{kf_h},$$

where t is rise time (10 to 90%) in seconds; f_h is frequency on the sine wave response curve where the response has fallen to 70%; and k depends on the circuit configuration, hence the rate at which the high-frequency response decreases with increasing frequency (high-frequency rolloff). In many cir-

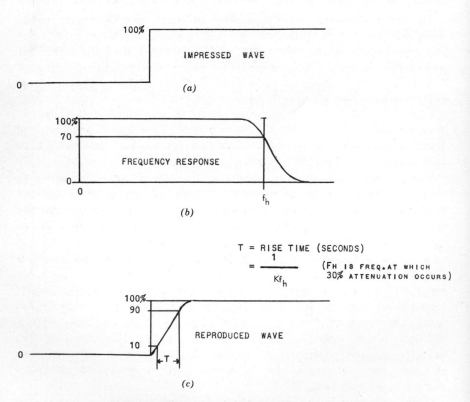

Figure 13-8. The effect of high-frequency response on the reproduction of a step function.

cuits, k varies between 2 and 3. From this it is obvious that increasing f_h—that is, improving the high-frequency response—shortens the rise time. Figure 13-9 summarizes how low-frequency and high-frequency responses affect the reproduction of a step function.

From this discussion it is readily apparent that the sharp portions of a complex wave dictate the high-frequency response required for its faithful reproduction. The required low-frequency response is determined by the fundamental frequency of the complex wave and by the presence or absence of an average value. If the complex waveform possesses an average value, the required low-frequency response must extend to 0 Hz (i.e., the system must provide dc response) if baseline information is to be retained.

13-4. DAMPED RESONANT SYSTEMS

Frequently in the course of measuring physiological events, the phenomenon of resonance is encountered. Basic to this phenomenon is the presence of at least two real or apparent energy-storage elements between which energy is continuously transferred. In the case of electrical components, capacitance and inductance are the real storage elements. It is also possible for the resonance phenomenon to exist in amplifier circuits that contain no inductive elements. Systems of this type show "ringing," or a tendency toward oscillation at a frequency for which there is a component of positive feedback around all or part of the circuit.

Resonance may also be purely mechanical, as in the case of devices possessing elasticity and mass. Two examples of such mechanical devices are blood pressure manometers, in which an elastic diaphragm or Bourdon tube is distorted by pressure, and moving-coil recorders, in which a torsion rod or spring returns the movement to its baseline when the signal is removed. The actual motion of the moving element (hence its capabilities as a transducer or reproducer) depends on three factors—inertia, elasticity or stiffness, and damping—and is described in mathematical terms by the interrelationship between them. *Inertia* is a measure of the force required to set the mass in motion or to alter its direction once it is in motion. *Stiffness* describes the rigidity of the system. It is defined in terms of the force required to deflect the moving member unit distance from its position of equilibrium. *Damping* is a measure of the frictional force acting on the mass. The frictional force is directed opposite to the direction of displacement of the mass. It is usually assumed that the magnitude of the frictional force varies directly with velocity; that is, the damping is viscous. Damping may be present as fluid resistance or it may exist as an electrically induced force.

Simple mechanical systems can be described in terms of one-to-one

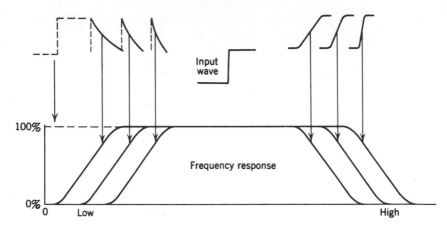

Figure 13-9.   The effect of low- and high-frequency responses on the reproduction of a step function.

electrical analogs because the behavior of both systems is expressed by the same mathematical equations. Inertia, damping, and stiffness determine the behavior of mechanical systems. In a series electrical circuit these quantities correspond to inductance, resistance, and capacitance, respectively.

Because the dynamic behavior of mechanical systems is so important in physiological measurements, the interrelationship between inertia, damping, and stiffness must be appreciated to understand how the characteristics of a given system can be altered under various conditions of measurement. Many devices can be well represented by a simple system involving only one degree of freedom (i.e., a system that can be completely characterized in terms of a single variable). Two simple mechanical models can be used to illustrate the behavior of most of these devices under the influence of a unit step of force and a constant-amplitude variable-frequency sinusoidal force.

Consider a mass M free to move on a frictionless horizontal surface coupled to a fixed support by a spring. Connected to the mass is a rod terminated by a vane dipping into a reservoir of fluid, providing viscous damping. Figure 13-10a is a sketch of such a system in which the mass M is free to move in a left- or righthand direction only. If a force is applied to move the weight from its position of equilibrium and then is removed, the mass will return to its original position slowly or rapidly and may overshoot and oscillate about the position of equilibrium several times before coming to rest, as shown. The type of motion executed depends on the relationship between the mass, stiffness, and damping.

Another simple example of the same phenomenon (Fig. 13-10*b*) illustrates the essential components of a recording pen or galvanometer having a mass with a given moment of inertia coupled to an elastic torsion rod. If a deflecting torque is applied to cause rotation and is then removed, the system will return to its position of equilibrium slowly or rapidly, as in the previous case, depending on the relationship between the same three quantities. The example of Fig. 13-10*a* deals with translation and describes the operation of blood pressure transducers and similar devices; that of Fig. 13-10*b* illustrates devices such as recording galvanometers in which rotary motion exists. Nonetheless, if the mass, stiffness, and coefficient of damping are time invariant, the displacement in both cases is described by a linear differential equation of the second order and first degree. The

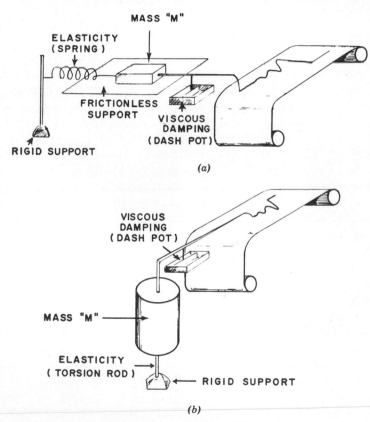

Figure 13-10.   Transient response of lightly damped systems.

following expressions describe the resultant motion:

Translation $M\dfrac{d^2x}{dt^2} + K_1\dfrac{dx}{dt} + K_2x$ = sum of applied forces.

Rotation $I\dfrac{d^2\phi}{dt^2} + K_1\dfrac{d\phi}{dt} + K_2\phi$ = sum of applied torques.

In these equations M and I are the mass-inertial components; M is the mass, and I is the moment of inertia; K_1 is the viscous damping force, K_2 is the stiffness or restoring force (usually represented by a spring constant), x is the linear displacement, ϕ is the angular displacement, and t is time.

Note the similarity between the two expressions just given and the following equation, which represents the sum of the voltage drops across an inductance L, resistance R, and capacitance C in a series circuit:

$$L\frac{d^2q}{dt^2} + R\frac{dq}{dt} + \frac{q}{C} = \text{applied voltage,}$$

where q is the charge, dq/dt is the rate of change of charge which is current i, and $d^2q/dt^2 = di/dt$.

Because the behavior of the mechanical systems is described by the same form of mathematical expression as that representing the electrical circuit, the electric circuit is called an analog of either mechanical system. Thus the behavior of these simple mechanical systems, and of others more complicated, can be investigated by the use of simple electrical components. The inertial components (M and I) are represented by the inductance L, the damping force K_1 by resistance R, and the stiffness of the mechanical systems K_2 by the reciprocal of capacitance. The displacement (x or ϕ) has as its analog the charge q. Hence in the electrical simulation, the voltage across the capacitance describes x or ϕ.

Because these equations are of similar form, the solutions are the same except for the letter designation of terms. A mathematical solution to the equations may be difficult to carry out, depending on the time function required to describe the applied force. A graphic solution, however, is easily obtained from the electrical analog if the desired forcing function can be generated. The electrical analog also provides a convenient means of changing parameters, thus permitting the behavior of such systems under a variety of conditions to be demonstrated easily. Hence the mathematical ability necessary to solve the equations directly is not essential for an appreciation of the importance of the individual circuit elements in determining the response of the system to many different inputs. A description of the response to two different applied forces—(1) a step function and (2) a variable-frequency sine wave—will enable the reader to understand the behavior of a simple system under a variety of operating conditions.

The first and probably most important condition is the particular inter-relationship between the quantities which provides just enough damping to render the motion nonoscillatory when a step force is applied or removed; that is, the moving element deflects or returns to its position of equilibrium as rapidly as possible without overshoot. Such a condition is called critical damping. Less damping results in a more rapid motion with overshoot. If the damping is reduced to zero, an oscillatory condition is produced. Although in practice it is never possible to achieve zero damping, a lightly damped system will oscillate for a long time before coming to rest. The frequency of forcefree oscillation is called the natural frequency of the system.

When damping is made greater than critical, there is no overshoot, but the time taken to reach the position of equilibrium is considerably longer. The types of response encountered with critical damping ($D = 1$) and damping less than critical are summarized in Fig. 13-11. With a step force applied or removed instantly, the response (curve a) is nonoscillatory for critical damping. With light damping ($D = 0.2$), the response (curve b) is partially oscillatory. Increasing the damping to 0.5 (curve c) results in an overshoot of approximately 15% followed by a heavily damped oscillation.

The time axis of Fig. 13-11 is in percentage of the undamped period T_0 (equal to the reciprocal of the resonant frequency with zero damping, i.e., the natural frequency). The resonant frequency with zero damping (f_0) is

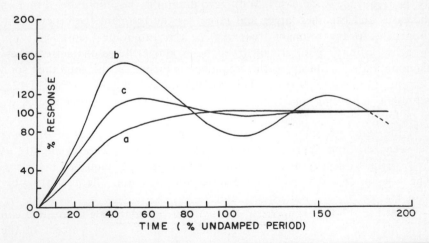

Figure 13-11. Transient response with various degrees of damping: (a) $D = 1.0$ (critical damping); (b) $D = 0.2$; (c) $D = 0.5$.

dependent on the relationship between the inertial component M or I and the stiffness K_2. It can easily be shown that

for the translational case $\qquad f_0 = \dfrac{1}{2\pi} \sqrt{\dfrac{K_2}{M}}$,

for the rotational case $\qquad f_0 = \dfrac{1}{2\pi} \sqrt{\dfrac{K_2}{I}}$,

for the electrical case $\qquad f_0 = \dfrac{1}{2\pi} \sqrt{\dfrac{1/C}{L}}$.

Thus, specifying the system constants permits calculation of values for the abscissa of Fig. 13-11. As the damping is decreased, the time for the system to rise from 0 to 100% becomes shorter and the overshoot is greater. Accordingly, the price of elimination of transient overshoot is prolongation of rise time. Therefore, to obtain more rapid response without excessive overshoot, it is necessary to use a stiffer or lighter system, that is, one with a higher resonant frequency. Thus the undamped resonant frequency of a system, along with the coefficient of damping, determines the rise time.

Intimately associated with the response to a step input is the behavior of such systems when subjected to sinusoidal forces. Figure 13-12a illustrates the normalized response A_f/A_k when tested with a constant-amplitude, variable-frequency sine wave of force A_f. With critical damping ($D = 1$), the frequency-response curve has a characteristic form, falling progressively as the frequency is increased. With zero damping, the amplitude of motion increases and becomes larger and larger as the resonant frequency is approached. At the resonant frequency f_0, the amplitude theoretically approaches infinity. With driving frequencies above the resonant frequency, the amplitude is reduced; as the frequency is increased, the amplitude soon becomes immeasurably small. This condition (dashed curve in Fig. 13-12a) represents a limiting condition under which all operating characteristics are to be found.

If the same procedure is carried out with various degrees of damping between zero and approximately 0.7, the amplitude increases slightly at first, rising to a peak and then falling rapidly as the frequency increases. The cases of $D = 0.2$ and $D = 0.5$ illustrate this point. The interesting behavior when $D = 0.7$ is discussed later.

From Fig. 13-12 it is apparent that with critical damping the system can respond fully only to sine wave frequencies up to a few percent of the resonant frequency. With light damping (0.2) there is a pronounced rise in the frequency-response curve at approximately 95% of the undamped natural resonant frequency. When the damping is increased to 0.5, the fre-

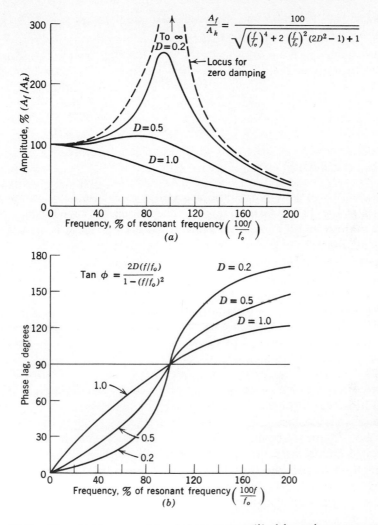

$$\frac{A_f}{A_k} = \frac{100}{\sqrt{\left(\frac{f}{f_o}\right)^4 + 2\left(\frac{f}{f_o}\right)^2 (2D^2 - 1) + 1}}$$

$$\text{Tan}\ \phi = \frac{2D(f/f_o)}{1 - (f/f_o)^2}$$

Figure 13-12.   Sinusoidal frequency (*a*) and phase response (*b*) of damped resonant systems.

quency-response curve is more uniform and exhibits a less pronounced resonant rise. The frequency at a resonant rise is less than that for the undamped condition. In both cases as the frequency is increased beyond the maximum response, the amplitude falls progressively. The foregoing discussion shows that by assigning various values to the damping coefficient, a family of amplitude-versus-frequency curves is determined. Those of most interest fall between zero and critical damping and assume a contour appropriate for their proximity to either of these curves.

When a periodic sine wave of force is presented to such systems, there is a time lag between the displacement of the mass and the applied force. This time lag is expressed in terms of degrees of a full cycle and is designated as phase shift. Damping has a pronounced effect on the phase characteristic of such systems. This relationship is presented in Fig. 13-12b. It is apparent from inspection of this figure that with some damping, between 0.5 and 1.0, phase shift can be nearly linear with frequency up to the natural resonant frequency f_0.

In deciding what degree of damping should be specified to obtain the best phase characteristic, it is useful to recall the three criteria for the faithful reproduction of an event: (a) linearity of amplitude, (b) adequate bandwidth of sine wave frequency response, and (c) linearity of phase shift. Because amplitude linearity is usually easy to achieve, the following discussion deals with the effect of damping on the sine wave frequency and phase response.

Figure 13-13 shows the amplitude of the resonant rise in the sine wave frequency-response curve as damping is increased. On the basis of uniform sine wave frequency response, a damping of 0.7 results in no resonant peak in the curve. Although not shown in Fig. 13-13, but certainly indicated by Fig. 13-12b, it can be stated that this degree of damping provides a linear phase shift up to and slightly beyond the undamped resonant frequency. It is logical then to conclude that this degree of damping fulfills the requirements for faithful reproduction of an event. Although this is true, it must be remembered that the reproduction of a step input by a system having

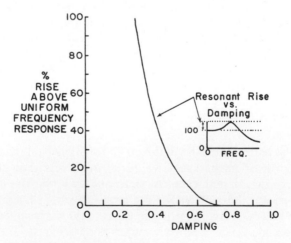

Figure 13-13. The effect of damping on the uniformity of the sine wave frequency response.

RESPONSE TO STEP FUNCTION

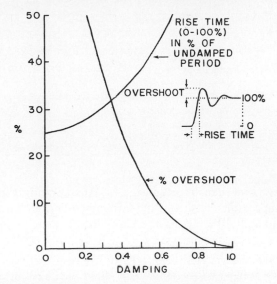

Figure 13-14. The effect of damping on rise time and overshoot in terms of the response to a step function.

these constants is slightly compromised. Under these conditions the rise time (0 to 100%) is approximately half the undamped period. Moreover, a 5% overshoot is present. It is to be recalled that decreasing the damping shortens the rise time at the expense of overshoot. Since with 0.7 damping some overshoot must exist, it is logical to investigate the improvement in rise time as damping is further decreaed to obtain a more rapid response from the system. Just what degree of damping is to be specified usually depends on the penalty that can be paid in terms of overshoot and rise time for a step function, along with the loss produced in the sine wave frequency response.

From Fig. 13-14, which relates rise time and overshoot to the various degrees of damping, it is seen that if the damping is reduced from 0.7 to 0.65, the response time shortens by about 3 to 47% of the undamped period, while the overshoot increases by 2%, giving a total overshoot of 7%. Under these conditions sine wave characteristics are not excessively compromised, since for 0.65 damping the resonant rise in the frequency response curve is slightly more than 1% and the phase error is approximately 4 degrees.

If a larger overshoot to the step function can be tolerated, a further

Table 13-2   Characteristics of a Resonant System with 0.65 Damping:
Undamped Resonant Frequency = f_0

Step Function	
	$\dfrac{1}{2.1 f_0}$ sec
Rise time (0 to 100% of terminal amplitude)	
Overshoot (% over terminal amplitude)	7%
Sine Wave	
Bandwidth (to 70% of uniform amplitude response)	(0 to 108%) f_0
Resonant peak (above uniform response)	1.3%
Maximum phase error over (0 to 100%) f_0 range	4%

decrease in rise time can be attained. At 0.6 damping the rise time is shortened to approximately 45% of the undamped period, but the overshoot is increased to about 10%. Under these conditions the resonant rise in the sine-wave curve is approximately 5%.

Thus it is apparent that with devices in which resonance can occur, a shorter response time can be attained if a small degree of overshoot can be tolerated when a step input is applied. The improvement in rise time simulates to some extent the characteristics of a stiffer system, that is, one with a higher natural frequency. With knowledge of the undamped resonant frequency and the degree of damping, the entire behavior of a system having one degree of freedom can be predicted. When the response to a step function (rise time and overshoot) is known, the sine wave frequency and phase characteristics can be deduced. Conversely, knowledge of the sine wave frequency and phase response characteristics makes it possible to predict the response to a step function or a square wave.

In practice, to obtain a good compromise between all the factors discussed, the damping of dynamic systems is usually adjusted to about 0.65. The characteristics of a system with one degree of freedom and this damping coefficient are given in Table 13-2.

13-5.   CONCLUSION

It is apparent that for a system to reproduce a complex wave faithfully, consideration must be given to its harmonic spectrum. Then the sine wave frequency and phase characteristics of the reproducing system must be examined for their suitability for reproduction of all the components of the complex wave. From such an investigation it is possible to determine the degree of fidelity of reproduction that can be expected.

REFERENCES

Geddes, L. A. 1951. A note on phase distortion. *EEG Clin. Neurophysiol.* 3:517–8.

Hansen, A. T. 1949. *Pressure Measurement in the Human Organism.* Technisk Forlag., Copenhagen.

Saunders, M. G., and R. M. Jell. 1959. Time distortion in electroencephalograph amplifiers. *EEG Clin. Neurophysiol.* 11:814–816.

Terman, F. E. 1943. *Radio Engineers Handbook.* McGraw-Hill, New York.

Valley, G. E., and H. Wallman. 1948. *Vacuum Tube Amplifiers.* McGraw-Hill, New York.

Index

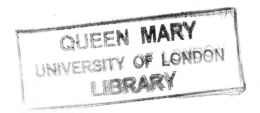